The GALE
ENCYCLOPEDIA *of*
NURSING &
ALLIED HEALTH

The GALE ENCYCLOPEDIA of NURSING & ALLIED HEALTH

VOLUME 3
I-O

Kristine Krapp, Editor

GALE GROUP

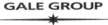

THOMSON LEARNING

Detroit • New York • San Diego • San Francisco
Boston • New Haven, Conn. • Waterville, Maine
London • Munich

The GALE ENCYCLOPEDIA of NURSING AND ALLIED HEALTH

STAFF

Kristine Krapp, *Coordinating Senior Editor*
Christine B. Jeryan, *Managing Editor*
Deirdre S. Blanchfield, *Associate Editor (Manuscript Coordination)*
Melissa C. McDade, *Associate Editor (Photos and Illustrations)*
Stacey L. Blachford, *Associate Editor*
Kate Kretschmann, *Assistant Editor*
Donna Olendorf, *Senior Editor*
Ryan Thomason, *Assistant Editor*

Mark Springer, *Technical Specialist*
Andrea Lopeman, *Programmer/Analyst*

Barbara Yarrow, *Manager, Imaging and Multimedia Content*
Robyn V. Young, *Project Manager, Imaging and Multimedia Content*
Randy Bassett, *Imaging Supervisor*
Dan Newell, *Imaging Specialist*
Pamela A. Reed, *Coordinator, Imaging and Multimedia Content*
Maria Franklin, *Permissions Manager*
Margaret A. Chamberlain, *Permissions Specialist*

Kenn Zorn, *Product Manager*
Michelle DiMercurio, *Senior Art Director*
Cynthia Baldwin, *Senior Art Director*

Mary Beth Trimper, *Manager, Composition, and Electronic Prepress*
Evi Seoud, *Assistant Manager, Composition Purchasing, and Electronic Prepress*
Dorothy Maki, *Manufacturing Manager*

Indexing provided by Synapse, the Knowledge Link Corporation.

ISBN 0-7876-4934-1 (set)   0-7876-4937-6 (Vol. 3)
0-7876-4935-X (Vol. 1)   0-7876-4938-4 (Vol. 4)
0-7876-4936-8 (Vol. 2)   0-7876-4939-2 (Vol. 5)

Printed in Canada
10 9 8 7 6 5 4 3 2 1

Library of Congress Cataloging-in-Publication Data
The Gale encyclopedia of nursing and allied health / Kristine Krapp, editor.
  p. cm.
  Includes bibliographical references and index.
  ISBN 0-7876-4934-1 (set : hardcover : alk. paper)
    ISBN 0-7876-4935-X (v. 1 : alk. paper) —
      ISBN 0-7876-4936-8 (v.2 : alk. paper) —
        ISBN 0-7876-4937-6 (v. 3 : alk. paper) —
          ISBN0-7876-4938-4 (v. 4 : alk. paper) —
            ISBN 0-7876-4939-2 (v. 5 : alk. paper)
1. Nursing Care—Encyclopedias—English. 2. Allied Health Personnel—Encyclopedias—English.
3. Nursing—Encyclopedias—English. WY 13 G151 2002]
RT21 .G353 2002
610.73'03—dc21
                                        2001040910

CONTENTS

PLEASE READ—IMPORTANT INFORMATION

The *Gale Encyclopedia of Nursing and Allied Health* is a medical reference product designed to inform and educate readers about a wide variety of diseases, treatments, tests and procedures, health issues, human biology, and nursing and allied health professions. The Gale Group believes the product to be comprehensive, but not necessarily definitive. While the Gale Group has made substantial efforts to provide information that is accurate, comprehensive, and up-to-date, the Gale Group makes no representations or warranties of any kind, including without limitation, warranties of merchantability or fitness for a particular purpose, nor does it guarantee the accuracy, comprehensiveness, or timeliness of the information contained in this product. Readers should be aware that the universe of medical knowledge is constantly growing and changing, and that differences of medical opinion exist among authorities.

INTRODUCTION

The *Gale Encyclopedia of Nursing and Allied Health* is a unique and invaluable source of information for the nursing or allied health student. This collection of over 850 entries provides in-depth coverage of specific diseases and disorders, tests and procedures, equipment and tools, body systems, nursing and allied health professions, and current health issues. This book is designed to fill a gap between health information designed for laypeople and that provided for medical professionals, which may be too complicated for the beginning student to understand. The encyclopedia does use medical terminology, but explains it in a way that students can understand.

SCOPE

The *Gale Encyclopedia of Nursing and Allied Health* covers a wide variety of topics relevant to the nursing or allied health student. Subjects covered include those important to students intending to become biomedical equipment technologists, dental hygienists, dieteticians, health care administrators, medical technologists/clinical laboratory sciencists, registered and licensed practical nurses, nurse anesthetists, nurse practitioners, nurse midwives, occupational therapists, optometrists, pharmacy technicians, physical therapists, radiologic technologists, and speech-language therapists. The encyclopedia also covers information on related general medical topics, classes of medication, mental health, public health, and human biology. Entries follow a standardized format that provides information at a glance. Rubrics include:

Diseases/Disorders

Definition
Description
Causes and symptoms
Diagnosis
Treatment
Prognosis

Health care team roles
Prevention
Resources
Key terms

Tests/Procedures

Definition
Purpose
Precautions
Description
Preparation
Aftercare
Complications
Results
Health care team roles
Resources
Key terms

Equipment/Tools

Definition
Purpose
Description
Operation
Maintenance
Health care team roles
Training
Resources
Key terms

Human biology/Body systems

Definition
Description
Function
Role in human health
Common diseases and disorders
Resources
Key terms

Nursing and allied health professions

Definition
Description
Work settings
Education and training
Advanced education and training
Future outlook
Resources
Key terms

Current health issues

Definition
Description
Viewpoints
Professional implications
Resources
Key terms

INCLUSION CRITERIA

A preliminary list of topics was compiled from a wide variety of sources, including nursing and allied health textbooks, general medical encyclopedias, and consumer health guides. The advisory board, composed of advanced practice nurses, allied health professionals, health educators, and medical doctors, evaluated the topics and made suggestions for inclusion. Final selection of topics to include was made by the advisory board in conjunction with the Gale editor.

ABOUT THE CONTRIBUTORS

The essays were compiled by experienced medical writers, including physicians, pharmacists, nurses, and allied health care professionals. The advisers reviewed the completed essays to ensure that they are appropriate, up-to-date, and medically accurate.

HOW TO USE THIS BOOK

The *Gale Encyclopedia of Nursing and Allied Health* has been designed with ready reference in mind.

- Straight **alphabetical arrangement** of topics allows users to locate information quickly.

- **Bold-faced terms** within entries direct the reader to related articles.

- **Cross-references** placed throughout the encyclopedia direct readers from alternate names and related topics to entries.

- A list of **Key terms** is provided where appropriate to define terms or concepts that may be unfamiliar to the student.

- The **Resources** section directs readers to additional sources of medical information on a topic.

- Valuable **contact information** for medical, nursing, and allied health organizations is included with each entry. An Appendix of Nursing and Allied Health organizations in the back matter contains an extensive list of organizations arranged by subject.

- A comprehensive **general index** guides readers to significant topics mentioned in the text.

GRAPHICS

The *Gale Encyclopedia of Nursing and Allied Health* is enhanced by over 400 black and white photos and illustrations, as well as over 50 tables.

ACKNOWLEDGMENTS

The editor would like to express appreciation to all of the nursing and allied health professionals who wrote, reviewed, and copyedited entries for the *Gale Encyclopedia of Nursing and Allied Health*.

Cover photos were reproduced by the permission of Delmar Publishers, Inc., Custom Medical Photos, and the Gale Group.

ADVISORY BOARD

A number of experts in the nursing and allied health communities provided invaluable assistance in the formulation of this encyclopedia. The advisory board performed a myriad of duties, from defining the scope of coverage to reviewing individual entries for accuracy and accessibility. The editor would like to express appreciation to them for their time and their expert contributions.

Dr. Isaac Bankman
Principal Scientist
Imaging and Laser Systems Section
Johns Hopkins Applied Physics Laboratory
Laurel, Maryland

Martha G. Bountress, M.S., CCC-SLP/A
Clinical Instructor
Speech-Language Pathology and Audiology
Old Dominion University
Norfolk, Virginia

Michele Leonardi Darby
Eminent Scholar, University Professor
Graduate Program Director
School of Dental Hygiene
Old Dominion University
Norfolk, Virginia

Dr. Susan J. Gromacki
Lecturer in Ophthalmology and Visual Sciences
University of Michigan Medical School
Ann Arbor, Michigan

Dr. John E. Hall
Guyton Professor and Chair
Department of Physiology and Biophysics
University of Mississippi Medical Center
Jackson, Mississippi

Lisa F. Harper, B.S.D.H., M.P.H., R.D., L.D.
Assistant Professor
Baylor College of Dentistry
Dallas, Texas

Robert Harr, M.S. MT (ASCP)
Associate Professor and Chair
Department of Public and Allied Health
Bowling Green State University
Bowling Green, Ohio

Dr. Gregory M. Karst
Associate Professor
Division of Physical Therapy Education
University of Nebraska Medical Center
Omaha, Nebraska

Debra A. Kosko, R.N., M.N., FNP-C
Instructor, Faculty Practice
School of Nursing, Department of Medicine
Johns Hopkins University
Baltimore, Maryland

Timothy E. Moore, Ph.D., C Psych
Professor of Psychology
Glendon College
York University
Toronto, Ontario, Canada

Anne Nichols, C.R.N.P.
Coordinator, Family Nurse Practitioner Program
School of Nursing
Widener University
Chester, Pennsylvania

Judith B. Paquet, R.N.
Medical Communications Specialist
Paquet Associates
Clementon, New Jersey

Lee A. Shratter, M.D.
Radiologist
Healthcare Safety and Medical Consultant
Kentfield, California

Linda Wheeler, C.N.M., Ed.D.
Associate Professor
School of Nursing
Oregon Health and Science University
Portland, Oregon

CONTRIBUTORS

Lisa Maria Andres, M.S., C.G.C
San Jose, California

Greg Annussek
New York, New York

Maia Appleby
Boynton Beach, Florida

Bill Asenjo, M.S., C.R.C.
Iowa City, Iowa

Lori Ann Beck, R.N., M.S.N., F.N.P.-C.
Berkley, Michigan

Mary Bekker
Willow Grove, Pennsylvania

Linda K. Bennington, R.N.C., M.S.N., C.N.S.
Virginia Beach, Virginia

Kenneth J. Berniker, M.D.
El Cerrio, California

Mark A. Best
Cleveland Heights, Ohio

Dean Andrew Bielanowski, R.N., B.Nurs.(QUT)
Rochedale S., Brisbane, Australia

Carole Birdsall, R.N. A.N.P. Ed.D.
New York, New York

Bethanne Black
Buford, Georgia

Maggie Boleyn, R.N., B.S.N.
Oak Park, Michigan

Barbara Boughton
El Cerrito, California

Patricia L. Bounds, Ph.D.
Zurich, Switzerland

Mary Boyle, Ph.D., C.C.C.-S.L.P., B.C.-N.C.D.
Lincoln Park, New Jersey

Rachael Tripi Brandt, M.S.
Gettysburg, Pennsylvania

Peggy Elaine Browning
Olney, Texas

Susan Joanne Cadwallader
Cedarburg, Wisconsin

Barbara M. Chandler
Sacramento, California

Linda Chrisman
Oakland, California

Rhonda Cloos, R.N.
Austin, Texas

L. Lee Culvert
Alna, Massachusetts

Tish Davidson
Fremont, California

Lori De Milto
Sicklerville, New Jersey

Victoria E. DeMoranville
Lakeville, Massachusetts

Janine Diebel, R.N.
Gaylord, Michigan

Stéphanie Islane Dionne
Ann Arbor, Michigan

J. Paul Dow, Jr.
Kansas City, Missouri

Douglas Dupler
Boulder, Colorado

Lorraine K. Ehresman
Northfield, Quebec, Canada

L. Fleming Fallon, Jr., M.D., Dr.P.H.
Bowling Green, Ohio

Diane Fanucchi-Faulkner, C.M.T., C.C.R.A.
Oceano, California

Janis O. Flores
Sebastopol, Florida

Paula Ford-Martin
Chaplin, Minnesota

Janie F. Franz
Grand Forks, North Dakota

Sallie Boineau Freeman, Ph.D.
Atlanta, Georgia

Rebecca Frey, Ph.D.
New Haven, Connecticut

Lisa M. Gourley
Bowling Green, Ohio

Meghan M. Gourley
Germantown, Maryland

Jill Ilene Granger, M.S.
Ann Arbor, Michigan

Elliot Greene, M.A.
Silver Spring, Maryland

Stephen John Hage, A.A.A.S., R.T.(R), F.A.H.R.A.
Chatsworth, California

Clare Hanrahan
Asheville, North Carolina

Robert Harr
Bowling Green, Ohio

Daniel J. Harvey
Wilmington, Delaware

Katherine Hauswirth, A.P.R.N.
Deep River, Connecticut

David L. Helwig
London, Ontario, Canada

Lisette Hilton
Boca Raton, Florida

René A. Jackson, R.N.
Port Charlotte, Florida

Nadine M. Jacobson, R.N.
Takoma Park, Maryland

Randi B. Jenkins
New York, New York

Michelle L. Johnson, M.S., J.D.
Portland, Oregon

Paul A. Johnson
San Marcos, California

Linda D. Jones, B.A., P.B.T.(A.S.C.P.)
Asheboro, New York

Crystal Heather Kaczkowski, M.Sc.
Dorval, Quebec, Canada

Beth Kapes
Bay Village, Ohio

Monique Laberge, Ph.D.
Philadelphia, Pennsylvania

Aliene S. Linwood, B.S.N., R.N., D.P.A., F.A.C.H.E.
Athens, Ohio

Jennifer Lee Losey, R.N.
Madison Heights, Michigan

Liz Marshall
Columbus, Ohio

Mary Elizabeth Martelli, R.N., B.S.
Sebastian, Florida

Jacqueline N. Martin, M.S.
Albrightsville, Pennsylvania

Sally C. McFarlane-Parrott
Mason, Michigan

Beverly G. Miller, M.T.(A.S.C.P.)
Charlotte, North Carolina

Christine Miner Minderovic, B.S., R.T., R.D.M.S.
Ann Arbor, Michigan

Mark A. Mitchell, M.D.
Bothell, Washington

Susan M. Mockus, Ph.D.
Seattle, Washington

Timothy E. Moore, Ph.D.
Toronto, Ontario, Canada

Nancy J. Nordenson
Minneapolis, Minnesota

Erika J. Norris
Oak Harbor, Washington

Debra Novograd, B.S., R.T.(R)(M)
Royal Oak, Michigan

Marianne F. O'Connor, M.T., M.P.H.
Farmington Hills, Michigan

Carole Osborne-Sheets
Poway, California

Cindy F. Ovard, R.D.A
Spring Valley, California

Patience Paradox
Bainbridge Island, Washington

Deborah Eileen Parker, R.N.
Lakewood, Washington

Genevieve Pham-Kanter
Chicago, Illinois

Jane E. Phillips, Ph.D.
Chapel Hill, North Carolina

Pamella A. Phillips
Bowling Green, Ohio

Elaine R. Proseus, M.B.A./T.M., B.S.R.T., R.T.(R)
Farmington Hills, Michigan

Ann Quigley
New York, New York

Esther Csapo Rastegari, R.N., B.S.N., Ed.M.
Holbrook, Massachusetts

Anastasia Marie Raymer, Ph.D.
Norfolk, Virginia

Martha S. Reilly, O.D.
Madison, Wisconsin

Linda Richards, R.D., C.H.E.S.
Flagstaff, Arizona

Toni Rizzo
Salt Lake City, Utah

Nancy Ross-Flanigan
Belleville, Michigan

Mark Damian Rossi, Ph.D, P.T., C.S.C.S.
Pembroke Pines, Florida

Kausalya Santhanam
Branford, Connecticut

Denise L. Schmutte, Ph.D.
Shoreline, Washington

Joan M. Schonbeck
Marlborough, Massachusetts

Kathleen Scogna
Baltimore, Maryland

Cathy Hester Seckman, R.D.H.
Calcutta, Ohio

Jennifer E. Sisk, M.A.
Havertown, Pennsylvania

Patricia Skinner
Amman, Jordan

Genevieve Slomski
New Britain, Connecticut

Bryan Ronain Smith
Cincinnati, Ohio

Allison Joan Spiwak, B.S., C.C.P.
Gahanna, Ohio

Lorraine T. Steefel
Morganville, New Jersey

Margaret A. Stockley, R.G.N.
Boxborough, Massachusetts

Amy Loerch Strumolo
Bloomfield Hills, Michigan

Liz Swain
San Diego, California

Deanna M. Swartout-Corbeil, R.N.
Thompsons Station, Tennessee

Peggy Campbell Torpey, M.P.T.
Royal Oak, Michigan

Mai Tran, Pharm.D.
Troy, Michigan

Carol A. Turkington
Lancaster, Pennsylvania

Judith Turner, D.V.M.
Sandy, Utah

Samuel D. Uretsky, Pharm.D.
Wantagh, New York

Michele R. Webb
Overland Park, Kansas

Ken R. Wells
Laguna Hills, California

Barbara Wexler, M.P.H.
Chatsworth, California

Gayle G. Wilkins, R.N., B.S.N., O.C.N.
Willow Park, Texas

Jennifer F. Wilson
Haddonfield, New Jersey

Angela Woodward
Madison, Wisconsin

Jennifer Wurges
Rochester Hills, Michigan

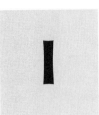

Ibuprofen *see* **Nonsteroidal anti-inflammatory drugs**

Ice packs *see* **Cooling treatments**

Icterus *see* **Jaundice**

Ileostomy *see* **Enterostomy**

IM injection *see* **Intramuscular injection**

Immovable joint

Definition

An immovable joint is an articulation between bones in which no movement occurs. It is also referred to as synarthrotic (meaning immovable).

Description

An immovable joint can be either one of two types of joints, fibrous or cartilaginous. In a fibrous joint, there are two types of articulations that are considered immovable, suture and gomphosis.

A suture is a type of articulation in which the bones that make up the joint are close together. An analogy to this is the interlocking fashion exhibited by placing puzzle pieces together. In a suture, the union of bones is bound by connective tissue.

A gomphosis is a type of joint in which one bone fits into another bone. The articulating edges are bound together by connective tissue. Similar to the suture, the bony surfaces in the articulation are close together. An analogy to this is a wooden dowel fitting into a hole and held together by glue, with the dowel and hole representing the bony structures and the glue representing the connective tissue.

In a cartilaginous type of joint, there is one type of articulation that is considered immovable, the synchondrosis.

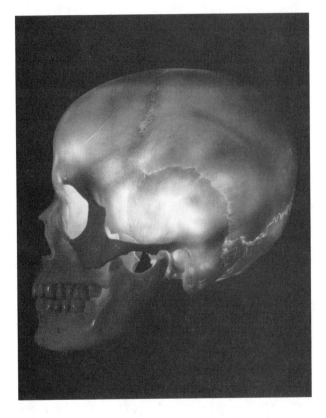

The immovable joints of the skull are joined by sutures. The coronal suture is along the top of the skull, and the lambdoidal suture is seen toward the back of the skull. *(Photograph by Simon Brown. Science Source/Photo Researchers. Reproduced by permission.)*

A synchondrosis is a joint in which the articulating surfaces are close together but are bound by hyaline cartilage. In a synchondrosis, the hyaline cartilage eventually converts to either bone or fibrocartilage.

Function

The function of the immovable or synarthrotic joint is to provide a stable union between bony surfaces. The suture and synchondrosis actually become more stable when ossification of the joint takes place.

KEY TERMS

Cartilaginous joint—A joint that represents the connection of two bones bound by either hyaline fibro or elastic cartilage.

Connective tissue—Tissue that has pliable fibers, which provide strength to the tissue.

Diaphysis—The center or shaft of a bone that is ossified.

Epiphysis—Considered a secondary center of ossification. This secondary center of ossification appears at the ends of long bone.

Fibrocartilage—Connective tissue made up of collagen fibers with less ground substance compared to hyaline cartilage.

Fibrous joint—Surfaces of two bones that are connected by fibrous tissue, which consists mainly of collagen fibers.

Hyaline cartilage—A mesh of collagen fibers and ground substance.

Proximal—The closest portion of a bone, structure, or other element that is close to the head of the body.

Synarthrosis—An immovable joint.

Role in human health

An example of a suture in the human body is the fibrous joints between the bones of the **skull**. Before birth the suture is fibrous tissue that forms soft spots on the skull. The common medical term is fontanelle. The fibrous joint between the bones of the skull allows the skull to be more pliable during birth as the head passes through the vagina. During infancy the pliable nature of the skull, secondary to fibrous sutures, allows for growth of the **brain**. As growth and development occurs the sutures become ossified.

An example of a gomphosis in the human body is the joining of the root of a tooth with the mandible or jaw bone. The fibrous union between the tooth and the bone secures the tooth in its position. This allows the teeth to function as grinders during chewing.

An example of synchondrosis in the human body is two distinct portions of long bone that are separated by a hyaline cartilaginous plate. This typically occurs at the ends of long bones where a cartilaginous plate separates the diaphysis from the epiphysis. This plate allows the

end of bones to grow throughout early human development. As growth and development continue, the hyaline cartilage ossifies. By adulthood the joint is gone. Another example of a synchondrosis in the human body is the articulation between the first rib and the manubrium or the upper portion of the sternum. Initially, the connection between the manubrium and first rib is hyaline cartilage. Through adulthood the hyaline cartilage is replaced by fibrocartilage. This process allows the superior portion of the thorax to be more secure and stable.

Common diseases and disorders

The most common disorder of sutures or fontanelles of the skull is the disruption of the bony components, thus compromising the integrity of the fibrous attachment. This could occur as a result of **head injury** from a blow to the head or a fall. Common disorders of the teeth that compromise the integrity of the fibrous attachment of tooth to bone are: fracture of the jaw bone, fracture of the tooth, avulsion of the tooth, loosening of the tooth secondary to decay, or a blow to the head or jaw. The most common disorder associated with a synchondrosis is a disruption of the epiphyseal hyaline cartilage plate. This is particularly evident in the proximal femur, specifically related to the hip. This disorder occurs mainly in young children as a result of a fall or other trauma. This disruption to the plate can lead to fracture, disruption of **blood** supply, and, if not treated appropriately, deformity of the hip. The medical term for this disorder is slipped capital femoral epiphysis.

Resources

BOOKS

Hall C.M., L.T. Brody. *Therapeutic Exercise Moving Toward Function.* Philadelphia: Lippincott, Williams & Wilkins, 1998.

Lehmkuhl L.D., L. K. Smith. *Brunnstroms Clinical Kinesiology.* Philadelphia: F.A. Davis Co., 1996.

Magee D. J. *Orthopedic Physical Assessment.* Philadelphia: W.B. Saunders Co., 1997.

Moore K.L., A.F. Dalley. *Clinically Oriented Anatomy.* Baltimore: Lippincott, Williams & Wilkins, 1999.

Rosse C., P. Gaddum-Rosse, W. Hollinshead. *Hollinshead's Textbook of Anatomy.* Baltimore: Lippincott, Williams & Wilkins, 1997.

Mark Damian Rossi, Ph.D., P.T.

Immune response

Definition

The action taken by the body to defend itself from pathogens or abnormalities is called the immune response. With the aid of the **immune system**, the body monitors constant exposure to harmful elements in the external and internal environment and provides a means of defense. Pathogens that are able to cause immune responses included **bacteria**, **viruses**, and parasites. The immune system must be able to determine what is a normal part of the body or "self," as opposed to that which is foreign or "non-self." The development of cancers, for example, represents a part of "self" that has been abnormally changed such that it is recognized as foreign to the immune system.

Description

The immune response can be roughly divided into two broad categories, innate (natural) immunity and adaptive (acquired) immunity. Innate immunity is the first line of defense against invasion by pathogens. This response is not directed against any one particular pathogen but is a capable of destroying many different invaders. If the pathogen is able to conquer this initial protection, an adaptive immune response will follow. In this response, lymphocytes arise that can specifically kill the invader and prevent re-infection. These lymphocytes recognize specific antigens on pathogens (substances that are foreign to the host cell and cause the production of antibodies to fight the disease).

Innate (natural) immunity

Innate immunity refers to those parts of the immune system that are normally present and do not given an elevated response upon a second exposure to a pathogen (without immunological **memory**). This immunity is non-specific and is not directed against one type of pathogen. It is more generalized to allow the recognition of common elements that may be shared among pathogenic microorganisms.

Anatomical or physical barriers provide innate protection. The skin provides a protective barrier and contains substances that are antimicrobial (against bacterial growth) such as lactic acid, ammonia, and uric acid. The bacteria (microflora) that normally inhabit the skin do not cause disease under normal conditions. These organisms also contribute to innate immunity. The competition of the microflora with pathogens for resources and nutrients limits the growth of pathogens. If the skin is broken due to **wounds** or **burns**, pathogenic bacteria may enter to cause disease. In the urinary and biliary tracts, the increased flow of secretions provides protection against the establishment of harmful organisms.

Physiologic barriers are also a part of the innate immune system. **Stomach** acid can kill and inhibit the growth of many microorganisms and degrade potentially harmful **proteins**. A rise in body temperature can create an environment that is no longer suitable for the growth of some bacteria. Saliva, nasal secretions, tears, and mucus also contain substances that block viruses and help in the destruction of harmful bacteria.

Some cells of the immune system are able to attack and engulf pathogens, molecules, or particles by a process known as phagocytosis. The Russian immunologist Eli Metchnikoff observed that some pathogenic microorganisms were destroyed by phagocytic cells he called macrophages. These phagocytic cells originate in the bone marrow, are called monocytes in the bloodstream, and become macrophages in the tissue. These phagocytic macrophages in the tissue are able to ingest and destroy some pathogens even though they have not previously encountered them. These cells are capable of migration and are found in many sites throughout the body, including the lymph nodes, spleen, **liver**, **lungs**, as well as the peritoneal lining that surrounds the organs and the lungs. Macrophages in the bone are called osteoclasts, in the **central nervous system** they are called microglia, and in the connective tissue they are known as histiocytes. The neutrophils (polymorphonuclear leukocytes or PMNs) are another type of phagocytic cell that is critically important for innate immunity. These cells are found in great numbers and are one of the most important types of white **blood** cells found in the bloodstream. They are quickly recruited to the site of **infection** to engulf pathogens. Both neutrophils and macrophages contain enzymes that break down the engulfed material.

Natural killer (NK) cells are a type of lymphocyte in the blood that can detect and destroy cells infected by certain viruses. Viruses attack host cells and use them to facilitate viral replication and production of more viruses. Infected host cells must be rapidly destroyed to prevent this replication and spread of disease. It has been observed that natural killer cells play an especially important role in the early defense against herpes viruses. They also are involved in the killing of some tumors. Natural killer cells may kill by activating a process called apoptosis, the programmed cell death that is present in all cells and is responsible for their self-destruction.

The plasma contains a group of proteins called complements that act in a coordinated manner to attack pathogens. When some pathogens bind with a complement protein called C3b, a series of reactions in the alternative complement pathway occur. The surface of the pathogen is changed so that phagocytic cells can ingest them, a process called opsinization.

If the pathogen is able to effectively cross the barriers of innate immunity, an early induced, non-adaptive response will occur. This response serves to stop pathogens or slow them down until the body can initiate an adaptive immune response. Additional phagocytic cells and molecules are summoned to the site of infection by cytokines, a group of proteins that affect the actions of other cells. Some cytokines can cause an increase in the number of neutrophils in the circulation and **fever**, an elevation in body temperature. As most pathogenic bacteria have optimal growth at lower temperatures, this temperature rise helps to inhibit their growth. The fever also enhances the adaptive immune responses that follow. Local effects from injury or infection give rise to inflammation as white blood cells, fluid, and plasma proteins gather at the site. This is evident clinically at the site by redness, **pain**, heat, and swelling. The **blood vessels** in the site of injury or infection increase in diameter and allow more blood to flow into the area at a slower rate. Immune cells arrive quickly to the site and move into the tissue from the bloodstream. Small proteins called chemokines assist in this process and enhance the migration and activation of cells. Other special proteins called interferons are produced by virally infected cells and may stop the virus from multiplying within other cells, preventing the spread of infection.

Adaptive (acquired) immunity

In adaptive immunity, the immune response is specific for a particular antigen, causes lymphocytes that recognize the antigen to multiply (clonal expansion), and imparts the quality of immunological memory of prior encounters with the antigen. Specificity is an essential component of adaptive immunity as many organisms have evolved to evade the innate immune system. A system of defense is needed to specifically eliminate these elusive invaders, of which there are countless numbers. Two parts of adaptive immunity meet this challenge: cellular-mediated immunity and humoral (antibody-mediated immunity).

CELL-MEDIATED IMMUNITY. Once a pathogen has evaded the innate immune system, the cellular immune response mechanisms are initiated. In the lymphoid tissues, naive lymphocytes that have not been exposed to the pathogen encounter pathogen antigens for the first time. Dendritic cells, macrophages, and B cells take up the antigens that have been trapped in the lymphoid tissue and present them to naïve T cells. These T cells become activated, recognizing specific antigens from the pathogen and become effector cells; helper T cells (TH1 or TH2) and cytotoxic T cells. The TH1 cells produce interferons and cytokines that assist in the activation of macrophages that have ingested pathogens. They also help B cells make antibodies that are used to opsinize pathogens and secrete cytokines that draw phagocytic cells to the site of infection. The TH2 cells produce B cell growth factors that activate the B cells, causing them to multiply and produce antibodies that give rise to a humoral (antibody) response. A delicate balance exists between the TH1 and TH2 cells and is directed by cytokines. Cytotoxic T cells are involved in the killing of pathogens that live inside host cells (cytosolic pathogens) such as viruses and some bacteria. These pathogens hide within cells, and cannot be reached with antibodies. Cytotoxic T cells cause infected cells to undergo programmed cell death or apoptosis and also secrete cytokines that assist in the immune response.

HUMORAL (ANTIBODY-MEDIATED) IMMUNITY. The humoral immune response uses antibodies produced by B cells to destroy pathogens. Pathogens travel in the extracellular fluid (outside of the cell) during the spread of infection. Antibodies specific for foreign pathogen antigens combine with them and neutralize the pathogen, preventing the spread of infection. Toxins secreted by bacteria, such as those from diphtheria and tetanus, are harmful to the body may also be neutralized by antibodies. Bacterial surfaces may be coated with antibody such that phagocytic cells can recognize them and ingest them (opsinization). When antibodies bind with pathogen antigens, the complement system of plasma proteins is activated. This results in opsinization and draws phagocytes to the site of infection.

The B cells are activated upon exposure to antigen, such as that which occurs in the lymphoid tissue. B cell surfaces contain immunoglobulin proteins (antibody) that bind with antigens from pathogens. With the aid of antigen-specific helper T cells, the B cells begin to multiply and produce cells that make antibody (plasma cells). This antibody is directed against the same specific antigen that was recognized by the helper T cell. Memory B cells are also produced and are involved in the protection of the body upon a second exposure to the pathogen at another time. Some pathogens can also cause the B cells to become activated without the help of T cells.

Role in human health

Pathogens have evolved over time such that they can avoid detection by the immune system. Bacteria may change their antigens to escape recognition by immune cells. Such mechanisms occur in the case of bacteria that cause **pneumonia**, **food poisoning**, and gonorrhea. The

influenza virus may undergo a similar process, hence the reason that new flu vaccines are continually under development. The protozoans that cause **malaria** and sleeping sickness also use such methods to escape detection. Epstein-Barr and herpes simplex viruses enter a period of latency within the cells in which the virus does not multiply. The disease is "hidden" from immune surveillance, yet persists in the system to become active at a later time.

In opportunistic infections, a microorganism that is normally present as part of the microflora is no longer controlled by the host and seizes an opportunity to establish infection. This occurs in HIV infection due to suppressed immunity in the body. Opportunistic infections may arise following medical or surgical treatments. Such is the case with urinary tract infections when *Esherichia coli* that are normally found on the gut enter the urinary tract during catheterization or yeast infections following the administration of **antibiotics**.

Immune responses are particularly important during the process of organ transplantation where the recipient may perceive donor antigens as "non-self." Careful matching of donor and recipient tissues and the use of immunosuppressive agents that diminish the immune response minimize rejection. Graft-vs-host disease occurs during bone marrow transplants when the T cells of the donor recognize antigens in the recipient as "foreign."

Directions in immunotherapy

Humans have tried to understand the immune response and prevent the spread of disease throughout history. In ancient China and Asia Minor, attempts were made to inoculate against the smallpox virus by a process called variolization. In 1774 a farmer, Benjamin Jesty, used the cowpox virus to protect his children from smallpox. Edward Jenner began studies using cowpox virus in 1796 and demonstrated that immunization with cowpox protected a child from developing a smallpox infection. He published his results, calling this process **vaccination**. Efforts to refine this process ultimately lead to the declaration by the World Health Organization 1979 that the disease had been eradicated. Research directions for 2000 and beyond include vaccine development for HIV, tumors, schitosomiasis (a parasitic disease), and malaria.

Advances in cytokine therapy are another promising area of research and development. This approach involves boosting the body's own immune modulators to initiate an increased response. The use of cytokines has been explored in bone marrow transplantation, sepsis trials, and treatment of leprosy.

KEY TERMS

Adaptive immunity—The immune response is specific for a particular antigen, causes lymphocytes that recognize the antigen to multiply (clonal expansion), and imparts the quality of immunological memory of prior encounters with the antigen.

Apoptosis—The programmed cell death that is present in all cells and is responsible for their self-destruction.

Innate immunity—Parts of the immune system that are normally present, non-specific, and do not given an elevated response upon a second exposure.

Phagocytosis—The process whereby a cell engulfs particles or materials.

Resources

BOOKS

Anderson, William L. *Immunology.* Madison, CT: Fence Creek Publishing, 1999.

Janeway, Charles A., et al. *Immunobiology: The Immune System in Health and Disease.* London and New York: Elsevier Science London/Garland Publishing, 1999.

Levine, M., et al.,eds., *New Generation Vaccines.* New York: Marcel Dekker, 1997.

Roitt, Ivan, and Arthur Rabson. *Really Essential Medical Immunology.* Malden: Blackwell Science, 2000.

Sharon, Jacqueline. *Basic Immunology.* Baltimore, MD: Williams and Wilkins, 1998.

Widmann, Frances K., and Carol A. Itatani *An Introduction to Clinical Immunology and Serology.* Philadelphia, PA: F.A. Davis Company, 1998.

Wier, Donald M., and John Stewart. *Immunology.* New York: Churchchill Livingstone, Inc., 1997.

OTHER

Mayo Clinic Website. <http://www.mayoclinic.com>.

Med Web, Emory University. <http://www.medweb.emory.edu/MedWeb/>.

Med Web, Medem. <http://www.medem.com>.

The Vaccine Page. <http://www.vaccines.com>.

Jill Ilene Granger, M.S.

Immune system

Definition

The immune system is composed of cells, organs, tissues, and molecules that protect the body from disease. The term "immunity" comes from the Latin word *immunitas*.

Description

Physical barriers

Anatomic barriers provide protection against invading bacterial and viral pathogens. The skin is composed primarily of keratin, which cannot be digested by most microorganisms. The skin is usually dry with a high salt concentration due to sweat. These conditions are not favorable for bacterial growth. Sweat and sebaceous skin secretions also contain substances that kill **bacteria**. Some types of bacteria inhabit the skin surface and do not cause disease under normal conditions (microflora). These bacteria may produce substances that kill other more pathogenic bacteria. The microflora may also consume nutrients required by pathogens. This gives rise to a competitive relationship that limits the growth of the pathogens. If the skin is broken, due to injuries or **burns**, harmful bacteria may enter and give rise to **infection**. The cilia of the **lungs** protect this organ from inhaled pathogens, transporting secretions to the throat so that they can be swallowed and destroyed by **stomach** acid. Secretions in the nose, saliva, and components of tears also contain substances that protect against bacteria and **viruses**.

Cells of the immune system

LYMPHOCYTES. There are two major types of lymphocytes, the T-cells and B-cells, which comprise 20–50% of the white **blood** cells in normal adult human circulation. T-cells mature and differentiate in the thymus gland and assist in cellular immune responses. These cells are responsible for the recognition of antigens (materials that give rise to an **immune response**, such as components of pathogenic bacteria). There are three major types of T-cells that are classified according to their function: cytotoxic T cells (Tc) that kill abnormal cells, helper T cells (Th) that enhance an immune response, and suppressor T-cells (Ts) that diminish the immune response. The B-cells mature in the bone marrow and recognize antigens with the help of T-cells. Upon activation, these cells give rise to plasma cells, which produce antibodies (immunoglobulins). Antibodies bind with toxic pathogen **proteins** or antigens and interact with other cells to remove the invader from the system. Plasma cells are found in the lymph nodes, spleen and bone marrow. B-cells also give rise to **memory** cells that remain alive for long periods of time and assist in a more effective immune response upon the next exposure to the same antigen.

The natural killer cells (NK) are a third type of lymphocyte and comprise approximately 3% of normal blood circulation. These large cells are responsible for the killing of some tumors and virus-infected cells. Additionally, some cells can be induced to kill their targets in a non-specific manner under the appropriate conditions. These cells are called lymphokine activated killer (LAK) cells.

GRANULOCYTES. The granulocytes or polymorphonuclear leukocytes (PMNs) are a group of cells that display a characteristic staining of granules in blood smears, hence their name. These cells have a short life span in the blood (about two or three days), and make up the majority of the white blood cells under normal conditions. They are usually found in greater numbers during an immune response to injury or infection. The neutrophils are a very important type of granulocyte and demonstrate phagocytosis (ingestion of particles by cells, such as particles of bacteria, with ultimate destruction by lysosomal enzymes). These cells are critical in the development of the immune response to pathogens and can migrate from the blood to the tissues during infection by a process known as chemotaxis (the movement of cells in response to and external chemical stimulation). They comprise approximately 40–75% of the blood. The eosinophils are mainly involved in an immune response to parasitic infection and also play a role in the allergic response, and comprise only 1–6% of the blood. The basophils, normally present in low numbers in the circulation (less than 1% of the blood), are thought to play a role in the inflammation and damage to tissue associated with allergic reactions.

MONOCYTES, MACROPHAGES, AND MAST CELLS. Monocytes are a type of cell that circulates in the bloodstream, comprising 2–10% of the blood. Upon migration into the tissues, these cells differentiate into macrophages that are capable of ingesting microorganisms by phagocytosis and have a critical role in the host defense to pathogens. They also produce substances called monokines that are a type of secreted protein (cytokine) that affects the actions of other cells.

Mast cells are distributed in the connective tissues, especially in the skin and mucosal surfaces of the respiratory, gastrointestinal, and urogenital tracts as well as the eye. These cells are also involved in the allergic response.

PLATELETS. Platelets are cell fragments in the blood that are involved in blood clotting and inflammation.

DENDRITIC CELLS. Dendritic cells are potent stimulators of immune responses. These cells play an important role in the increased immune response upon a second exposure to an antigen. Dendritic cells are distributed throughout the body, especially in the T-cell areas of lymphoid organs. In the lymphoid tissue, dendritic cells are involved in the stimulation of T-cell responses.

Central lymphoid tissues

The central lymphoid organs include the bone marrow and thymus. At these sites, the lymphocytes interact with other cells to enhance their development or increase their ability to assist in an immune response. They also acquire the ability to recognize specific antigens before they actually become exposed to them, and are antigen-independent. At this stage the lymphocytes are called naïve lymphocytes because they have not yet been exposed to antigens. The bone marrow is the site of hematopoiesis. Both B-lymphocytes and T-lymphocytes come from this site, but only the B cells undergo maturation in this area (hence the name *B*-cell T-cell).

Peripheral lymphoid tissues

The peripheral lymphoid tissues include the lymphatic vessels, lymph nodes, various lymphoid tissues, and spleen. The events that occur in these areas require exposure to an antigen, and are called antigen-dependent events.

Lymphatic vessels

The filtration of the blood results in the production of extracellular fluid called lymph. The lymphatic vessels that carry the fluid back to the bloodstream also carries cells with antigens. These antigens come from other sites within the body where infection may be present. The fluid passes through the lymph nodes. This fluid is eventually returned to the blood via lymphatic vessels. All the lymph from the body is carried back to the **heart** by way of the thoracic duct.

Lymph nodes and lymphoid tissue

Lymph nodes are distributed along lymphatic vessel pathways and act as a filter for the lymph. The lymph nodes are distributed throughout the **lymphatic system**, and are especially prominent in the neck, axilla (underarm), and groin. These fibrous nodes contain immune cells such as lymphocytes, macrophages, and dendritic cells. Dendritic cells have long, filamentous cytoplasmic processes. These processes have the ability to bind antibodies such that the antibodies can also bind with their specific antigens. This creates a web that traps antigens. The macrophages in the lymph nodes degrade debris and

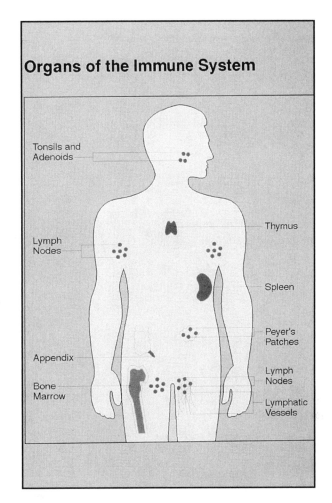

The organs of the immune system are located throughout the body. (*National Institutes of Health. Reproduced by permission.*)

extract material that contains antigens, such as those from pathogenic bacteria. The structure of the lymph nodes is such that both T- and B-cells are exposed to this antigenic material. The cells that recognize this material are held in the lymphoid nodes and tissues where they multiply and differentiate. These cells become effector cells that are capable of fighting disease. The node may enlarge during this process, giving rise to the clinical observation of swollen glands.

Lymphocytes can also be found in several other areas throughout the body. The gut-associated lymphoid tissue is a broad term that describes lymphoid tissue found in the Peyer's patches of the intestine, appendix, adenoids, and tonsils. Cells that protect the respiratory tract are called bronchial-associated lymphoid tissue (BALT). Other mucosal areas are protected as well, and are collectively known as mucosal-associated lymphoid tissue (MALT).

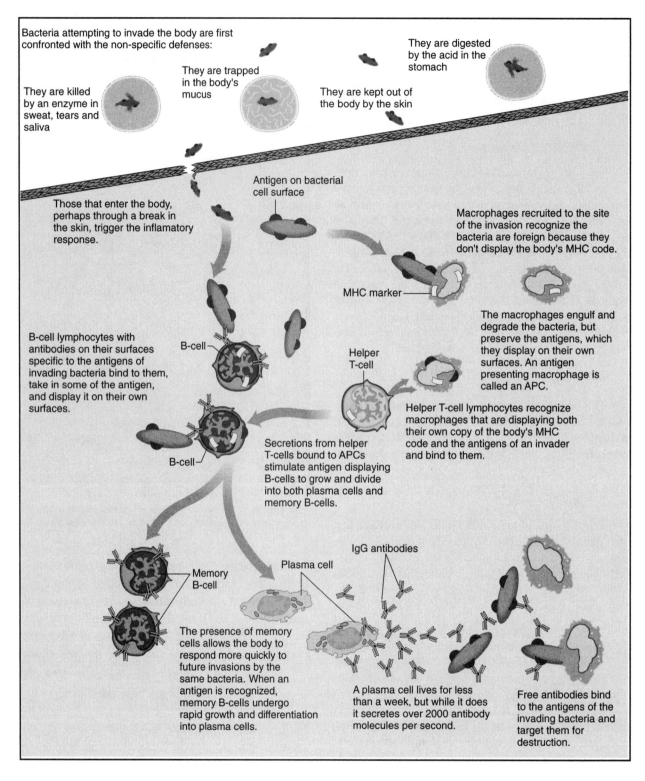

Bacteria attempting to invade the body are first confronted with the non-specific defenses:

They are killed by an enzyme in sweat, tears and saliva

They are trapped in the body's mucus

They are kept out of the body by the skin

They are digested by the acid in the stomach

Those that enter the body, perhaps through a break in the skin, trigger the inflamatory response.

Antigen on bacterial cell surface

Macrophages recruited to the site of the invasion recognize the bacteria are foreign because they don't display the body's MHC code.

MHC marker

B-cell lymphocytes with antibodies on their surfaces specific to the antigens of invading bacteria bind to them, take in some of the antigen, and display it on their own surfaces.

B-cell

Helper T-cell

The macrophages engulf and degrade the bacteria, but preserve the antigens, which they display on their own surfaces. An antigen presenting macrophage is called an APC.

Helper T-cell lymphocytes recognize macrophages that are displaying both their own copy of the body's MHC code and the antigens of an invader and bind to them.

B-cell

Secretions from helper T-cells bound to APCs stimulate antigen displaying B-cells to grow and divide into both plasma cells and memory B-cells.

Memory B-cell

Plasma cell

IgG antibodies

The presence of memory cells allows the body to respond more quickly to future invasions by the same bacteria. When an antigen is recognized, memory B-cells undergo rapid growth and differentiation into plasma cells.

A plasma cell lives for less than a week, but while it does it secretes over 2000 antibody molecules per second.

Free antibodies bind to the antigens of the invading bacteria and target them for destruction.

Immune system. *(Illustration by Hans & Cassidy. Courtesy of Gale Group.)*

Spleen

Blood is filtered in the spleen, where damaged or dead red blood cells are removed from the blood as well as antigens. This organ also serves as a site for storage of erythrocytes and platelets. In the fetus, it is the site of erythropoiesis (formation of red blood cells). Within this organ reside B-cells, T-cells, macrophages, and dendritic cells. As in the lymph nodes, lymphocytes are trapped in this organ. Antibodies and effector cells are produced in the spleen.

Common disorders and diseases

Hypersensitivity reactions result from an immune-mediated inflammatory response to an antigen that would normally be innocuous (causing no harm to the body). Examples include allergic reactions, such as hay **fever**, **asthma**, reactions to insect bites, and the systemic anaphylactic **shock** that occurs in response to bee stings, **allergies** to **antibiotics**, and foods.

Delayed-type hypersensitivity reactions are due to the release of lymphokines. These lymphokines are small polypetides produced by lymphocytes that have been stimulated by an antigen, affecting other cells. This hypersensitivity reaction may occur as part of the normal immune response to infection by bacteria and viruses. This effect is responsible for the tissue damage in the lungs due to **tuberculosis**, the skin lesions that occur in leprosy and herpes, and rashes associated with chicken pox and measles. This may also occur via skin exposure to cosmetics, poison ivy, and allergy to metals in jewelry, resulting in contact dermatitis.

Autoimmune diseases occur when the immune system begins to attack the body or "self." In Grave's disease, antibodies are produced against the thyroid-stimulating hormone (TSH) receptor. In **multiple sclerosis** (MS), antibodies are produced against elements of the myelin sheaths in the **brain** and **spinal cord**. The effects of myasthenia gravis are traced to antibodies directed against the acetylcholine receptor. Following a heart attack, antibodies may form against heart muscle antigens resulting in autoimmune myocarditis. Rheumatoid arthritis (RA) develops from complexes pf antibodies to immunoglobulin G (IgG) in the joints and connective tissue. In systemic lupus erythematosus, the body produces antibodies directed against nuclear antigens and DNA.

In acquired **immunodeficiency** syndrome (**AIDS**), the HIV retrovirus attacks T-cells (CD4), dendritic cells, and macrophages. The number of CD4 T-cell in the blood eventually declines and the body can no longer resist the HIV infection. With the immune system compromised, constitutional disease can develop with fever, weight loss, or **diarrhea**. Neurological disease can occur, resulting in **dementia** and effects to the peripheral nervous system. Pathogenic microorganisms may cause opportunistic infections in this compromised immune state, such as **pneumonia**, diarrhea, skin and mucous membrane infections, and **central nervous system** infections. Cancers may also arise, such as lymphomas. Death from HIV is due to one of these complications or a combination of effects.

Immune system

KEY TERMS

Antibodies (immunoglobulins)—Proteins that bind to their corresponding specific antigen.

Antigen—A material that gives rise to an immune response.

Autoimmune disease—An immune response that occurs when the immune system begins to attack the body or self.

B lymphocyte—A lymphocyte that contains an immunoglobulin on the surface (the B-cell receptor). B cells mature in the bone marrow.

Effector cells—Mature lymphocytes that assist in the removal of pathogens from the system and do not require further differentiation to perform this function.

Hypersensitivity—An immune reaction that results from an immune mediated inflammatory response to an antigen that would normally be innocuous.

Macrophages—Cells that are capable of ingesting microorganisms by phagocytosis and have a critical role in the host defense to pathogens.

Pathogen—A microorganism that has the potential to cause a disease.

T cytotoxic cells (Tc)—T lymphocytes that kill abnormal cells.

T helper cells (Th)—T lymphocytes that enhance an immune response.

T lymphocyte—A lymphocyte that matures in the thymus and has receptors related to CD3 complex proteins.

T suppressor cells (Ts)—T lymphocytes that diminish the immune response.

Resources

BOOKS

Anderson, William L. *Immunology.* Madison, CT: Fence Creek Publishing, 1999.

Janeway, Charles A., et al. *Immunobiology: The Immune System in Health and Disease.* New York: Elsevier Science London/Garland Publishing, 1999.

Roitt, Ivan, and Arthur Rabson. *Really Essential Medical Immunology.* Malden: Blackwell Science, 2000.

Sharon, Jacqueline. *Basic Immunology.* Baltimore: Williams and Wilkins, 1998.

Widmann, Frances K., and Carol A. Itatani. *An Introduction to Clinical Immunology and Serology*. Philadelphia: F. A. Davis Company, 1998.

Wier, Donald M., and John Stewart. *Immunology*. New York: Churchchill Linvingstone, Inc., 1997.

ORGANIZATIONS

American Autoimmune Related Disease Association. <http://www.aarda.org>.

OTHER

Mayo Clinic <http://www.mayoclinic.com>.

Med Web, Emory University. <http://www.medweb.emory.edu/MedWeb/>.

Jill Ilene Granger, M.S.

Immunoassay tests

Definition

Immunoassays are chemical tests used to detect or quantify a specific substance, the analyte, in a **blood** or body fluid sample using an immunological reaction. Immunoassays are highly sensitive and specific assays. Their high specificity results from the use of antibodies and purified antigens as reagents. An antibody is a protein (immunoglobulin) produced by B lymphocytes in response to stimulation by an antigen. Immunoassays measure the formation of antibody-antigen complexes and detect them via an indicator reaction. This may be done by precipitation of the immune complexes and measurement of turbidity or light scattering or by labeling either the antibody or antigen with a radioactive tag, enzyme, fluorescent, or chemiluminescent molecule. High sensitivity is achieved by using an indicator system (e.g. enzyme label) that results in amplification of the measured product.

Immunoassays may be qualitative or quantitative. An example of a qualitative assay is an immunoassay test for **pregnancy**. Pregnancy tests detect the presence of human chorionic gonadotropin (hCG) in urine or serum. In a typical **pregnancy test**, two antibodies are used. The hCG molecule, a protein hormone produced by the trophoblast, is the antigen. One antibody is directed against the alpha polypeptide chain of hCG and the other against the beta polypeptide chain. The sample is added to a support medium containing immobilized antibody to the alpha subunit of hCG. If hCG is present in the sample, it will bind to the antibody. The support is washed to remove all unbound molecules, and an antibody to the beta subunit is added. This second antibody is conjugat-

ed to an enzyme. After washing away any unbound antibody-conjugate, a substrate is added that changes color when acted on by the enzyme. Therefore, the presence of color at the end of the test indicates that hCG was present in the sample. With the use of highly purified antibodies and the enzyme indicator system, pregnancy can be detected within two days after fertilization.

Quantitative immunoassays are performed by measuring the signal produced by the indicator reaction. This same test for pregnancy can be made into a quantitative assay of hCG by measuring the concentration of product formed using a spectrophotometer. A calibration curve is produced by measuring several standards of known hCG concentration, and the curve is used to calculate the concentration of hCG in the sample after measuring the amount of product formed.

Purpose

The purpose of an immunoassay is to measure (or in a qualitative assay detect) an analyte. Immunoassay is the method of choice for measuring analytes normally present at very low concentrations which cannot be determined accurately by less expensive colorimetric tests. Common uses include measurement of drugs, hormones, specific **proteins**, tumor markers, and markers of cardiac injury. Qualitative immunoassays are often used to detect antigens on infectious agents and antibodies produced against them. For example, immunoassays are used to detect antigens on *Hemophilus, Cryptococcus*, and *Streptococcus* organisms in the cerebrospinal fluid of **meningitis** patients. They are also used to detect antigens associated with organisms that are difficult to culture such as hepatitis B virus and *Chlamydia trichomatis*. Immunoassays for antibodies produced in viral hepatitis, HIV, and Lyme disease are commonly used to identify patients with these diseases.

Immunoassay methods

Immunoprecipitation

The reaction of antibodies with protein antigens is a two-phase reaction. The first phase results in the formation of an antibody-antigen complex and takes place within seconds. This is followed by cross linking of individual immune complexes to form a macromolecular aggregate which precipitates out of the solution or gel. This second reaction is slow and often requires overnight incubation to reach completion. The simplest immunoassay method measures the quantity of precipitate which forms after the reagent antibody (precipitin) has incubated with the sample and reacted with its respective antigen to form an insoluble aggregate. Immunoprecipitation reactions may be qualitative or quantitative. In quantitative assays, the immune complexes can be measured by turbidimetry or by performing the reaction in an agarose gel. In gel assays, an excess of the specific antibody is usually poured into the gel. The sample is placed in a well cut into the gel and is allowed to diffuse into the gel. The result will be a ring of precipitated immune complexes which grows larger with time until the endpoint is reached. At the endpoint, the diameter of the ring is proportional to antigen concentration. There will be insufficient antigen beyond the ring to form a visible reaction. Inside the ring, antigen concentration is in excess resulting in small invisible antibody-antigen complexes. The ring position represents the equivalence point or optimal molar ratio of antibody to antigen for the visible reaction. An alternative and more rapid immunoprecipitation method is the Laurel rocket electrophoresis or electroimmunoassay method. In this procedure the antigen is added to wells on one side of the gel which contains a specific antibody throughout. The gel is electrophoresed, and the antigen migrates toward the anodal side of the gel (see Electrophoresis tests). This results in an immunoprecipitation reaction in the shape of a rocket (peak). The height of the peak is logarithmically proportional to antigen concentration.

Particle immunoassays

Immunoprecipitation reactions can be direct or indirect. In direct assays the union of antibody with antigen occurs without attaching the antibody or antigen to a solid phase. In passive or indirect assays, the visible phase of the reaction is enhanced by binding one of the reactants to a solid phase such as latex, red blood cells, or suspension of colloidal gold particles. Particle immunoassays add sensitivity by enhancing surface area and visibility. By linking several antibodies to the particle, the particle is able to bind many antigen molecules simultaneously. This greatly accelerates the speed of the visible reaction. Particle assays may also be performed using antigens bound to the particle. This allows rapid and sensitive detection of antibodies that are markers of diseases such as infectious mononucleosis and rheumatoid arthritis.

Immunonephelometry

The immediate union of antibody and antigen forms immune complexes that are too small to precipitate. However, these complexes will scatter incident light and can be measured using an instrument called a nephelometer. These instruments measure the rate at which the immune complexes form. Incident light from a high intensity monochromatic light source is passed through the reaction cuvet. A photomultiplier tube is placed at an angle (e.g. 70 degrees) to the incident light beam. The

amount of light striking the tube is proportional to antigen concentration. The antigen concentration can be determined within minutes of the reaction. A calibration curve based on a nonlinear model such as a cubic spline plot is used to calculate the antigen concentration from the reaction rate.

Radioimmunoassay (RIA)

RIA is a method employing radioactive isotopes to label either the antigen or antibody. Isotopes are atoms that have unstable nuclei and emit radiation in order to transform into stable atoms. Most RIA methods employ 125 iodine (^{125}I) as the radiolabel. This isotope emits gamma rays. It has a high specific activity so that a very small mass of isotope is needed, and a short half-life (60 days). These properties result in minimal disposal problems with leftover or spent reagents. Gamma rays emitted by the immune complexes are usually measured following removal of unbound (free) radiolabel. Since background radiation is very low and the counting time can be extended if needed to generate more counts, RIA is the most sensitive of all immunoassay methods.

There are two types of RIA, competitive and immunoradiometric (sandwich) assays. Competitive assays use radiolabeled antigen. The labeled antigen "competes" with non-radioactive antigen in the sample for a limited number of binding sites on the reagent antibody. Following incubation, the free radiolabeled antigens are removed by decanting or washing and the radioactivity of the antibody-bound antigens is measured. The radioactivity of the antibody-antigen complexes is inversely proportional to antigen concentration. In the immunoradiometric (IRMA) or sandwich assay, two antibodies are used and one is radiolabeled. In the test system, the sample is incubated with a specific antibody usually attached to a solid phase such as a plastic bead or the wall of a plastic test tube. After washing to remove unbound sample components, a radioactively labeled antibody is added. The second antibody may be directed against a different part of the antigen molecule, or it may be directed against the first antibody (e.g. anti-human immunoglobulin). The second antibody binds to the immune complexes making an antibody-antigen-antibody "sandwich." After washing to remove the unbound radiolabeled antibody, the radioactivity is measured. The amount of radioactivity is directly proportional to antigen concentration.

As with immunonephelometric assays, the calibration curve for RIA is nonlinear. The reagent antibodies reacting with different parts of the antigen have different binding affinities causing the curve to be hyperbolic. Various methods are used to transform the plot so that result can be more accurately determined. Concentration is plotted on the x-axis and radioactivity on the y-axis. In competitive assays, radioactivity is usually expressed as %B/Bo where B is the count per minute of the sample and Bo is the count per minute of the zero calibrator. This keeps the slope of the curve from changing each day as the amount of radioactivity of the reagent decreases naturally. The most common plotting method converts the concentration (x-axis) to log10 and the %B/Bo to logit B/Bo (the natural log of B/Bo divided by 1-B/Bo). This produces a linear plot from which the concentration of unknown can be easily determined.

The major advantages of RIA when compared to other immunoassays are higher sensitivity, easy signal detection, and well-established, rapid assays. The major disadvantages are the health and safety risks posed by use of radiation and the time and expense associated with maintaining a licensed radiation safety and disposal program. For this reason, RIA has been largely replaced in routine clinical laboratory practice by enzyme immunoassay. It is still the gold standard to which other immunochemical methods are compared and is still performed in reference laboratories for analytes such as 11-deoxycortisol, which are not available by other methods.

Enzyme immunoassay (EIA)

Enzyme immunoassay was developed as an alternative to RIA. These methods use an enzyme to label either the antibody or antigen. As for RIA, the EIA methods may be divided into competitive or sandwich type assays. Competitive assays use enzyme labeled antigen, and sandwich assays use an enzyme labeled antibody. The steps performed in RIA and EIA are similar. However, EIA requires an additional step, the addition of substrate which follows the immunological reaction. The sensitivity of EIA approaches that for RIA because a single enzyme molecule can catalyze the conversion of many molecules of substrate to product. Therefore, the enzyme label amplifies the reaction by producing many colored, fluorescent, or chemiluminescent molecules for each antibody-antigen reaction. As with RIA, the relationship between enzyme activity and concentration is nonlinear, and curve-fitting methods such as the cubic spline plot or the four-parameter logistic curve are used to calculate concentration. Many EIA assays use monoclonal antibodies as reagents to increase the sensitivity and lot to lot reproducibility of the assay. Monoclonal antibodies are made by fusing the immunoglobulin genes from a B lymphocyte, which produces the desired antibody specificity with a malignant plasmacytoma cell line. This results in a malignant cell line called a hybridoma that secretes large quantities of the desired antibody. Since the antibodies are derived from identical cells, the antibody molecules are identical and all have the same binding affinity for the antigen.

In addition to safety, another advantage of EIA is that light (versus) radiation is measured. This obviates the need for a scintillation counter that is more expensive than a light measuring instrument. In addition, some competitive EIA methods do not require the separation of antibody-bound and free antigen. These methods are called homogenous assays. Examples of homogenous EIAs are the enzyme multiplied immunoassay technique (EMIT), fluorescence polarization immunoassay (FPIA), and cloned enzyme donor immunoassay (CEDIA).

One of the most widely used EIA methods for detection of infectious diseases is the enzyme-linked immunosorbent assay (ELISA). The ELISA method is a heterogenous sandwich immunoassay, which means that separation of bound and free enzyme label is required. The term ELISA refers to the use of a solid phase to which the antibody (or antigen) is bound in order to facilitate the separation. ELISA methods are usually performed using a microtiter plate containing 96 wells rather than in test tubes. Incubation, washing, and signal reading steps are performed as with EIA sandwich assays described above.

Fluorescent immunoassay (FIA)

FIA refers to immunoassays that utilize a fluorescent label or an enzyme label that acts on the substrate to form a fluorescent product. In fluorescence measurements short wavelength light (usually near ultraviolet light) is used to excite the molecules. Fluorescent molecules stabilize by losing part of the absorbed light energy as heat and part as longer wavelength (visible) light. Fluorescent measurements are inherently more sensitive than colorimetric (spectrophotometric) measurements. Therefore, FIA methods have greater analytical sensitivity that EIA methods which employ absorbance (optical density) measurement.

Chemiluminescent immunossay

Chemiluminescent immunosassays utilize a chemiluminescent label. Chemiluminescent molecules produce light when they are excited by chemical energy. The energy usually comes from an oxidation-reduction reaction. These molecules can be conjugated directly to antigens, or they can be used as substrates for enzyme labels. The most commonly used chemiluminescent labels are acrodinium, luminol, and dioxetane. Acrodinium and luminol are excited by peroxidase enzyme reactions and can be used with EIAs that employ a horseradish peroxidase label. Dioxetane-phosphate can be excited by hydrolysis of the phosphate bond using the enzyme alkaline phosphatase as the label. Consider this example of a competitive binding assay for thyroxine (T4) based on chemiluminescence. The sample is mixed with T4 labeled with alkaline phosphatase (ALP) in a plastic tube containing anti-T4 conjugated to the tube wall. T4 in the sample competes with the ALP-labeled T4 for the antibody. After the reaction, the tube is washed to remove any unbound T4 and dioxetane-phosphate is added. The enzyme hydrolyzes the phosphate ester bond exciting the dioxetane which releases flashes of light. These emissions are measured by a light detector and are inversely proportional to the T4 concentration of the sample.

Precautions

Blood samples are collected by venipuncture using standard precautions for reducing exposure to blood-borne pathogens. It is not necessary to restrict fluids or food prior to collection. Blood should be collected in tubes containing no additive. Risks of venipuncture include bruising of the skin or bleeding into the skin. Random urine samples are acceptable for drug assays; however, 24-hour urine samples are preferred for hormones and other substances which show diurnal or pulse variation.

Special safety precautions must be observed when performing radioimmunoassay (RIA) methods. RIA tests use radioactive isotopes to label antigens or antibodies. Pregnant females should not work in the area where RIA tests are being performed. Personnel handling isotope reagents must wear badges which monitor their exposure to radiation. Special sinks and waste disposal containers are required for disposal of radioactive waste. The amount of radioisotope discarded must be documented for both liquid and solid waste. Leakage or spills of radioactive reagents must be measured for radioactivity; the amount of radiation and containment and disposal processes must be documented.

Results

Immunoassays that are qualitative are reported as positive or negative. Quantitative immunoassays are reported in mass units along with reference intervals (normal ranges) for the test. Normal ranges may be age and gender dependent. Immunoassays that measure antibody concentration may be reported as an antibody titre. The titre is the reciprocal of the highest dilution of sample that gives a positive (detectable) result. Positive immunoassay test results for HIV and drugs of abuse generally require confirmatory testing.

Although immunoassays are both highly sensitive and specific, false positive and negative results may

---

KEY TERMS

Antibody—A protein produced by B lymphocytes in response to stimulation by an antigen.

Antigen—Any substance which induces an immune response.

Chemiluminescent immunoassay—An immunoassay in which the label is a molecule that emits light when excited by a chemical reaction.

Enzyme immunoassay—An immunoassay using an enzyme as the label. The enzymatic reaction product is measured to determine the concentration of the analyte in the sample.

Fluorescent immunoassay—An immunoassay that uses a fluorescent label or produces a fluorescent product.

Immunoassay—A method that measures antibody-antigen complexes formed by reacting purified antibody or antigen with the sample.

Nephelometry—A method for measuring the light scattering properties of a sample.

Radioimmunoassay—A method that uses a radioisotope label in an immunoassay.

---

occur. False negative results may be caused by improper sample storage or treatment, reagent deterioration, or improper washing technique. False positive results are sometimes seen in persons who have heterophile antibodies, especially to mouse immunoglobulins that may be used in the test. False positive results have been reported for samples containing small fibrin strands that adhere to the solid phase matrix. False positives may also be caused by substances in the blood or urine that cross react or bind to the antibody used in the test.

Preparation

Generally, no special instructions need be given to patients for immunoassay testing. Some assays require a timed specimen collection while others may have special dietary restrictions.

Aftercare

When blood testing is used for the immunoassay, the venipuncture site will require a bandage or light dressing to accomplish hemostasis.

Complications

Immunoassay is an *in vitro* procedure, and therefore not associated with complications. When blood is collected slight bleeding into the skin and subsequent bruising may occur. The patient may become lightheaded or queasy from the sight of blood.

Health care team roles

Immunoassay tests are ordered by physicians and samples may be collected by a physician, physician assistant, nurse, or phlebotomist. Simple immunoassay tests (e.g. pregnancy tests and rapid Strep tests) may be performed by medical personnel without special laboratory training. More complex testing is preformed by clinical laboratory scientists CLS(NCA) or medical technologists, MT(ASCP) or by clinical laboratory technicians, CLT(NCA) or medical laboratory technicians, MLT(ASCP).

Resources

BOOKS

Bishop, M.L., J.L. Duben-Engelkirk, and E.P. Fody. *Clinical Chemistry Principles, Procedures, Correlations, 4th ed.* Lippincott, Williams, and Wilkins, 2001.

Burtis, C.A. and E.R. Ashwood, eds. *Tietz Fundamentals of Clinical Chemistry, 5th ed.* Philadelphia: W.B. Saunders, 2001.

Henry, J.B., ed. *Clinical Diagnosis and Management by Laboratory Methods, 20th ed.* Philadelphia: W.B. Saunders, 2001.

Kaplan, L.A. and A.J. Pesce. *Clinical Chemistry Theory, Analysis, Correlation, 3rd ed.* St. Louis: Mosby, 1996.

Law, B. *Immunoassay: A Practical Guide.* London: Taylor and Francis, 1996.

Wild, D., ed. *Immunoassay Handbook, 2nd Ed.* London: Nature Pulishing Group, 2000.

Robert Harr
Paul Johnson

Immunodeficiency

Definition

Immunodeficiency disorders are characterized by an **immune system** that is lacking, impaired, or defective. As a result, patients with immunodeficiency disorders have increased susceptibility to **infection** and neoplasia (**cancer** development). They have more frequent infections that are generally more severe and last longer than those experienced by persons with healthy, functioning immune systems. Patients with immunodeficiency disorders also are susceptible to infection with organisms that do not normally infect healthy people.

Description

The immune system is the body's primary defense against infections. Any defect in the immune system decreases the body's ability to combat infections. Patients with immunodeficiency disorders may suffer more frequent infections, heal more slowly, and have a higher incidence of some cancers.

The normal immune system involves a complex interaction of cells and molecules that can recognize and attack invaders such as **bacteria**, **viruses**, and **fungi**. It also plays a role in fighting cancer. The immune system has both innate and adaptive components. Innate immunity is the immune protection present at birth. Adaptive immunity develops throughout life and has two components, humoral immunity and cellular immunity.

The innate immune system consists of the skin (which serves as a barrier to prevent organisms from entering the body), white **blood** cells called phagocytes, a system of **proteins** called the complement system, and chemicals called interferon. When phagocytes encounter an invading organism, they surround and engulf it to destroy it. The complement system attacks bacteria. The elements of the complement system create a hole in the outer layer of the target cell, which leads to the death of the cell.

The adaptive component of the immune system is extremely complex and is still not entirely understood. Basically, it has the ability to recognize a foreign organism, tumor cell, or foreign chemical as an invader, and to develop a response to attempt to eliminate it.

The humoral response of adaptive immunity involves a type of cell called B lymphocytes that manufacture proteins called antibodies (also called immunoglobulins). Antibodies attach themselves to the foreign substance allowing phagocytes to begin engulfing and destroying the invading organism. The action of antibodies also activates the complement system. The humoral response is particularly useful for attacking bacteria.

The cellular response of adaptive immunity is useful for attacking viruses, some parasites, and possibly cancer cells. The main type of cell in the cellular response is the T lymphocyte. There are helper T lymphocytes and killer T lymphocytes. Helper T lymphocytes play a role in recognizing invading organisms and help killer T lympho-

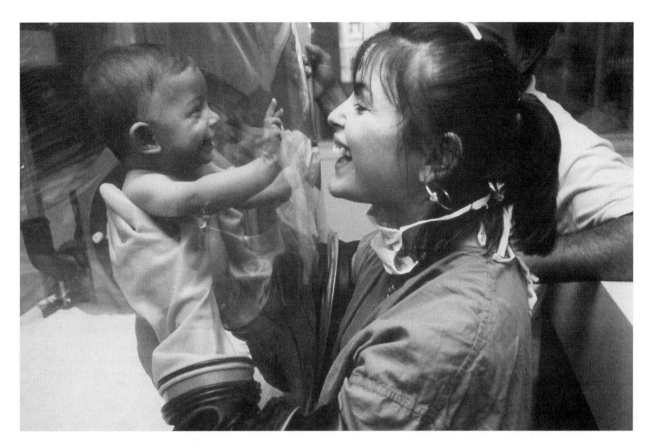

A nurse holds a baby with immunodeficiency, who must be treated in a sterile environment. *(Science Source/Photo Researchers. Reproduced by permission.)*

cytes to multiply. As the name suggests, killer T lymphocytes destroy the target cell or organism.

Defects can occur in any component of the immune system. They can also occur in several components simultaneously, and are then referred to as combined immunodeficiency. Defects can be congenital or acquired.

Congenital immunodeficiency disorders

Congenital immunodeficiency is present at the time of birth and is the result of genetic defects. Though more than 70 different types of congenital immunodeficiency disorders have been identified, they are rare. They may be caused by defects in either B lymphocytes or T lymphocytes, or both, and can also occur in the innate immune system.

B LYMPHOCYTE DEFICIENCY. If there is an abnormality in either the development or function of B lymphocytes, then the ability to make antibodies is impaired. Impaired antibody production results in increased susceptibility to recurrent infections. Bruton's agammaglobulinemia, also known as X-linked agammaglobulinemia, is one of the most common congenital immunodeficiency disorders. The defect results in a decrease or absence of B lymphocytes and therefore a decreased ability to produce antibodies. Patients with this disorder are particularly susceptible to infections of the throat, skin, middle ear, and **lungs**. It is seen only in males because it is caused by a genetic defect on the X chromosome. Since males have only one X chromosome, they always have the disorder if the defective gene is present. Females may have the defective gene; however, since they have two X chromosomes, only one will have the defective gene and the other will have a normal gene to counter the defective gene. Women may pass the defective gene to their male offspring.

Another type of B lymphocyte deficiency involves a group of disorders called selective immunoglobulin deficiency syndromes. There are five different types of immunoglobulins—IgA, IgG, IgM, IgD, and IgE. The most common type of immunoglobulin deficiency is selective IgA deficiency. Some patients with selective IgA deficiency experience no symptoms while others have occasional lung infections and **diarrhea**. In another immunoglobulin disorder, IgG and IgA antibodies are deficient and there is increased IgM. Patients with this disorder tend to develop severe bacterial infections.

Common variable immunodeficiency is another type of B lymphocyte deficiency. In this disorder production of one or more of the immunoglobulin types is decreased and the antibody response to infections is impaired. This disorder generally develops between the ages of 10 and 20 years. Symptoms vary among affected patients, however, most suffer frequent infections and some also experience anemia and rheumatoid arthritis. Many patients with common variable immunodeficiency develop cancer.

T LYMPHOCYTE DEFICIENCIES. Severe defects in the ability of T lymphocytes to mature results in impaired immune responses to infection with viruses, fungi, and certain types of bacteria. These infections are often severe and can be fatal. DiGeorge syndrome is a T lymphocyte deficiency that begins during **fetal development**, although it is not inherited. Children with DiGeorge syndrome either have no thymus or have an underdeveloped thymus. Since the thymus directs the production of T lymphocytes, people with this immunodeficiency have very low numbers of T lymphocytes. They are susceptible to recurrent infections and usually have physical abnormalities as well, which may include low-set ears, a small receding jawbone, and widely spaced eyes. In some cases no treatment is required for DiGeorge syndrome because T lymphocyte production spontaneously improves. Either an underdeveloped thymus begins to produce more T lymphocytes or organ sites other than the thymus compensate by producing more T lymphocytes.

COMBINED IMMUNODEFICIENCIES. Some types of immunodeficiency disorders affect both B lymphocytes and T lymphocytes. For example, severe combined immunodeficiency disease (SCID) is caused by defective development or function of both of these types of lymphocytes. It results in impaired humoral and cellular immune responses. SCID is usually recognized during the first year of life. It tends to cause thrush (a fungal infection of the mouth), diarrhea, failure to thrive, and other serious infections. Treatment requires bone marrow transplant and, if left untreated, children with SCID generally die from infections before the age of two years.

DISORDERS OF INNATE IMMUNITY. Disorders of innate immunity affect phagocytes or the complement system. These disorders also result in recurrent infections.

Acquired immunodeficiency disorders

Acquired immunodeficiency is more common than congenital immunodeficiency. It is the result of an infectious process or other disease. For example, the human immunodeficiency virus (HIV) is the virus that causes acquired immunodeficiency syndrome (**AIDS**). It is not, however, the most common cause of acquired immunodeficiency.

Acquired immunodeficiency often occurs as a complication of other conditions and diseases. For example, the most common causes of acquired immunodeficiency are malnutrition, some types of cancer, and infections such as chickenpox, cytomegalovirus, German measles, measles, **tuberculosis**, infectious mononucleosis (Epstein-Barr virus), chronic hepatitis, lupus, and bacterial and fungal infections.

Sometimes, acquired immunodeficiency is a side effect or consequence of drugs used to treat another condition. For example, organ transplant patients are given drugs to suppress the immune system so the body will not reject the transplanted organ. Some **chemotherapy** drugs, given to combat cancer, have the side effect of killing immune system cells. The risk of infection increases significantly while these drugs are being taken and usually returns to normal one the patient is off the drugs.

Causes and symptoms

Congenital immunodeficiency is caused by genetic defects, which generally occur while the fetus is developing in the womb. These defects affect the development and/or function of one or more components of the immune system. Acquired immunodeficiency is the result of a disease process and occurs later in life. The causes can be disease, infection, or side effects of drugs given to treat other conditions.

Patients with an immunodeficiency disorder tend to become infected by organisms that do not usually cause disease in healthy people and they suffer repeated infections that resolve slowly and cause symptoms that persist for long periods of time. Patients with chronic infections tend to be pale and thin and may have skin rashes. Their lymph nodes tend to be larger than normal and their **liver** and spleen may also be enlarged. Broken **blood vessels**, especially near the surface of the skin, may be apparent and they may develop alopecia (hair loss) and/or conjunctivitis (inflammation of the lining of the eye).

Diagnosis

One of the first signs that a patient may have an immunodeficiency disorder is failure to improve rapidly when given **antibiotics** to treat an infection. Another strong indicator is if a person becomes ill from organisms that do not normally cause diseases. When this occurs in very young children, it may indicate a genetic defect responsible for the immunodeficiency disorder. Among older children or young adults, their medical history helps determine if childhood diseases may have caused an immunodeficiency disorder. Other possibilities to consider are recently acquired infections such as HIV, hepatitis, or tuberculosis.

Laboratory tests are used to determine the exact nature of an immunodeficiency. Most tests are performed on blood samples. A blood cell count will determine if the number of phagocytic cells or lymphocytes is below normal. Lower-than-normal counts of either of these cell types indicate the presence of immunodeficiency. The blood cells are also examined for their appearance. Some patients may have normal cell counts but their blood cells may be structurally defective. If the lymphocyte cell count is low, further testing is performed to determine whether any particular type of lymphocyte is lower than normal. A lymphocyte proliferation test determines if the lymphocytes can respond to stimuli. The failure to respond to stimulants correlates with immunodeficiency. Antibody levels may be measured by a process known as electrophoresis, while complement levels can be determined by immunodiagnostic tests.

Treatment

There is no cure for congenital or most acquired immunodeficiency disorders. Therapy is aimed at controlling infections and, for some disorders, replacing defective or absent cellular components. Patients with Bruton's agammaglobulinemia must be given periodic injections of gamma globulin throughout their lives to compensate for their decreased ability to produce antibodies. The gamma globulin preparation contains antibodies against common invading bacteria. Untreated, the disease is usually fatal.

Common variable immunodeficiency also is treated with periodic injections of gamma globulin throughout life. Additionally, antibiotics are given when necessary to treat infections.

Patients with selective IgA deficiency usually do not require any treatment for the deficiency. Instead, antibiotics are given for infections.

In some cases, no treatment is required for DiGeorge syndrome because T lymphocyte production increases spontaneously. However, in some severe cases, bone marrow transplant or thymus transplant may be performed.

For patients with SCID, bone marrow transplantation is essential. In this procedure, healthy bone marrow is removed from a compatible donor (one with a similar tissue type, usually a brother or sister). The bone marrow of the patient receiving the transplant is destroyed and replaced with the bone marrow from the donor.

Treatment of the HIV infection that causes AIDS consists of drugs called antiretrovirals. Several of these drugs, used in various combinations, can prolong the period of time before the disease becomes symptomatic. However, these drugs do not produce a cure. Other treatments for patients with AIDS are aimed at the particular infections that arise as a result of the impaired immune system. In most cases immunodeficiency caused by malnutrition is reversible. The health of the immune system is directly linked to the nutritional status of the patient. Among the essential nutrients required by the immune system are proteins, **vitamins**, **iron**, and **zinc**. Among cancer patients, periodic relief from chemotherapy drugs can restore the function of the immune system.

In general, patients with immunodeficiency disorders should be counseled to maintain a healthy diet. This is because malnutrition can aggravate immunodeficiencies. Patients should also be advised to avoid exposures to sick people because they can easily acquire new infections. For the same reason, patients should be instructed to practice good personal hygiene, especially dental care. Patients with immunodeficiency disorders should also avoid eating undercooked food because it might contain bacteria that could cause infection. Also, they should be given antibiotics at the first indication of an infection.

Prognosis

Prognosis for individuals with immunodeficiency disorders depends upon the type of disorder. Patients with Bruton's agammaglobulinemia who are given injections of gamma globulin generally live into their 30s or 40s and death is usually from chronic pulmonary infections. Patients with selective IgA deficiency generally live normal lives. They may experience allergic reactions to a blood transfusion, however, and should therefore wear a Medic Alert bracelet or have some other way to alert healthcare professionals about their disorder.

SCID is a serious immunodeficiency disorder. Without successful bone marrow transplant, a child with this disorder usually will not live beyond two years of age.

Although people with HIV/AIDS are living longer than in the past because of **antiretroviral drugs**, AIDS remains a fatal disease. AIDS patients usually die of opportunistic infections—viral and bacterial infections that occur because the impaired immune system is unable to fight them.

Health care team roles

Diagnosis and effective management of immunodeficiency disorders involves cooperation and collaboration between the patient and an interdisciplinary team of

KEY TERMS

Agammaglobulinemia—The lack of gamma glob-ulins in the blood. Antibodies are the main gamma globulins of interest, so this term means a lack of antibodies.

Humoral immune response—Immune system response to antigens found in body fluids. This response is mediated by antibodies, which are secreted by B lymphocytes circulating in the blood.

Lymphocytes—White blood cells that fight infec-tion and disease.

health care professionals. The patient's primary care physician or pediatrician, immunologist, nurses, labora-tory technologists, respiratory therapists, pharmacists, pharmacy assistants, and health educators are involved in helping patients and families gain an understanding of how to prevent infections and effectively manage them when they occur or recur.

Patient education

Nurses and health educators help patients learn how to prevent infection. They teach patients how to identify early symptoms of infection that require prompt medical attention. Pharmacists and pharmacy assistants may offer additional instruction about antibiotic therapy and the importance of adhering to prescribed treatment.

Prevention

There is no way to prevent a congenital immunode-ficiency disorder. Physicians and health care providers should recognize symptoms as early warning signs and implement appropriate treatment as soon as possible. People with congenital immunodeficiency disorders may want to consider **genetic counseling** before having chil-dren to determine if there is a chance they will pass the defect on to their children.

Some infections associated with acquired immunod-eficiency can be prevented or treated before they cause problems. For example, there are effective treatments for tuberculosis and most bacterial and fungal infections. HIV infection can be prevented by practicing "safe sex," and by not using illegal intravenous drugs. These are the primary routes of transmitting the virus.

Malnutrition can be prevented by obtaining adequate **nutrition**. Although it does exist in the United States,

malnutrition is considered a problem of greater magni-tude in developing countries.

Resources

BOOKS

Abbas, A.K., A.H. Lichtman, and J.S. Pober. *Cellular and Molecular Immunology.* Philadelphia: W.B. Saunders Company, 1997.

Berkow, Robert, Editor in Chief. *Merck Manual of Medical Information.* Whitehouse Station: Merck Research Laboratories, 1997.

Roitt, Ivan M. *Roitt's Essential Immunology.* Oxford: Blackwell Science Ltd., 1997.

The Washington Manual of Medical Therapeutics, 30th ed. Philadelphia: Lippincott Williams & Wilkins., 2001.

Barbara Wexler

Impacted stool removal *see* **Fecal impaction removal**

Impacted tooth

Definition

An impacted tooth is a dental disorder in which a tooth fails to fully emerge through the gums.

Description

Teeth emerge through the gums during infancy and also when primary (baby) teeth are replaced by the per-manent teeth. If a tooth fails to emerge or emerges only partially, it is considered impacted. The teeth most com-monly impacted are the wisdom teeth (or third molars). These teeth are the last to develop, but don't begin break-ing through the bone and gum tissue until the later teen years. By this time, the upper and lower jaws have stopped growing and may be too small to accommodate these four additional teeth. As the wisdom teeth continue to grow, one or more may become impacted. If there is not enough room in the mouth to accommodate these teeth, they will remain trapped in the jawbone.

Impacted teeth can take many positions in the bone as they attempt to find a pathway that will allow them to erupt. According to the American Board of Oral and Maxillary Surgeons nine out of every ten people have an impacted tooth. Impacted tooth surgery is the leading surgical problem faced by general dentists and oral sur-geons.

Causes and symptoms

An impacted tooth may be caused by overcrowding of the teeth often because the jaw is too small. Teeth may also become twisted, tilted, or displaced as they try to emerge. Less common symptoms of an impacted tooth may be:

- **pain** and tenderness of the gums
- visible gap where a tooth has not emerged
- redness and swelling of the gums around the impacted tooth area
- swollen lymph nodes of the neck
- difficulty opening the mouth
- prolonged headaches or jaw ache
- unpleasant **taste** when biting down on or near the impacted area
- raised gum tissue where impacted tooth lies under the gum tissue

Diagnosis

Upon visual examination, the dentist may find signs of **infection** or swelling in the area where the tooth is absent or only partially erupted. **Dental x rays** are essential in diagnosing an impacted tooth. The dentist may also see signs of enlargement of the tissue over the area where a tooth has not emerged, or has emerged only partially. The impacted tooth may also be pressing on an adjacent tooth causing pain.

Treatment

The goal of treatment is to relieve irritation of the mouth and remove pain caused by the impacted tooth. If the impacted tooth is not causing infection or inflammation, or is not affecting the alignment of the other teeth, no treatment may be necessary. Warm, salt-water rinses may be advised to aid in soothing the swollen gums.

A dentist may perform an extraction with forceps and local anesthetic agent if the tooth is exposed and appears to be easily removable. Extracting an impacted tooth typically requires making an incision through gum tissue to expose the tooth and may require removing portions of bone to free the tooth. The tooth may have to be removed in pieces to minimize destruction to the surrounding bone and tissue. The extraction site may require one or more stitches to aid healing.

Another type of treatment called ligation is performed on impacted teeth in conjunction with orthodontics. A small portion of the crown of an impacted tooth is exposed through the gum tissue and a small orthodontic

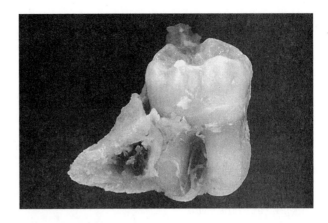

This impacted wisdom tooth, attached to part of the jaw bone, was broken during extraction. *(Photograph by James Stevenson, Photo Researchers, Inc. Reproduced by permission.)*

bracket is attached to the exposed area so that the tooth can be brought into alignment with the rest of the teeth while the patient is being orthodontically treated. An oral and maxillofacial surgeon commonly performs this type of treatment.

Antibiotics may be required after the extraction or ligation if the area is infected or there is a risk of infection. Over the counter pain medications, such as Tylenol, Advil, or Motrin may be taken to lessen the pain of the treated area. This pain will gradually decrease over two to three days.

Prognosis

The prognosis is very good for the removal or ligation of an impacted tooth. Potential complications include postoperative infection, temporary numbness from nerve irritation, jaw fracture, and jaw joint pain. A painful condition, which may develop after an extraction, is known as a dry socket, when a **blood** clot does not completely fill the empty tooth socket, or is disturbed by an oral vacuum, by drinking through a straw, or by smoking. The bone beneath the socket is painfully exposed to air. The general dentist will pack the socket with medication to allow healing to take place. One complication of the ligation process is that the bracket and chain may come off and will need to be replaced by the oral and maxillofacial surgeon.

Health care team roles

Extraction of a symptomatic impacted tooth is often treated in a general dental office. If the tooth is deeply impacted or more difficult to remove than expected the general dentist may refer the patient to an oral and maxillofacial surgeon.

KEY TERMS

Dry socket—A painful condition following tooth extraction in which a blood clot does not properly fill the empty socket, leaving the bone underneath exposed to air and food.

Eruption—The process of a tooth breaking through the hard and soft oral tissue to grow into place in the mouth.

Extraction—The surgical removal of a tooth from its socket in the bone.

Ligated—Where a small chain and wire are glued to the impacted tooth by an oral and maxillofacial surgeon. The wire is tightened during monthly visits with an orthodontist. This brings the tooth out of the bone and gum tissue and into alignment with the other teeth.

Oral and maxillofacial surgeon—A dentist specializing in oral and maxillofacial surgical procedures of the mouth.

Wisdom teeth—Also called third molars, the last teeth to erupt in the upper and lower jawbone.

Prevention

There is no way to prevent an impacted tooth. Heredity plays a role in the growth and development of the jaw, making it hard to prevent an impacted tooth from happening. Complications with an impacted tooth can be prevented by **patient education**, good **oral hygiene**, and proper care of the extraction area.

Resources

PERIODICALS

Frank, Charles A. "Treatment Options for Impacted Teeth." *Journal of The American Dental Association* (May 2000): 623.

ORGANIZATIONS

American Association of Oral and Maxillofacial Surgeons, 9700 West Bryn Mawr Avenue, Rosemont, IL 60018-5701. (847) 678-6200. <http://www.aaoms.org>.

American Board of Oral and Maxillofacial Surgeons, 625 North Michigan Avenue, Suite 1820, Chicago, Illinois 60611. (312) 642-0070. <http://www.aaoms.org>.

American Dental Association, 211 East Chicago Avenue, Chicago, IL 60611. (312) 440-2500. <http://www.ada.org>.

OTHER

Ashman, Steven G. "Impacted Tooth," July 1999. <http://dr.ashman.com/sg00059.htm>.

"Impacted Tooth." Adam.com Health Issues, <http://merckmedco.adam.com/ency/article/001057.htm>.

"Impacted Tooth." BIOME, April 9, 2001. <http://omni.ac.uk/browse/mesh/detail/C0040456L0040456.html>.

Cindy F. Ovard, RDA

Impedance phlebography *see* **Impedance plethysmography**

Impedance plethysmography

Definition

Impedance plethysmography, also called impedance test or **blood** flow or impedance **phlebography**, is a non-invasive test that uses electrical monitoring in the form of resistance (impedance) changes to measure blood flow in veins of the leg. Information from this test helps doctors detect deep vein thrombosis (blood clots or thrombophlebitis).

Purpose

Impedance plethysmography may be done in order to:

• detect blood clots lodged in the deep veins of the leg

• screen patients who are likely to have blood clots in the leg

• detect the source of blood clots in the **lungs** (pulmonary emboli)

Accurate diagnosis of deep vein thrombosis (DVT) is critical because blood clots in the legs can lead to more serious problems. If a clot breaks loose from a leg vein, it may travel to the lungs and lodge in a blood vessel in the lungs. Blood clots are more likely to occur in people who have recently had leg injuries, surgery, **cancer**, or a long period of bed rest.

Precautions

Because this test is not invasive, it can be done on all patients and is easy to perform. However, the accuracy of the results is affected if the patient does not breathe normally or keep the leg muscles relaxed. Compression of the veins because of pelvic tumors or decreased blood flow, due to **shock** or any condition that reduces the amount of blood the **heart** pumps, may also change the test results. Both false-positives (e.g. when thrombi are non-occulsive) and false-negatives have been reported using this technique, which justifies repeated testing over a period of seven to ten days for patients with initial negative results. Success rates for this test have been estimated at anywhere from 65–66% to 92–98%.

Description

Using conductive jelly, the examiner strategically places two to four electrodes on the patient's calf (the four-electrode configuration yields a more uniform and precise current density and consequent measurement result). These electrodes are connected to an instrument called a plethysmograph, which records the changes in electrical resistance that occur during the test and produces a graph of the results.

The patient must lie down and raise one leg at a 30° angle so that the calf is above the level of the heart. The examiner then wraps a pressure cuff around the patient's thigh and inflates it to a pressure of 45–60 cm of water for 45 seconds. The plethysmograph records the electrical impedance changes that correspond to changes in the volume of blood in the vein at the time the pressure is exerted and again three seconds after the cuff is deflated. This procedure is repeated several times in both legs.

This test takes 30-45 minutes, costs an estimated $50-$100 (as of 2001), and results can be available within a few minutes.

Impedance plethysmography works by measuring the resistance to the transmission of electrical energy (impedance). This resistance is dependent upon the volume of blood flowing through the veins. By graphing the impedance, the doctor or technician can tell whether a clot is obstructing blood flow.

Preparation

Patients undergoing this test do not need to alter their diet, change their normal activities, or stop taking any medications. They will wear a surgical gown during the test and should be asked to urinate before the test starts. If keeping the legs elevated causes discomfort, mild **pain** medication can be given.

Aftercare

The patient may resume normal or postoperative activities after the test.

Complications

Impedance plethysmography is painless and safe. It presents no risk to the patient.

Results

Normally, inflating the pressure cuff will cause a sharp rise in the pressure in the veins of the calf because blood flow is blocked. When the cuff is released, the pressure decreases rapidly as the blood flows away.

If a clot is present, the pressure in the calf veins will already be high. It does not become sharply higher when the pressure cuff is tightened. When the pressure cuff is deflated, the clot blocks the flow of blood out of the calf vein. The decrease in pressure is not as rapid as when no clot is present and the shape of the resulting graph is different, all of which is indicative of obstruction of major deep veins.

Health care team roles

Doctors, nurses, or well-trained technicians may perform all or part of the procedure, which includes application of electrodes and placement of cuffs as well as handling of the electronic equipment and analysis of results.

Training

Training for the procedure includes instruction on placement of electrodes and cuffs, facility with the electronic equipment, correct patient positioning during the procedure, and capability for accurate interpretation of resulting impedance graphs.

Resources

PERIODICALS

Aksamit, T. R. "Thromboembolism Occurrence and Diagnosis in the Medical Intensive Care Unit." *Seminars in Thrombosis and Hemostasis* 27, no. 1 (2001): 47-58.

Halek, J., "A Method of Local Skin Perfusion Detection." *Journal of Medical Systems* 24, no. 4 (2000): 257-264.

Kahn, S. R., L. Joseph, S. A. Grover, and J. R. Leclerc. "A Randomized Management Study of Impedance Plethysmography vs. Contrast Venography in Patients With a First Episode of Clinically Suspected Deep Vein Thrombosis." *Thrombosis Research* 102 (2001): 15-24.

OTHER

Griffith, H. Winter. *Complete Guide to Medical Tests.* Fisher Books. <http://www.mdadvice.com/library/test/medtest224.html>.

Bryan Ronain Smith

Implantable cardioverter-defibrillator

Definition

The implantable cardioverter-defibrillator (ICD) is a surgically implanted electronic device that directs an electric charge directly into the **heart** to treat life-threatening heartbeat irregularities.

Purpose

The implantable cardioverter-defibrillator is used to detect and stop serious arrhythmias and restore a normal heartbeat. The exact indications for the implantation of the device are controversial, but patients suffering from ventricular fibrillation (unproductive heartbeat), ventricular tachycardia (abnormally fast heartbeat), long QT syndrome (an inherited heart disease), or others at risk for sudden cardiac death are potential candidates for this device. A study by the National Institute for Heart, Lung, and Blood of the National Institutes of Health indicated a significant increase in survival for patients suffering from ventricular arrhythmias when ICD implant is compared to medication. Several follow-up studies indicate that this may be due to the marked increase in survival for the sickest patients, generally defined as those having a heart weakened to less than 50% of normal, as measured by the ability of the left side of the heart to pump blood. Overall, studies have documented a very low mortality rate of 1–2% annually for persons implanted with the device, compared to approximately 15–25% for patients on drug therapy.

Description

Similar in structure to a pacemaker, an ICD has three main components: a generator, leads, and an electrode. The generator is encased in a small rectangular container, usually about 2 in (5 cm) wide and around 3 oz (85 g) in weight. Even smaller generators have been developed, measuring 1 in (2.54 cm) in diameter and weighing about half an ounce (14.17 g). The generator is powered by lithium batteries and is responsible for generating the electric shock. The generator is controlled by a computer chip that can be programmed to follow specific steps according to the input gathered from the heart. The programming is initially set and can be changed using a device (called a wand programmer) that communicates by radio waves through the chest of the patient after implantation.

One or two leads, or wires, are attached to the generator. These wires are generally made of platinum with an insulating coating of either silicone or polyurethane. The leads carry the electric shock from the generator. At the tip of each lead is a tiny device called an electrode that delivers the necessary electrical shock to the heart. Thus, the electric shock is created by the generator, carried by the leads and delivered by the electrodes to the heart. The decision of where to put the leads depends on the needs of the patient, but they can be located in the left ventricle, the left atrium, or both.

According to the American College of Cardiology, more than 100,000 persons worldwide currently have an ICD. The battery-powered device rescues the patient from a life-threatening arrhythmia by performing a number of functions in order to reestablish normal heart rhythm, which varies with the particular problem of the patient. Specifically, if encountered with ventricular tachycardia, many devices will begin treatment with a pacing regimen. If the tachycardia isn't too fast, the ICD can deliver several pacing signals in a row. When those signals stop, the heart may go back to a normal rhythm. If the pacing treatment is not successful, many devices will move onto cardioversion. With cardioversion, a mild shock is sent to the heart to stop the fast heartbeat. If the problem detected is ventricular fibrillation, a stronger shock called a defibrillation is sent. This stronger shock can stop the fast rhythm and help the heartbeat go back to normal. Finally, many ICDs can also detect heartbeats that are too slow. It can act like a pacemaker and bring the heart rate up to normal.

ICDs that defibrillate both the ventricles and the atria have also been developed. Such devices not only provide dual-chamber pacing but also can distinguish ventricular from atrial fibrillation. Patients that experience both atrial and ventricle fibrillation or atrial fibrillation alone that would not be controlled with a single chamber device are candidates for this kind of ICD.

Operation

ICD insertion is considered minor surgery and can be performed in either an operating room or an electrophysiology laboratory. The insertion site, in the chest, will be cleaned, shaved and numbed with the injection of a medication (local anesthetic). Generally, left handed persons have ICDs implanted on the right side and visa versa, to speed return to normal activities. Two small cuts (incisions) are made, one in the chest wall and one in a vein just under the collarbone. The wires of the ICD are passed through the vein and attached to the inner surface of the heart. The other ends of the wires are connected to the main box of the ICD, which is inserted into the tissue under the collarbone and above the breast. Once the ICD is implanted, the physician will test it several times before the anesthesia wears off by causing the heart to fibrillate and making sure the ICD responds properly. The doctor then closes the incision with sutures (stitches), staples or surgical glue. The entire procedure takes about an hour.

Immediately following the procedure, a **chest x ray** will be taken to confirm the proper placement of the wires in the heart. The ICD's programming may be adjusted by passing the programming wand over the chest. After the initial operation, the physician may induce ventricular fibrillation or ventricular tachycardia one more time prior to the patient's discharge, although recent studies suggest that this final test is not generally necessary.

A short stay in the hospital is usually required following ICD insertion but this varies with the patient's age and condition. If there are no complications, complete recovery from the procedure will take about four weeks. During that time, the wires will firmly take hold where they were placed. In the meantime, the patient should avoid heavy lifting or vigorous movements of the arm on the side of the ICD, or else the wires may become dislodged.

After implantation, the implantable cardioverter-defibrillator is programmed to respond to rhythms above the patient's **exercise** heart rate. Once the device is in place, many tests will be conducted to ensure that the device is sensing and defibrillating properly. About 50% of patients with ICDs require a combination of drug therapy and the ICD.

Safety

Environmental conditions that can affect the functioning of the ICD after installation include:

- strong electromagnetic fields, such as those used in arc-welding
- contact sports
- shooting a rifle from the shoulder nearest the installation site
- cell phones used on that side of the body
- magnetic mattress pads, such as those believed to treat arthritis
- some medical tests such as **magnetic resonance imaging** (MRI)

Environmental conditions often erroneously thought to affect ICDs include:

- microwave ovens (the waves only affect old, unshielded **pacemakers** and do not affect ICDs)
- airport security (although metal detector alarms could be set off, so patients should carry a card stating they have an ICD implanted)
- anti-theft devices in stores (although patients should avoid standing near the devices for prolonged periods)

Patients should also be instructed to memorize the manufacturer and make of their ICD. Although manufacturing defects and recalls are rare, they do occur and a patient should be prepared for that possibility.

Maintenance

In general, if the condition of the patient's heart, drug intake, and metabolic condition remain the same, the ICD requires only periodic checking every two months or so for battery strength and function. This is done by placing a special device over the ICD that allows signals to be sent over the telephone to the doctor, a process called trans-telephonic monitoring.

If changes in medications or physical condition occur, the doctor can adjust the ICD settings using a programmer, which involves placing the wand above the pacemaker and remotely changing the internal settings. One relatively common problem is the so-called "ICD storm," where the machine inappropriately interprets an arrhythmia and gives a series of shocks. Reprogramming can sometimes help alleviate that problem.

When the periodic testing indicates that the battery is getting low, an elective ICD replacement operation is

KEY TERMS

Arrhythmia—A variation of the normal rhythm of the heartbeat.

Cardioverter—A device to apply electric shock to the chest to convert an abnormal heartbeat into a normal heartbeat.

Defibrillation—An electronic process which helps re-establish a normal heart rhythm.

Ventricles—The two large lower chambers of the heart which pump blood to the lungs and the rest of the human body.

Ventricular fibrillation—An arrhythmia in which the heart beats very fast but blood is not pumped out to the body that can become fatal if not corrected.

Ventricular tachycardia—An arrhythmia in which the heart rate is more than 100 beats per minute.

scheduled. The entire signal generator is replaced because the batteries are sealed within the case. The leads can often be left in place and reattached to the new generator. Batteries usually last about four to eight years.

Health care team roles

Electrophysiologists are specially trained cardiologists or thoracic surgeons who study and treat problems with the heart conduction system. They often implant the ICD system and oversee the programming or reprogramming of the device. They are assisted in the operating room by specially trained nurses, who can help with the testing of the ICD, and the anesthesiologist, who is responsible for numbing the area of the incision and keeping the patient comfortable. ICD manufacturers often send representatives to be present for the implantation and initial programming.

The maintenance of the ICD can be overseen by the electrophysiologist or cardiologist and associated staff, which can include specially trained cardiac medical assistants as well as nurses.

Training

The training for implantation of ICDs and their use occurs during medical training (medical or nursing school) and on the job. Physicians, nurses, and other allied health professionals can also receive training about ICDs as part of their continuing education courses.

Continuing education concerning ICD tends to be in specific subject areas, such as the psychological effects of ICD firing, the interpretation of clinical trials in the area, or comparisons between appropriate and inappropriate firing rates.

Resources

BOOKS

Gersh, Bernard J., ed. *Mayo Clinic Heart Book.* New York: William Morrow and Company, Inc., 2000.

PERIODICALS

Moss, A. "Implantable Cardioverter-defibrillator Therapy: The Sickest Patients Benefit Most." *Circulation.* 101 (April 2000): 1638–1640.

Sears, Samuel F. Jr. et al. "Fear of Exertion Following ICD Storm: Considering ICD Shock and Learning History." *Journal of Cardiopulmonary Rehabilitation.* 21 (January/February 2001): 47.

ORGANIZATIONS

American Heart Association. National Center. 7272 Greenville Avenue, Dallas, TX, 75231-4596. (214) 373-6300. <http://www.americanheart.org>.

North American Society of Pacing and Electrophysiology. 6 Strathmore Road, Natick, MA, 01760-2499. (508) 647-0100. <http://www.naspe.org/index.html>.

OTHER

"Implantable Cardioverter-Defibrillator." *American Academy of Family Physicians* <http://www.familydoctor.org/handouts/270.html> (May 7, 2001).

"Implantable Cardioverter-Defibrillators (ICDs)" *North American Society of Pacing and Electrophysiology* 2000. <http://www.naspe.org/your_heart/treatments/icds.html&>. (May 7, 2001).

Michelle L. Johnson, M.S., J.D.

Incentive spirometry *see* **Ventilation assistance**

Incontinence, fecal *see* **Fecal incontinence**

Infant nutrition

Definition

Infant **nutrition** is the feeding behavior of an infant during the first year after birth.

Purpose

Due to the tremendous amount of growth during infancy, adequate nutrition after birth is essential for the development and nourishment of children. Proper nutrition can be obtained from the use of breast milk, infant formulas, and adequate diet related to age.

Precautions

When assessing the nutritional status of infants, it is important to consider the differences in the bodily functions of infants. The gastrointestinal functions of newborns are much slower than that of older infants, especially gastric emptying, which may account for the regurgitation, or spitting up, in newborns.

Passage through the **small intestine** is slower for infants, which helps ensure proper absorption and digestion of nutrients. However, the **large intestine** has a much faster transit time, which puts infants at an increased risk of **dehydration** if resorption of water and electrolytes is compromised.

The digestion of fat is also limited in infancy due to the decreased amount of pancreatic lipase, an enzyme secreted by the **pancreas** to digest fat. However, other lipases present in breast milk compensate for the lack of this enzyme and aid in fat digestion. Thus, the fat in human milk is more readily absorbed than the fat in prepared formulas.

Renal function is also limited in newborns because their **kidneys** are not fully developed until one month of age. The immature kidneys and other factors limit the newborns' ability to cope with fluid and electrolyte loads. Infants fed breast milk or properly prepared formulas normally do not have problems with renal solute load, although problems may occur with **fever**, **diarrhea**, or a reduction in the volume of fluids consumed.

Infants who sleep through the night may need to be woken up mid-way through the night to feed if they are underweight or not consuming enough. It is important to have routine check-ups with the doctor or dietitian to ensure that infants are eating adequately. Honey should also not be given to infants because it may contain spores that cause botulism.

Description

During the first six months of life, infants can receive adequate nutrition through either breast milk or fortified formula. An infant who is breastfeeding will need to nurse on demand or usually about eight to 12 times per day, while babies who are formula fed need to eat about six to eight times per day. In both breastfed and formula-fed infants, the number of feedings decreases as they get older, but the amount of milk the baby consumes at each feeding increases.

Prior to four months of age, an infant's **digestive system** has not developed well enough to tolerate solid foods. But at about four to six months of age, solid foods can start to be introduced into the infant's diet. It is important to look for signs that an infant is developmentally ready to handle solid foods. Once infants can hold their head up, sit up with minimal support, and begin to show an interest in food, solid feedings of iron-fortified baby cereal can be started. Mixing it with breast milk or formula to get a thin consistency is recommended until the infant can control its mouth better to handle a thicker consistency.

At six to eight months of age, the introduction of fruit juices and strained fruits and vegetables can begin. Use unsweetened juices that contain large amounts of **vitamin C**, such as orange, apple, or grape, but avoid putting an infant to sleep with a bottle of juice as this can lead to tooth decay. Introduce fruits and vegetables one at a time and wait a few days in between introductions to make sure the infant has no allergic reactions. Use plain fruits and vegetables such as carrots, squash, beans, bananas, applesauce, and pears. Introducing vegetables into the diet before fruits is often recommended because the sweet **taste** of fruit may make vegetables less appealing to the infant. Finger foods may also be introduced at this time, but avoid foods that may cause choking, such as grapes, hotdogs, nuts, and seeds. Breast milk or fortified formula should still be given about three to five times a day.

At eight to 12 months of age, an infant should still be receiving breast milk or formula three to four times a day, but also should start eating strained or finely chopped meat. Introduce different meat every week and include strained and ground meats and hotdogs. If eggs are given, only the yolk should be used until one year of age in case the infant is sensitive to egg whites.

If an infant still uses a bottle at one year of age, the bottle should only contain water, or whole (**vitamin D**) milk can be used instead of breast milk or formula. Low-fat milk should not be used until at least two years of age because infants need the extra calories for adequate development. Thereafter, no less than 2% milk should be fed to a young child.

Breastfeeding versus formula feeding

During the first year of life, breast milk is the best source of nutrition for infants. Breast milk provides several health benefits for both the mother and infant beyond the benefits of adequate nutrition. Nutritionally, breast milk provides the appropriate amounts of carbohydrate, protein, and fat for infants, along with essential **vitamins**, **minerals**, and digestive enzymes. It also provides antibodies that help increase the infant's **immune system**, decrease gastrointestinal distress, reduce the risk of allergy, and promote the development of the jaws and teeth. Colostrum is the milk secreted from the mother's breasts during the first few days after giving birth. This milk adequately provides the infant's needs during its first week of life as it is characterized by high protein and antibody content. For the mother, breastfeeding facilitates a faster recovery from labor, allows the mother to rest more often, and saves money that would have been spent on formula.

If breastfeeding is not the chosen method of feeding, iron-fortified formulas can be used to provide adequate nutrition. Infant formula has more protein and more **iron** than human milk, but it lacks antibodies. The American Academy of Pediatrics recommends that all formula-fed infants be given iron-fortified formula. Formula feeding also allows the mother to receive help with feedings and sleep more during the night. Formulas are available for infants who may have **allergies** to milk protein or are lactose intolerant. There are also formulas available for **premature infants** and those who have **metabolism** disorders.

Preparation

Improperly prepared formulas can be a very common cause of infant illnesses. When preparing formula, it is recommended that it not be mixed with warm tap water as this can increase the amount of lead in the formula, which can be very harmful to the infant. Bottles should also not be heated in a microwave because this could cause the milk to scald or the bottle to explode. Lastly, adding sweetened beverages or cereals to bottles should also be avoided because they will only displace the more nutrient-dense formula.

Complications

Most women are capable of breastfeeding as long as they allow their infant to nurse, although there are special circumstances when formula must be used instead of breast milk. Galactosemia is a rare genetic disease in which newborns lack the enzyme needed to convert galactose to glucose. Galactose is a component of lactose, which is very abundant in breast milk. Without the enzyme to convert it to glucose, galactose accumulates in the **blood** causing tissue damage and possibly death. Therefore, it is essential that these infants receive a lactose-free soy-based formula.

Phenylketonuria is another genetic disorder in which newborns lack the enzyme needed to convert the essential amino acid phenylalanine to the amino acid tyrosine. Accumulation of phenylalanine in the blood can cause severe mental retardation. Therefore, it is necessary to start a low phenylalanine diet with a low phenylalanine formula.

Health care team roles

The dietitian plays a very important role in educating parents on the importance of adequate infant nutrition and proper feeding methods. Dietitians are also responsible for informing people of the proper preparation of formula and the advantages and disadvantages of both breastfeeding and formula feeding. While caring for an infant, it is important to have routine check-ups with the doctor to check the infant's height and weight to ensure that the infant is at the right stage of growth and receiving adequate nutrition.

Resources

BOOKS

Worthington-Roberts, Bonnie S., and Sue Rodwell Williams. *Nutrition Throughout the Life Cycle, 4th ed.* New York: McGraw-Hill, 2000.

PERIODICALS

Fein, Sara, and Christina D. Falci. "Infant Formula Preparation, Handling, and Related Practices in the United States." *Journal of the American Dietetic Association* (October 1999): 1234-40.

ORGANIZATIONS

La Leche League International. 1400 N. Meacham Road, Schaumburg, IL 60168-4079. (847) 519-7730. <http://www.lalecheleague.org/>.

Women, Infants, and Children. The Food and Nutrition Service Headquarters. 3101 Park Center Drive. Alexandria, VA 22302. (703) 305-2746.

OTHER

"Appropriate Diet for Age." *WebMD* 2001. <http://my.webmd.com/content/asset/adam_nutrition_diet_for_age>. (18 April 2001).

"Breastfeeding." *WebMD* 2001. <http://my.webmd.com/content/asset/adam_nutrition_nursing>. (18 April 2001).

"Infant Formulas." *WebMD* 2001. <http://my.webmd.com/content/asset/adam_nutrition_bottle_feeding>. (18 April 2001).

Lisa M. Gourley

Infant respiratory distress syndrome *see* **Respiratory distress syndrome**

Infarct avid imaging *see* **Technetium heart scan**

Infection

Definition

Infection is the invasion and replication of microorganisms—**viruses**, **bacteria**, protozoa, or **fungi**—in body tissues.

Description

There are thousands of infectious agents that can cause human disease. Although the body is extraordinarily adaptive in its responses to such agents, sometimes its

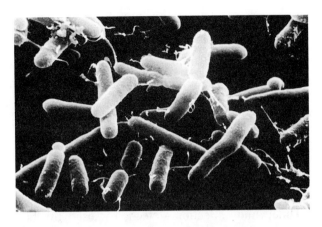

Salmonella **bacteria often cause infection through food contamination.** *(Photograph by Oliver Meckes. Photo Researchers, Inc. Reproduced by permission.)*

preventative measures fail, resulting in disease. A subclinical infection occurs when the body's defensive mechanisms are effective, resulting in no apparent clinical symptoms. When infection persists to cause disease, it is called an acute or chronic infection.

Infectious agents

There are four major classes of organisms that infect the human body:

- Viruses: microscopic agents that consist of genetic material coding for the virus's reproduction enclosed in a protective protein coat or lipid membrane. Viruses are obligate intracellular parasites; they cannot replicate without first infecting a cell and exploiting its reproductive capabilities.

- Bacteria: microscopic prokaryotic organisms (lacking a nuclear membrane, mitochondria, and other organelles). Two major classes include gram-positive bacteria (surrounded by a protective cell wall) and gram-negative bacteria (surrounded by an outer lipid membrane).

- Fungi: eukaryotic organisms (containing distinct organelles and a nucleus enclosed by a nuclear membrane). Fungi can be unicellular (e.g., yeast) or multicellular (e.g., mold).

- Parasites: eukaryotic organisms ranging from microscopic, unicellular protozoa to macroscopic arthropods and worms.

Infectious organisms are found everywhere on Earth—in extremes of hot and cold; in acidic and alkaline environments; in air, soil, and water; in our bodies, and on our skin. The human body is colonized by numerous types of bacteria (called normal flora) that reside in the **stomach**, intestines, colon, upper respiratory tract, and

KEY TERMS

B cells—White blood cells responsible for the production of antibodies.

Ciliated cells—Cells with hair-like structures that help flush out foreign particles from the human body.

Complement system—Proteins that activate inflammation response and recruit white blood cells to the site of infection.

Endogenous infection—Infection caused by the normal flora of the human body.

Eukaryote—An organism whose cells contain a true nucleus bound by a membrane.

Exogenous infection—Infection caused by microbes found external to the human body.

Normal flora—Types of bacteria and other organisms that colonize the human body without normally causing disease.

Obligate intracellular parasites—Microbes that must remain inside of a cell in order to survive and replicate.

Phagocytosis—Engulfment and digestion of foreign particles and cells by phagocytic cells such as neutrophils and macrophages.

Prokaryote—A cell that contains no true nucleus or membrane-bound organelles.

T cells—White blood cells responsible for activating and controlling immune response.

on the skin. Ordinarily, normal flora aids in food digestion, protection against disease, and various other functions. Exogenous infections occur when organisms found outside of the body cause disease, while endogenous infections are caused by the normal flora colonizing sterile tissue sites.

Transmission

There are countless ways in which an individual can become infected with an infectious organism. The mode of transmission depends largely on the type of organism, its size, its structure, its vector (who transmitted it), and other factors. Some common ways that infectious agents are transmitted (and examples of such agents) are:

- inhalation (*Mycobacterium tuberculosis;* **influenza** viruses; *Histoplasma capsulatum*, a fungus that causes pneumonia)

- ingestion (*Salmonella, Vibrio, Giardia* and *Listeria* species; *Escherichia coli*)

- penetration of skin (*Clostridium tetani*, causative agent of tetanus; *Staphylococcus aureus;* hepatitis C virus [HCV])

- sexual transmission (human **immunodeficiency** virus [HIV]; *Neisseria gonorrhoeae; Chlamydia trachomatis*)

- zoonoses or animal contact (flaviviruses; rabies virus; *Yersinia pestis*, causative agent of bubonic plague)

- mother-to-child (Rubella virus or German measles; herpes simplex virus [HSV]; varicella-zoster virus or chicken pox)

Role in human health

Response to infection

The human body has three basic means of defense against invading microorganisms: natural barriers, innate non-specific immunity, and antigen-specific immunity. Each protective measure acts at a different time point in infection and varies according to the type of infectious agent.

NATURAL BARRIERS. The first barriers against infection are the skin and mucous membranes (the inner lining of the mouth, nose, vagina, urethra, and upper respiratory tract). Besides providing a physical barrier against the entry of infectious agents, these tissues are inhospitable environments for invading microbes. For example, mucus (a secretion made of protein and sugar molecules) in the upper respiratory tract can trap infectious particles before they go on to colonize the lung; ciliated cells (with hair-like structures on their surface) help flush the particles out of the respiratory tract to be expelled. The gastrointestinal tract (including the stomach and intestines) and the urinary tract (including the bladder and **kidneys**) secrete fluids such as gastric juice and bile that create hostile conditions for infectious agents.

The temperature of the human body (normally 98.6°F or 37°C) is itself a mechanism of evading infection. A major elevation of body temperature (i.e., **fever**) can slow or prevent the colonization and spread of many microbes and increase the efficiency of **immune response**.

INNATE NON-SPECIFIC IMMUNE RESPONSE. When an infectious agent is able to evade natural barriers and enter the body, the first responses to its presence are non-specific protective responses. For example, the presence of certain microbial surface molecules activates the complement system (**proteins** that activate inflammation response and recruit white **blood** cells to the site of infection). The complement system attracts phagocytic cells such as neutrophils and macrophages, which engulf foreign particles and digest them. (Neutrophils circulate primarily in the blood stream, while machrophages reside in tissues.) Activation of the complement system leads to the classic symptoms of inflammation: **pain**, fever, erythema (redness), and **edema** (swelling).

ANTIGEN-SPECIFIC IMMUNE RESPONSE. If non-specific immunity fails to slow or prevent the spread of a microorganism, another line of defense may be used: antigen-specific immunity. Two classes of white blood cells have a large role in specific immune response; these are B cells (or B lymphocytes) and T cells (or T lymphocytes).

B cells are responsible for the production of antibodies, also called immunoglobulins. Antibodies bind specifically to a foreign particle (called an antigen) so that once antibodies have been produced against a particular invader, the **immune system** can react more rapidly if that invader enters the body again. Antibodies can also enhance phagocytosis, neutralize toxins, inhibit the binding of microorganisms to human cells, and activate the complement system.

There are two main types of T cells: helper T cells (CD4 type) and cytolytic and suppressor T cells (CD8 type). Helper T cells activate and control immune response by stimulating B cells to produce antibodies. Receptors on the surface of cytolytic T cells recognize cells with surface antigens; the cell is then killed. Suppressor T cells help regulate immune response.

In some cases immune response is over-stimulated, resulting in extensive tissue damage and systemic effects. An example is toxic shock syndrome (TSS), a disease that results from infection with *Staphylococcus aureus*. Upon infection the bacteria produces a toxin that over-stimulates immune response. The result is a proliferation of T cells and over-secretion of cytokines (small proteins that act as signals between cells of the immune system). The clinical manifestations of this disease are devastating: symptoms start with fever and hypotension (low **blood pressure**) and may progress to multiple organ failure and desquamation of the skin (extensive peeling or scaling).

Infection control

In the brochure "An Ounce of Prevention: Keeps the Germs Away," (2000) the Centers for Disease Control and Prevention (CDC) identified some simple and inexpensive means of preventing the spread of infectious diseases. These include:

• Wash hands frequently.

• Clean and disinfect.

• Handle and prepare foods safely.

• Get immunized.

• Do not take unnecessary **antibiotics** (e.g., for viral infections).

• Keep pets healthy.

• Avoid contact with wild animals.

Resources

BOOKS

Murray, P.R., K.S. Rosenthal, G.S. Kobayashi, and M.A. Pfaller. *Medical Microbiology.* St. Louis, MO: Mosby, Inc., 1998.

Nicklin, J., K. Graeme-Cook, T. Paget, and R. Killington. "Bacteria and their environment." In *Instant Notes in Microbiology.* Oxford, UK: BIOS Scientific Publishers, Inc., 1999, pp.161-71.

PERIODICALS

Delves, P.J., and I.M. Roitt. "The Immune System: First of two parts." *New England Journal of Medicine* (July 6, 2000): 27-49.

Delves, P.J., and I.M. Roitt. "The Immune System: Second of two parts." *New England Journal of Medicine* (July 13, 2000): 108-17.

Huston, David. "The Biology of the Immune System." *Journal of the American Medical Association* (December 1997): 1804-14.

ORGANIZATIONS

National Center for Infectious Diseases. Mailstop C-14, 1600 Clifton Road, Atlanta, GA 30333. <http://www.cdc.gov/ncidod/>.

OTHER

"Biology of Infectious Disease." In *The Merck Manual of Diagnosis and Therapy,* on-line. 2001. Merck & Co., Inc. <http://www.merck.com/pubs/ mmanual/section13/chapter150/150a.htm>.

Stephanie Islane Dionne

▎Infection control

Definition

Infection control is the protection of patients and health care workers by the prevention of **infection** in the health care setting in a cost-efficient manner.

Standard precautions for infection control

Environmental control	Follow hospital procedures for routine care, cleaning, and disinfection of all surfaces, beds, bedrails, bedside equipment, and other frequently touched surfaces.
Linen	Handle, transport, and process used linen soiled with blood, body fluids, secretions, or excretions in a manner that prevents exposures and contamination of clothing, and avoids transferring microorganisms to other patients and environments.
Occupational health and bloodborne pathogens	Prevent injuries when using needles, scalpels, and other sharp instruments or devices; when handling sharp instruments after procedures; when cleaning used instruments; and when disposing of used needles.
	Never recap used needles using both hands or any other technique that involves pointing the needle toward any part of the body; instead , use a one-handed "scoop" technique or a mechanical device designed for holding the needle sheath.
	Do not remove used needles from disposable syringes by hand, and do not bend, break, or otherwise manipulate used needles by hand. Place used disposable syringes and needles, scalpel blades, and other sharp items in puncture-resistant sharps containers located as close as practical to the area in which the items were used, and place reusable syringes and needles in a puncture-resistant container for transport to the processing area.
	Use resuscitation devices as an alternative to mouth-to-mouth resuscitation.
Patient-care equipment	Handle used patient-care equipment soiled with blood, body fluids, secretions, or excretions in a manner that prevents skin and mucous membrane exposures and contamination of other patients and environments. Ensure that reuasable equipment is not used for the care of another patient until it has been appropriately cleaned and reprocessed and single use items are properly discarded.
Patient placement	Use a private room for a patient who contaminates the environment or who does not (or cannot be expected to) assist in maintaining appropriate hygiene or environmental control. Consult Infection Control if a private room is not available.
Wash hands (plain soap)	Wash after touching blood, body fluids, secretions, excretions, and contaminated items.
	Wash immediately after gloves are removed and between patient contacts.
	Avoid transfer of microorganisms to other patients or environments.
Wear gloves	Wear when touching blood, body fluids, secretions, excretions, and contaminated items.
	Put on clean gloves just before touching mucous membranes and nonintact skin.
	Change gloves btween tasks and procedures on the same patient after contact with material that may contain high concentrations of microorganisms. Remove gloves promptly after use, before touching non-contaminated items and other surfaces, and before going to another patient, and wash hands immediately to avoid transfer of microorganisms to other patients or environments.
Wear gown	Protect skin and prevent soiling of clothing during procedures that are likely to generate splashes or sprays of blood, body fluids, secretions, or excretions. Remove a soiled gown as promptly as possible and wash hands to avoid transferring microorganisms to other patients or environments.
Wear mask and eye protection or face shield	Protect mucous membranes of the eyes, nose, and mouth during procedures and patient-care activities that are likely to generate splashes or sprays of blood, body fluids, secretions, or excretions.

SOURCE: CDC, 1996.

Purpose

The purpose of infection control is to reduce the risk of health care worker exposure and infection and nosocomial (hospital-acquired) infections, which can complicate existing diseases or injuries.

Description

Organized efforts at infection control began in the United States in the 1950s, along with the increase in intensive care units to care for critically ill patients and the emergence of nonsocomial **staphylococcal infections**. Many hospitals implemented programs in the 1960s and 1970s at the insistence of various organizations. In the 1980s, state and federal agencies, along with professional organizations, began to make recommendations for infection control and require adherence to regulations.

Infection control procedures are followed in hospitals, long term care facilities, rehabilitation units, outpatient facilities, and **home care**. All infection control programs should encourage actions that limit the spread of nosocomial infections. All healthcare institutions are mandated by the Joint Commission on Accreditation of Healthcare Organizations (JCAHO) to "develop specific objectives and outcome measures to determine whether or not its infection control goals have been achieved" (AJIC, 1998). Infection control programs must include the means to measure the effectiveness of procedures, policies, or programs to protect patients and health care providers and to determine if these activities are cost-effective.

Health care organizations must be in compliance with regulations and accreditation requirements by various federal and state agencies and governing bodies. JCAHO, for instance, has standards that are incorporated into many state licensing, as well as **Medicare** and **Medicaid**, regulations. The facility's administration is responsible for ensuring compliance. Ongoing education and training are an important part of an effective infection control program. Also, the monitoring of patient-care activities can identify areas of concern, and the data obtained is vital to improving the program and ensuring successes.

The Hospital Infections Program (HIP) of the National Center for Infectious Diseases, Centers for Disease Control and Prevention (CDC), is the focus for information, surveillance, investigation, prevention, and control of nosocomial infections for the U.S. Public Health Service, state and local health departments, hospitals, and professional organizations in the United States and around the world. Studies indicate that one-third of nosocomial infections can be prevented by well-organized infection control programs, yet only 6-9% are actually prevented. The Study of Efficacy of Nosocomial Infection Control (SENIC) carried out by HIP over ten years showed that, to be effective, nosocomial infection programs must include the following: 1) organized surveillance and control activities, 2) a ratio of one infection control practitioner for every 250 acute care beds, 3) a trained hospital epidemiologist, and 4) a system for reporting surgical wound infection rates back to surgeons (NNIS, 1996). The National Nosocomial Infections Surveillance (NNIS) System has been gathering information for 20 years regarding nosocomial infections. This information is being used to assist hospitals in conducting successful surveillance of these infections.

In 1987, the Centers for Disease Control (CDC) expanded previous recommendations to prevent the spread of human **immunodeficiency** virus (HIV), hepatitis B virus (HBV), and other bloodborne pathogens. Previously, certain isolation precautions were recommended only for those patients who were known or suspected to have bloodborne infectious diseases. Because of the growing number of persons infected with HIV and the high mortality rates associated with **AIDS**, Universal Blood and Body Fluids Precautions were developed. Under these new recommendations, all patients are considered potentially infectious for bloodborne infections. In 1991, the Occupational Safety and Health Administration's (OSHA) Bloodborne Pathogen Standard required the use of **universal precautions** and dictated that all staff must be trained annually on the risk of exposure to bloodborne pathogens. Preventing exposure is the best and safest way to reduce infection.

The effectiveness of infection control programs are evaluated in several ways: lower rates of infection for the patient, shorter periods of hospital stays, decreased morbidity, and reduction of on-the-job exposure of health

Methods of disinfection

Method	Use
Alcohols	Skin degerming.
Autoclaving	Sterilize instruments not harmed by heat and water pressure.
Boiling water	Kill non-spore-forming pathogenic organisms.
Chlorines	Water disinfection; food surface sanitization.
Ethylene oxide gas	Sterilization of heat-sensitive materials or those that must be kept dry.
Fiberglass filters	Air disinfection.
Formaldehyde (formalin)	Drastic disinfection.
Formaldehyde gas	Fumigation; sterilization of heat-sensitive materials.
Germicidal soaps (hexachlorophene)	Skin degerming.
Iodines, tincture	Skin degerming.
Iodines, iodophors	General disinfectant.
Ionizing	Sterilize medicines, some plastics, sutures, and biologicals.
Membrane filtration	Water purification.
Mercurials	Skin degerming.
Phenols	General disinfectant.
Quaternary ammonia compounds, tincture	Skin degerming.
Quaternary ammonia compounds, aqueous	General disinfectant.
Ultrasonic	Disinfect instruments.
Ultraviolet light	Air and surface disinfection.
Washing	Disinfect hands and surfaces.

SOURCE: Benarde, M.A., ed. *Disinfection: A Treatise.* New York: Marcel Dekker, 1970.

care workers to infection and contamination from patients. To do this, infection control policies focus on strategies for isolation, barrier precautions, case investigation, health care worker education, immunization services, and employee health programs. When healthcare institutions are successful in their infection control programs, it decreases the cost of care and has a positive impact on the institution's image within the community.

It is the responsibility of infection control to identify problems, collect and analyze data, change policies and procedures when necessary, and monitor data. The specific functions of an infection control program should be based on the needs of the individual healthcare institution. It is most important to monitor infection activity. Data is collected and disseminated based on the principles of epidemiology to implement quality-improvement activities and improve patient outcomes. Policies and procedures of the facility must be based on scientific and valid infection control prevention and be reviewed and updated frequently to reflect practice guidelines and standards.

SELECTED INFECTIOUS DISEASES AND CORRESPONDING TREATMENT

Disease	Symptoms	Transmittal	Treatment
Chicken pox	Rash, low-grade fever	Person to person	None
Common cold/ Influenza	Runny nose, sore throat, cough, fever, headache, muscle aches	Person to person	None
Hepatitis	Jaundice, flu-like symptoms	Sexual contact with an infected person, contaminated blood, food, or water	None
Legionnaire's Disease	Flu symptoms, pneumonia, diarrhea, vomiting, kidney failure, respiratory failure	Air conditioning or water systems	Antibiotics
Measles	Skin rash, runny nose and eyes, fever, cough	Person to person	None
Meningitis	Neck pain, headache, pain caused by exposure to light, fever, nausea, drowsiness	Person to person	Antibiotics for bacterial meningitis, hospital care for viral meningitis
Mumps	Swelling of salivary glands	Person to person	Anti-inflammatory drugs
Ringworm	Skin rash	Contact with infected animal or person	Antifungal drugs applied topically
Tetanus	Lockjaw, other spasms	Soil infection of wounds	Antibiotics, antitoxins, muscle relaxers

(Public Domain.)

Transmission of infection within a health care organization requires three elements: a source of infecting microorganisms, a susceptible host, and a means of transmission for the microorganism. The skin of patients and personnel can function as a reservoir for infectious agents and as a vehicle for transfer of infectious agents to susceptible persons. The microbial flora of the skin consists of resident and transient microorganisms. Resident microorganisms persist and multiply on the skin. Transient microorganisms are contaminants that can survive for only a limited period of time. Most resident microorganisms are found in superficial skin layers, but about 10-20% inhabit deep epidermal layers. Handwashing with plain soaps is effective in removing many transient microorganisms. Resident microorganisms in the deep layers may not be removed by hand-

washing with plain soaps, but usually can be killed or inhibited by antimicrobial products. *Handwashing is the single most important measure for preventing nosocomial infections.*

Hand-washing indications

Health care workers should wash their hands:

• after removing gloves

• when coming on duty

• when hands are soiled, including after sneezing, coughing, or blowing the nose

• between patient contacts

• before medication preparation

• after personal use of the toilet

- before performing invasive procedures
- before taking care of particularly susceptible patients, such as those who are severely immunocompromised and newborns
- before and after touching wounds
- before and after eating
- after touching inanimate objects that are likely to be contaminated with pathogenic microorganisms, such as urine-measuring devices and secretion collection apparatuses
- after taking care of infected patients or patients who are likely to be colonized with microorganisms of special clinical or epidemiologic significance; for example, **bacteria** that are resistant to multiple antibiotics

Preparation

Routine hand-washing is accomplished by vigorously rubbing together all surfaces of lathered hands followed by thorough rinsing under a stream of water. This should take 10-15 seconds to complete. The hands should be dried with a paper towel. Immediate recontamination of the hands by touching sink fixtures may be avoided by using a paper towel to turn off faucets.

Universal precautions recommend that all health care workers who come into contact with a patient's blood or body fluids that contain visible blood should wear an appropriate type of barrier to prevent the spread of blood-borne pathogens. Other body fluids for which barrier protection is recommended include semen, vaginal secretions, cerebrospinal fluid (CSF), synovial fluid, pleural fluid, pericardial fluid, and amniotic fluid. The type of exposure determines the specific barrier that should be used. Universal precautions are designed to augment, not replace, standard infection control procedures such as hand washing and the use of gloves when touching obviously infected materials.

Adequate routine cleaning and removal of soil should be the environmental sanitation procedure for all healthcare facilities. Microorganisms are normal contaminants of the environment. A healthcare facility's environmental services department should maintain schedules for routine cleaning in all rooms and include equipment and working surfaces. General and infectious wastes are disposed of on a regular schedule. All departments, though, are responsible for implementing infection control policies.

Complications

Health care workers must not be complacent about implementing their facility's infection control policies.

Perhaps due to long-time exposure to occupationally acquired infections, they have the tendency to minimize or ignore the ramifications. Infections oftentimes go undetected, underreported, or overlooked by health care workers.

Results

If infection control programs are successful, the result will be a reduction in the risk of infection and related adverse outcomes in the healthcare setting, achieved in a cost-efficient manner.

Health care team roles

Much of the responsibility for infection control rests on the shoulders of the clinical staff providing care at the bedside. Because nurses are close to the patient physically, they are able to prevent the spread of infection, but they can also be a means of transmitting infection. Therefore they need to foster compliance with infection control policies to ensure a high quality outcome for the patient. Infection control practices should have a positive effect on not only the clinical staff, but the patient as well.

Resources
BOOKS

Jennings, J., and F. Manian. *APIC Handbook of Infection Control.* Washington, D.C.: Association for Professionals in Infection Control and Epidemiology, 1999.

PERIODICALS

Barrs, A. "Infection Control Across the Board." *Nursing Homes Long Term Care Management* 49, Issue 11 (November 2000):38.

Henderson, D. "Raising the Bar: The Need for Standardizing the Use of "Standard Precautions" as a Primary Intervention to Prevent Occupational Exposures to Bloodborne Pathogens." *Infection Control and Hospital Epidemiology* 22 (February 2001):6.

Heseltine, P. "Why Don't Doctors and Nurses Wash Their Hands?" *Infection Control and Hospital Epidemiology* 22 (April 2001):4.

Hood, R., and D. Olesen. "Re-evaluating the Role of the Clinical Nurse in Minimizing Health Care Related Infection." *Australian Nursing Journal* (8 October 2000):1.

Rello, J. "Impact of Nosocomial Infections on Outcome: Myths and Evidence." *Infection Control and Hospital Epidemiology* 20 (June 1999):6.

"Requirements For Infrastructure and Essential Activities of Infection Control and Epidemiology in Hospitals: A Consensus Panel Report." *Infection Control and Epidemiology* 19 (1998):114-124.

Shimkins, J. "Making the Grade." *Health Facilities Management* 1 (January 1999):18.

Stratton, C. "Occupationally Acquired Infections: A Timely Reminder." *Infection Control and Hospital Epidemiology* (January 2001):22.

ORGANIZATIONS

Hospital Infections Program. Center for Disease Control and Prevention. 1600 Clifton Road, Atlanta, GA 30333. <http://www.cdc.gov/ncidod/publications/brochures/hip.htm>.

OTHER

Infection Control: Hand-Washing and Antisepsis. Johns Hopkins University. 2001.

René A. Jackson, RN

Infectious mononucleosis test

Definition

Infectious mononucleosis (IM) tests detect the presence or absence of antibodies in the **blood** stream directed against **proteins** of the Epstein-Barr Virus (EBV), the cause of IM.

Purpose

Infectious mononucleosis tests are used to diagnose infectious mononucleosis in patients with symptoms compatible with the disease. Initial testing is based on the demonstration of heterophile antibodies produced in infectious mononucleosis. Heterophile antibodies are those that react with the cells from a different (nonhuman) species. A positive result from a rapid slide (Monospot) test for IM specific heterophile antibodies is diagnostic, and no further testing is necessary. The Monospot test will be positive in more than 90% of adults or adolescents with IM, but is more frequently negative in young children. When the Monospot test results are negative, an EBV antibody panel may be needed to differentiate EBV infections from mononucleosis-like illnesses induced by cytomegalovirus, adenovirus, or *Toxoplasma gondii*. The EBV antibody panel can differentiate persons who have never been infected with EBV, acute infections, and past infections. EBV antibody tests are not needed when the doctor believes that a person has IM and the Monospot test is positive.

Precautions

Blood for this test is collected by venipuncture. The nurse or phlebotomist performing the procedure should observe **universal precautions** for the prevention of transmission of bloodborne pathogens. False positive Monospot results occur in a small percentage of the patient population. False negative Monospot results occur in 10% to 15% of patients, primarily in children under the age of 10. With the EBV panel false positive results may occur in patients with rheumatoid arthritis, leukemia, lymphoma, or HIV.

Description

The Epstein-Barr Virus (EBV) is one of the most common human **viruses**, and most of the world's population is infected at sometime during their lives. According to the CDC, when an EBV **infection** occurs during adolescence or young adulthood, it causes infectious mononucleosis 35–50% of the time. The virus is believed to be transmitted primarily via salivary exchange, including intimate kissing, sharing toothbrushes, cups, or eating utensils..

Symptoms of infectious mononucleosis include **fever**, **sore throat**, swollen lymph glands lasting for two to three weeks, and fatigue and a swollen spleen or **liver** typically lasting for approximately one month. While the infection is rarely fatal and usually resolves in one or two months, the course is more chronic in some persons, and the virus may remain dormant in some throat and blood cells for the rest of the person's life.

The clinical diagnosis of infectious mononucleosis is suggested on the basis of the symptoms of fever, sore throat, swollen lymph glands, and the age of the patient. Laboratory tests are needed for confirmation. Laboratory findings suggestive of infectious mononucleosis include an elevated white blood cell count, an increased lymphocyte count, and the presence of a significant number of atypical lymphocytes (seen when viewing a stained blood smear under the **microscope**). Diagnosis is usually made by demonstrating a positive reaction to a rapid slide test (usually referred to as a Monospot test) for the specific heterophile anibodies seen in IM.

Heterophile antibodies may be of two types, called Forssman and nonForssman. Infectious mononucleosis causes production of nonForssman heterophile antibodies. Testing for heterophile antibodies must distinguish these from the Forssman type which are not produced by IM and are present in the blood of many persons without IM. The Monospot test is based upon the principle that IM heterophile antibodies will agglutinate horse red blood cells (because they are nonForssman). First, the serum is mixed with two different antigen suspensions, guinea pig kidney antigen and beef red blood cell stroma, prior to testing with the horse red cells. The guinea pig kidney antigen absorbs (removes) Forssman heterophile antibodies while the beef red cell stroma removes nonForssman IM antibodies. After mixing the serum with these two suspensions, the serum is mixed with the horse red cells. In infectious mononucleosis, agglutination should be seen in the serum mixed with guinea pig antigen. Little or no agglutination should be seen in the serum mixed with the beef red cell stroma.

An EBV antibody panel can be used to confirm a negative Monospot result or rule out a false positive Monospot result. The panel includes four antibody measurements: IgM viral capsid antigen (VCA), IgG VCA, Early Antigen (EA), and Epstein-Barr nuclear antigen (EBNA), which help determine the stage of the patient's EBV infection.

Preparation

To obtain the 2 mLs of blood required for this test, a nurse or phlebotomist ties a tourniquet on the person's upper arm, locates a vein in the inner elbow region, and inserts a needle into that vein. Vacuum action draws the blood through the needle into an attached tube. Collection of the sample takes only a few minutes.

Aftercare

Discomfort or bruising may occur at the puncture site. Applying pressure to the puncture site until the bleeding stops reduces bruising; warm packs relieve discomfort. Some people feel dizzy or faint after blood has been drawn and should be treated accordingly.

Complications

There are no risks beyond those of having blood drawn for any other purpose.

Results

Results of the rapid slide test are determined as positive or negative. According to the CDC, the confirmatory diagnosis of EBV infection is summarized as follows:

• Susceptibility: If antibodies to the VCA are not detected.

• Primary infection: If IgM antibody to the VCA is present in the absence of antibody to EBNA. A rising or high IgG antibody titre to the viral capsid antigen and a negative antibody test to EBNA after at least four weeks of illness are strongly suggestive of primary infection.

• Past infection: If antibodies to both the VCA and EBNA are present, then past infection (from four to six months to years earlier) is indicated.

• Reactivation: In the presence of antibodies to EBNA, an elevation of antibodies to early antigen suggests reactivation.

KEY TERMS

Heterophile antibodies—Antibodies created against one species that cross react with another.

Lymphocyte—White blood cell that fights viral and some bacterial infections by direct attack or the production of antibodies.

• Chronic EBV infection: Reliable laboratory evidence for continued active EBV infection is very seldom found in patients who have been ill for more than four months.

If the results are difficult to interpret, it may be necessary to retest later, after waiting one to three weeks. The change in the amounts of antibody detected between the two tests can be particularly useful, at times, in helping to make a diagnosis.

The **complete blood count** (CBC) in a patient with infectious mononucleosis typically reveals:

• a white blood cell count (WBC) of 10,000 to 20,000 cells per microliter

• more than 4,500 lymphocytes per microliter and more than 50% lymphocytes in the differential

• atypical lymphocytes (Downey cells) accounting for more than 10% of total leukocytes

Health care team roles

Physicians order and interpret the IM tests. Nurses or phlebotomists usually draw the blood needed for these tests. Clinical laboratory scientists/medical technologists or clinical laboratory technicians/medical laboratory technicians perform the antibody tests in clinical laboratories. Interpretation of EBV antibody tests is somewhat complex and requires familiarity with EBV testing and access to all the patient's clinical information.

Resources

BOOKS

Bailey, R. Eugene. "Infectious Mononucleosis." In *Current Diagnosis,* edited by Rex B. Conn, William Z. Borer, and Jack W. Snyder. Philadelphia: W. B. Saunders, 1997.

Chernecky, Cynthia C., and Barbara J. Berger. *Laboratory Tests and Diagnostic Procedures.* 3rd ed. Philadelphia, PA: W. B. Saunders Company, 2001.

Kee, Joyce LeFever. *Handbook of Laboratory and Diagnostic Tests.* 4th ed. Upper Saddle River, NJ: Prentice Hall, 2001.

PERIODICALS

Henle, G., W. Henle, and C. A. Horowitz. "Epstein-Barr Virus Specific Diagnosis: Tests in Infectious Mononucleosis." *Human Pathology* 5 (1997): 551-558.

OTHER

Centers for Disease Control. National Center for Infectious Diseases: Epstein-Barr and Infectious Mononucleosis. Updated Sept 1999. <http://www.cdc.gov/ncidod/diseases/ebv.htm>.

Victoria E. DeMoranville

Infertility

Definition

Infertility is the failure to conceive a **pregnancy** after attempting for at least one full year. In primary infertility, pregnancy has never occurred. In secondary infertility, one or both members of the couple have previously conceived, but are unable to conceive again after a full year of attempting.

Description

Currently, in the United States, about one in five couples struggles with infertility at any given time. Infertility has increased as a problem over the last 30 years. Some studies assign the blame for this increase on social phenomena, including the tendency for marriage to occur at a later age. Fertility in women decreases with increasing age, as illustrated by the following statistics. In one year of trying to become pregnant:

- Infertility in women at age 20 is 4%.
- Infertility in women at age 30 is 7%.
- Infertility in women at age 35 is 12%.
- Infertility in women over the age of 40 is 75%.

Many individuals have multiple sexual partners before marriage. This increase in numbers of sexual partners has led to a rise in sexually transmitted diseases. Scarring from these infections, especially from pelvic inflammatory disease (PID, a serious **infection** of the female reproductive organs, most commonly caused by chlamydia and gonorrhea), seems to be partially responsible for increases in infertility. Furthermore, use of some forms of a contraceptive called the intrauterine device (IUD) contributed to an increased rate of pelvic inflammatory disease. However, the newer IUDs do not cause infections.

To understand issues of infertility, it is first necessary to understand the basics of human reproduction. Fertilization occurs when a sperm from the male merges with an egg (ovum) from the female, creating a zygote that contains genetic material (DNA) from both the father and the mother. If pregnancy is then established, the zygote will develop into an embryo, then a fetus, and ultimately a baby will be born.

The male contribution to fertilization and the establishment of pregnancy is the sperm. Sperm are small cells that carry the father's genetic material, which is contained within the oval head of the sperm. The sperm are mixed into a fluid called semen that is discharged from the penis during sexual intercourse. The whip-like tail of sperm allows them to swim up the female reproductive tract in search of an egg (ovum).

The female makes many contributions to fertilization and the establishment of pregnancy. The ovum is the cell that carries the mother's genetic material; ova (plural of ovum) develop within the ovaries. Once a month, a single mature ovum is produced, and leaves the ovary in a process called ovulation. This ovum enters a tube leading to the uterus (the fallopian tube). If fertilization is to occur, the ovum must encounter the sperm in the fallopian tube.

When fertilization occurs, the resulting cell is called a zygote. This single cell will multiply within the fallopian tube, and the resulting cluster of cells, a blastocyst, will then move into the womb (uterus). The uterine lining (endometrium) has been preparing itself to receive a pregnancy by growing thicker. If the blastocyst successfully reaches the inside of the uterus and attaches itself to the wall of the uterus, then pregnancy has been achieved.

Causes and symptoms

Unlike most medical problems, infertility is an issue requiring the careful evaluation of two separate individuals, as well as an evaluation of their interactions with each other. In about 3–4% of couples, no cause for their infertility will be discovered.

The main factors involved in causing infertility, ranging from the most to the least common, include:

- male problems: 30-40%
- ovulation problems: 10-15%
- pelvic disease: 30-40%
- cervical factors: 10-15%
- undiagnosed: 5-10%

Diagnosis

Diagnosis of infertility involves examination of both male and female partners.

Male factors

Male infertility can be caused by a number of different characteristics of sperm. To check for these characteristics, a sample of semen is obtained and examined under a **microscope (semen analysis)**. Four basic characteristics are usually evaluated:

• Sperm count refers to the number of sperm present in a semen sample. The typical number of sperm present in just one milliliter (ml) of semen is more than 20 million. A male with only 5–20 million sperm per ml of semen is considered subfertile, while a male with less than 5 million sperm per ml of semen is considered to be infertile.

• Sperm are examined to determine how well they swim (sperm motility) and to ensure that most have normal structure (morphology). Not all sperm within a specimen of semen will be perfectly normal. Some may be immature, and others may have abnormalities of the head or tail. A typical semen sample will contain no more than 25% abnormal forms of sperm.

• Volume of the semen sample is important; an abnormal amount of semen could adversely affect the ability of the sperm to successfully fertilize an ovum.

• The ability of the sperm to penetrate the outer coat of the ovum is also evaluated. This is accomplished by observing whether sperm in a semen sample can penetrate the outer coat of a hamster ovum. Fertilization cannot occur, of course, but this test is useful in predicting the ability of an individual's sperm to penetrate a human ovum.

Any number of conditions result in abnormal findings in the semen analysis. Men can be born with testicles that have not descended properly from the abdominal cavity into the scrotal sac, or may be born with only one testicle, instead of the normal two. Testicle size might be smaller than normal. Past infection (including mumps) can affect testicular function, as can a past injury. The presence of abnormally large veins (varicocele) in the testicles can increase testicular temperature, which decreases sperm count.

History of having been exposed to various toxins, drug use, excessive alcohol use, use of anabolic steroids, certain medications, diabetes, thyroid problems, or other endocrine disturbances can have direct effects on the formation of sperm (spermatogenesis). Problems with the male anatomy can cause sperm to be ejaculated into the bladder, or scarring from past infections can interfere with ejaculation.

Female factors

OVULATORY PROBLEMS. The first step in diagnosing ovulatory problems is to make sure that an ovum is being produced each month. A woman's body temperature in the morning is slightly higher around the time of ovulation. A woman can measure and record her temperatures daily, and a chart can be drawn to show whether or not ovulation has occurred. Luteinizing hormone (LH) is released just before ovulation. A simple urine test can be done to check if LH has been released around the time that ovulation is expected.

PELVIC ADHESIONS AND ENDOMETRIOSIS. Pelvic adhesions and endometriosis can cause infertility by preventing the sperm from reaching the egg or interfering with fertilization.

Pelvic adhesions are fibrous scars. These scars can be the result of past infections, such as pelvic inflammatory disease, or infections following abortions or prior births. Previous surgeries can also leave behind scarring. Pelvic adhesions cause infertility by blocking the fallopian tubes. The ovum may be prevented from traveling down the fallopian tube from the ovary or the sperm may be prevented from traveling up the fallopian tube from the uterus.

A hysterosalpingogram (HSG) can show if the fallopian tubes are blocked. This is an x-ray exam that tests whether dye material can travel through a woman's fallopian tubes. Scarring also can be diagnosed by examining the pelvic area through the use of a scope that can be inserted into the abdomen through a tiny incision made near the navel. This technique is called **laparoscopy**.

Endometriosis may lead to pelvic adhesions. Endometriosis is the abnormal location of uterine tissue outside of the uterus. When uterine tissue is implanted elsewhere in the pelvis, it still bleeds on a monthly basis with the start of the normal menstrual period. This leads to irritation within the pelvis around the site of this abnormal tissue and bleeding, and may cause scarring.

CERVICAL FACTORS. The cervix is the opening from the vagina into the uterus through which the sperm must pass. Mucus produced by the cervix helps to transport the sperm into the uterus. Cervical mucus can be examined under a microscope to diagnose whether cervical factors are contributing to infertility. An injury to the cervix or scarring of the cervix after surgery or infection can result in a smaller than normal cervical opening, which would make it difficult for sperm to enter. Injury or infection can also decrease the number of glands in the cervix, leading to a smaller amount of cervical mucus. In other situations, the mucus produced might be the wrong consistency to allow sperm to travel through. In addition, some women produce antibodies (immune cells) that identify sperm as foreign invaders and kill them. Finally, cervical stenosis is a rare cause of infertility.

Treatment

Treatment of infertility first involves addressing underlying conditions in the male and female partners. If these fail to produce a pregnancy, additional steps can be undertaken to assist pregnancy.

Treatment of male infertility includes first addressing known reversible factors such as discontinuing any medication known to have an effect on spermatogenesis or ejaculation, decreasing alcohol intake, or treating thyroid or other endocrine disease. Varicoceles can be treated surgically. Testosterone in low doses can improve sperm motility.

Other treatments of male infertility include collecting semen samples from multiple ejaculations, after which the semen is put through a process that allows the most motile sperm to be sorted out. These motile sperm are pooled together to create a concentrate that can be deposited into the female partner's uterus at ovulation. In cases where the male partner's sperm is proven unviable, with the consent of both partners, donor sperm may be used. Depositing the male partner's sperm or donor sperm by mechanical means into the female partner is a form of artificial insemination.

Treatment of ovulatory problems depends on the cause. If a thyroid or pituitary problem is responsible, treating that problem can restore fertility. Medication such as Clomid and Pergonal can be used to stimulate fertility. These drugs may increase the risk of multiple births (twins, triplets, etc.).

Pelvic adhesions can be excised with laparoscopy. Endometriosis can be treated with certain medications, but may also require surgery to repair any obstruction caused by adhesions.

Treatment of cervical factors includes **antibiotics** in the case of an infection, steroids to decrease production of anti-sperm antibodies, and artificial insemination techniques to completely bypass the cervical mucus.

Assisted reproductive techniques include in vitro fertilization (IVF), gamete intrafallopian transfer (GIFT), and zygote intrafallopian tube transfer (ZIFT). These are usually used after other techniques to treat infertility have failed.

IVF involves the use of a drug to induce the simultaneous release of many eggs from a female's ovaries. These are surgically retrieved. Meanwhile, several semen samples are obtained from the male partner, and a sperm

concentrate is prepared. The ova and sperm are then combined in a laboratory, where several of the ova may be fertilized. **Cell division** is allowed to take place up to the embryo stage. While this takes place, the female may be given drugs to prepare her uterus to receive an embryo. Three or four of the embryos are transferred to the female's uterus, and the wait begins to see if any or all of them implant and result in an actual pregnancy.

Success rates of IVF are still rather low. Most centers report pregnancy rates between 10–20%. Since most IVF procedures put more than one embryo into the uterus, the chance for a multiple birth is greatly increased in couples undergoing IVF.

GIFT involves retrieval of both multiple ova and semen, and the mechanical placement of both within the female partner's fallopian tubes. ZIFT involves the same retrieval of ova and semen and the fertilization and growth in the laboratory up to the zygote stage, at which point the zygotes are placed in the fallopian tubes. Both GIFT and ZIFT have higher success rates than IVF.

Prognosis

It is very difficult to obtain statistics regarding the prognosis of infertility because many different problems may exist within an individual or couple trying to conceive. In general, of all couples who undergo a complete evaluation of infertility followed by treatment, about half will ultimately have a successful pregnancy. Of those couples who do not choose to undergo evaluation or treatment, about 5% will go on to conceive after a year or more of infertility.

Health care team roles

Gynecologists who specialize in infertility lead most investigations. Registered nurses (RNs) assist throughout investigations and other associated procedures. Laboratory technicians conduct laboratory tests and evaluations of ova and sperm. Other technicians may assist in preparing eggs and sperm for IVF, or readying women for GIFT or ZIFT. Pharmacists dispense the many drugs that are required for GIFT, ZIFT, or IVF.

Prevention

Prevention of infertility involves avoiding many of the various problems that can cause infertility. Since sperm count declines with age, insemination is more likely to occur with younger men than older men. Males can preserve maximal fertility by maintaining optimal temperatures in their testicles by wearing non-binding undergarments. People should avoid exposure to coal-based products such as tar and soot as they are associated with infertility. Protecting the testicles from trauma helps to preserve fertility. Immunization for mumps is important.

Women are maximally fertile in the beginning of their third decade of life. Thereafter, conception becomes more difficult. Avoiding or promptly treating sexually transmitted diseases lessens the possibility of endometriosis and pelvic adhesions. Limiting the number of male partners improves fertility as antibodies against sperm will not be formed. Hasty decisions to perform tubal ligations as a means of birth control may be regretted if marital arrangements change. Although tubal ligations can be reversed, subsequent pregnancy rates are not 100%.

Resources

BOOKS

Aronson, Diane. *Resolving Infertility.* New York: Harper Resource, 1999.

Peoples, Debby, and Harriet R. Ferguson. *Experiencing Infertility: An Essential Resource.* New York: Norton, 2000.

Speroff, Leon, Robert H. Glass, and Nathan G. Kase. *Clinical Gynecologic Endocrinology and Infertility, 6th ed.* Philadelphia: Lippincott, 1999.

Treiser, Susan, and Robin K. Levinson. *Infertility. A Woman Doctor's Guide.* New York: Kensington Publishing Corp, 2001.

PERIODICALS

Mastroianni, Luigi, et al. "Helping Infertile Patients." *Patient Care* (October 15, 1997): 103+.

ORGANIZATIONS

American College of Obstetricians and Gynecologists. 409 12th St., S.W., P.O. Box 96920, Washington, D.C. 20090-6920. <http://www.acog.org>.

American Infertility Association. 666 Fifth Avenue, Suite 278, New York, NY 10103. (718) 621-5083. <http://www.americaninfertility.org>. info@americaninfertility.org.

American Society for Reproductive Medicine. 1209 Montgomery Highway, Birmingham, AL 35216-2809. (205) 978-5000. <http://www.asrm.com>.

International Council on Infertility Information Dissemination, Inc. P.O. Box 6836, Arlington, Virginia 22206. (703) 379-9178. <http://www.inciid.org>.

Resolve: The National Infertility Association. 1310 Broadway, Somerville, MA 02144. (617) 623-0744. <http://www.resolve.org.> resolveinc@aol.com.

OTHER

Internet Health Resources. <http://www.ihr.com/infertility>.
IVF.com. <http://www.ivf.com>.

KEY TERMS

Blastocyst—A cluster of cells representing multiple cell divisions that have occurred in the fallopian tube after successful fertilization of an ovum by a sperm.

Cervix—The opening from the vagina that leads into the uterus.

Embryo—The stage of development of a baby between the second and eighth weeks after conception.

Endometrium—The lining of the uterus.

Fallopian tube—The tube leading from the ovary into the uterus; there are two fallopian tubes.

Fetus—A baby developing in the uterus from the third month to birth.

Ovary—The female organ in which eggs (ova) are stored and mature.

Ovum (plural: ova)—The reproductive cell of the female that contains genetic information and participates in the act of fertilization. Also popularly called the egg.

Semen—The fluid that contains sperm that is ejaculated by the male.

Sperm—The reproductive cell of the male that contains genetic information and participates in the act of fertilization of an ovum.

Spermatogenesis—The process by which sperm develop to become mature sperm, capable of fertilizing an ovum.

Zygote—The result of sperm successfully fertilizing an ovum, the zygote is a single cell that contains the genetic material of both the mother and the father.

National Library of Medicine. <http://www.nlm.nih.gov/medlineplus/infertility.html>.

"Trying for a Year." WebMd.com <http://my.webmd.com/content/article/3606.512>. Accessed July 30, 2001.

Worldwide Infertility Network. <http://www.ein.org>.

L. Fleming Fallon, Jr., M.D., Ph.D., Dr.P.H.

Infertility therapies *see* **Fertility treatments**

Influenza

Definition

Usually referred to as the flu or grippe, influenza is a highly infectious respiratory disease caused by certain strains of influenza virus. When the virus is inhaled it attacks cells in the upper respiratory tract causing typical flu symptoms such as fatigue, **fever** and chills, hacking cough, and body aches. Influenza victims are also susceptible to potentially life-threatening secondary infections. Although the **stomach** or intestinal upsets and **diarrhea** are commonly called "flu," the influenza virus rarely causes gastrointestinal symptoms. Such symptoms are most likely due to other organisms such as rotavirus, *Salmonella*, *Shigella*, or *Escherichia coli*.

Description

Influenza is considerably more debilitating than the **common cold**. Influenza outbreaks occur suddenly and **infection** rapidly spreads. The annual death toll attributable to influenza and its complications averages 20,000 in the United States alone.

Influenza outbreaks occur on a regular basis. Pandemics, the most serious outbreaks, affect millions of people worldwide and last for several months. The 1918–1919 influenza outbreak serves as the primary example of an influenza pandemic. In that Spanish flu pandemic, the death toll reached a staggering 20–40 million people worldwide. Approximately 500,000 of these fatalities occurred in the United States. Pandemics also occurred in 1957 and 1968 with the Asian flu and Hong Kong flu, respectively. The Asian flu was responsible for 70,000 deaths in the United States, while the Hong Kong flu killed 34,000 people.

Epidemics are widespread regional outbreaks that occur every two to three years and affect 5–10% of the population. The Russian flu in the winter of 1977 is an example of an epidemic. A regional epidemic is shorter lived than a pandemic, lasting only several weeks. Finally, there are smaller outbreaks each winter that are confined to specific locales.

The earliest existing descriptions of influenza were written nearly 2,500 years ago by the ancient Greek physician, Hippocrates. Historically, influenza was ascribed to a number of different agents, including "bad air" and several different **bacteria**. It was not until 1933 that the causative agent was identified as a virus.

There are three types of influenza **viruses**, identified as A, B, and C. Influenza A can infect a range of species, including humans, pigs, horses, and birds, but only humans are infected by types B and C. Influenza A is responsible for most flu cases, while infection with types B and C viruses are less common and cause a milder illness.

Causes and symptoms

Approximately one to four days after infection with the influenza virus, a person is hit with an array of symptoms. "Hit" is an appropriate term, because symptoms are sudden, harsh, and followed by overall bodily aches and a fever that may run as high as 104°F (40°C). As the fever subsides, nasal congestion and a **sore throat** become noticeable. Persons with the flu feel extremely tired and generally miserable. Typical influenza symptoms include the abrupt onset of a headache, dry cough, and chills, and a rapid onset of physical weakness. Normal energy levels typically do not return for several days, but this can extend up to two weeks.

Influenza complications usually arise from secondary bacterial infections of the lower respiratory tract. Signs of a secondary respiratory infection often appear just as a person seems to be recovering. These signs include high fever, intense chills, chest pains associated with breathing, and a productive cough with thick, yellowish-green sputum. If these symptoms appear, medical treatment is necessary. Other secondary infections, such as sinus or ear infections, may also require medical intervention. **Heart** and lung problems and other chronic diseases can be aggravated by influenza. This is a particular concern among elderly people.

With children and teenagers, it is advisable to be alert for symptoms of Reye's syndrome, a rare but serious complication of the flu. Symptoms of Reye's syndrome are nausea and vomiting, and—more seriously—neurological problems such as confusion or delirium. Among children Reye's syndrome can be fatal. The syndrome has been associated with the use of aspirin to relieve flu symptoms.

Diagnosis

Although specific laboratory tests can be performed on respiratory samples to identify a flu virus strain, doctors typically rely on a set of symptoms and the presence of influenza in the community for diagnosis. Specific tests are useful to determine the type of flu in the community, but they do little to influence individual treatment. Doctors may administer tests, such as throat cultures, to identify and treat secondary bacterial infections.

Treatment

Essentially, little can be done for a case of influenza an it must simply run its course. Symptoms can be relieved with bed rest and by keeping well hydrated. A steam vaporizer may make breathing easier, and **pain** relievers such as ibuprofen and acetaminophen will relieve most aches and pains. Food may not seem appetizing, but an effort should be made to consume nourishing food. Returning to normal activities too quickly invites a possible relapse or complications.

Drugs

Since influenza is a viral infection, **antibiotics** are not an effective treatment. However, antibiotics are frequently used to treat secondary infections. Over-the-counter medications are used to treat symptoms, but it is not necessary to purchase a product marketed specifically for flu symptoms. Any medication designed to relieve pain and coughing will provide some relief. Products containing alcohol, however, should be avoided because of the dehydrating effects of alcohol. The best medicine for symptoms is simply an analgesic, such as acetaminophen or ibuprofen. Without a doctor's approval, aspirin is generally not recommended for people under the age of 18 years owing to its association with Reye's syndrome. As a precaution against the syndrome, children should receive acetaminophen or ibuprofen to treat their symptoms.

There are two **antiviral drugs** marketed for use in the United States against the influenza virus. These may be useful in treating individuals who have weakened immune systems or who are at risk for developing serious complications of influenza but may be allergic to the flu vaccine. The first is amantadine hydrochloride, which is marketed under the names Symmetrel (syrup), Symadine (capsule), and Amantadine-hydrochloride (capsule and syrup). The second antiviral is rimantadine hydrochloride, marketed under the trade name Flumandine (tablet and syrup). These two drugs are chemically related and are only effective against type A influenza viruses. Both drugs can cause side effects such as nervousness, **anxiety**, lightheadedness, and nausea. Side effects are more likely to occur with amantadine. Severe side effects include seizures, delirium, and hallucinations. These are rare and are nearly always limited to people who have kidney problems, seizure disorders, or psychiatric disorders.

Alternative treatment

There are several alternative treatments that may help in fighting off the virus, easing symptoms, and promoting recovery:

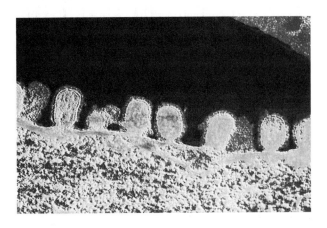

A transmission electron micrograph (TEM) of influenza viruses budding from the surface of an infected cell. *(Photo Researchers, Inc. Reproduced by permission.)*

- Acupuncture and **acupressure**. Both are said to stimulate natural resistance, relieve nasal congestion and headaches, fight fever, and calm coughs, depending on the acupuncture and acupressure points used.

- Aromatherapy. Aromatherapists recommend gargling daily with one drop each of the essential oils of tea tree (*Melaleuca* spp.) and lemon mixed in a glass of warm water. If the patient is already suffering from the flu, two drops of tea tree oil in a hot bath may help ease the symptoms. Essential oils of eucalyptus (*Eucalyptus globulus*) or peppermint (*Mentha piperita*) added to a steam vaporizer may help clear chest and nasal congestion.

- Herbal remedies. Herbal remedies such as echinacea can be used to stimulate the **immune system**; as antivirals, goldenseal (*Hydrastis canadensis*) and garlic (*Allium sativum*) can be used. They can also be used to alleviate whatever symptoms arise as a result of the flu. For example, an infusion of boneset (*Eupatroium perfoliatum*) may counteract aches and fever, and yarrow (*Achillea millefolium*) or elderflower tinctures may combat chills.

- Homeopathy. To prevent flu a homeopathic remedy called *Oscillococcinum* may be taken at the first sign of flu symptoms and repeated for a day or two. Other recommended homeopathic remedies vary according to the specific flu symptoms present. *Gelsemium* (*Gelsemium sempervirens*) is recommended to combat weakness accompanied by chills, headache, and nasal congestion. *Bryonia* (*Bryonia alba*) may be used to treat muscle aches, headaches, and a dry cough. For restlessness, chills, hoarseness, and achy joints, poison ivy (*Rhus toxicodendron*) is recommended. Finally, for bodily aches and a dry cough or chills, *Eupatorium perfoliatum* is suggested.

- Hydrotherapy. A hot bath to induce a fever will speed recovery from the flu by creating an environment in the body where the flu virus cannot survive. Taking a bath in water as hot as can be tolerated, and remain in the bath for 20–30 minutes, is recommended. While in the bath, drinking a cup of yarrow or elderflower tea helps induce sweating. However, a cold cloth should be held on the forehead or the nape of the neck to keep down the temperature of the **brain**. In case dizziness or weakness occurs, the patient should be assisted when getting out of the bath. The individual should then go to bed and cover up with layers of blankets to induce more sweating.

- Vitamins. For adults, 2–3 grams of **vitamin C** daily may help prevent the flu. Increasing the dose to 5–7 grams per day if infected by the flu can help overcome the infection. The dose of vitamin C should be reduced if diarrhea develops.

Prognosis

Following proper treatment guidelines, healthy people under the age of 65 years of age usually suffer no long-term consequences associated with influenza infections. While the elderly and the chronically ill are at greater risk for secondary infection and other complications, they can also recover completely. While most people fully recover from an influenza infection, the flu should not be viewed with complacency. Influenza is a serious disease. Approximately one in every 1,000 cases proves fatal.

Health care team roles

Family physicians, internists, and pediatricians most often diagnose influenza in people who seek medical attention. Nurse practitioners and physician assistants may also make such diagnoses. A physician usually prescribes over-the-counter products for symptomatic relief. Occasionally, antiviral products are prescribed for people at particular risk. Nurses administer vaccines to prevent influenza, providing education and information to those contemplating or receiving the vaccine.

Prevention

The Centers for Disease Control and Prevention recommend that people—particularly the at-risk population such as children, individuals with other diseases or disorders or a compromised immune system, and the elderly—get an influenza vaccine injection each year before the flu season starts. In the United States the flu season typically runs from late December to early March. Vaccines should be received two to six weeks prior to the beginning of the flu season to allow people's bodies enough time to establish immunity. Adults need only one dose of the yearly vaccine, but children under nine years of age who have not previously been immunized should receive two doses with a month between each dose.

Each season's flu vaccine contains three virus strains that are the most likely to be encountered in the coming flu season. When there is a good match between the anticipated flu strains and the strains used in the vaccine, the vaccine is 70–90% effective in people younger than 65 years of age. Because **immune response** diminishes somewhat with age, people older than 65 years may not receive the same level of protection from the vaccine as do younger people. Even if they do contract the flu, the elderly benefit from vaccines, which diminish severity and help prevent complications.

The virus strains used to make the vaccine are inactivated and will not cause a case of influenza. In the past, flu symptoms following **vaccination** were associated with vaccine preparations that were not as highly purified as modern vaccines, not to the virus itself. In 1976 there was a slightly increased risk of developing Guillain-Barré syndrome, a very rare disorder associated with the swine flu vaccine. This association occurred only with the 1976 swine flu vaccine preparation and has never recurred.

Serious side effects with modern vaccines are extremely unusual. Some people experience a slight soreness at the point of injection, which resolves within a day or two. People who have never been exposed to influenza, particularly children, may experience one to two days of a slight fever, tiredness, and muscle aches. These symptoms start within 6 to 12 hours after vaccination.

It should be noted that certain people should not receive an influenza vaccine. Infants six months and younger have immature immune systems and will not benefit from the vaccine. Since the vaccines are prepared using hen eggs, people who have severe **allergies** to eggs or other vaccine components should not receive the influenza vaccine. As an alternative, they may receive a course of amantadine or rimantadine, which are also used as protective measures against influenza. Other people who might receive these drugs are those who have been immunized after the flu season has started or who are immunocompromised, such as people with advanced HIV disease. Amantadine and rimantadine are 70–90% effective in preventing influenza.

Members of certain groups are strongly advised to be vaccinated because they are at-risk for influenza-related complications:

- all people 65 years and older

/>

- residents of **nursing homes** and chronic-care facilities, regardless of age

- adults and children who have chronic heart or lung problems, such as asthma

- adults and children who have chronic metabolic diseases, such as diabetes and renal dysfunction, as well as severe anemia or inherited hemoglobin disorders

- children and teenagers receiving long-term aspirin therapy

- pregnant women who will be in the second or third trimester during flu season, or women who are nursing

- anyone who is immunocompromised, including HIV-infected people with CD4 count over 200; people with **cancer**; organ transplant recipients; and people receiving steroids, **chemotherapy**, or radiation therapy

- anyone in contact with people in these groups, such as teachers, care givers, health-care personnel, and family members

- travelers to foreign countries

An individual need not be in one of the at-risk categories listed above, however, to receive a flu vaccination. Anyone who wants to avoid the discomfort and inconvenience of a case of influenza should receive the vaccine.

Resources

BOOKS

Craighead, John E. *Pathology and Pathogenesis of Human Viral Disease.* New York: Academic Press, 2000.

Dolin, Raphael. "Influenza." In *Harrison's Principles of Internal Medicine,* 14th ed. Ed. Anthony S. Fauci et al., New York: McGraw-Hill, 1998, 1096-1098.

Hayden, Frederick G. "Influenza." In *Cecil Textbook of Medicine,* 21st ed. Ed. Lee Goldman and J. Claude Bennett. Philadelphia: W.B. Saunders, 2000, 1797-1800.

Kolata, Gina B. *Flu: The Story of the Great Influenza Pandemic of 1918 and the Search for the Virus That Caused It.* Carmichael, CA: Touchstone Books, 2001.

Ramen, Fred. *Influenza.* New York: Rosen Publishing Group, 2001.

Wright, Peter. "Influenza Viruses." In *Nelson Textbook of Pediatrics,* 16th ed. Ed. Richard E. Behrman et al., Philadelphia: Saunders, 2000, 987-990.

PERIODICALS

Berry, B B, D.A. Ehlert, R.J. Battiola, and G. Sedmak. "Influenza Vaccination Is Safe and Immunogenic when Administered to Hospitalized Patients." *Vaccine* 19, nos. 25–26 (2001): 3493-3498.

Chisholm, J.C., T. Devine, A. Charlett, C.R. Pinkerton, and M. Zambon. "Response to Influenza Immunization During

---

KEY TERMS

Common cold—A mild illness caused by an upper respiratory virus. Usual symptoms include nasal congestion, coughing, sneezing, throat irritation, and a low-grade fever.

Epidemic—A widespread regional disease outbreak.

Guillain-Barré syndrome—Also called acute idiopathic polyneuritis, this condition is a neurologic syndrome that can cause numbness in the limbs and muscle weakness following certain viral infections.

Pandemic—Worldwide or multiregional outbreak of an infection afflicting millions of people.

Reye's syndrome—A syndrome of nausea, vomiting, and neurological problems such as confusion or delirium. It can be fatal in children.

Treatment for Cancer." *Archives of Diseases of Children* 84, no. 6 (2001): 496-500.

Fleming, D.M., and M. Zambon. "Update on Influenza and Other Viral Pneumonias." *Current Opinions on Infectious Diseases* 14, no. 2 (2001): 199-204.

Fleming, D.M. "Managing Influenza: Amantadine, Rimantadine and Beyond." *International Journal of Clinical Practice* 55, no. 3 (2001): 189-195.

Green, M.S. "Compliance with Influenza Vaccination and the Health Belief Model." *Israel Medical Association Journal* 2, no. 12 (2001): 912-913.

Hak, E., T.J. Verheij, G.A. van Essen, A. B. Lafeber, D.E. Grobbee, and A.W. Hoes. "Prognostic Factors for Influenza-Associated Hospitalization and Death During an Epidemic." *Epidemiology of Infections* 126, no. 2: 261-268.

James, J.S. "Flu Epidemic: Shots, New Treatments Available." *AIDS Treatment News* no 335 (21 Jan. 2000): 2-4.

Michaeli, D. "Influenza Vaccination." *Israel Medical Association Journal* 2, no. 12 (2000): 914-915.

Wareing, M.D., and G.A. Tannock. "Live Attenuated Vaccines Against Influenza; An Historical Review." *Vaccine* 19, nos. 25, 26 (2001): 3320-3330.

ORGANIZATIONS

American Academy of Emergency Medicine. 611 East Wells Street, Milwaukee, WI 53202. (800) 884-2236. <http://www.aaem.org>.

American Academy of Pediatrics. 141 Northwest Point Boulevard, Elk Grove Village, IL 60007-1098. (847) 434-4000. <http://www.aap.org/default.htm>.

OTHER

Centers for Disease Control and Prevention. <http://www.cdc.gov/ncidod/diseases/flu/fluvirus.htm>.

Food and Drug Administration. <http://www.fda.gov/cder/drug/advisory/influenza.htm>.

National Coalition for Adult Immunization. <http://www.nfid.org/factsheets/influadult.html>.

National Foundation for Infectious Diseases. <http://www.nfid.org/library/influenza>.

National Institute of Allergy and Infectious Diseases. <http://www.niaid.nih.gov/publications/flu.htm>.

National Library of Medicine. <http://www.nlm.nih.gov/medlineplus/influenza.html>.

World Health Organization. <http://www.who.int/emc/diseases/flu/>.

L. Fleming Fallon, Jr., M.D., Dr.P.H.

Informed consent

Definition

Informed consent is a legal document in all 50 states, prepared as an agreement for treatment, nontreatment, or for an invasive procedure that requires physicians to disclose the benefits, risks, and alternatives to said treatment, nontreatment, or procedure. It is the method by which a fully informed, rational patient may be involved in choices about his or her health care.

Description

Informed consent stems from the legal and ethical right the patient has to decide what is done to his or her body, and from the physician's ethical duty to make sure that the patient is involved in decisions about his or her own health care. The process of securing informed consent has three phases, all of which involve information exchange between doctor and patient and are part of **patient education**. First, in words the patient can understand, the physician must convey the details of a planned procedure or treatment, its potential benefits and serious risks, and any feasible alternatives. The patient should be presented with information on the most likely outcomes of the treatment. Second, the physician must evaluate whether or not the person has understood what has been said, must ascertain that the risks have been accepted, and that the patient is giving consent to proceed with the procedure or treatment with full knowledge and forethought. Finally, the patient must sign the consent form, which documents in generic format the major points of

consideration. The only exception to this is securing informed consent during extreme emergencies.

It is critical that the patient receive enough information on which to base informed consent, and that the consent is wholly voluntary and has not been forced in any way. It is the responsibility of the physician who discusses the particulars with the patient to detail the conversation in the patient's record. A physician may, at his or her discretion, appoint another member of the health care team to obtain the patient's signature on the consent form, with the assurance that the physician has satisfied the requirements of informed consent.

Paul H. Ting, M.D., Assistant Professor of Anesthesiology at the University of Virginia and editor of the "About Anesthesiology" web site discusses why patients are apprehensive. "I think that people's greatest concerns are...whether they will live or die...whether they will feel any **pain** or be uncomfortable...whether they will be well taken care of (and I include in this whether their care will lead to a successful result and whether they will be treated with dignity)...."

"The boilerplate consent form has good intentions; it is comprehensive and therefore should reflect that a comprehensive discussion was completed," said Dr. Ting. "The actual form itself is in place to protect the hospital and the physician. Legally, it is proof that things have been covered and the patient agrees to the procedure, risks, benefits, options, etc. However, the informed consent process (which the form merely is supposed to document) is in place for the protection of the patient. The process is in place to make sure that everything is discussed with the patient—all of the options, all of the common risks, the worst thing that can happen, etc."

The law requires that a reasonable physician standard be applied when determining how much information is considered adequate when discussing a procedure or treatment with the patient. There are three approaches to making this discussion: what the typical physician would say about the intervention (the reasonable *physician* standard); what the average patient would need to know to be an informed participant in the decision (the reasonable *patient* standard); and what the patient would need to know/understand to make a decision that is informed (*subjective* standard).

Viewpoints

There is a theory that the practice of acquiring informed consent is rooted in the post-World War II Nuremberg Trials. At the war crimes tribunal in 1949, 10 standards were put forth regarding physicians' requirements for experimentation on human subjects. This established a new standard of ethical medical behavior for the post-WW II human rights age, and the concept of voluntary informed consent was established. A number of rules accompanied voluntary informed consent. It could only be requested for experimentation for the gain of society, for the potential acquisition of knowledge of the pathology of disease, and for studies performed that avoided physical and mental suffering to the fullest extent possible.

As of 2001, most of the 50 United States had legislation that spells out the required standards for informed consent. For example, the State of Washington employs the second approach outlined as the *reasonable patient* standard. This ensures that the doctor fulfills all professional responsibilities and provides the best care possible and that the patient has a choice in decisions about his or her health care. However, the patient's competence in making a decision is considered. This points to the issue of the patient's "capacity." Anyone suffering from an illness, anticipating surgery, or undergoing treatment for a disease is under a great deal of **stress** and **anxiety**. It may be natural for a patient to be confused or indecisive. When the attending physician has serious doubts about the patient's understanding of the intervention and its risks, the patient may be referred for a psychiatric consultation. This is strictly a precaution to ensure that the patient understands what has been explained; declining to be treated or operated on does not necessarily mean the person is incompetent. It could mean that the person is exercising the right to make his or her own health care decisions.

Although it is the law to formally present the procedure or treatment to the patient, physicians do express doubt as to its wisdom. Some believe that informing patients of the risks of treatment might scare them into refusing it when the risks of non-treatment are even greater. But patients might have a different view. Without the complete story, for example, a patient might consent to beginning a particular course of **chemotherapy**. Convinced by the pressures from a pharmaceutical company, it is conceivable that a doctor will use an agent less effective than a newer treatment. By withholding information about treatment alternatives, the physician may be denying the patient a choice and a chance of an extended life of greater quality.

The international community has also had much to say in this regard. Martin Tattersall, professor at the Sydney University Cancer Medicine Department, and Alan Langslands, professor in Radiation Oncology at Westmead, said in the August 1995 issue of the *Medical Journal of Australia*, "Our findings indicate the extent of variation in the practice of providing information to **cancer** patients commencing treatment.... The current dou-

ble standard between former clinical trials (where ethics committees require that patients be given a 'plain language statement,' as well as giving their signed consent) and the 'usual' practice outside such trials, is apparently narrowing. The reasons for this may relate to the fear of litigation, rather than recognition of the need to provide full information." A litigious society such as the United States might be plagued by an even greater number of lawsuits than at present if informed consent were not legally mandated.

Professional implications

Undeniably, physicians in surgery, anesthesia, oncology, infectious disease—the list is endless—are faced with issues regarding Informed Consent. As the federal government takes a more active role in deciding the extent to which patients must be informed of treatments, procedures, and clinical trials in which they voluntarily become enrolled, more and more health care providers must become educated in what needs to be conveyed to patients. This is emphasized by the report of a case in which a federal court (Hutchinson vs. United States [91 F2d 560 (9th Cir. 1990)]) ruled in favor of the physician, despite his failure to advise his asthmatic patient (for whom he had prescribed the steroid, prednisone), of the well-known risk of developing aseptic necrosis (bone death), which did occur. The practitioner neglected to inform the patient that there were other drugs available with a much less serious side effect profile that could have treated the **asthma**. However, and despite this "neglect," a higher, appellate court reversed the ruling and found the physician guilty. Apparently the patient had used more conservative drugs in the past with good results. The court believed that if the physician had merely advised the patient of the more serious side effects of prednisone and offered the patient more conservative treatment, the physician would have avoided liability.

Nursing professionals have a greater role in evaluating whether the consent is informed or not than they might believe. When a nurse witnesses the signature of a patient for a procedure, or surgery, he or she is not responsible for providing its details. Rather, the role is to be the patient's advocate; to protect the patient's dignity; identify any fears; and determine his or her degree of comprehension and approval of care to be received. Each patient is an individual, and each one will have a different and unique response depending on his or her personality, level of education, emotions, and cognitive status. If the patient can restate the information that has been imparted to him or her, then that will help to confirm that he or she has received enough information and has understood it. The nurse is obligated to report any doubts about the patient's understanding regarding what has been said, or any concerns about his or her capacity to make decisions.

Resources

PERIODICALS

Dunn, Debra. "Exploring the Gray Areas of Informed Consent." *Nursing* (1999). <http://www.findarticle.com>.

Lehman, C. M., and G. M. Rodgers. "To IRB or Not to IRB?" *American Journal of Clinical Pathology* 115, no. 2(2001):187-191.

Lutz, S., and S. J. Henkind. "Recruiting for Clinical Trials on the Web." *Healthplan* 41, no. 5(2000):36-43.

"Nuremberg Code (1947): standards for medical experimentation." *British Medical Journal* 7070, no. 313 (1996). Circumcision Information and Responses Position?...<http://www.cirp.org/library/ethics/nuremberg>.

Wirshing D. A., W. C. Wirshing, S. R. Marder, R. P. Liberman, and J. Mintz. "Informed Consent: assessment of comprehension." *American Journal of Psychiatry* 155, no. 11 (1998):1508-11.

OTHER

"Cancer treatment and informed consent." Sydney University Cancer Medicine Department. <http://jinx.sistm.unsw.edu/au/~greenlft/1996/216/216p13.htm>.

"Health Information for surgical procedures, family health, patient education...." <http://www.docs4patients.com/informed-consent.asp>.

"Informed consent." <http://www.nocirc.org/consent>.

"Informed Consent." The University of Washington. <http://eduserv.hscer.washington.edu/bioethics/topics/consntc1.html>.

"Informed Consent." *Risk Management Handbook*. Yale-New Haven Hospital & Yale University School of Medicine. <http://info.med.yale.edu/cim/risk/handbook/rmh_informed_consent.html>.

"Medical-Legal Issues in HIV Treatment." <http://www.medscape/SCP/TAR4/2001>.

"Risk Management Issues: Improved Informed Consent." <http://www.rmf.harvard.edu/rmLibrary/rmissues/infconsent/body.html>.

Randi B. Jenkins

Inheritance, principles of

Definition

The patterns governing how genetic information is transmitted from generation to generation are collectively known as the principles of inheritance.

Description

Single-gene inheritance

Genes are composed of DNA (deoxyribonucleic acid), whose building blocks, the nucleotides, code for the multitude of **proteins** in the human body, including enzymes and structural proteins. In 2001, estimates place the number of human protein-coding genes between 25,000 and 35,000. A single-gene disorder is one caused by an alteration (mutation) in a specific gene that normally plays an important role in the human body. The protein product of a mutated gene is either abnormal in function, reduced in amount, or missing entirely.

Genes are passed down from parent to child in predictable patterns, discussed below. Knowledge of these patterns allows health care providers to explain to patients why a certain genetic disease is present in members of the family, and to predict the possibility that another family member will also be affected. As of 2001 more than 10,000 traits or diseases had been identified as following a single-gene pattern of inheritance. These are catalogued in the Online Mendelian Inheritance in Man (OMIM) at <http://www.ncbi.nlm.nih.gov/omim/>. In the following discussion, the MIM numbers associated with each disease example are the OMIM catalogue numbers.

In order to understand single-gene inheritance, it is necessary to be familiar with several terms and concepts. With some exceptions, discussed later, genes are present in pairs. Each member of the pair is termed an allele. An individual is said to be homozygous (a homozygote) at a certain gene locus if the two alleles of a pair are the same (i.e., if both alleles are either normal or carry the same mutation). In contrast, if the two alleles are different, the person is heterozygous (a heterozygote). For example, a person is heterozygous if he or she has one normal and one mutant allele; or if he or she has two abnormal alleles, each of which has a different mutation. The word "genotype" refers to an individual's allelic makeup at a gene. "Phenotype" refers to the observable result of having a certain genotype. Hair color is an example of a phenotype. Phenotype can be affected by other genes or by environmental influences.

Genetic traits caused by single genes are often referred to as Mendelian traits, in tribute to the Austrian monk Gregor Mendel, who in 1865 reported the results of his painstaking work on the transmission of traits such as color and shape in the garden pea. His three laws of heredity are:

- Unit inheritance. Prior to Mendel, many believed that traits were blended as they were passed from generation to generation. Although genes would not be "discovered" until the next century, Mendel clearly spelled out that inheritance is a matter of passing on discrete traits.

- Segregation. The two alleles of a gene are never transmitted together from one parent to an offspring. This means that, in humans, an individual egg or sperm is formed with only one allele of each gene.

- Independent assortment. Alleles of different genes pass randomly to offspring. This law was later found to have important exceptions: If two genes are very close to each other on a chromosome, they tend to be passed down together.

Mendel's laws went unnoticed until 35 years later, when they were simultaneously and independently discovered by Hugo De Vries in the Netherlands, Erich von Tschermak in Austria, and Carl Correns in Germany. These rediscoveries marked the real beginning of genetics as a science. Over the years many other scientists and physicians have contributed to our current understanding of inheritance in humans.

AUTOSOMAL INHERITANCE. The transmission of single-gene traits from generation to generation follows one of several basic patterns, depending on the location of the particular gene. A gene on one of the 22 pairs of autosomes—that is, the non-sex-determining chromosomes—is called an autosomal gene. Similarly, a trait or disease associated with that gene is an autosomal trait. Autosomal conditions are the most common and are equally likely to occur in males or females. Autosomal traits are further classified as either dominant or recessive.

Autosomal-dominant inheritance. Dominant conditions are those that are expressed in heterozygotes. For example, in a dominant disorder, if the two alleles of the gene are labeled A for the mutant (disease-producing) copy and B for the normal copy, an individual who is AB at that gene locus will have the disease, as will the individual who is AA. However, because a mutant allele is much less common than its normal counterpart, it is very unlikely that an affected individual would be AA.

The inheritance pattern of dominant traits is distinctive. If one parent has a particular dominant trait (e.g., an AB genotype), he or she has a 50% chance of passing the mutant allele (A) to each offspring, and, similarly, a 50% chance of passing the normal allele. Since most mutant alleles are very rare, there is usually little chance that the other parent would have the same mutant allele. Therefore, the total risk of having a child with the same disorder is 50% with each **pregnancy**. However, depending on the particular trait or disease, there are often circumstances in which the actual risk is less than 50%. For example, whether or not a person with the mutant gene

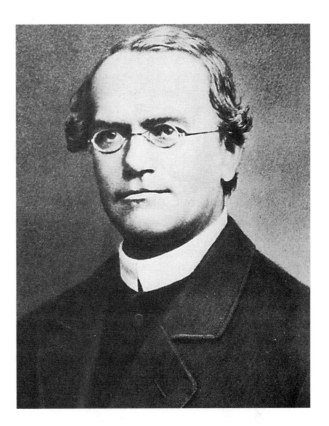

Gregor Mendel. *(Archive Photos, Inc. Reproduced by permission.)*

exhibits the trait may depend on a phenomenon called penetrance. If an autosomal-dominant disorder is fully penetrant, every individual with a mutant copy of the gene will have the disease. An allele is said to have reduced penetrance if only some individuals with the allele ever develop signs of the disorder. Similarly, expressivity refers to the degree to which someone who has inherited the mutant gene will be affected. For example, one person with a particular mutant allele might be severely affected, while another will have only mild features of the disease. The degree to which penetrance and expressivity play a role in autosomal-dominant disorders varies with the particular gene. In addition, some mutant alleles cause disease only later in life; these are the so-called adult-onset single-gene disorders.

Of the 10,000 genetic traits and diseases currently known, more than half are autosomal-dominant. When considered individually, the majority are rare, with the most common being present in only 1 in 500 to 1,000 individuals. However, taken together, they have an important impact on health. One of the most common is familial hypercholesterolemia (MIM 143890), a cause of early-onset **heart** disease. Mutations in the gene for this condition disrupt the normal **metabolism** of **fats** in the body and lead to a significant buildup of cholesterol deposits in the arteries. Huntington disease (MIM 143100), a progressive neurological disorder affecting approximately 1 in 20,000 individuals, is an example of an autosomal-dominant disorder that does not usually appear until well into adulthood. Individuals with a mutant copy of this gene typically begin to show symptoms between ages 30 and 50, with death occurring approximately 15 years later. Neurofibromatosis (von Recklinghausen disease, MIM 162200), a commonly encountered autosomal-dominant condition (1 in 3,000 individuals), is a good example of a disease exhibiting variable expressivity. Signs and symptoms can vary from extremely mild ones such as pigmentary changes of the skin (cafe-au-lait spots) to more severe complications (including learning disabilities and multiple disfiguring tumors).

Autosomal-recessive inheritance. The genes for autosomal-recessive traits are also located on the autosomes, but the mutant, disease-causing alleles are recessive to the normal alleles; thus, if one normal allele is present, it is usually sufficient to prevent any expression of the disease. If the normal allele is designated A and the mutant allele is designated a, individuals who are AA or Aa will be phenotypically normal. Only those with an aa genotype will exhibit signs of the disease. Aa individuals are termed carriers, because they carry one mutant copy without showing symptoms themselves. Except for extremely rare cases of new mutations, both parents of an individual (aa) with an autosomal recessive disorder are carriers (Aa). Each time they make a germ cell (egg or sperm), that germ cell can receive only one allele. Thus, each parent always has a 50% (1 in 2) chance of passing on the mutant allele. If both parents pass the mutant allele to their germ cells, at fertilization the resulting embryo will have two mutant alleles (aa) and no normal allele. Thus, the chance that two parents who are both carriers of a mutant allele at the same gene locus will have a child with the disease is 25% (50% x 50%), or 1 in 4 with each pregnancy. Similarly, the probability of their having a child who is a carrier (Aa) is 50%, and the chance of having a child (AA) who did not inherit the disease allele from either parent is 25%.

Because an individual who carries one copy of a gene for an autosomal-recessive disorder is usually symptom-free, he or she can unknowingly transmit the disease allele to offspring. However, because of the rarity of most autosomal-recessive disorders, it is unlikely that both members of a couple will be carriers for the same disease gene and have a risk for producing children with the disorder. An exception to this is when parents are consanguineous (**blood** relatives), because they are both at risk of being carriers for the same disease allele present in their family. Consanguinity is a hallmark of autosomal-recessive traits, and couples who are related may be at an increased risk over nonconsanguineous couples for an autosomal-recessive disorder in their offspring if a disease allele is carried in their family.

X-LINKED INHERITANCE. In addition to the 22 pairs of autosomes, humans have two sex chromosomes, X and Y, which determine an individual's sex (gender). Females have two X chromosomes (XX) and males have an X and a Y (XY). Because the smaller Y chromosome has only a very few genes as compared to the larger X, X-linked inheritance is often referred to as sex-linked inheritance. The pattern of inheritance of X-linked traits is very different from that of autosomal conditions. A distinguishing feature is the lack of male-to-male transmission, because a father transmits only his Y chromosome, not his X, to his sons. There are examples of both X-linked recessive and X-linked dominant diseases, although the former are far more common.

X-linked recessive inheritance. Another hallmark of X-linked recessive traits is that they are almost exclusively seen in males, while females are the carriers. This is explained by the fact that males only have one X chromosome and females have two Xs. The rarity of an particular mutant allele (Xm) in the general population means that a female's other allele at that gene locus is likely to be normal (Xn). Because the mutant allele is recessive, females with one mutant allele and one normal allele (Xm Xn) are rarely affected. However, on average, one half, or 50%, of the sons of a carrier female will have the particular disease as a result of inheriting the mother's X chromosome with the mutant allele (XmY). Similarly, half of a carrier female's daughters will be carriers. Since a male with an X- linked recessive trait has only one X chromosome and he transmits that X to all of his daughters, all of his daughters will be carriers.

X-linked dominant inheritance. An X-linked disease is considered dominant if is expressed in heterozygotes (Xm Xn). All of the daughters of an affected male, but none of his sons, will have the disease. All offspring, female or male, of an affected female will be affected. However, because of a phenomenon called X-inactivation, some females may have a milder disease. In all females, one X in each cell is normally inactivated, and most genes on that X are nonfunctioning in that cell. The process is usually random, meaning that in females with one mutant and one normal allele, approximately half of the cells will have an active normal allele, which is often enough to ensure a milder course of the disease. In some severe X-linked disorders, most affected individuals are females, and it is rare to see a male with the disease. This is explained by the fact that males do not have another X with a normal allele. Rett syndrome (MIM 312750), a severe mental-retardation syndrome, is an X-linked dominant disorder seen only in females. It is proposed that male fetuses with the abnormal Rett syndrome gene do not survive to birth.

MITOCHONDRIAL INHERITANCE. The above-described patterns of inheritance are applicable to genes present on the chromosomes in the nucleus of the cell. However, cells have additional genes in their mitochondria, the energy-producing organelles in the cytoplasm, the non-nuclear portion of the cell. Leber hereditary optic atrophy (MIM 535000), a severe type of midlife **vision** loss, is one of the rare disorders traced to mutations in mitochondrial DNA. Because mitochondria are almost exclusively passed from parent to child in the egg and not in the sperm, a hallmark of mitochondrial inheritance is transmission from an affected woman to all of her children. Although mitochondrial diseases are single-gene disorders, they are not considered Mendelian.

Chromosome abnormalities

In humans, the 35,000 or so nuclear genes are located on 46 chromosomes: 22 pairs of autosomes and 1 pair of sex chromosomes. Unlike single-gene diseases that are due to mutations in the DNA, chromosomal disorders are the result of too little or too much normal DNA. These disorders are usually divided into two types, numerical and structural.

NUMERICAL CHROMOSOME ABNORMALITIES. Numerical disorders are the result of either a missing or an extra whole chromosome. Although classified as genetic disorders, they are not transmitted through families. Rather, they are usually the result of an error in the specialized cell divisions (meiosis) that produce eggs and sperm. **Down syndrome**, a condition involving mental retardation and characteristic physical features, with an incidence of approximately 1 in 800 live births, is perhaps the most familiar example of a chromosome disorder. In 95% of individuals with Down syndrome, the condition is due to an extra, free-standing chromosome 21 (trisomy 21). More than 90% of trisomy 21 is due to an extra chromosome being packaged into the egg. In less than 10% of individuals, the sperm is the source of the extra 21. The only known risk factor for trisomy 21 is the age of the mother. Women have an increasingly greater risk for having a child with trisomy 21 as they get older. The reason for this is not known. Other examples of clinically important conditions that result from either a missing or an extra chromosome are Turner syndrome, Klinefelter syndrome, trisomy 13, and trisomy 18.

STRUCTURAL CHROMOSOME ABNORMALITIES. Structural chromosome abnormalities are caused by chromosome breakage and rearrangement. Among the more common types are inversions, translocations, dele-

tions, and duplications. If the rearrangement preserves all of the genetic material, it is called balanced. Individuals who carry balanced rearrangements are not affected themselves, but their altered chromosomes are at risk for further breakage and rearrangement during egg and sperm formation. This can result in offspring with extra or missing portions of chromosomes. In approximately 5% of individuals with Down syndrome, the extra chromosome 21 is not free-standing, as in trisomy 21, but is attached to another chromosome as the result of a unbalanced translocation. Often one parent will carry the balanced form of the translocation and be at risk for having other children with Down syndrome. Unbalanced structural chromosome abnormalities are found in about 1 in 17,000 live births. In the majority of cases, the resulting imbalance in the amount of genetic material results in serious physical and developmental abnormalities.

Multifactorial inheritance

Instead of one single gene being of paramount importance in producing disease, a multifactorial disorder results from the interaction of a number of genes plus influences in the environment. Despite the fact that multifactorial disorders are among the most common causes of disease in humans, the specific genes and environmental factors are still poorly understood. In contrast to single-gene disorders, multifactorial diseases do not exhibit a clear-cut pattern of inheritance within families. After one affected individual in the family, the risk of a second affected with the disorder may be somewhat increased, but that increase is more in the range of 2–10% percent than the 25–50% seen in single-gene disorders.

Nontraditional inheritance

In addition to the well-known patterns of inheritance described above, some important clinical disorders exhibit variations on these patterns. Several of these nontraditional types of inheritance are introduced briefly here. The reader is referred to other sources listed in the references for more detailed treatments.

• Triplet-repeat disorders. These are caused by genes that change in size and function from parent to child. Fragile X syndrome (MIM 309550), primarily affecting males, is caused by a gene on the X chromosome that can expand when passed from parent to child. The expansion disrupts gene function and results in mental retardation, characteristic facial features, and enlarged testes. There are a number of other triplet-repeat disorders, including the autosomal-dominant Huntington disease.

KEY TERMS

Allele—A member of a pair of genes.

Autosomes—Non-sex-determining chromosomes.

Chromosomes—Structures in the nucleus of a cell consisting of a thread of DNA containing the genetic information (genes). Humans have 46 chromosomes in 23 pairs.

Enzyme—A protein catalyst that promotes chemical reactions within the body.

Hemoglobin—The iron-containing protein of the red blood cells. Its function is to carry oxygen from the lungs to the tissues.

- Imprinting disorders. Most genes are expressed the same in an individual whether that gene was contributed by the mother or the father. However, there are exceptions in which the allele from one parent is normally imprinted and inactive. If the allele from the other parent is missing, for example, due to a deletion of a portion of the chromosome containing the gene, the individual is left with no functioning gene. Two very different conditions involving mental retardation, Prader-Willi syndrome (MIM 176270) and Angelman syndrome (MIM 105830), have been found to involve the phenomenon of imprinting.

- Uniparental disomy. This is the presence of both members of a chromosome pair from one parent and no copy from the other parent. The reader is referred to other sources for a more detailed treatment of this rare phenomenon. Uniparental disomy in combination with imprinting can also result in clinically important disorders, including some cases of Prader-Willi and Angelman syndromes.

Role in human health

Although genetics plays a role in the majority of human diseases, the contribution of genes may be primary or secondary in the pathophysiology of diseases. A British Columbian survey of more than one million individuals estimated that by age 25, at least 53 of 1,000 will have a disease with a significant genetic component.

Common diseases and disorders

Most genetic disorders fall into one of three main types; single gene, chromosomal, and multifactorial. Each type has its important hallmarks, and a basic knowl-

edge of the distinguishing factors of each is important for those who work in a clinical setting.

Single-gene disorders

Cystic fibrosis (CF, MIM 602421) is a typical autosomal-recessive disease. CF is often said to be the most common serious autosomal-recessive condition in the Caucasian population, with a frequency of about 1 in 2,000 children. Its clinical features include chronic respiratory disease, pancreatic insufficiency, and a decreased life expectancy. At present there is no cure, but because a great deal is being learned about the function of the CF gene, CF is a disease for which treatment at the gene level (also known as gene replacement or **gene therapy**) is being considered. Carrier parents who have had one child with CF have a 25% risk, with each subsequent pregnancy, of having another affected child. It is customary to offer these couples the option of prenatal diagnosis in future pregnancies to determine if the fetus is affected.

Sickle-cell anemia (MIM 603903), another autosomal-recessive disorder, is due to a specific mutation in one of the genes that codes for hemoglobin. The resulting abnormalities in the hemoglobin-rich red blood cells lead to multiple clinical symptoms in affected (aa) individuals, including increased risks for infections, blood clots, strokes, and painful swelling of the joints. Sickle cell is more common in those who can trace their ancestry to the African continent. About 1 in 500 African Americans is born with this disease. Approximately 8% are carriers (Aa) but remain symptom-free.

Perhaps the best-known example of an X-linked recessive disease is **hemophilia** A (MIM 306700). Seen almost exclusively in males, this is a failure of the blood to clot normally because of a mutation in the gene for one of the clotting factors, factor VIII. Affected males require life-long treatment with blood transfusions and factor VIII concentrates. In recent years research has been directed toward being able to offer gene therapy for males with this disorder. Duchenne **muscular dystrophy** (DMD, MIM 310200) is another X-linked recessive condition affecting the muscle fibers; it results in death usually by age 20. Since most males with DMD do not survive to reproduce, their abnormal genes are not passed on. Nevertheless, the frequency of DMD does not decline over time, because approximately one third of all cases are due to new mutations and not to the transmission of the gene from a carrier mother.

Multifactoral inherited disorders

Spina bifida, or open-spine defect, is a multifactorial birth defect, as are many cases of cleft lip/palate.

Recent studies have suggested that a deficiency of **folic acid**, one of the B **vitamins**, may play a role in causing spina bifida, and women who are planning a pregnancy are urged to take supplemental folic acid. Not withstanding the important part that multifactorial inheritance plays in the etiology of birth defects, perhaps its greatest role is in the common diseases that are adult-onset. For example, most coronary heart disease is thought to be multifactorial, with genes plus dietary habits playing a part in determining an individual's risk for atherosclerosis, a narrowing of the arteries of heart caused by lipid (fat) deposits. A variety of cancers are also thought to be due to a combination of genetic and environmental factors. An enormous challenge awaits the next generation of geneticists as they attempt to unravel the complex interactions of genes and environment in these clinically important multifactorial disorders.

Resources

BOOKS

Jorde, L. B., J. C. Carey, M. J. Bamshad, and R. L. White. *Medical Genetics, Second Edition.* New York: Mosby, 1999.

Rimoin, D. L., J. M. Connor, and R. E. Pyeritz, editors. *Emery and Rimoin's Principles and Practice of Medical Genetics, Third Edition.* New York: Churchill Livingstone, 1997.

PERIODICALS

Baird, P. A., T. W. Anderson, H. B. Newcombe, and R. B. Lowry. "Genetic Disorders in Children and Young Adults: A Population Study." *American Journal of Human Genetics* 42: 677- 693.

Wolfsberg, T. G., J. McEntyre, and G. D. Schuler. "Guide to the Draft Human Genome." *Nature* (February 15, 2001), 409: 824-825.

OTHER

Medicine and the New Genetics: Human Genome Project Information. <http://www.ornl.gov/hgmis/medicine>.

OMIM (Online Mendelian Inheritance in Man). <http://www3.ncbi.nlm.nih.gov/htbin- post/Omim>.

Sallie Boineau Freeman, Ph.D.

Integumentary system

Definition

The integumentary system includes the skin and the related structures that cover and protect the body. The human integumentary system is composed of the skin, and includes glands, hair, and nails. The largest organ in the body, the skin protects the body, prevents water loss, regulates body temperature, and senses the external environment.

Description

The integumentary system serves many protective functions for the body. It acts as a mechanical barrier, simultaneously preventing water from entering the body and excessive water loss. It also limits access of microorganisms that could cause illness, and protects underlying tissues from mechanical damage. Pigments in the skin called melanin, give skin its color, and absorb and reflect the sun's harmful ultraviolet radiation.

Function

In addition to serving as a protective barrier, the skin helps to regulate the body temperature by several mechanisms. If heat builds up in the body, sweat glands in the skin produce more sweat that evaporates and cools the skin. When the body overheats, **blood vessels** in the skin dilate (expand), bringing more **blood** to the surface, and allowing body heat to dissipate. When the body is too cold, the blood vessels in the skin constrict, shunting blood away from the body surface, thus conserving heat. Along with temperature regulation, the skin serves as a minor excretory organ, since sweat removes small, clinically insignificant amounts of nitrogenous wastes produced by the body. The skin also functions as a sense organ since it contains millions of nerve endings that detect touch, heat, cold, **pain** and pressure. Finally, the skin produces **vitamin D** in the presence of sunlight, and renews and repairs damage to itself.

In an adult, the skin covers about 21.5 sq. ft (2 sq. m), and weighs about 11 lb. (5 kg). Depending on location, the skin thickness ranges from 0.02-0.16 in (0.5-4.0 mm). Skin is composed of an outer layer, or epidermis, and a thicker inner layer, the dermis. A subcutaneous layer of fatty or adipose tissue is immediately below the dermis. Fibers from the dermis attach the skin to the subcutaneous layer, and the underlying tissues and organs also connect to the subcutaneous layer.

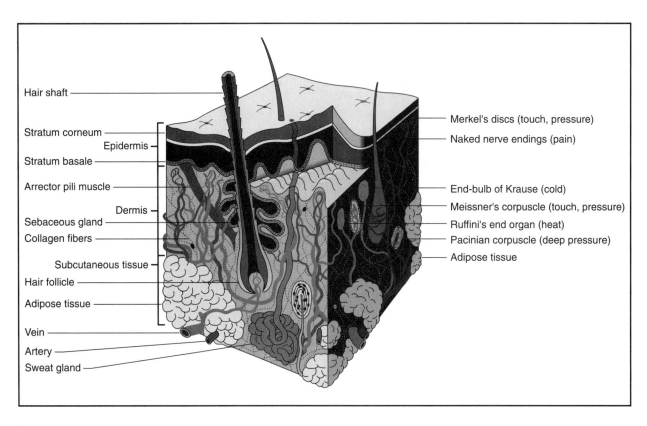

Hair shaft

Stratum corneum
Epidermis
Stratum basale

Arrector pili muscle
Dermis
Sebaceous gland
Collagen fibers

Subcutaneous tissue
Hair follicle
Adipose tissue

Vein
Artery
Sweat gland

Merkel's discs (touch, pressure)
Naked nerve endings (pain)

End-bulb of Krause (cold)
Meissner's corpuscle (touch, pressure)
Ruffini's end organ (heat)
Pacinian corpuscle (deep pressure)
Adipose tissue

Human skin. *(Diagram by Hans & Cassidy. Courtesy of Gale Group.)*

The epidermis

Ninety percent of the epidermis, including the outer layers, contains keratinocytes, cells that produce keratin, a protein that helps waterproof and protect the skin. Melanocytes are pigment cells that produce melanin, a brown-black pigment that adds to skin color and absorbs ultraviolet light, thereby shielding the genetic material in skin cells from damage. Merkel's cells disks are touch-sensitive cells found in the deepest layer of the epidermis of hairless skin.

In most areas of the body, the epidermis consists of four layers. On the soles of the feet and palms of the hands where there is considerable friction, the epidermis has five layers. Calluses, abnormal thickenings of the epidermis, occur on skin subject to constant friction. At the skin surface, the outer layer of the epidermis constantly sheds the dead cells containing keratin. The uppermost layer consists of about 25 rows of flat dead cells that contain keratin.

The dermis

The dermis is made up of connective tissue that contains protein, collagen, and elastic fibers. It also contains blood and lymph vessels, sensory receptors, related nerves, and glands. The outer part of the dermis has fin-gerlike projections, called dermal papillae, that indent the lower layer of the epidermis. Dermal papillae cause ridges in the epidermis above it, which in the digits give rise to fingerprints. The ridge pattern of fingerprints is inherited, and is unique to each individual. The dermis is thick in the palms and soles, but very thin in other places, such as the eyelids.

The blood vessels in the dermis contain a volume of blood. When a part of the body, such as a working muscle, needs more blood, blood vessels in the dermis constrict, shifting blood from the skin to supply muscles and other body parts. Sweat glands with ducts that pass through the epidermis and open on the skin surface through pores are embedded in the deep layers of the dermis. Hair follicles and hair roots also originate in the dermis, and the hair shafts extend from the hair root through the skin layers to the surface. The dermis also contains sebaceous glands associated with hair follicles. Sebaceous glands produce an oily substance called sebum. Sebum softens the hair and prevents it from drying, but if sebum blocks a sebaceous gland, a whitehead appears on the skin. A blackhead results if the material oxidizes and dries. Acne pimples are caused by infections of the sebaceous glands.

The skin is an important sense organ and as such includes a number of types of nerves, which are mainly in the dermis, with a few reaching the epidermis. Nerves carry impulses to and from hair muscles, sweat glands, and blood vessels, and receive messages from touch, temperature, and pain receptors. Some nerve endings are specialized such as sensory receptors that detect external stimuli. The nerve endings in the dermal papillae, known as Meissner's corpuscles, detect light touch, or the feel of clothing on the skin. Pacinian corpuscles, located in the deeper dermis, are stimulated by stronger pressure on the skin. Receptors near hair roots detect displacement of the skin hairs by stimuli such as touch or wind. Bare nerve endings throughout the skin supply information to the **brain** about temperature change (both heat and cold), texture, pressure, and trauma.

Role in human health

Along with its vital roles as shield against microorganisms and regulating body temperature, skin often provides information about overall health and a variety of medical conditions. The color, texture, temperature, and elasticity of skin can aid in diagnosing a variety of disorders. For example, patients with hepatitis may have a characteristic yellow tinge to their skin. Similarly, cold sores and **fever** blisters are indications of **infection** with herpes simplex virus, and warts (intraepidermal skin tumors) result from infection with human papilloma virus (HPV).

Skin testing is an important diagnostic tool in the evaluation of **allergies**. Skin testing involves a series of superficial injections of one or more suspected allergens. A positive response, such as redness, or inflammation, at the site of the skin test, helps to pinpoint the culprit.

Common diseases and disorders

Acne, caused by clogged pores and bacterial infection, is commonly diagnosed in teenagers and young adults. Acne may be mild, moderate, or severe and is characterized by blackheads, whiteheads, papules, pustules, and cysts on the face, shoulders, chest, and back. Mild acne may be treated with topical antimicrobial agents to kill the **bacteria** on the skin and topical retinoids to open the pores. Moderate and severe acne often respond to treatment with systemic **antibiotics** such as tetracycline or doxycycline.

Common bacterial skin infections are impetigo, folliculitis, and cellulitis. Impetigo is a contagious skin infection caused by streptococci or staphylococcus. It produces crusty patches on the skin. Local outbreaks may be treated with antibacterial ointment, and patients with widespread infections are given oral antibiotics. Infectious folliculitis produces erythema (redness) and pustules. It is caused by staphylococcus and treated with oral antibi-

otics. Cellulitis is swelling, erythema, warmth, and pain caused by infection of the dermis and subcutaneous tissue often near a wound site. Cellulitis is usually caused by Group A streptococci or staph aureus and is treated with a course of anti-strep or anti-staph antibiotics.

Common viral skin disorders include infection with herpes simplex or herpes zoster. Herpes simplex is responsible for cold sores, fever blisters, and lesions on the genitals and buttocks. Herpes zoster produces a painful rash characterized by vesicles. Both conditions are treated with acyclovir, or other orally administered anti-viral agent.

Skin reactions include eczema, allergic contact dermatitis (rashes), such as those resulting from contact with poison ivy, sumac, or oak, and **hives**. Contact dermatitis, an eruption of itchy skin vesicles, is an allergic skin reaction. Patients are advised to avoid contact with the suspected allergen, and mild cases may be treated with warm soaks and topical ointments to reduce inflammation and soothe inflamed skin.

Cosmetic damage as well as potentially fatal skin disorders may result from overexposure to the ultraviolet (UV) rays in sunlight. At first, overexposure to sunlight results in injury known as sunburn. UV rays damage skin cells, blood vessels, and other dermal structures. Continual overexposure produces leathery skin, wrinkles, and discoloration and may also lead to skin **cancer**. Anyone excessively exposed to UV rays runs a risk of skin cancer, regardless of the amount of pigmentation normally in the skin. Seventy-five percent of all skin cancers are basal cell carcinomas that arise in the epidermis and rarely metastasize (spread) to other parts of the body. Physicians can surgically remove basal cell cancers. Squamous cell carcinomas also occur in the epidermis, and these may metastasize. Malignant melanomas are life-threatening skin cancers that metastasize rapidly. There can be a 10 to 20 year delay between exposure to sunlight and the development of skin cancers.

Dermatology is the medical specialty devoted to the diagnosis and treatment of skin disorders. In addition to the disorders previously described, primary care physicians and dermatologists are frequently called upon to diagnose and treat the following conditions:

- alopecia (hair loss)

- athlete's foot (fungus infection)

- moles

- psoriasis (scaly skin on the scalp, trunk, arms and legs)

- rosacea (symmetrically distributed papules and pustules on the nose and cheeks)

KEY TERMS

Chitin—Polysaccharide that forms the exoskeleton of insects, crustaceans, and other invertebrates.

Dermis—Thicker layer of skin lying below the epidermis.

Epidermis—Thinner outermost layer of the skin.

Keratin—Insoluble protein found in hair, nails, and skin.

Melanin—Brown-black pigment found in skin and hair.

• scabies (skin infestation with mites that produces inflammatory papules in the wrists, web spaces, and sides of feet)

• seborrheic dermatitis (facial redness and scaling)

• spider veins, varicose veins

• vitiligo (loss of skin color on patches of skin, usually affects the face and extremities)

Today, many dermatologists also provide a range of cosmetic services to reduce the signs of aging, such as wrinkles, sagging skin and discoloration, and reverse some of the effects of sun damage to skin. Microdermabrasion, laser skin resurfacing, and injections of collagen are among the techniques used to improve the appearance of skin.

Resources

BOOKS

Freedberg, Irwin, et al. *Fitzpatrick's Dermatology In General Medicine, Fifth Edition.* Vols. I, II, and III. New York, NY: McGraw-Hill, 1999.

Odom, Richard B., et al. *Andrew's Diseases of the Skin.* Philadelphia, PA: W.B. Saunders Company, 2000.

OTHER

Skin Deep. Video and videodisc. Princeton, NJ: Films for the Humanities and Sciences, 1995.

Barbara Wexler

Intensive care unit equipment

Definition

Intensive care unit (ICU) equipment includes patient monitoring, respiratory and cardiac support, **pain man-agement**, emergency resuscitation devices, and other life support equipment designed to care for patients who are seriously injured, have a critical or life-threatening illness, or have undergone a major surgical procedure, thereby requiring 24-hour care and monitoring.

Purpose

An ICU may be designed and equipped to provide care to patients with a range of conditions, or it may be designed and equipped to provide specialized care to patients with specific conditions. For example, a neuromedical ICU would care for patients with acute conditions involving the nervous system or for patients who have just had neurosurgical procedures and would require equipment for monitoring and assessing the **brain** and **spinal cord**. A neonatal ICU is designed and equipped to care for infants who are ill, born prematurely, or have a condition requiring constant monitoring.

Patient monitoring equipment

Patient monitoring equipment includes the following:

• Acute care physiologic monitoring system—Continuously measures and displays data on **vital signs**, such as **heart** rate, **blood pressure**, cardiac output, and **blood** oxygen levels.

• Pulse oximeter—Monitors the oxygen saturation in the blood.

• Intracranial pressure monitor—Measures the pressure of fluid in the brain in patients with head trauma or other conditions affecting the brain (such as tumors, **edema**, or hemorrhaging).

• Apnea monitor—Continuously monitors breathing to detect cessation in infants and adults at risk of respiratory failure.

Life support and emergency resuscitative equipment

ICU equipment for life support and emergency resuscitation include the following:

• Ventilator (also called a respirator)—Assists with or controls pulmonary ventilation in patients who cannot breathe on their own.

• Infusion pump—Device that delivers fluids intravenously or epidurally, including continuous anesthesia, drugs, and blood infusions.

• Crash cart—Portable cart containing emergency resuscitation equipment for patients who are "coding" (that is, their vital signs are in a dangerous range), including a defibrillator, airway intubation devices, resuscitation bag/mask, and medication box.

- Intra-aortic balloon pump—A device that helps reduce the heart's workload and helps blood flow to the coronary arteries for patients with unstable angina, **myocardial infarction**, or patients awaiting transplants.

The use of diagnostic equipment is also required in the ICU. Mobile x-ray units are used for bedside radiography, particularly of the chest. Portable clinical laboratory devices, called point-of-care analyzers, are used for blood analysis at the bedside to provide results much faster than if samples were sent to the central laboratory.

Disposable ICU equipment includes urinary (Foley) catheters, catheters used for arterial and central venous lines, Swan-Ganz catheters, chest and endotracheal tubes, gastrointestinal and nasogastric feeding tubes, and monitoring electrodes.

Description

ICU equipment includes patient monitoring, life support and emergency resuscitation devices, and diagnostic devices.

Patient monitoring equipment

- Acute care physiologic monitoring systems are comprehensive patient monitoring systems that can be configured to measure and display various parameters, such as an electrocardiogram (ECG), respiratory rate, blood pressure (noninvasive and invasive), body temperature, cardiac output, arterial hemoglobin oxygen saturation, mixed venous oxygenation, and end-tidal carbon dioxide, via electrodes and sensors connected to the patient. Each patient bed in an ICU has a physiologic monitor, and all monitors are networked to a central nurses' station.

- Pulse oximeters measure the arterial hemoglobin oxygen saturation of the patient's blood with a sensor clipped over the finger or toe. Pulse oximetry is usually a capability included in a physiologic monitoring system, but the ICU also uses dedicated pulse oximeters for some patients.

- Intracranial pressure monitors are connected to sensors inserted into the brain through a cannula or bur hole. These devices warn of elevated pressure and record or display pressure trends. Intracranial pressure monitoring may be a capability included in a physiologic monitor.

- Apnea monitors use electrodes or sensors placed on the patient to detect cessation of breathing, display respiration parameters, and trigger an alarm if a certain amount of time passes without a patient's breath being detected. Apnea monitoring may be a capability included in a physiologic monitor.

Life support and emergency resuscitative equipment

- **Ventilators** consist of a flexible breathing circuit, gas supply, heating/humidification mechanism, monitors, and alarms. They are microprocessor-controlled and programmable, and regulate the volume, pressure, and flow of patient respiration. Ventilator monitors and alarms may be interfaced to a central monitoring system or information system.

- Infusion pumps employ automatic, programmable pumping mechanisms to supply the patient with fluids intravenously or epidurally through a catheter. The pump is hung on an intravenous pole, which is located next to the patient's bed.

- Crash carts, also called resuscitation carts or code carts, are strategically located in the ICU for immediate availability when a patient experiences cardiorespiratory failure. The cart holds a defibrillator, which is used to apply an electric shock to a patient in ventricular fibrillation. Two paddles are placed on the patient's chest and buttons are pressed to discharge an electrical shock of approximately 2,000 to 4,000 volts. The cart also holds a resuscitator, which is inserted into the patient's airway, and a bag is pressed to push air into the **lungs**.

- Intra-aortic balloon pumps use a balloon placed in the patient's aorta to help the heart pump. The balloon is on the end of a catheter that is connected to the pump's console, which displays heart rate, pressure, and ECG readings. The patient's ECG is used to time the inflation and deflation of the balloon.

Diagnostic devices most commonly used in the ICU are mobile x-ray units, which can be pushed to the patient's bedside to take x rays using a battery-operated generator that powers an x-ray tube, and point-of-care blood analyzers, which are handheld devices that require a small amount of whole blood and display blood chemistry parameters.

Operation

The ICU is a demanding environment due to the critical condition of patients and the variety of equipment necessary to support and monitor patients. Therefore, when operating ICU equipment, staff should pay attention to the types of devices and the variations between different models of the same type of device, so as not to make an error in operation or adjustment. Although many

KEY TERMS

Apnea—Cessation of breathing.

Arterial line—A catheter inserted into an artery and connected to a physiologic monitoring system to allow direct measurement of oxygen, carbon dioxide, and invasive blood pressure.

Edema—An abnormal accumulation of fluids in intercellular spaces in the body; causes swelling.

Central venous line—A catheter inserted into a vein and connected to a physiologic monitoring system to directly measure venous blood pressure.

Chest tube—A tube inserted into the chest to drain fluid and air from around the lungs.

Endotracheal tube—A tube inserted through the patient's nose or mouth that functions as an airway and is connected to the ventilator.

Gastrointestinal tube—A tube surgically inserted into the stomach for feeding a patient unable to eat by mouth.

Nasogastric tube—A tube inserted through the nose and throat and into the stomach for direct feeding of the patient.

Ventricular fibrillation—An irregular cardiac rhythm characterized by contractions of the ventricular muscle of the heart and signaling impending cardiac arrest; treated by using a defibrillator and medications.

hospitals make an effort to standardize equipment, for example, using the same manufacturer's infusion pumps or patient monitoring systems, older devices and non-standardized equipment may still be used, particularly when the ICU is busy. Clinical staff should be sure to check all devices and settings to ensure patient safety.

ICU patient monitoring systems are equipped with alarms that sound when the patient's vital signs deteriorate, for instance, when breathing stops, blood pressure is too high or too low, or when heart rate is too fast or too slow. Usually, all patient monitors connect to a central nurses' station for easy supervision. ICU staff should be sure that all alarms are functioning properly and that the central station is staffed at all times.

For reusable patient care equipment, clinical staff should be sure to properly disinfect and sterilize devices that contact patients. Disposable items, such as catheters and needles, should be disposed of in an appropriately labeled container.

Maintenance

Since ICU equipment is used continuously on critically ill patients, it is essential that equipment be properly maintained, particularly those devices used for life support and resuscitation. ICU staff should perform daily checks on equipment and inform **biomedical engineering** staff when equipment needs maintenance, repair, or replacement. For mechanically complex devices, service and preventive maintenance contracts are available from the manufacturer or third-party servicing companies.

Health care team roles

ICU equipment is used by an ICU care team, which consists of a critical care attending physician, ICU nurses, respiratory therapists, pharmacists, physical therapists, and nutritionists. Physicians trained in other specialties, such as anesthesiology, cardiology, radiology, surgery, neurology, pediatrics, and orthopedics, may be consulted and called to the ICU to treat patients who require their expertise. Radiologic technologists perform mobile x-ray examinations (bedside radiography). Either nurses or clinical laboratory personnel perform point-of-care blood analysis. ICU equipment is maintained and repaired by the hospital biomedical engineering staff and/or the equipment manufacturer.

Some studies have shown that patients in the ICU following high-risk surgery are at least three times as likely to survive when cared for by "intensivists," physicians trained in critical care medicine.

Training

Manufacturers of more sophisticated ICU equipment, such as ventilators and patient monitoring devices, provide clinical training for all involved staff when the device is purchased. All ICU staff must have undergone specialized training in the care of critically ill patients and must be trained to respond to life-threatening situations, since ICU patients are in critical condition and may experience respiratory or cardiac emergencies.

Resources

BOOKS

Merck Manual of Diagnosis and Therapy, 17th ed. Beers, Mark H. and Robert Berkow, eds. Merck Research Laboratories, 1999.

PERIODICALS

Savino, Joseph S., C. William Hanson III, and Timothy J. Gardner. "Cardiothoracic Intensive Care: Operation and Administration." *Seminars in Thoracic and Cardiovascular Surgery* 12 (October 2000): 362–70.

ORGANIZATIONS

American Association of Critical Care Nurses. 101 Columbia, Aliso Viejo, CA 92656. (800) 809-2273. <http://www.aacn.org>.

National Association of Neonatal Nurses. 4700 West Lake Ave., Glenview, IL 60025-1485. (847) 375-3660. <http://www.nann.org>.

Society of Critical Care Medicine. 701 Lee St., Suite 200, Des Plaines, IL 60016. (847) 827-6869. <http://www.sccm.org>.

OTHER

Committee to Establish Recommended Standards for Newborn ICU Design. *Recommended Standards for Newborn ICU Design. Report of the Fourth Consensus Conference.* January 28-29, 1999.

ICU Personnel Guide. July 2001. <http://www.waiting.com/icupersonnel.html>.

"Intensive Care Units." July 2001. <http://www.pulmonologychannel.com/icu/index.html>. <http://www.pulmonologychannel.com/icu/equipment.shtml>.

"ICU Equipment Guide." July 2001. <http://www.waiting.com/icuequipment.html>.

"Intensivists in the ICU Linked to Vastly Reduced Patient Deaths." Johns Hopkins University. April 13, 1999. <http://www.hopkinsmedicine.org/press/1999/April99/990414.htm>.

Jennifer E. Sisk, M.A.

Intermittent positive-pressure breathing unit *see* Ventilators

Internal fetal monitoring *see* Electronic fetal monitoring

Intestinal culture *see* Stool culture

Intestine, large

Definition

The large intestine is located in the abdominal cavity. It is the site of the last phases of digestion and consists of three segments: the cecum, the colon, and the rectum. The colon divides into ascending colon, transverse colon, descending colon, and sigmoid colon. The large intestine is called large because its diameter is considerably greater than the diameter of the **small intestine**.

Description

The large intestine is the terminal part of the **digestive system**. This important system is responsible for the ingestion and digestion of foodstuffs. Along the digestive tract, food is broken down into nutrient molecules small enough to pass into the bloodstream. Nutrient molecules are mostly absorbed in the small intestine, with the remainder being absorbed in the large intestine, which also prepares waste for elimination from the body through the anus.

The large intestine is called the ascending colon as it starts from the cecum, which marks the end of the small intestine. The caecum contains the worm-shaped appendix. The ascending colon then passes along the right abdominal wall to the inferior surface of the **liver** and bends sharply at a right angle to the left at a curve called the hepatic flexure. At this point, it crosses the abdominal cavity, passing to the left abdominal wall and is known as the transverse colon. Under the spleen, it bends again at the splenic flexure, and is known as the descending colon, passing along the left abdominal wall to the pelvic region. The colon then forms an S-shaped curve and is called the sigmoid colon. The rectum marks the end of the colon. It is a storage site for solid waste which can then exit the body through an external opening called the anus, controlled by muscles called sphincters.

The large intestine is about 6 ft (1.8 m) long and about 2 in (5 cm) wide in the average, normal adult.

Function

The large intestine has three major functions:

- Recovery of water and essential ions. When the partially digested foodstuffs reach the end of the small intestine (ileum), roughly 80% of their water contents has been absorbed, but considerable water and small ions, such as sodium and chloride, still remain and must be recovered by further absorption. The colon then absorbs most of the remaining water and ions and additionally secretes bicarbonate ions as well as mucus, an important lubricant that protects the intestinal lining.

- Formation and storage of feces. As matter moves through the colon, it is dehydrated, mixed with **bacteria** and mucus, and formed into feces for subsequent storage and elimination. The composition of normal feces is approximately 75% water and 25% solid waste, mostly consisting of bacteria and roughage, that is, undigested protein, fat, fibers, dried digestive juices, and dead cells. Its typical brown color is due to pigments resulting from the bacterial degradation of bilirubin and fecal odor results from gases released by bacteria.

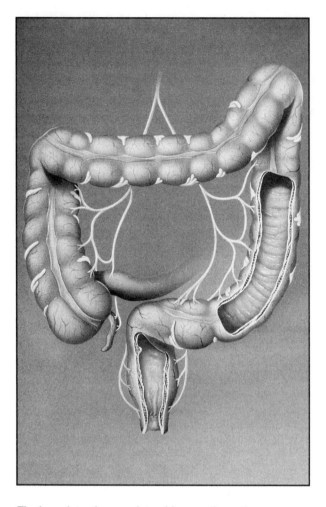

The large intestine consists of four sections: the ascending (left), transverse (top), descending (right), and sigmoid (bottom) colon. *(Photograph by John Bavosi. Science Source/Photo Researchers. Reproduced by permission.)*

- Bacterial fermentation. Fermentation refers to the enzymatic decomposition and utilization of foodstuffs by bacteria. The large intestine has a rich bacterial life that produces a wide variety of enzymes capable of fermenting many of the nutrient molecules that would otherwise not be absorbed. A normal adult harbors some 450 different species of bacteria in the colon and most of these are anaerobes, meaning bacteria that survive only in oxygen-free environments. Bacterial populations in the large intestine digest **carbohydrates, proteins**, and **lipids** that escape digestion and absorption in the small intestine and they also manufacture **vitamin K** and certain B vitamins.

The movement of bulk matter in the colon is referred to as large intestinal motility and it consists of four different types of muscle-assisted contractions:

- Segmentation contractions. These contractions mash and mix the partially digested foodstuff, exposing it to the mucous membrane where nutrient absorption occurs.

- Peristaltic contractions. These contractions are wave-like contractions that allow material to advance from the small intestine through the colon.

- Antiperistaltic contractions. These contractions occur in a backwards direction toward the ileum, so as to slow down the forward movement of matter through the colon. This provides more residence time for the absorption of nutrients.

- Giant migrating contractions. These contractions represent a type of motility only seen in the colon. Giant migrating contractions are a type of very intense and prolonged peristaltic contraction that can strip a large segment of colon free of contents.

Following the ingestion of food, large intestinal motility increases significantly, triggered by the duodenocolic reflex, which is stimulated by the presence of fat in the small intestine. Additionally, giant migrating contractions push feces into the empty rectum. Stretching of the rectum in turn stimulates the defecation reflex. This is a reflex controlled by the pelvic nerves, and it results in relaxation of the ring-like internal anal sphincter, the muscle that constricts or closes the anus. This is followed by voluntary relaxation of the external anal sphincter and defecation.

Role in human health

The importance of the large intestine in human health is mostly derived from its role in removing water from food residues and transporting it into the bloodstream. Along with this water, dissolved **minerals** and ions, notably sodium, potassium, and chlorine, are also transported to the bloodstream. Without these chemicals, the **blood** is chemically unbalanced, a condition that can lead to serious illness and even death.

Common diseases and disorders

- **Appendicitis**. Appendicitis is an inflammation of the appendix. It occurs due to accumulated waste material that cannot move out of the appendix easily because it only has one opening. The symptoms of appendicitis are muscular rigidity, sharp **pain** in the right lower abdomen, and vomiting.

- Colitis. Colitis is commonly known as irritable bowel or spastic colon. It refers to the inflammation of the inner lining of the colon. Colitis is related to **stress** and

KEY TERMS

Abdomen—A part of the body that lies between the thorax and the pelvis. It contains a cavity (abdominal cavity) that holds organs such as the pancreas, stomach, intestines, liver, and gallbladder. It is enclosed by the abdominal muscles and the vertebral column (spine).

Abdominal cavity—The hollow part of the body located between the diaphragm, which is the thin muscle below the lungs and heart, and the pelvis, the basin-shaped cavity that contains the reproductive organs, bladder, and rectum. The abdominal cavity contains the abdominal organs.

Anaerobes—Bacteria that live only in environments that are virtually oxygen-free.

Anal sphincter—The ring-like band of muscle that constricts or closes the anus.

Anus—The terminal opening of the digestive tract.

Appendix—A worm-shaped structure projecting from the cecum.

Bilirubin—A waste product from the breakdown of heme, the active group of hemoglobin, the molecule that carries oxygen in the blood. Bilirubin is produced in the liver and excreted in bile.

Cecum—The pouch-like start of the large intestine that links it to the small intestine.

Colon—Part of the large intestine, located in the abdominal cavity. It consists of the ascending colon, the transverse colon, the descending colon, and the sigmoid colon.

Digestion—The conversion of food in the stomach and in the intestines into substances capable of being absorbed by the blood.

Digestive system—Organs and paths responsible for processing food in the body. These are the mouth, the esophagus, the stomach, the liver, the gallbladder, the pancreas, the small intestine, the large intestine, and the rectum.

Feces—Waste product of digestion formed in the large intestine. About 75% of its mass is water, the remainder is protein, fat, undigested roughage, dried digestive juices, dead cells, and bacteria.

Fermentation—Enzymatic breakdown and utilization of foodstuffs by bacteria, as occurs in the large intestine.

Goblet cells—Mucus-secreting cells found scattered among other cells in the epithelium of many organs, especially in the intestinal and respiratory tracts. They are most abundant in the colon.

Hepatic flexure—Sharp right-angle bend of the ascending colon under the liver as it becomes the transverse colon.

Ion—Elements consist of positively charged nuclei surrounded by negatively charged electrons. These charges are balanced and the overall charge of an element is zero. An element becomes an ion, that is a charged species, if it gains or losses electrons. Many small ions are essential for the functioning of the body. The major ones include: the potassium ion (K+), the sodium ion (Na+), the chlorine ion (Cl), and the HCO_3^- ion.

Large intestinal motility—Muscle-assisted contractions occurring in the colon to facilitate movement of intestinal contents. There are four type of motility: segmentation contractions, peristaltic contractions, antiperistaltic contractions and giant migrating contractions.

Large intestine—The terminal part of the digestive system, site of water recycling, nutrient absorption, and waste processing located in the abdominal cavity. It consists of the caecum, the colon, and the rectum.

Mucous membrane—The lubricated lining of several body organs that contains mucus-secreting glands.

Mucus—The slimy secretion of glands found on mucous membranes composed of various proteins, salts, and white blood cells.

Pelvis—The basin-shaped cavity located below the abdomen that contains the reproductive organs, the bladder, and rectum.

Peristalsis—A pattern of wave-like muscle contractions that allows material to advance through the digestive tube.

Peritoneum—The thin membrane that lines the abdominal and pelvic cavities, and covers most abdominal organs.

Rectum—The rectum is a short, muscular tube that forms the lowest portion of the large intestine and connects it to the anus.

can lead to ulcerative colitis, in which open sores appear in the mucous membrane of the colon.

- Colorectal cancers. Colorectal cancers start in the innermost layer of the tissues of the large intestine and can grow through some or all of the layers. They can develop in any of the four sections of the colon or in the rectum.

- Constipation. Constipation is caused primarily by insufficient fiber in the diet, lack of **exercise**, or not drinking enough fluids. As a result, fecal matter hardens and large intestinal motility is impaired.

- **Diarrhea**. Diarrhea is a condition characterized by frequent, loose, watery stools that range from yellowish to light brown to green in color. If enough water is lost, **dehydration** occurs.

- Diverticulosis. Diverticulosis is characterized by outward ballooning (diverticula) of the large intestine wall caused by chronic constipation.

- Dysentery. Dysentery is a general term for various disorders characterized by severe diarrhea, inflamed intestines, and intestinal bleeding. Some forms of dysentery may clear up by themselves, while other forms may continue for years without treatment.

- Hemorrhoids. Hemorrhoids are commonly known as piles. They are dilated veins in the anus and rectum.

- Peritonitis. Peritonitis refers to inflammation of the peritoneum, the membrane that lines the abdominal and pelvic cavities. It can occur as a result of a ruptured appendix, which empties its contents of fecal matter and waste into the abdominal cavity. This condition is extremely serious.

- Ptosis of the colon. Also known as prolapsed colon, this is a common condition that occurs when the colon falls from its normal position to a lower position.

Resources

BOOKS

Ballard, Carol. *The Stomach & Digestive System.* Toronto: Britnell Book Wholesalers, 1997.

Janowitz, Henry D. *Your Gut Feelings: A Complete Guide to Living Better With Intestinal Problems.* New York: Taylor & Francis, 1995.

Johnson, L.R., and T.A. Gerwin, eds. *Gastrointestinal Physiology.* St. Louis: Mosby, 2001.

ORGANIZATIONS

American Gastroenterology Society. 7910 Woodmont Ave., Seventh Floor, Bethesda, MD 20814. (310) 654-2055. Fax: (310) 652-3890. mgoslin@gastro.org. <http://www.gastro.org>.

OTHER

Gross and Microscopic Anatomy of the Large Intestine. <http://biology.about.com/science/biology/library/organs/bldigestlargeint.htm>.

"The Large Intestine." <http://www.medic-planet.com/MP_article/internal_reference/large_intestine>.

Monique Laberge, PhD

Intestine, small

Definition

The small intestine is a long coiled tube located in the abdominal cavity. It is the major site of chemical digestion and absorption of nutrients by the body and consists of three sections: the duodenum, the jejunum, and the ileum.

Description

The small intestine is the longest section of the **digestive system**. This important body system digests food by breaking it down into nutrient molecules small enough to pass into the bloodstream. Nutrient molecules are absorbed in the small intestine and sent into the **blood** circulatory system. The digestive system also eliminates solid waste, recycles water, and absorbs **vitamins** from nutrients in the large intestines. Even though some starch breakdown takes place in the mouth and some breakdown of protein is done in the **stomach**, most of the digestion occurs in the duodenum.

The small intestine is a coiled, tube-like organ held in place by two membrane sheets attached to the walls of the abdominal cavity and referred to as the mesentery. Nerves, blood and lymph vessels to and from the small

KEY TERMS

Abdomen—A part of the body that lies between the thorax and the pelvis. It contains a cavity (abdominal cavity) that holds organs such as the pancreas, stomach, intestines, liver, and gallbladder. It is enclosed by the abdominal muscles and the vertebral column (spine).

Abdominal cavity—Hollow part of the body located between the diaphragm, which is the thin muscle below the lungs and heart, and the pelvis, which is the basin-shaped cavity that contains the reproductive organs, the bladder, and the rectum. The abdominal cavity contains the abdominal organs.

Acid—Refers to a compound that is acid or sour. When dissolved in water, acids yield hydrogen ions.

Amino acids—Organic compounds containing mostly the elements carbon, nitrogen, and oxygen that combine to form peptides and proteins.

Base—Refers to a compound that is caustic (soda, lime). Bases dissolve in alcohol and in water, and can combine with fats.

Bile—A greenish yellow fluid produced by the liver and stored in the gallbladder that is secreted in the small intestine to assist in the absorption of fats.

Bile ducts—Passages external to the liver for the transport of bile.

Digestion—The conversion of food in the stomach and in the intestines into substances capable of being absorbed by the blood.

Digestive system—Organs and paths responsible for processing food in the body. These are the mouth, the esophagus, the stomach, the liver, the gallbladder, the pancreas, the small intestine, the colon (large intestine), and the rectum.

Duodenum—The first section of the small intestine, extending from the stomach to the jejunum, the next section of the small intestine.

Epithelial cells—Cells covering the surface of the body and the lining of its cavities. In the small intestine, the epithelial cells cover the villi and contain microvilli.

Epithelium—The covering of the internal and external surfaces of the body and of the lining of blood vessels and small cavities. It consists of cells joined by cementing substances.

Gastric juice—An acidic secretion of the stomach that breaks down the proteins contained in the ingested food, prior to digestion.

Gland—An organ that produces and releases substances for use in the body, such as fluids or hormones.

Ileum—The last section of the small intestine located between the jejunum and the large intestine.

Jejunum—The section of the small intestine located between the duodenum and the ileum.

Lymph—Colorless liquid that bathes body tissues and circulates in the lymph vessels.

Mesentery—The membrane that connects the jejunum and the ileum to the abdominal cavity walls.

Mucosal folds—Mucosal folds are circular folds found on the inner surface of the small intestine. They increase surface area and help mix the partially broken down foods by acting as baffles.

Mucous membrane—The lubricated lining of several body organs that contains mucus-secreting glands.

Mucus—Slimy secretion of glands found on mucous membranes composed of various proteins, salts, and white blood cells.

Pancreas—The pancreas is a flat, glandular organ lying below the stomach. It secretes the hormones insulin and glucagon that control blood sugar levels and also secretes pancreatic enzymes in the small intestine for the breakdown of fats and proteins.

Peritoneum—Thin membrane that lines the abdominal and pelvic cavities and covers most abdominal organs.

Pylorus—The opening from the stomach into the small intestine.

Small intestine—The part of the digestive tract located between the stomach and the large intestine.

Villi intestinales—Microscopic hair-like structures covered with epithelial cells measuring 1–1.5 mm that line the mucous inner membrane of the small intestine. The epithelial cells of the villi contain microvilli and are responsible for the absorption of nutrients. Being so small and numerous, they effectively increase the absorptive surface area of the small intestine.

intestine lie between the two sheets of the mesentery. In the adult, the small intestine measures on average about 22 ft (6.7 m) with a diameter of 1–2 in (2.5–5 cm). It consists of three segments: the short duodenum, the jejunum, which represents 40% of the small intestine, and the terminal ileum, which accounts for the remaining 60% and which empties into the **large intestine**. The small intestine thus forms a passage going from the pylorus (opening from the stomach) to the large intestine.

The inner mucous membrane of the small intestine is not flat and uniform but folded to such a great extent that its inner lining is referred to as the mucosal folds. The mucosal folds are covered with approximately 20,000 tiny hair-like projections called villi that are lined with epithelial cells studded with microvilli. One villus contains about 500 microvilli and in one square inch of small intestine, there are some ten billion microvilli.

Function

Together, the intestines process 2–3 gal (7.6–11.4 l) of food, liquids, and bodily waste every day. The small intestine is the major site of absorption of almost all nutrients into the blood.

The stomach delivers foodstuffs to the duodenum that it has reduced to a liquid pulp with gastric juices, called the chyme, for further breakdown. The duodenum also receives pancreatic enzymes from the **pancreas** and bile from the **liver** via the pancreatic and common bile ducts. The pancreatic enzymes are required for the chemical breakdown of **fats**, sugars, and **proteins**, and the bile plays an important role in the absorption of fats. To assist the process, the villi sway constantly so as to stir up the chyme for nutrient removal and transport across their membranes into the blood and lymph vessels. The fatty molecules are transferred to the lymph, while sugar (glucose) and amino acids go into the blood and are carried to the liver. The muscles that encircle the small intestine constrict about seven to twelve times a minute to shake, knead, and mix the chyme with its secretions and the gastric juices of the stomach. The small intestine also absorbs enormous quantities of water. Normal water intake for an adult is about 0.5 gal (2 l) of dietary fluid per day. An additional 1.6–1.8 gal (6–7 l) of fluid is delivered to the small intestine by secretions from salivary glands, stomach, pancreas, liver, and its own secretions. Of these 2.1–2.3 gal (8–9 l), the small intestine absorbs 80% on a daily basis.

The absorption of nutrients across the epithelial cell boundary of the small intestine is made possible by maintaining a "sodium electrochemical gradient." The interior of all cells maintains a low concentration of sodium. The epithelial cells lining the small intestine (enterocytes)

achieve this using a large number of enzymes (Na_+/K_+ ATPases), called sodium pumps. These pumps export sodium ions from the cell in exchange for potassium ions, thus establishing a gradient of both charge and sodium concentration across the cell membrane that facilitates transport. This constant flow of sodium is ultimately responsible for the absorption of water, amino acids, and **carbohydrates** by the small intestine. It is known that each intestinal enterocyte has some 150,000 such sodium pumps, which allow each cell to transport about 5 billion sodium ions out of each cell per minute.

Role in human health

The passage of foodstuffs through the small intestine results in the absorption of most of the water and electrolytes (sodium, chloride, potassium) as well as almost all nutrient molecules, such as glucose, amino acids, and fatty acids. The small intestine not only provides the nutrients required for the functioning of the body, but also plays a critical role in water and acid-base equilibrium. Acid-base equilibrium refers to a condition by which the net rate of acid or base production by the body is balanced by the net rate of acid or base elimination from the body, resulting in stable amounts of hydrogen ions in body fluids.

Common diseases and disorders

The common diseases and disorders of the small intestine include:

• Adenocarcinoma. Adenocarcinomas are cancers of the gland cells that line the small intestine. They tend to occur in the duodenum.

• Adenomas. Adenomas are non-cancerous gland cell tumors often found in the intestinal villi.

• Atresia of small intestine. Atresia of the small intestine is characterized by the absence or closure of parts of the small intestine. Duodenal atresia is diagnosed in 1:5,000 live births and is frequently associated with **Down syndrome**. Jejuno-ileal atresia occurs less frequently (1:1,500 to 1:20,000 live births).

• Carcinoid tumors. Carcinoid tumors develop from the neuroendocrine cells that are found in the numerous secretions entering the intestine. About 2,500 carcinoid tumors are diagnosed each year in the United States and they account for about one-third of all tumors that develop in the small intestine and appendix.

• **Crohn's disease**. Crohn's disease causes inflammation in the small intestine. It usually occurs in the ileum.

• Cytomegalovirus (CMV). CMV is a herpes-type virus that can infect the epithelial cells of the small intestine.

- Duodenal ulcer. Gastric and duodenal ulcers afflict approximately 4 million people in the United States. They are associated with **alcoholism**, chronic lung and kidney disease, and thyroid disorders.

- Dysentery. Dysentery is a general term for various disorders characterized by severe **diarrhea**, inflamed intestines, and intestinal bleeding. Some forms of dysentery may clear up by themselves while other forms may continue for years without treatment.

- Protein-losing enteropathy. Disease of the small intestine characterized by excessive loss of plasma proteins.

- Gastrointestinal stromal tumor (GIST). GIST is most commonly diagnosed in the muscular wall of the jejeunum and ileum.

- Gluten sensitive enteropathy. Disease of the small intestine characterized by impaired absorption of nutrients due to loss of villi because of an adverse immune reaction to gluten, a protein found in wheat and other related foods.

- Small intestinal hemorrhages. The major causes of small intestinal hemorrhage are infections, vascular anomalies, and bleeding disorders.

- Small intestinal infarction. Small intestinal infarction is caused by the partial or complete obstruction to blood flow. It usually occurs in people over age 50–55.

Resources

BOOKS

Ballard, Carol. *The Stomach & Digestive System.* Toronto: Britnell Book Wholesalers, 1997.

Janowitz, Henry D. *Your Gut Feelings: A Complete Guide to Living Better With Intestinal Problems.* New York: Taylor & Francis, 1995.

Johnson, L.R., and T.A. Gerwin, eds. *Gastrointestinal Physiology.* St. Louis: Mosby, 2001.

ORGANIZATIONS

American Gastroenterology Society. 7910 Woodmont Ave., Seventh Floor, Bethesda, MD 20814. (310) 654-2055. Fax: (310) 652-3890. mgoslin@gastro.org. <http://www.gastro.org>.

OTHER

Diseases of the Small Intestine. <http://radiology.uchc.edu/eAtlas/nav/msSmall.htm>.

"Small Intestine Cancer." University of Pennsylvania Oncolink. <http://cancer.med.upenn.edu/pdq_html/1/engl/101175.html>.

Monique Laberge, PhD

Intracranial ultrasound *see* **Ultrasonic encephalography**

Intradermal injections

Definition

Intradermal injections are injections given to a patient in which the goal is to empty the contents of the syringe between the layers of the skin.

Purpose

Intradermal injection is often used for conducting skin **allergy tests** and testing for antibody formation.

Precautions

This is a painful procedure and is used only with small amounts of solution. The nurse should ensure that the needle is inserted into the epidermis, not subcutaneously, as absorption would be reduced. It is imperative that the following information is reviewed prior to administration of any medication: the right patient, the right medicine, the right route, the right dose, the right site, and the right time. Because this method of injection is often used in allergy testing, it is important that latex-free syringes are used.

Description

With the intradermal injection, a small thin needle of 25 or 27 gauge and 3/8 to 3/4 inch (1-2 cm) is inserted into the skin parallel with the forearm, with the bevel facing upward. These injections are normally given in the inner palm-side surface of the forearm, with the exception of the human diploid cell rabies vaccine, which is given in the deltoid muscle.

Preparation

After washing his or her hands, the nurse should put on latex-free gloves to complete the procedure. A sterile syringe and a needle should be prepared. If a sterile multiple-dose vial is used, the rubber-capped bottle should be rubbed with an antiseptic swab. The needle is then inserted through the center of the cap, and some air from the syringe inserted to equalize the pressure in the container. Slightly more of the required amount of drug is should then be removed. The syringe should be held vertically at eye level, then the syringe piston should be pushed carefully to the exact measurement line.

If a small individual vial containing the correct amount of drug is used, the outside should be wiped with an antiseptic swab and held in the swab while the top is snapped off. The needle is then inserted into the vial, tak-

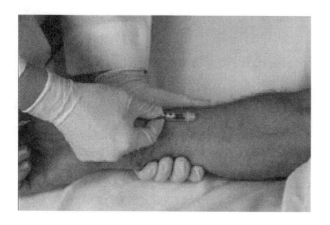

Skin must be spread taut for an intradermal injection.
(Delmar Publishers, Inc. Reproduced by permission.)

ing care that the tip of the needle does not scratch against the sides of the vial, thereby becoming blunt.

The **syringe and needle** containing the drug should be placed on a tray with sterile cotton swabs and cleaning disinfectant. If the patient is unfamiliar with the procedure, the nurse should explain what he or she is about to do, and let the patient know that the medication was prescribed by the doctor. As with all drugs prescribed for a patient, the dose on the patient's prescription sheet should be checked prior to administration.

A screen should be drawn around the patient to ensure privacy. The injection site is then rubbed vigorously with a swab, and disinfectant applied to cleanse the area and increase the **blood** supply. With the bevel of the needle facing upwards, the needle is inserted into the skin, parallel with the forearm. The syringe piston should then be pushed in steadily and slowly, releasing the solution into the layers of the skin. This will cause the layers of the skin to rise slightly.

Aftercare

Monitor the patient's reaction and provide reassurance, if required. Dispose of all waste products carefully and place the syringe and needle in a puncture-resistant receptacle.

Complications

If the circulation is depleted, absorption of the drug administered may be slow.

Results

Check for any adverse reactions if the drug is being administered for the first time.

Health care team roles

As this procedure is often used as a diagnostic tool, the process should be explained fully to the patient.

The health care team should record any side effects or negative reactions to the drug that has been injected; medical staff should be notified.

Resources

PERIODICALS

Advisory Committee on Immunization Practices. *Recommendation of Advisory Committee on Immunization Practices.* (January 28, 1994): 43 (RRO1); 1-38.

Guide to Good Prescribing, Annex 4: The Use of Injections. World Health Organization.

ORGANIZATIONS

American Academy of Nurse Practitioners, AANP, PO Box 12846, Austin, Texas, 78711. (512) 442 4262. E-mail: admin@aanp.org.

OTHER

American College of Allergy, Asthma, and Immunology. *Latex Allergy Home Page.* <http://allergy.mcg.edu/advice/latex.html>.

"Guidance on the content of premarket notification [510(K)] submissions for piston syringes." <http://www.fda.gov/cdrh/ode/odegr821.html>.

"How to protect yourself from needlestick injuries." DHHS 9NIOSH) publication No. 2000-135. NIOSH <http://www.cdc.gov/niosh/homepage.html>.

Margaret A Stockley, R.G.N.

Intramuscular injection

Definition

An intramuscular injection is an injection given directly into the central area of a specific muscle. In this

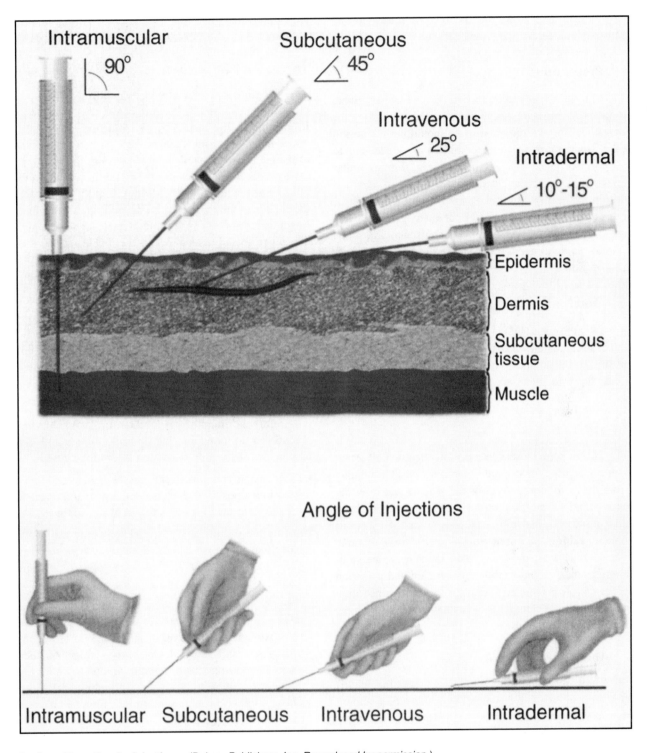

Angles of insertion for injections. *(Delmar Publishers, Inc. Reproduced by permission.)*

way, the **blood vessels** supplying that muscle distribute the injected medication via the **cardiovascular system**.

Purpose

Intramuscular injection is used for the delivery of certain drugs not recommended for other routes of administration, for instance intravenous, oral, or subcutaneous. The intramuscular route offers a faster rate of absorption than the subcutaneous route, and muscle tissue can often hold a larger volume of fluid without discomfort. In contrast, medication injected into muscle tissues is absorbed less rapidly and takes effect more slowly that medication that is injected intravenously. This is favorable for some medications.

Precautions

Careful consideration in deciding which injectable route is to be used for the prescribed medication is essential. The intramuscular route should not be used in cases where muscle size and condition is not adequate to support sufficient uptake of the drug. Intramuscular injection should be avoided if other routes of administration, especially oral, can be used to provide a comparable level of absorption and effect in any given individual's situation and condition. Intramuscular injections should not be given at a site where there is any indication of **pain**.

Description

Intramuscular (IM) injections are given directly into the central area of selected muscles. There are a number of sites on the human body that are suitable for IM injections; however, there are three sites that are most commonly used in this procedure.

Deltoid muscle

The deltoid muscle located laterally on the upper arm can be used for intramuscular injections. Originating from the Acromion process of the scapula and inserting approximately one-third of the way down the humerus, the deltoid muscle can be used readily for IM injections if there is sufficient muscle mass to justify use of this site. The deltoid's close proximity to the radial nerve and radial artery means that careful consideration and palpation of the muscle is required to find a safe site for penetration of the needle. There are various methods for defining the boundaries of this muscle.

Vastus lateralis muscle

The vastus lateralis muscle forms part of the quadriceps muscle group of the upper leg and can be found on the anteriolateral aspect of the thigh. This muscle is more commonly used as the site for IM injections as it is generally thick and well formed in individuals of all ages and is not located close to any major arteries or nerves. It is also readily accessed. The middle third of the muscle is used to define the injection site. This third can be determined by visually dividing the length of the muscle that originates on the greater trochanter of the femur and inserts on the upper border of the patella and tibial tuberosity through the patella ligament into thirds.

Palpation of the muscle is required to determine if sufficient body and mass is present to undertake the procedure.

Gluteus medius muscle

The gluteus medius muscle, which is also known as the ventrogluteal site, is the third commonly used site for IM injections. The correct area for injection can be determined in the following manner. Place the heel of the hand of the greater trochanter of the femur with fingers pointing towards the patient's head. The left hand is used for the right hip and vice versa. While keeping the palm of the hand over the greater trochanter and placing the index finger on the anterior superior iliac spine, stretch the middle finger dorsally palpating for the iliac crest and then press lightly below this point. The triangle formed by the iliac crest, the third finger and index finger forms the area suitable for intramuscular injection.

Determining which site is most appropriate will depend upon the patient's muscle density at each site, the type and nature of medication you wish to administer, and of course the patient's preferred site for injections.

Preparation

Before **administering medication**, a health care practitioner verify the medication order for accuracy and prepare the medication from the vial or ampule.

- First, ensure you have identified the patient and assist them into a position which is comfortable and practical for access to the injection site you have chosen.

- Locate the correct area for injection using the above guidelines or those taught during medical training. Clean the site with an alcohol swab or other cleansing agent.

- Prepare the syringe by removing the needle cover, inverting the syringe, and expelling any excess air. Approximately 0.1–0.2 ml of air should be left in the syringe so that the air in the top of the syringe chamber, when the **syringe and needle** are pointing down, forces the entire amount of medication to be delivered. This also prevents medication residue from being left in the needle, where it can leak into the subcutaneous and dermal layers when the syringe and needle are removed from the muscle.

- When ready to inject, spread the skin using the fingers of the non-dominant hand. Holding the syringe with the thumb and forefinger of the dominant hand, pierce the skin and enter the muscle. This process should be done quickly with sufficient control so as to lessen the discomfort of the patient. If there is little muscle mass, particularly in infants or the elderly, then you may need to pinch the muscle to provide more volume of tissue in which to inject.

- Aspirate at the injection site (while syringe and needle are within the muscle) by holding the barrel of the syringe with the non-dominant hand and pulling back on the syringe plunger with the dominant hand. If **blood** appears in the syringe, it is an indication that a blood vessel may have been punctured. The needle and syringe should be immediately withdrawn and a new injection prepared. If no blood is aspirated, continue by slowly injecting the medication at a constant rate until all medication has been delivered.

- Withdraw the needle and syringe quickly to minimize discomfort. The site may be briefly massaged, depending on the medication given. Some medication manufacturers advise against massaging the site after injection, as it reduces the effect and intention of the medication by dispersing it too readily or over too large an area. Manufacturers' recommendations should be checked.

- Discard the used syringe and needle intact as soon as possible in an appropriate disposal receptacle.

- Check the site at least once more a short time after the injection to ensure that no bleeding, swelling or any other signs of reaction to the medication are present. Monitor the patient for other signs of side effects, especially if it is the first time the patient is receiving the medication.

- Document all injections given and any other relevant information.

Aftercare

Monitor for signs of localized redness, swelling, bleeding, or inflammation at injection site. Observe the patient for at least 15 minutes following the injection for signs of reaction to the drug.

Complications

Most complications of intramuscular injections are a result of the drug injected and not the procedure. However, it is possible that localized trauma of the injection site may result as part of the process. Minor discomfort and pain is common for a short period following the injection, but usually resolves within a few hours.

Results

The optimal outcome is a situation in which the medication is safely and effectively delivered to the patient via intramuscular injection without signs of com-

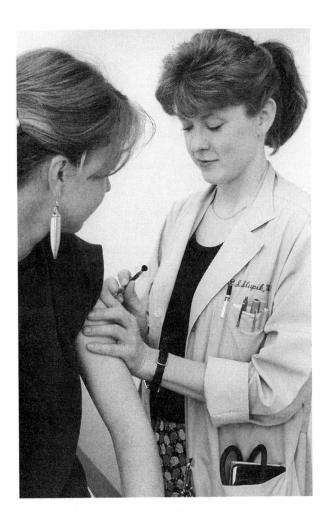

A doctor gives a vaccine by intramuscular injection.
(Custom Medical Stock Photo. Reproduced by permission.)

plications or discomfort. Safety for the health care provider is also paramount.

Health care team roles

The health care provider is obliged to undertake the following when administering an intramuscular injection:

- Inform and educate the patient on the need and effect of the medication being delivered.

- Ensure the correct identification and verification procedures are followed.

- Provide privacy for the patient during the procedure.

- Understand the theory behind selecting appropriate injection sites.

- Demonstrate correct technique when undertaking the procedure.

- Monitor for complications.

- Document all relevant information and ensure safe disposal of equipment.

Resources

BOOKS

Elkin M.K., Perry A.G., and Potter P.A. *Nursing Interventions and Clinical Skills*. Missouri: Mosby-Year Book, Inc., 1996.

Kozier B., et al. *Techniques in Clinical Nursing*. Canada: Addison-Wesley Nursing, 1993.

Dean Andrew Bielanowski, R.N.

Intraoperative care

Definition

The term "intraoperative" refers to the time during surgery. Intraoperative care is patient care during an operation and ancillary to that operation.

Activities such as monitoring the patient's **vital signs**, **blood** oxygenation levels, fluid therapy, medication transfusion, anesthesia, radiography, and retrieving samples for laboratory tests, are examples of intraoperative care. Intraoperative care is provided by nurses, anesthesiologists, nurse anesthetists, surgical technicians, surgeons, and residents, all working as a team.

Purpose

The purpose of intraoperative care is to maintain patient safety and comfort during surgical procedures. Some of the goals of intraoperative care include maintaining homeostasis during the procedure, maintaining strict sterile techniques to decrease the chance of cross-infection, ensuring that the patient is secure on the operating table, and taking measures to prevent hematomas from safety strips or from positioning.

Precautions

Patients undergoing surgery most often are given some type of anesthesia. The administration of **general anesthesia** has a relaxing effect on the patient's body, which can suppress cardiovascular function or heighten cardiovascular irritability. It may also result in respiratory depression, loss of consciousness, **paralysis**, and lack of sensation. These effects, some of which are intentional for the period of the surgery, mean the patient is in a very vulnerable position. It is the responsibility of the health care team in the operating room to maintain the patient's safety and yet facilitate surgery.

In 1992 the American Association of Nurse Anesthetists (AANA) established guidelines for monitoring patients undergoing general anesthesia. The guidelines call for continuous observation of the patient by the nurse assigned to the patient. Ventilation should be assessed by continuous auscultation of breath sounds, and oxygenation should be monitored by continuous pulse oximetry. Continuos electrocardiograph (ECG) showing the patient's cardiac function should be in place, and the patient's **heart** rate and **blood pressure** should be monitored at least every five minutes. A means to monitor the patient's temperature must be available immediately for use. In case of an emergency backup personnel who are experts in **airway management**, emergency intubation, and advanced cardiac life support (ACLS) must be available. An emergency cart containing the necessary supplies and equipment must be immediately accessible. The ACLS equipment should be checked daily to ensure proper function.

Total analgesia is a goal of general anesthesia in order to facilitate surgery. This means that the patient does not have the normal "pain" sensations that warn of potential injury. The health care team must keep this in mind when they are positioning the patient for a surgical procedure. Although it may be necessary for a patient to be positioned in an unusual way for access to a particular area during surgery, care must be taken to ensure that the patient's body is in proper alignment and that joints and muscles are not in such an unnatural position that they will be damaged if they remain in that position for a lengthy procedure. Areas of the operating table that come into contact with the patient's bony prominences must be padded to prevent skin trauma and hematomas.

During a surgical procedure many instruments, drapes, and sponges are used. Also, a multitude of care providers may be working in the operative field performing different tasks. These factors, combined with the complexity and length of some surgical procedures, may provide extensive opportunity for patient trauma from equipment malfunction or the failure of the surgical team to avoid using full weight on the sedated patient. Additionally, it is the responsibility of the nurses working in the operating room to maintain an accurate count of all sponges, instruments, and sharps that may become **foreign bodies** upon incision closure. Nurses who fail to make accurate counts can be held legally liable.

Most surgical procedures are invasive and compromise a patient's skin integrity. This increases the risk of infection. To decrease the risk, strict asepsis (sterile technique) must be followed at all times. It is recommended that the ventilation system in an operative area provide a minimum of fifteen exchanges of filtered air per hour. The temperature in the intraoperative area should be maintained at 68–73°F (20–23°C), and the relative humidity should be maintained at 30%–60%. Health care personnel who work in the operating room must not be permitted to work if they have open lesions on the hands or arms, eye infections, **diarrhea**, or respiratory infections. Scrub attire must be worn by all personnel entering the operating room. Fresh scrub attire must be donned daily and, if heavily soiled during one case, should be changed before the next case. Most facilities provide personnel with scrub attire that is professionally laundered. Shoe covers are required and should be changed often. Head and facial hair must be completely contained in a lint-free cap or hood. Properly fitting disposable surgical masks must be worn at all times and discarded immediately after use. Sterile gloves and sterile gowns must be worn by those working in, and in proximity to, the sterile field. Careful skin preparation with appropriate antiseptic solutions is preformed on the patient's arrival to the operating area.

Patients who have a known or suspected allergy to latex should be scheduled for surgery as the first case of the day whenever possible to avoid contact with airborne latex particles (often attached to powder granules from the gloves) that may be in the room from a previous surgery. These patients should also be identified (some facilities use special colored identification bands and colored tapes on the patient's medical record) so that all health care personnel can recognize them. Special care must be taken to limit the uses of equipment containing latex that will contact the patient's skin. This includes anesthesia masks, adhesive tape and dressings, injections drawn from multidose vials with rubber stoppers, adhesive ground plates for electrocautery or diathermy, and pad coverings on the operating table and arm extensions.

Description

Intraoperative care includes the activities performed by the health care team during surgery that ensure the patient's safety and comfort, implement the surgical procedure, monitor and maintain vital functions, and document care given. The intraoperative time period can vary greatly from less than one hour to 12 hours or more, depending on the complexity of the surgery being performed.

Preparation

Prior to surgery the patient or legal guardian must have the surgical procedure explained to them in great detail, including the expected outcomes and all possible complications, in order to give **informed consent**. The explanation should be given to the patient at a time when he or she is relaxed, but when judgment is not clouded by the use of any **pain** medication or anesthesia, which would invalidate the consent. A consent form must be signed by the patient or guardian and witnessed by a staff member as well as the surgeon performing the procedure. It is the duty of the RN admitting the patient to the surgical suite to check the patient's ID band and ensure that all records are intact and accounted for.

After consent is given the patient may be taken to a holding area where a large-bore intravenous catheter is inserted into the patient's arm for use in fluid replacement and to infuse medications during the procedure. The area of the body where the incision will be made is meticulously prepared using drapes, and a skin preparation that is antiseptic and may include the use of alcohol solutions and iodophor. Monitoring devices such as continuous ECG nodes, pulse oximetry probes, and a blood pressure cuff are usually applied prior to skin preparation. Anesthesia, also, is begun before skin prep. Surgery is then ready to begin.

Aftercare

The time after surgery is referred to as the postoperative period and includes the recovery and convalescence phases. The recovery phase is the time immediately after surgery when the effects of anesthesia are wearing off and the patient is waking up. The convalescence phase is spent either in the hospital, in an interim care facility, or at home—depending on the procedure and the preferences of the physician and patient.

Complications

Intraoperative complications are surgery related, anesthesia related, or position related. One complication occurring during the intraoperative period that is not common but can be life threatening is an anaphylactic (allergic) reaction to anesthesia. The intraoperative staff is trained extensively in the treatment of such a reaction, and emergency equipment should always be available in the event it is needed for this purpose. Another anesthesia-related complication is called "awareness under anesthesia." This occurs when the patient receives sufficient muscle relaxant (paralytic agent) to prohibit voluntary motor function but insufficient sedation and analgesia to block pain and the sense of **hearing**. Patients are aware

KEY TERMS

Anaphylactic reaction (anaphylaxis)—A hypersensitive reaction to an antigen resulting in life-threatening, progressive symptoms.

Anesthesia—A classification of medications that are intended to cause the loss of normal sensation.

Aseptic technique—Strict sterile procedures instilled to decrease the risk of contamination of a surgical site or open wound.

ECG—Abbreviation for electrocardiograph. Electro-cardiograph is a tracing of the electrical activity of the heart obtained through electrodes placed on a person's skin in certain areas where electrical activity can be easily be detected.

Hypovolemic shock—A state of shock caused by the sudden loss of large amounts of blood.

Informed consent—Written or oral permission given by a patient or guardian for medical or surgical treatment after a complete explanation is given and any questions the patient has are answered. If consent is given orally, documentation must have two witnesses.

Intraoperative care—Care provided to a patient during surgery that is ancillary to the surgery.

Malignant hyperthermia—A chain reaction triggered in susceptible people by commonly used general anesthetics. Signs include greatly increased body metabolism, muscle rigidity, and eventual hyperthermia which may exceed 110°F (43.3°C). Death may be caused by cardiac arrest, brain damage, internal hemorrhage, or failure of other body systems.

Pulmonary function tests—Tests used to determine ventilation and perfusion capabilities of the lungs.

Pulse oximetry—A method of measuring a patient's blood oxygenation status. A measure of 100% is optimal.

of being "awake" because they hear the sounds and conversation in the room and, in some cases, can feel the pain associated with the skin incision and surgery. However, they cannot respond to these sensations in a way—not even with so small a motion as blinking the eyelid—that will tell someone what they are sensing. This condition creates an exaggerated fear response that can affect hemodynamics and vital signs. Another com-

plicating reaction may be that of malignant hyperthermia. This is a chain reaction triggered in susceptible people by commonly used general anesthetics. Signs include greatly increased body **metabolism**, muscle rigidity, and eventual hyperthermia which may exceed 110°F (43.3°C). Death may be caused by cardiac arrest, **brain** damage, internal hemorrhage, or failure of other body systems.

Complications of surgery include, but are not limited to, hypovolemic **shock** (due to blood loss during surgery), injuries from poor positioning during surgery, infection of the surgical wound, fluid and electrolyte imbalances, aspiration **pneumonia**, blood clots, and paralytic ileus (paralysis of the intestines, causing distention).

Results

The results of a surgical procedure depend greatly on the procedure preformed, the skill of the surgeon, the general health of the patient preoperatively, and the ability of the patient's body to recover from the procedure. Some surgeries cure a condition (e.g., an appendectomy for an inflamed appendix). Others are only one step in a long process to cure a disease or repair an injury (e.g., discectomy for a patient suffering from back pain). Still others are performed as palliative measures rather than as a cure. An example of palliative surgery would be the removal of a metastatic abdominal tumor to relieve abdominal pressure. In this example removing the abdominal tumor is not going to cure the **cancer** that exists in other parts of the patient's body; it is simply going to relieve the discomfort caused by the abdominal mass.

Health care team roles

Nurses may fill two different roles in the operating room. The scrub nurse is responsible for providing the surgeon with instruments and supplies and maintaining the sterile field. This role also may be assumed by a scrub or surgical technician. The second role nurses have in the operating room is that of circulating nurse. The circulating nurse is first the patient's advocate, with primary concern and responsibility for the patient's safety and welfare. In addition, the circulating nurse is responsible for anything related to the patient that is not directly contingent to the sterile field. That means all activities necessary to prepare the patient and the operative site for surgery, and assistance required by anesthesia personnel. Of crucial import is that the circulating nurse must be certified to give intravenous medication to the patient in case of an emergency. Finally, nurses must document and process tissue specimens for pathology.

Resources

BOOKS

Potter, Patricia A., and Anne G. Perry. *Fundamentals of Nursing Concepts, Process, and Practice.* 4th ed. St. Louis, Missouri: Mosby-Year Book, Inc., 1997.

PERIODICALS

Armstrong, D, and P. Bortz. "An Integrative Review of Pressure Relief in Surgical Patients." *AORN Journal* 73, no. 3 (March 2001): 645-8, 650-3, 656-7.

Byers, P.H., S.G. Carta, and H.N. Mayrovitz. "Pressure Ulcer Research Issues in Surgical Patients." *Advances in Skin Wound Care* 13, no. 3 (May-June 2000): 115-21.

Kleinveck, S.V., and M. McKennett. "Challenges of Measuring Intraoperative Patient Outcomes." *AORN Journal* 72, no. 5 (November 2000): 845-50, 853.

Truell, K.D., P.R. Bakerman, M.F. Teodori, and A. Maze. "Third-Degree Burns Due to Intraoperative Use of a Bair Hugger Warming Device." *Annals of Thoracic Surgery* 69, no. 6 (June 2000): 1933-4.

Wolfson, K.A., L. L. Seeger, B.M. Kadell, and J.J. Eckardt. "Imaging of Surgical Paraphernalia: What Belongs in the Patient and What Does Not." *Radiographics* 20, no. 6 (November-December 2000): 1665-73.

OTHER

Intraoperative Care Website. Jack Stem's Midwest Anesthesia Consultants, 2001. <http://www.jackstem.com/intraoperative_care.htm>.

Perioperative, Intraoperative, Postoperative Care *Infection Control Policy Manual* Henry Ford Health System, 1998. <http://www.hfhsmanuals.com/ICM/Invasive%20Procs/peroperative.htm>.

Jennifer Lee Losey, R.N.

Intravenous fluid regulation

Definition

Intravenous (IV) fluid regulation refers to the manual or automatic pump control of the rate of flow of IV fluids as they are delivered to a patient through a vein.

Purpose

The purpose of intravenous fluid regulation is to control the amount of fluid that a patient is receiving, usually within a given hour of IV therapy. Without fluid regulation, the IV would run in by gravity at a rapid rate and could cause fluid or drug overload.

Precautions

There are varied types of IV administration sets, and they deliver fluid at different amounts per drop. Nurses should always determine the type of drip chamber that they are using and calculate the IV flow per minute based upon the amount of fluid that the administration set delivers per drop.

There are varied types of IV pumps and IV tubing used to deliver IV fluids. Nurses should be sure to use the correct tubing for the pump selected. The specific directions for the use of each individual pump should be followed.

Description

Manual regulation of IV fluids is performed by adjusting the roller adaptor on the IV tubing until it reaches the appropriate drip rate per minute. To manually regulate the IV rate, the nurse looks at her watch and times the number of drops that fall into the drip chamber over one full minute. If the rate is too slow, the adapter should be rolled to a looser position to speed the dripping of the IV. If the rate is too fast, the roller adapter should be tightened to decrease the dripping of the IV. Nurses should adjust the roller until the IV rate is set at the correct amount of drops per minute to deliver the IV fluids as ordered. The IV rate must be checked every hour or more often according to the policy of the medical setting to be certain that the rate remains accurate.

To regulate the IV fluid to be delivered by an IV pump, the tubing should be threaded into the machine correctly. Nurses should dial in the hourly IV rate (cc to be delivered over an hour) and start the pump following the manufacturers guidelines. IVs must be checked hourly when on a pump to be sure that the rate remains accurate and that the correct amount of fluid is delivered. Most pumps have a reading that shows how much fluid has been delivered over the past hour.

Preparation

The physicians order for IV therapy should be reviewed. An IV therapy order will include the type of IV fluid to be delivered over a specific amount of time. Some physicians will order IV therapy in terms of an hourly rate. (Example: Lactated Ringers IV, run at 125 cc/hour.) More commonly the physician will order IV therapy in terms of eight, 12, or 24 hour time periods. (Example: One liter of D5W IV over the next eight hours.)

If the fluid is ordered by the shift (every eight hours) or for a 24-hour period, the first calculation must be to

KEY TERMS

Diaphoresis—Profuse sweating.

Phlebitis—An inflammation of a vein.

Tachycardia—A condition where the heart rate is faster than normal, usually over 100 beats a minute in an adult.

determine how much fluid is ordered per hour. This can be determined by dividing the total amount of fluid by the total time ordered for delivery. For example, if the doctor ordered 1000 cc to be given over eight hours, divide the 1000 cc by the time (eight hours) to obtain the rate per hour. The hourly rate for the IV would be 125 cc for each hour. Another example would be that the doctor orders 3 liters of IV fluid to be given over 24 hours. Divide 3 liters (3000 cc) by the time (24 hours) to obtain the hourly rate of 125 cc per hour. When using an IV pump, the only calculation needed is the rate per hour because IV pumps when set will deliver an hourly rate of IV fluid automatically. The machine does the calculation and drip control. Nurses should be sure to select the specific tubing that the manufacturer recommends for use with each pump.

When not using an automatic IV pump, an administration set should be selected, and the nurse should look on the packaging for the calibration of the drip rate. Standard IV administration sets have a drip factor of 10, 15, or 20 drops/cc. A microdrip or minidrip administration set has a drip factor of 60 drops/cc and is used primarily for low IV rates, such as those used for pediatric clients. The calibration of the administration set must be known in order to calculate the flow of the IV fluids correctly.

The next step is to convert the drops per hour into drops per minute so that the nurse can literally count the drops delivered each minute to set the IV flow. To calculate the drops per minute, the drip factor of the administration set must be used. The nurse should divide the number of ccs to be delivered per hour by the number of minutes in an hour (60) and multiply by the drip factor of the IV administration set to find the drops per minute. For example, if the patient should receive 125 cc per hour using a set that delivers 10 drops/cc, the nurse would multiply the fraction 125/60 times 10 to get a drip rate per minute of 20.8 drops/minute. The number should be rounded to 21 drops per minute. Another example would be if the patient should receive 150 cc per hour using a set that delivers 20 drops/cc, the nurse would multiply the fraction 150/60 times 20 to get a drip rate of 50 drops

per minute. The easiest calculation is using an administration set that delivers 60 drops/cc, because the drops and the minutes cancel each other out. For example, to give 50 cc/hr using a 60 drops/cc administration set, the fraction 50/60 should be multiplied by 60 to get a drip rate per minute of 50. Once the drip rate per minute is determined, the flow of the IV is ready to be regulated according to the doctor's order.

Aftercare

Regulating IV fluid is an ongoing process from the time that an IV is started until it is completed. Hourly checks of an IV should include assessing the client's response to the IV, the rate of the IV flow, how much fluid has infused, how much fluid remains to be infused, and the condition of the IV insertion site. Adjust the rate if the IV is not flowing at the rate that was ordered. If IV fluid is flowing in slowly, the nurse should check for a kink in the tubing or a positional problem. In addition, the IV could be out of the vein, or a small clot, phlebitis, or **infection** at the site could be slowing the IV down. If an IV is flowing too rapidly, it may be leaking out around the IV insertion site or may run faster when the patient extends the extremity. The whole system, from the insertion site to the IV bag, should be examined. The physician will assess IV fluid needs and reorder IV therapy daily according to client needs.

Complications

Circulatory overload can occur if an IV is not regulated and IV fluids infuse too rapidly for the patient's body to handle. Signs of fluid overload include tachycardia, elevated **blood pressure**, headache, **anxiety**, wheezing or other signs of respiratory distress, diaphoresis, restlessness, distended neck veins, or chest **pain**. If these signs occur, slow the IV rate and contact the physician.

Sluggish IV flow or mechanical failure can also occur, which results in the IV fluid not being delivered as ordered. The sign of sluggish IV flow is an IV rate that is persistently behind in spite of constant regulation. Sluggish IV flow can be caused by kinked tubing; small clots, phlebitis, or infection at the site; infiltration of the IV cannula; or a problem with the needle leaning against the wall of the vessel and cutting off IV flow. If the problem is not positional or equipment related, the IV will need to be restarted in a new vein in order to deliver the IV therapy safely and effectively.

Results

IV fluids when regulated to flow according to the physicians orders have positive therapeutic effects such as rehydration, restoration of **electrolyte balance**, restoration of **acid-base balance**, replacement of **vitamins**, **proteins**, and calories, and safe rapid medication administration.

Health care team roles

IV fluid regulation is delegated to registered nurses in most medical settings. Paramedics, LPNs, and IV team technicians who have received special IV training may regulate IV flow rates according to the policies in some medical settings. Patients and their families can be trained to use IV therapy in the home setting. The equipment for home IV therapy, however, will usually include a pump that automatically controls the IV rate. This setting is usually locked so that it cannot be accidentally altered. Patients are taught the signs of complications and learn to trouble-shoot IV alarms. IV nurses visit daily or every few days to change the IV tubing and are on-call to assist the patients and their families 24 hours a day when problems arise.

Resources

BOOKS

"Intravenous Administration." In *Medication Administration. Nurse's Clinical Guide*. Pennsylvania: Springhouse Corporation, 2000.

OTHER

"Basics of IV Therapy." *Baxter Online.* Baxter, Inc. June 1999.
<http://www.baxter.com/doctors/iv_therapies/index.html/>.

"Calculating IV Flow Rates." *Medical CEUs Online.* 2001.
<http://www.medceu.com/tests/ivflow.htm>.

Clark, B., R.N., M.S. and Houser, C. "IV Flow Rates." *Dosage Calculations for Nurses Online.* 2001.
<http://home.sc.rr.com/nurdosagecal/IV%20Flow%20Rates%20and%20Duration.htm/>.

"IV Therapy." Chapter 6. *Lippincott Manual of Nursing Practice*. Books at Ovid Online. 2001.
<http://pco.ovid.com/lrppco/>.

Mary Elizabeth Martelli, R.N., B.S.

Intravenous medication administration

Definition

Intravenous (IV) medication administration refers to the process of giving medication directly into a patient's vein. Methods of administering IV medication may include giving the medication by rapid injection (push) into the vein using a syringe, giving the medication intermittently over a specific amount of time using an IV secondary line, or giving the medication continuously mixed in the main IV solution. IV medications are most often given through a peripheral line or saline IV lock, but may also be administered direct IV, through an implanted vascular access port or through a central line.

Purpose

The primary purpose of giving IV medications is to initiate a rapid systemic response to medication. It is one of the fastest ways to deliver medication. The drug is immediately available to the body. It is easier to control the actual amount of drug delivered to the body by using the IV method and it is also easier to maintain drug levels in the **blood** for therapeutic response. The IV route for medication administration may be used if the medication to be delivered would be destroyed by digestive enzymes, is poorly absorbed by the tissue, or is painful or irritating when given by intra-muscular (IM) or subcutaneous (SQ) injection.

Precautions

Proper IV administration should follow the five "rights" of medication administration to avoid medication errors: be sure it is the right patient, the right drug, the right dose, the right time, and the right route before giving any medication.

The IV line must be intact before any IV medication can be administered. Some IV medications can cause severe tissue damage if injected into the tissue through an infiltrated IV site.

Some IV push medications must be diluted before injection. The health care professional must check the directions for giving the specific drug IV before performing the injection. Administration guidelines for giving IV medications must be followed to avoid serious complications from the drug injection. Most medical settings have an approved IV drug list and instructions for injecting each drug IV. Other resources include the PDR guide, drug administration handbooks, or printed inserts from the pharmaceutical company.

The drug delivery rate is an important factor when administering IV medication. Some IV drugs are meant to be delivered rapidly over several minutes to obtain therapeutic effect. Other drugs are most effective when delivered slowly and intermittently throughout the day. Each drug delivery rate is unique. Administration guide-

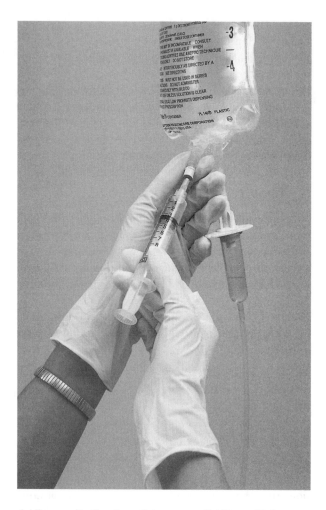

Adding medication to an intravenous fluid bag. *(Delmar Publishers, Inc. Reproduced by permission.)*

lines for giving IV medications must be followed to achieve the therapeutic effect desired.

IV drugs may not be compatible with certain IV fluids or other drugs. Drug incompatibility is a true risk to the patient because it can cause crystallization of the medication that may at the least clog the IV line or at the worst have an embolus effect on the patient. The health care professional must check compatibility warnings that are included in IV drug administration guidelines. The line must be flushed with saline before and after giving medications IV to avoid contact of incompatible solutions or medications.

The effects of medication appear rapidly after an IV injection. The health care professional must know the indications, actions, and adverse effects of the medication that is to be delivered and must observe the patient closely for adverse medication reactions or allergic reactions and be prepared to respond with supportive therapy or drug reversing agents.

Description

IV push medication techniques deliver a bolus (a dose of medication injected all at once intravenously) of medication directly into a vein or access port to produce an immediate peak drug level in the patient's bloodstream. Large quantities of fluid IV push can cause severe complications; follow the recommendations of the drug administration guidelines. To deliver an IV bolus medication, draw the appropriate amount of medication that has been prepared, diluted, and/or reconstituted according to IV drug administration guidelines into a syringe. A bolus injection is most often given through a peripheral IV line, a saline lock, directly into a vein, or through a vascular access port.

When giving an IV bolus medication through a peripheral line with compatible fluid, the health care professional must shut off the IV line using the control clamp. The Y-port closest to the insertion site is cleaned with an alcohol or povidone-iodine pad to prevent bacterial contamination. The health care professional must then connect the medication needle or needle-less system connector to the port. The medication is injected over the period of time ordered, after which the syringe is disconnected and removed. The IV line is reopened using the control clamp and the IV flow is reset to the appropriate setting. If the peripheral line fluid is not compatible with the IV bolus medication, two syringes with 3cc of normal saline are prepared before giving the medication. The line is flushed before and after the IV medication administration with the prepared saline syringes. The Y-port is quite vulnerable to contamination when switching syringes. After the IV line is flushed the second time, the line can be reopened and the IV flow rate reset to the appropriate setting.

A saline (heparin) lock is a peripheral IV device. It is a short IV line that has been locked off to prevent venous fluid from flowing out. It is primarily used to access a vein for intermittent IV drug therapy. A latex cap that can be accessed by a needle or needle-less system connector to deliver drugs or IV fluids intermittently covers the distal tip. When giving an IV bolus medication through a saline lock, prepare two syringes with 3 cc of normal saline as well as the IV bolus medication syringe. (The health care professional should check the medical institution policy because some institutions require the use of heparin to flush IV locks.) The health care professional wipes off the cap of the saline lock with an alcohol or povidone-iodine swab to prevent bacterial contamination. The needle or needle-less system connector is connected to the latex cap of the lock and the patency of the lock is checked by pulling back on the syringe. A flashback of blood into the tubing indicates that the IV

Flow rates for intravenous infusions

Drop factor of tubing (drops/ml)	1000 ml/6 hr (drops/min)	1000 ml/10hr (drops/min)	1000ml/12hr (drops/min)	1000 ml/24hr (drops/min)
10	28	17	14	7
15	42	25	21	10
20	56	34	28	14
60	167	100	84	42

SOURCE: Smith-Temple, J. and J.Y. Johnson. *Nurses' Guide to Clinical Procedures*. 3rd ed. Philadelphia: Lippincott-Raven Pub., 1998.

catheter or needle is in the vein. If no blood appears, a tourniquet is applied above the IV site for about one minute and then the line is aspirated again. Medication should not be given unless the IV is patent (open and unblocked). To continue, the saline is injected into the lock and the insertion site is examined for signs of leaking or puffiness. If the IV lock appears intact, the saline syringe is removed. The medication syringe is connected to the cap using a needle or needle-less connector and the IV push medication is administered over the amount of time that was ordered. The medication syringe is removed and then the second saline syringe is connected to flush the line. Care is taken not to contaminate the cap when switching syringes. Finally the saline syringe is removed and the saline lock apparatus is left well secured to the patient's skin.

In an emergency when a patient has no IV line in and an IV bolus medication needs to be given, the nurse or physician may elect to insert a temporary butterfly IV apparatus connected to a needle. This is not a common situation. In most cases the staff will attempt to insert a regular IV catheter line to enable them to have a stable line for follow-up infusions of medications or fluids. To insert a temporary butterfly IV apparatus, the health care professional washes his/her hands and puts on gloves. A tourniquet is applied and a large vein is selected. The skin over the vein is swabbed with a povidone-iodine swab and the needle is inserted into the skin and then into the vein. When the IV is in place and a blood flashback is visible in the tubing, the tourniquet is removed and the distal end of the line is connected to a syringe of normal saline. The wings of the apparatus are secured with a piece of tape, and the line is aspirated with a syringe to assure proper line placement. If a blood return occurs, the line is slowly injected with 3 cc of normal saline to flush it. The insertion site is checked for puffiness or signs of leakage. Then the saline syringe is removed and rapidly replaced with the medication syringe. The prepared bolus of medication is given over the amount of time ordered. When the medication administration is complete, the syringe is removed and quickly replaced with another 3cc syringe filled with normal saline. The line is flushed

with the saline and the butterfly apparatus is removed from the vein. Pressure is applied to the site using a sterile 2 x 2 gauze pad. This method is not recommended for more than one dose of medication because of the temporary nature of the apparatus. If a patient may require further IV therapy a regular IV catheter should be inserted and connected to an IV line or capped off for use as a saline lock.

IV bolus medication may be given through a vascular access port that has been surgically implanted in the chest. When giving IV medication into an access port follow the procedures for accessing and giving IV medications through the port that are defined by the medical setting. A special needle apparatus is required that will not damage the port or the skin over the port. PICC line and mid-line catheters are not usually used for IV bolus medications because of the length of their tubing. Central lines must be used cautiously when giving IV bolus medication. Since the bolus will be pouring into a large central vein, the effect of the medication will be immediate and can be overwhelming to the patient's body.

IV medication may be given intermittently using a larger amount of fluid to be administered over a longer period of time (such as 50 cc over 20 minutes). Intermittent infusions may be administered through a secondary IV set (piggy back set) using an IV pump or a volume control set using an automatic IV syringe pump. There are many types of tubing and apparatus that can be used to deliver intermittent IV therapy. When administering intermittent IV therapy the instructions as defined on the administration set or in the medical center's IV policies are followed. The basic principles include: ensuring that the IV secondary set (piggy back) is positioned into the correct port on the main IV line and verifying that the pump is set to deliver the IV medication over the correct amount of time that was ordered by the physician. All lines are primed before they are connected to the IV to avoid delivering air through the lines. If the IV medication to be given is not compatible with the IV solution that is hanging, the line is flushed with normal saline before and after running the IV medication. The patient is observed carefully as the medication is delivered for signs of medication reaction or allergic reaction. When the IV medication has run in, the main IV solution is switched back on and the pump is reset for the maintenance rate as ordered by the physician.

Some IV medications, such as potassium chloride, are mixed into the main IV solution bag and run continuously. These medications are injected into the IV bag by the pharmacy or the nurse prior to hanging the IV solution. They run continuously at the rate of flow ordered by the physician.

Preparation

The patient is placed in a comfortable position, the procedure is explained, and the patient is told the name of the drug to be administered. The patient also should be instructed to alert the health care professional immediately if he/she has unusual feelings or discomfort after medication administration. The patency of the IV line is checked to insure that the line is intact and not leaking. The physician's order is reviewed and the five rights of medication administration are checked. The label on the medication is checked to be sure that it is not outdated. (Outdated medication should not be given.) The IV administration guidelines for the specific drug are reviewed, and the health care professional verifies that the drug is approved for IV administration according to the policies of the medical setting. After washing his/her hands, the health care professional calculates and prepares the drug according to drug administration guidelines. Any necessary equipment is assembled and ready access to emergency response equipment (such as contained in a crash cart) is verified.

The health care professional determines the amount of time over which the drug should be delivered according to the physician's order and/or the IV drug administration guidelines. For IV push medications this is calculated in cc to be delivered per minute. This number is calculated by dividing the amount to be delivered (in cc) by the time over which the drug should be delivered (in minutes). For example, if the order is to give 10 mg of drug X over 5 minutes, first determine that 10 mg of drug X comes prepared in 6 cc of liquid. Divide 6 cc by 5 minutes to determine that the rate of IV injection should be 1.2 cc per minute. If the drug must be reconstituted, the rate is calculated using the total amount of drug in cc after reconstitution. For example, give 25 mg of drug Y over 5 minutes. Drug Y is a powder that is reconstituted with 5 cc of sterile water. When reconstituted, the medication has a fluid volume of 6 cc. Divide 6 cc by 5 minutes to determine that the drug should be given at 1.2 cc per minute. Intermittent IV drug doses are usually calculated in cc per hour. They are given in larger amounts of fluid that are usually given with an IV pump and most IV pumps are set in cc per hour, not cc per minute. To calculate the cc per hour rate, the cc per minute rate is multiplied by 60. For example, if the order reads give drug Z in 50 cc of normal saline over 20 minutes, calculate the cc to be delivered per minute by dividing 50 cc by 20 minutes and then multiply times 60 minutes. The rate would be 150 cc per hour to deliver the IV medication in 20 minutes.

Aftercare

After an IV medication has been delivered, the patient is observed for adverse or allergic reactions. Used needles are discarded without recapping them in a puncture proof, contaminated needle container. Used IV tubing, bags, gloves, and disposable supplies are discarded in a plastic bag that can be sealed and discarded in the contaminated trash. The health care professional washes his/her hands and documents that the medication that has been given. If reverting to a primary IV line, the health care professional must be sure to reset the IV flow rate to the correct hourly rate that is ordered for the IV fluids.

Complications

Complications of IV medication administration may include:

- infiltration of the IV line when a drug is injected IV bolus

- tissue necrosis when drugs are injected into infiltrated IV sites

- thrombophlebitis of the vein

- injection of air embolism

- serious adverse drug reactions such as hypotension, cardiac arrhythmias, and cardiac arrest

- allergic reaction to the medication

- venous thrombosis
- pain at the IV site

Results

When administered according to the physicians orders, following drug administration guidelines, and using the correct technique and IV apparatus, IV medications can have immediate positive therapeutic effects. The effects of the medication will vary depending upon the type of medication given.

Health care team roles

IV medication administration is delegated to registered nurses in most medical settings. Paramedics, LPNs, and IV team technicians who have received special IV training may give certain medications IV according to the policies of some medical settings. Patients and their families can be trained to use IV therapy pumps that automatically deliver IV medications in the home setting. IV nurses visit the home daily or every few days to change the medication cartridge and check the status of the IV line. The settings for the IV pump delivering IV medications are usually locked so that they cannot be accidentally altered. Patients are taught the signs of complications and learn to trouble-shoot IV alarms. IV nurses remain on-call to assist the patient and the family 24 hours a day when problems arise.

Resources

BOOKS

"Intravenous Administration." In *Medication Administration: Nurse's Clinical Guide.* Springhouse, PA: Springhouse Corporation, 2000.

OTHER

"Basics of IV Therapy." *Baxter Online,* June 1999. <http://www.baxter.com/doctors/iv_therapies/index.html/>.

Clark, B., and C. Houser. "IV Push." *Dosage Calculations for Nurses Online,* 200l. <http://home.sc.rr.com/nurdosagecal/IV%20Push.htm>.

"IV Therapy." In *Lippincott Manual of Nursing Practice.* Books at Ovid Online, 2001. <http://pco.ovid.com/lrppco/>.

Trimble, Tom. "IV Starts...Improving Your Odds." *Emergency Nursing World Online,* 2001. <http://enw.org/IVStarts.htm>.

Mary Elizabeth Martelli, R.N., B.S.

Intravenous nutrition *see* **Parenteral nutrition**

Intravenous tubing and dressing change

Definition

Intravenous (IV) infusion is the process whereby fluids, medications, **blood** products, and nutritional substances are administered into a vein by means of an intravascular device. The most commonly used device is the short peripheral venous catheter, which is usually inserted into the veins of the forearm or hand. IV fluids are supplied in plastic bags and delivered via an administration set, i.e., tubing. The fluid to be infused and the flow rate are prescribed by a physician or nurse practitioner.

Purpose

IV infusion is a method of fluid replacement used most often to maintain fluid and **electrolyte balance**, or to correct fluid volume deficits after excessive loss of body fluids, or in patients unable to take sufficient volumes by mouth. Many medications are also given by IV infusion and it is used for prolonged nutritional support of patients with gastrointestinal dysfunction.

Precautions

The insertion of an IV access device creates an open wound and the continued presence of the catheter within the wound keeps it "open," which provides easy access for opportunistic **bacteria.** These bacteria may be present on a patient's skin or may come from touch contamination by a practitioner. Technically, the administration of IV solutions takes place within a "closed-system," but the delivery system usually has a number of connections, which may allow entry of bacteria. Strict adherence to handwashing and **aseptic technique** must always be followed while obtaining venous access and the equipment must be handled carefully to prevent contamination. Before using any materials, the practitioner must ensure that all packaging is intact prior to opening, that expiration dates have not passed, and that there are no visible signs of contamination. The site at which a catheter is placed has been shown to influence the subsequent risk of catheter-related infections; and in adults, hand vein insertions have a lower risk of problems than do upper arm or wrist vein insertions. Similarly, there is a greater risk with insertions in the legs than the arms, but the choice of a site may be limited by patient factors, e.g., preexisting catheters, anatomic deformity, present illness, or trauma. The practitioner must also be aware of any patient **allergies** to latex, iodine, or other substances. For

KEY TERMS

Catheter—A hollow tube that is flexible and used for withdraw or introduce fluids into the body.

Dehydration—A condition that results from a loss of water in the body.

Intravascular—Within a vessel, as a blood vessel.

Semipermeable—Permitting passage of only certain molecules.

Peripheral—That portion of the body that is outside the main region, as arms or legs.

Povidone—A synthetic polymer used as a dispersing and suspending agent as in povidone-iodine, a topical anti-infective agent.

selection of catheters, the Centers for Disease Control (CDC) recommend the use of a Teflon catheter, a polyurethane catheter, or a steel needle. The choice depends on the intended purpose, duration of use, and known complications. Transparent, semipermeable, polyurethane dressings reliably secure the site, permit continuous visual inspection of it, allow patients to bathe or shower without saturating the dressing, and require less frequent changes than standard gauze and tape dressings. Research has shown no clinically important differences between the two with regard to rate of **infection** or occurrence of inflammation.

Description

The initial insertion of a catheter with transparent dressing or sterile gauze should be labeled as to the time and date of insertion in an obvious location near the site (e.g. on dressing or on the bed) and the IV administration set should likewise be labeled as to time and date of hanging. CDC recommendations for care and management of peripheral venous catheter sites, IV administration sets, and dressing changes include the following:

- Hands must be washed before and after palpating, inserting, replacing, or changing dressing.

- The catheter site must be visually inspected and palpated for redness, tenderness, or warmth (phlebitis) daily.

- Sites must be replaced and rotated every 48–72 hours to minimize risk of phlebitis. Catheters inserted under emergency conditions must be replaced with new catheters within 24 hours due to possible break-in aseptic technique. Heparin locks must be replaced within 96 hours. Catheters with signs of phlebitis should be removed immediately or as soon as its use is no longer

clinically indicated. Do not routinely apply topical antimicrobial ointment to site.

- When the catheter is removed or replaced, the site dressing should be replaced. The dressing should also be replaced when it becomes damp, loosened, or soiled. Dressings are changed more frequently for patients that sweat. Avoid touching the site when dressing is replaced.

- The IV tubing, including piggyback tubing and stopcocks, is replaced no more frequently than at 72-hour intervals, unless clinically indicated. Tubing used to infuse blood, blood products, or lipid emulsions is replaced within 24 hours of initiation.

- Injection ports are cleaned with 70% alcohol or povidone-iodine before accessing the system. Heparin locks require a routine flush with normal saline solution, unless they are used to obtain blood specimens, in which case a dilute heparin (10 units/ml) flush solution should be used.

Preparation

- All needed materials must be assembled prior to approaching the patient for catheter insertion or IV tubing and dressing change.

- Hands must be washed before and after the procedure.

- The procedure is explained to the patient and he/she is encouraged to ask questions.

- If the patient's veins are difficult to access, warm soaks can be applied to the area prior to attempted insertion to increase blood flow to that area and facilitate the process.

- Nonlatex or latex gloves are worn for insertion of the catheter and for changing the dressing.

- The site or dressing should be marked with labels carrying the date, time, and initials of the individual performing the procedure.

Aftercare

Follow-up care includes:

- The site is inspected and palpated daily.

- IV fluids and additives are monitored to ensure that they are those ordered by the physician or nurse practitioner.

- The infusion rate is checked to make sure that it is correct as ordered.

Complications

The use of IV devices is frequently complicated by a variety of local or systemic infectious complications to include:

• bloodstream infection

• inflammation and/or infection of the lining of the cavities of the heart

• inflammation of the vein sometimes associated with a clot

• infections in other areas of the body

The risk of complications in IV therapy is actually higher on the second day of therapy and was believed to increase with time, which made routine restarts after three days a common practice. Recent research has shown, however, that a restarted catheter has a significantly higher risk of complication in its first 24 hours than does an initial catheter. Thus, restarting catheters routinely at 72 hours does not reduce the risk of complication in the next 24 hours when compared to simply continuing therapy with the original catheter, provided the site or the original has no signs of inflammation. Once additional studies confirm these data, the recommendations may change.

Results

The results obtained from IV therapy should primarily serve to improve the condition of the patient. A dehydrated patient's fluid volume and electrolyte balance should improve. Any patient ill from an infection should feel improved with IV antibiotic therapy. The purpose of an IV is to alleviate symptoms and assist with enhancing well-being.

Health care team roles

The **registered nurse** is the primary provider of IV catheter insertion, IV fluids, tubing, and dressings. It is the role of this nurse to ensure that the recommended procedures, protocols, and written orders for IV therapy are followed. It is also the duty of the nurse to maintain her skills for IV therapy and keep updated on any changes in recommendations in providing care. Available data suggest that personnel specially trained or designated with the responsibility for insertion and maintenance of IV devices provide a service that reduces the rate of infections and overall costs.

Resources

BOOKS

Hankins, J., et al., eds. *Infusion Therapy in Clinical Practice.* Fort Worth, TX: Harcourt Health Sciences Publishers, 2001.

PERIODICALS

Holmes, K. R., and L. D. Homer, "Risks Associated with 72–96-hour Peripheral Intravenous Catheter Dwell Times." *Nursing* 21 (September/October 1998).

ORGANIZATIONS

Infusion Nurses Society, 220 Norwood Park Rd., Norwood, MA 02062. (781) 440-9408. <http://www.ins1.org>.

League of Intravenous Therapy Education, Empire Building, Suite 3, 3001 Jacks Run Road, White Oak, PA 15131. (412) 678-5025. <http://www.lite.org>.

OTHER

Pearson, Michele L., and the Hospital Infection Control Practices Advisory Committee. "Guidelines for Prevention of Intravascular Device-related Infections." Centers for Disease Control, April 1995. <http://www.cdc.gov/ncidod/hip/iv/iv.htm>.

Linda K. Bennington, CNS

▌Intravenous urography

Definition

Intravenous urography is a radiographic study of the **urinary system** using an intravenous contrast agent (dye).

Of the many ways to obtain images of the urinary system, the intravenous injection of a contrast agent has been traditionally considered the best, although other modalities, such as computed tomography (CT) or ultrasound, are better for some disease processes. The **kidneys** excrete the contrast into the urine, which becomes visible when x rayed (radiopaque), creating images of the urinary collection system.

The procedure has several variations and many names, including:

• Intravenous pyelography (IVP).

• Intravenous urography (IVU).

• Pyelography.

• Antegrade pyelography differentiates this procedure from retrograde pyelography, which injects the contrast agent directly into the lower end of the system. The contrast agent flows backward, hence the name "retrograde." Retrograde pyelography is used to better define problems in the lower ureters and is the only way to get x rays if the kidneys are non-functional.

• Nephrotomography, or tomographic slices of the kidneys, is taken by a moving x-ray source emitting x rays onto a film moving in the opposite direction. Images above and below the level of the kidneys are blurred, allowing a more detailed image of the kidneys with no overlying material, such as gas or fecal material.

There are numerous exams available for detecting kidney abnormalities, with varying risks and costs.

• Nuclear renal scans rely on the radiation given off by certain atoms (isotopes), which are injected into the bloodstream. They reach the kidneys, where images are constructed by measuring the radiation emitted. The radiation is no more dangerous than standard x rays. This exam has limited applications, including the evaluation of reflux, chronic obstruction, and renal function. It is also used to evaluate high **blood pressure** that is refractory to treatment, and is commonly used to evaluate the kidney of a renal transplant patient for early rejection where renal artery stenosis is suspected as the cause.

• Ultrasound is a quick, safe, simple, and inexpensive way to obtain views of internal organs. Renal size can be measured as well as the visualization of hydronephrosis, cysts, tumors, and renal calculi. Small stones in the ureters are not as well visualized and the function of the kidneys can not be determined.

• Retrograde pyelography is better able to define problems in the lower part of the ureters, and is the only way to completely opacify the ureters in patients with reduced kidney function. This exam is performed in an operating room by a urologist. A cystoscope is placed into the bladder and a catheter is placed into each ureter to inject the contrast agent. The advantage of this method is that small stones can be removed immediately by the urologist.

• Computed tomography scans (CT or CAT scans) use a fine beam of x rays creating images at precise levels in the body. The information is processed by a computer and imaged onto film with a laser printer. Three-dimensional images can be constructed from this method of imaging. An injection of a contrast agent is necessary to visualize the kidneys in detail. The CT scan is done without IV contrast to look for stones (calculi). In some centers, this modality has replaced IVPs and ultrasound for this application. Special equipment is necessary and the exam can be costly.

• Magnetic resonance imaging (MRI) uses magnetic fields and radio frequency signals instead of ionizing radiation to create computerized images. This form of energy is entirely safe as long as the patient has no metal in his or her body. It has limited applications and usually is not done for common problems, such as **pain** and hematuria (**blood** in the urine). MRI usually is done if other tests are inconclusive. MRA (magnetic resonance **angiography**) may be done to evaluate the renal arteries, particularly is renal artery stenosis is suspected as a cause of **hypertension** that is refractory to treatment. MRI requires special apparatus and installation and is a very costly exam.

Purpose

An intravenous urogram is ordered to demonstrate the structure and function of the kidneys, ureters, and bladder. Patients complaining of abdominal pain radiating to the back may require this exam to rule out **kidney stones**. Hematuria may also be an indication of kidney stones, **infection**, or tumors. Patients with high blood pressure (hypertension) and recurrent bladder infections may also require an intravenous urogram (but hypertension usually is imaged with MRA or nuclear medicine imagery and this exam is done when renal artery stenosis is the suspected cause of refractory hypertension). Sometimes the exam is ordered to evaluate the function of the kidney in a renal transplant patient. The transplanted kidney is located in the iliac fossa, so special films of the pelvis area are done instead of the normal routine views. The radiographic technologist may also be required to take x rays in the operating room when a retrograde pyelogram is ordered by a urologist during a C and P (**cystoscopy** and pyelography).

Emergency patients with blunt abdominal trauma are usually evaluated with a CT scan or occasionally ultrasound instead of an intravenous urogram.

Precautions

A serious complication of an intravenous urogram is an allergic reaction to the iodine-containing contrast agent. Severe reactions are rare, but can be dramatic and even lethal. For this reason all radiology departments performing this exam are equipped with emergency drugs and oxygen in the x-ray room itself.

Description

The patient will be required to change into a hospital gown and empty his or her bladder. The x-ray technologist will verify that the patient has followed the bowel preparation and complete a detailed questionnaire on the current medical history of the patient. This includes previous contrast reactions, known **allergies**, risks of **pregnancy**, and current medications. The x-ray technologist will explain the exam in detail to the patient as well as the risks of the contrast material that will be injected intravenously. All departments require that the patient sign a consent form before the examination is started. The x-ray technologist will relay this information to the radiologist who will decide on what type of contrast will be used. Patients who have had an injection with no reaction can be given less expensive iodine-based contrast, whereas patients who take various **heart** medications or those with known allergies or **asthma** will be injected with a more expensive contrast agent (known as non-ionic contrast) that has fewer side effects. Some departments use the non-ionic contrast exclusively.

The patient will be instructed to lie supine (face-up) on the x-ray table and a preliminary KUB will be done. This is an abdominal view of the kidneys, ureter, and bladder used to verify patient preparation, centering, and the radiographic technique needed to demonstrate all the required structures.

Kidney stones may or may not be visualized on the preliminary film. The x-ray technologist prepares the required amount of contrast to be used depending on the weight of the patient (1 ml per pound). This is normally 50–75 cc of contrast for an average-sized patient. The contrast will be injected all at once (bolus injection) or in some cases, through an intravenous drip. Some radiologists prefer to start an intravenous drip with saline as a precautionary measure while others inject with a small butterfly needle. The needle usually remains in place for 10–15 minutes, in case more contrast is needed or in case drugs need to be administered because of an allergic reaction. Most reactions occur immediately but some can take place 10 or 15 minutes after the injection.

The first film is taken immediately after the injection to see a detail of the renal outline (nephrogram). Films are usually taken at five-minute intervals depending on the routine of the radiologist. Compression may be applied to the lower abdomen with a wide band to keep the contrast material in the kidneys longer. This creates a more detailed image of the renal collecting system. When the compression is released after approximately 10 minutes the contrast material drains quickly and a detailed, filled image of the ureters is obtained. Films done in the upright or prone (face-down) position may also be ordered to better visualize the lower ureters. Some departments require routine renal tomographic images to be done as well when the kidneys are well visualized. This allows the kidneys to be seen free of gas or fecal shadows. Sometimes the radiologist requires oblique views of the kidneys or bladder to determine the exact location of calculi (stones). At approximately 20 minutes after the injection a film centered on the bladder may be

required. The x-ray tube is angled slightly caudad (towards the feet) so that there is no superimposition of the pubic area of the pelvis over the bladder. The films are shown to the radiologist and if no further films are necessary the patient will be asked to void (urinate) and a post-void film will be taken. The exam can take from 30 minutes to one hour depending on the number of films required. If the kidney is obstructed, delayed films may be required to complete the exam.

Preparation

In order to obtain the best visualization of the kidneys, ureters, and bladder, the intestines must be free of gas and fecal material. Every radiology department has their own specific requirements. Most include a laxative such as X-Prep or Dulcolax tablets taken around 4 p.m. the day preceeding the exam. This is followed with a light fat-free dinner which includes lean meats, noodles, white rice, bread with no butter, and tea or black coffee. Fluids are permitted until midnight, after which no food or liquid is allowed until after the intravenous urogram is completed. Patients who are diabetic are sometimes done early in the morning to avoid any complications. Patients who have had a previous reaction to a contrast material can be given a series of steroids and **antihistamines** the day before the exam as well as the morning of the exam. The patient must consult with their physician before this is administered. In patients with known or suspected renal failure, lab tests, including BUN and creatinine, may be ordered prior to the IVP.

Complications

An allergic reaction to the contrast agent is the primary risk, although kidney damage is also a potential complication. Patients with a possible iodine allergy or a previous reaction to a radiographic contrast agent should inform the x-ray technologist. A detailed history of known allergies, risk of pregnancy, and current medications is required before an intravenous urogram. All radiology departments have consent forms that must be signed by the patient before starting the exam. Emergency equipment and specific drugs such as antihistamines (Benadryl), adrenaline, and atropine are kept in the x-ray room. All radiography technologists must have specific training and education on the various signs and symptoms of an allergic reaction. A mild reaction consists of a skin rash or **hives**, whereas a more serious reaction includes swelling of the larynx, difficulties in breathing, asthmatic attacks, and a severe drop in blood pressure (hypotension).

Since x-rays are involved during this procedure, there is a minimal risk due to radiation. This exam is not done on pregnant women or women who think they may be pregnant.

Results

A normal intravenous urogram indicates no visible abnormality in the structure or function of the urinary system. The radiologist looks for a smooth non-lobulated outline of each kidney, no clubbing or other abnormality of the renal calyces (collecting system), and no abnormal fluid collection in the kidneys that could suggest obstruction. The ureters must contain no filling defects (stones) or deviations due to an adjacent tumor. The bladder must have a smooth outline and empty normally as visualized on the post-void film.

Abnormal results include hydronephrosis (distension of the renal pelvis and calices due to obstruction) as a result of tumors or calculi (stones). Cysts or abscesses may also be present in the urinary system. A delay in renal function can also indicate renal disease. An abnormal amount of urine in the bladder after voiding may indicate prostate or bladder problems.

Intravenous urograms are often done on children to rule out a rapid developing tumor in the kidneys, called a Wilm's tumor. Children are also prone to infections of the bladder and kidneys due to urinary reflux (return backflow of urine).

Health care team roles

The x-ray technologist must work in conjunction with the doctors and nurses in making sure the patient has not had a previous allergic reaction to a contrast agent. All hospitals have an emergency team ready to react in such a situation, so the technologist must be aware of the procedure to follow when assistance is necessary due to a severe reaction. Details of patient preparation must also be communicated to the hospital wards. In some hospitals the radiologic technologists are trained to give injections, but if this is not the case nurses may be asked to install an intravenous drip before the patient is brought to the radiology department.

Patient education

The x-ray technologist must explain the risks of an allergic reaction to each patient even though severe reactions are extremely rare due to the advances made in the preparation of contrast agents. The x-ray technologist explains to the patient that a warm, flushed feeling or a metallic **taste** in the mouth are normal reactions in some patients. Breathing instructions are also important since the kidneys change position depending on the phase of respiration and to prevent motion artifacts. Sometimes an emergency patient with renal colic (acute abdominal pain) is asked to urinate through a special filter used to trap small stones. All radiographic technologists must be certified and registered with the American Society of Radiologic Technologists or an equivalent organization. Continued education credits are mandatory to remain registered.

Resources

BOOKS

Ballinger, Frank, et al.. *Merrill's Atlas of Radiographic Positioning.* 9th ed. St. Louis, MO: Mosby, 1999.

Schull, Patricia, ed. *Illustrated Guide to Diagnostic Tests.* 2nd ed. Springhouse, PA: Springhouse Corporation, 1998.

Lorraine K. Ehresman

Iodine *see* **Antiseptics**

Iodine deficiency *see* **Mineral deficiency**

Iodine uptake test *see* **Thyroid radionuclide scan**

Ipecac

Description

There are two categories of ipecac preparations—a syrup used in standard medical practice and a homeopathic remedy. They are given for different purposes. The medicinal effects of ipecac were recognized centuries ago by the Portuguese who settled in South America. They found a plant that can make people vomit and appropriately named it *Caephalis ipecacuanha*, meaning sick-making plant. Nowadays, ipecac is used to treat a variety of conditions. Its most widely accepted use is to induce vomiting in cases of accidental **poisoning**. When ipecac is swallowed, a substance in it called cephaeline irritates the **stomach** and causes vomiting. Syrup of ipecac is now considered the safest drug to treat poisoning and is often the most effective. There are different types of ipecac preparations that vary greatly in strength. Syrup of ipecac is best for use at home to treat accidental poisoning. Ipecac fluid extract and ipecac tincture should be avoided as they are much stronger compounds and can be toxic.

Ipecacuanha is a homeopathic remedy made from ipecac by a process of dilution and succussion (shaking). In contrast to syrup of ipecac, it is given to relieve vomiting.

General use

Treatment of poisoning

Standard medical practice uses ipecac to cause vomiting in cases of poisoning in order to remove the toxic substance from the stomach before absorption occurs. It can be used on animals as well as humans. Ipecac is safer and more effective than many other methods for inducing vomiting, such as sticking a finger down a child's throat or using salt water. There are times, however, when ipecac should not be used because it can make certain kinds of poisoning worse. Syrup of ipecac should not be used if the poison is one of the following.

• strychnine

• alkalis (lye)

• strong acids

• kerosene

• fuel oil

• gasoline

• coal oil

• paint thinner

• cleaning fluid

Poisoning is a potentially serious condition. It is best to contact a local poison control center, local hospital emergency room, or the family doctor for instructions before using syrup of ipecac.

Ipecac's reputation for inducing vomiting has encouraged some bulimics to take it on a regular basis in order to purge the contents of the stomach after an eating binge. This misuse of ipecac is extremely dangerous; it can cause **heart** problems, tears in the esophagus or stomach lining, vomiting **blood**, seizures, or even death.

Homeopathy

The homeopathic remedy made from ipecac is called *Ipecacuanha*. Homeopathic preparations are given for a reason completely opposite from that of standard allopathic treatment. In **homeopathy**, ipecac is given to stop

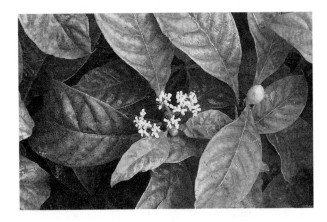

Ipecac plant *(Cephaelis ipecacuanha).* (PlantaPhile Germany. Reproduced by permission.)

vomiting rather than to induce it. According to Hahnemann's law of similars, a substance that would cause vomiting in large doses when given to a healthy person will stimulate a sick person's natural defenses when given in extremely dilute and carefully prepared doses. *Ipecacuanha* is a favorite homeopathic remedy for morning sickness associated with **pregnancy**. It is also given to stop nausea that is not relieved by vomiting; when the vomitus is slimy and white; when there is gagging and heavy salivation; when the tongue is clean despite the patient's feelings of nausea; and when the patient is not thirsty. The nausea may be accompanied by a headache, cough, or heavy menstrual bleeding. The modalities (circumstances) that suggest *Ipecacuanha* as the appropriate homeopathic remedy is that the patient feels worse lying down; in dry weather; in winter; and when exercising or moving about.

A homeopathic practitioner would not necessarily prescribe ipecac for all cases of nausea. *Arsenicum* would be given when the nausea is caused by **food poisoning** and accompanied by strong thirst, *Nux vomica* when the nausea is the result of overindulgence in food or alcohol and accompanied by gas or heartburn. A sick child might be given *Pulsatilla*, particularly if rich foods have been eaten.

On the other hand, a homeopathic practitioner may prescribe ipecac for any of the following conditions that are not related to nausea and vomiting:

• Nosebleeds producing bright red blood.

• Dental bleeding.

• Diarrhea with cramping abdominal **pain**. The stools are green with froth or foam.

KEY TERMS

Bulimia nervosa—An eating disorder characterized by episodic binge eating followed by self-induced vomiting or laxative abuse.

Cephaeline—A chemical compound found in ipecac that irritates the stomach lining and triggers the vomiting reflex.

Fluid extract—A concentrated preparation of a drug.

Law of similars—A principle of homeopathic treatment according to which substances that cause specific symptoms in healthy people are given to sick people with similar symptoms.

Modality—A factor or circumstance that makes a patient's symptoms better or worse. Modalities include such factors as time of day, room temperature, the patient's level of activity, sleep patterns, etc.

Tincture—An alcoholic solution of a chemical or drug.

- Asthma of sudden onset. The patient has to sit up in order to breathe, but cannot bring up any mucus in spite of violent coughing.

- Hoarseness or loss of voice following a cold.

- Physical or mental exhaustion.

Preparations

Syrup of ipecac

Syrup of ipecac is made from the dried roots and rhizomes (underground stems) of *Cephaelis ipecacuanha*. It is available over the counter in 0.5–1 oz bottles. Larger bottles require a doctor's prescription. The dosage for infants under 6 months old should be prescribed by the family doctor or poison control center. For children six months to one year, the usual dose is 5–10 ml or 1–2 tsp. One-half or one full glass (4–8 oz) of water should be taken immediately before or after the dose. The dose may be repeated once after 20–30 minutes if vomiting does not occur. For children one to 12 years of age, the usual dose is 15 ml (1 tbsp) to be taken with one full glass (8 oz) of water. Adults and teenagers should take 15–30 ml of ipecac with at least 1 full glass of water. Syrup of ipecac should not be taken with milk or soda drinks as these foods may prevent it from working properly. If vomiting does not occur within 20–30 minutes after the

first dose, a second dose may be needed. If the second dose fails to induce vomiting, the patient should be taken to a hospital emergency room.

If both activated charcoal and syrup of ipecac are recommended to treat poison, ipecac must be used first. Activated charcoal should not be taken until 30 minutes after taking syrup of ipecac, or until the vomiting caused by ipecac stops.

Homeopathic preparations

Ipecacuanha is available as an over-the-counter remedy in 30x potency. This is a decimal potency, which means that one part of ipecac has been mixed with nine parts of alcohol or water; 30x means that this decimal dilution has been repeated 30 times. The dilute solution of ipecac is then added to sugar tablets so that the remedy can be taken in tablet form.

Precautions

Syrup of ipecac

For inducing vomiting in cases of accidental poisoning, only the syrup form of ipecac should be used. Syrup of ipecac should not be mixed with milk or carbonated drinks as they may prevent vomiting.

Syrup of ipecac should not be used in the following situations (contact poison control center or family doctor for alternative treatments):

- Poisoning caused by strychnine; sustained-release theophylline; such corrosive substances as strong alkalis (lye); strong acids (such as toilet bowl cleaner); and such petroleum products as kerosene, gasoline, coal oil, fuel oil, paint thinner, or cleaning fluids.

- Overdoses of medications given for depression.

- Excessive vomiting.

- A serious heart condition.

- Timing. Do not give ipecac more than 4–6 hours after the poison was ingested.

- Pregnancy.

- Very young children (less than six months old). Infants and very young children may choke on their own vomit or get vomit into their lungs.

- Drowsy or unconscious patients.

- Seizures.

Homeopathic preparations

Ipecacuanha should not be given after *Arsenicum* or *Tabac* because these remedies will counteract it.

Side effects

The following side effects have been associated with the use of syrup of ipecac.

- Loose bowel movements.

- Diarrhea.

- Fast irregular heartbeat.

- Inhaling or choking on vomit.

- Stomach cramps or pains.

- Coughing.

- Weakness.

- Aching.

- Muscle stiffness.

- Severe heart problems often occur in cases of ipecac abuse. Because ipecac stays in the body for a long time, damage to the heart frequently occurs in persons who repeatedly take ipecac to induce vomiting.

- Seizures. These are most likely to occur in patients who accidentally swallow ipecac or in ipecac abusers.

- Death. Deaths have been reported due to ipecac abuse in bulimic persons.

Homeopathic *Ipecacuanha* has been highly diluted and is relatively nontoxic.

Interactions

Ipecac should not be given together with other drugs because it can decrease their effectiveness and increase their toxicity. If both syrup of ipecac and activated charcoal are needed to treat suspected poisons, ipecac should be given first. Activated charcoal should not be given until vomiting induced by ipecac has stopped. Soda pop should also be avoided because it can cause the stomach to swell. The person should lie on the stomach or side in case vomiting occurs.

Homeopathic *Ipecacuanha* is considered complementary to *Arnica* and *Cuprum*. It is counteracted by *Arsenicum* and *Tabac*.

Resources

BOOKS

Cummings, Stephen, MD, and Dana Ullman, MPH. *Everybody's Guide to Homeopathic Medicines*. New York: G. P. Putnam's Sons, 1991.

Ellenhorn's Medical Toxicology, 2nd ed. Baltimore: Williams & Wilkins, 1997.

Hammond, Christopher. *The Complete Family Guide to Homeopathy: An Illustrated Encyclopedia of Safe and Effective Remedies*. New York: Penguin Studio, 1995.

PDR Nurse's Drug Handbook. Montvale, NJ: Delmar Publishers, 2000.

ORGANIZATIONS

American Foundation for Homeopathy. 1508 S. Garfield. Alhambra, CA 91801.

Homeopathic Educational Services. 2124B Kittredge St. Berkeley, CA 94704. (510) 649-0294. Fax: (510) 649-1955.

Mai Tran

Iron-binding capacity test *see* **Iron tests**

Iron

Description

Iron is a mineral that the human body uses to produce the red **blood** cells (hemoglobin) that carry oxygen throughout the body. It is also stored in myoglobin, an oxygen-carrying protein in the muscles that fuels cell growth.

General use

Iron is abundant in red meats, vegetables, and other foods, and a well-balanced diet can usually provide an adequate supply of the mineral. But when there is insufficient iron from dietary sources, or as a result of blood loss in the body, the amount of hemoglobin in the bloodstream is reduced and oxygen cannot be efficiently transported to tissues and organs throughout the body. The resulting condition is known as iron-deficiency anemia, and is characterized by fatigue, shortness of breath, pale skin, concentration problems, dizziness, a weakened **immune system**, and energy loss.

Iron-deficiency anemia can be caused by a number of factors, including poor diet, heavy menstrual cycles, **pregnancy**, kidney disease, **burns**, and gastrointestinal disorders. Individuals with iron-deficiency anemia should always undergo a thorough evaluation by a physician to determine the cause.

Children two years old and under also need adequate iron in their diets to promote proper mental and physical development. Children under two who are not breastfeeding should eat iron-fortified formulas and cereals. Women who breastfeed need at least 15 mg of dietary or supplementary iron a day in order to pass along adequate amounts of the mineral to their child in breast milk. Parents should consult a pediatrician or other healthcare

KEY TERMS

Chelation—The use of a medication or herbal substances to inactivate toxic substances in the body. Chelation is used to treat iron overload in some patients.

Decoction—An herbal extract produced by mixing an herb in cold water, bringing the mixture to a boil, and letting it simmer to evaporate the excess water. The decoction is then strained and consumed hot or cold. Decoctions are usually chosen over infusion when the botanical in question is a root or berry.

Ferritin—An iron storage protein found in the blood. High levels of serum ferritin may indicate iron overload.

Hemochromatosis—Also known as iron overload; a genetic condition in which excess iron is stored in the tissues and organs by the body where it can build up to toxic amounts.

Homeopathic remedy—Used to treat illnesses that manifest symptoms similar to those that the remedy itself causes, but administered in extremely diluted doses to prevent any toxic effects.

Infusion—An herbal preparation made by mixing boiling water with an herb, letting the brew steep for 10 minutes, and then straining the herb out of the mixture. Tea is made through infusion.

Thalassemia—A group of several genetic blood diseases characterized by absent or decreased production of normal hemoglobin. Individuals who have thalassemia have to undergo frequent blood transfusions, and are at risk for iron overload.

Tincture—A liquid extract of an herb prepared by steeping the herb in an alcohol and water mixture.

professional for guidance on iron supplementation in children.

It has been theorized that excess stored iron can lead to atherosclerosis and ischemic **heart** disease. Phlebotomy, or blood removal, has been used to reduce stored iron in patients with iron overload with some success. Iron chelation with drugs such as desferrioxamine (Desferal) that help patients excrete excess stores of iron can be helpful in treating iron overload caused by multiple blood transfusions.

Iron levels in the body are measured by both hemoglobin and serum ferritin blood tests.

Normal total hemoglobin levels are:

- neonates: 17-22 g/dl
- one week: 15-20 g/dl
- one month: 11-15 g/dl
- children: 11-13 g/dl
- adult males: 14-18 g/dl (12.4-14.9 g/dl after age 50)
- adult females: 12-16 g/dl (11.7-13.8 g/dl after menopause)

Normal serum ferritin levels are:

- neonates: 25-200 ng/ml
- one month: 200-600 ng/ml
- two to five months: 50-200 ng/ml
- six months to 15 years: 7-140 ng/ml
- adult males: 20-300 ng/ml
- adult females: 20-120 ng/ml

Preparations

Iron can be found in a number of dietary sources, including:

- pumpkin seeds
- dried fruits (apricots)
- lean meats (beef and liver)
- fortified cereals
- turkey (dark meat)
- green vegetables (spinach, kale, and broccoli)
- beans, peas, and lentils
- enriched and whole grain breads
- molasses
- sea vegetables (blue-green algae and kelp)

Eating iron-rich foods in conjunction with foods rich in **vitamin C** (such as citrus fruits) and lactic acid (sauerkraut and yogurt) can increase absorption of dietary iron. Cooking food in cast-iron pots can also add to their iron content.

The recommended dietary allowances (RDA) of iron as outlined by the United States Department of Agriculture (USDA) are as follows:

- children 0–3: 6-10 mg/day
- children 4–10: 10 mg/day
- adolescent and adult males: 10 mg/day
- adolescent and adult females: 10-15 mg/day

- pregnant females: 30 mg/day
- breastfeeding females: 15 mg/day

A number of herbal remedies contain iron, and can be useful as a natural supplement. The juice of the herb stinging nettle (*Urtica dioica*) is rich in both iron and vitamin C (which is thought to promote the absorption of iron). It can be taken daily as a dietary supplement. Dandelion (*Taraxacum officinale*), curled dock (*Rumex crispus*), and parsley (*Petroselinum crispum*) also have high iron content, and can be prepared in tea or syrup form.

In Chinese medicine, dang gui (dong quai), or *Angelica sinensis*, the root of the angelica plant, is said to both stimulate the circulatory system and aid the **digestive system**. It can be administered as a decoction or tincture, and should be taken in conjunction with an iron-rich diet. Other Chinese remedies include foxglove root (*Rehmannia glutinosa*), Korean ginseng (*Panax ginseng*), and astragalus (*Astragalus membranaceus*).

Ferrum phosphoricum (iron phosphate), is used in homeopathic medicine to treat anemia. The remedy is produced by mixing iron sulfate, phosphate, and sodium acetate, which is administered in a highly diluted form to the patient. Other homeopathic remedies for anemia include *Natrum muriaticum*, *Chinchona officinalis*, *Cyclamen europaeum*, *Ferrum metallicum*, and *Manganum aceticum*. As with all homeopathic remedies, the type of remedy prescribed for iron deficiency depends on the individual's overall symptom picture, mood, and temperament. Patients should speak with their homeopathic professional or physician, or healthcare professional before taking any of these remedies.

Iron is also available in a number of over-the-counter supplements (i.e., ferrous fumerate, ferrous sulfate, ferrous gluconate, iron dextran). Both heme iron and non-heme iron supplements are available. Heme iron is more efficiently absorbed by the body, but non-heme iron can also be effective if used in conjunction with vitamin C and other dietary sources of heme iron. Some multivitamins also contain supplementary iron. Ingesting excessive iron can be toxic, and may have long-term negative effects. For this reason, iron supplements should only be taken under the recommendation and supervision of a doctor.

Precautions

Iron deficiency can be a sign of a more serious problem, such as internal bleeding. Anyone suffering from iron-deficiency anemia should always undergo a thorough evaluation by a healthcare professional to determine the cause.

Iron **overdose** in children can be fatal, and is a leading cause of **poisoning** in children. Children should never take supplements intended for adults, and should only receive iron supplementation under the guidance of a physician.

Individuals with chronic or acute health conditions, including kidney **infection**, **alcoholism**, liver disease, rheumatoid arthritis, **asthma**, heart disease, colitis, and **stomach** ulcer should consult a physician before taking herbal or pharmaceutical iron supplements.

If individuals taking homeopathic dilutions of *Ferrum phosphoricum* experience worsening of their symptoms (known as a homeopathic aggravation), they should stop taking the remedy and contact their healthcare professional. A homeopathic aggravation can be an early indication that a remedy is working properly, but it can also be a sign that a different remedy is needed.

Patients diagnosed with hemochromatosis, a genetic condition in which the body absorbs too much iron and stores the excess in organs and tissues, should never take iron supplements.

Side effects

Taking herbal or pharmaceutical iron supplements on an empty stomach may cause nausea. Iron supplementation may cause hard, dark stools, and individuals who take iron frequently experience constipation. Patients who experience dark bowel movements accompanied by stomach pains should check with their doctor, as this can also indicate bleeding in the digestive tract.

Other reported side effects include stomach cramps and chest **pain**. These symptoms should be evaluated by a physician if they occur.

Some iron supplements, particularly those taken in liquid form, may stain the teeth. Taking these through a straw, or with a dropper placed towards the back of the throat, may be helpful in preventing staining. Toothpaste containing baking soda and/or hydrogen peroxide can be useful in removing iron stains from teeth.

Signs of iron overdose include severe vomiting, racing heart, bloody **diarrhea**, stomach cramps, bluish lips and fingernails, pale skin, and weakness. If overdose is suspected, the patient should contact poison control and/or seek emergency medical attention immediately.

Interactions

Iron supplements may react with certain medications, including **antacids**, acetohydroxamic (Lithostat), Dimercaprol, Etidronate, Fluoroquinolones. In addition, they can decrease the effectiveness of certain tetracy-clines (**antibiotics**). Individuals taking these or any other medications should consult their healthcare professional before starting iron supplements.

Certain foods decrease the absorption of iron, including some soy-based foods, foods with large concentrations of **calcium**, and beverages containing **caffeine** and tannin (a substance found in black tea). These should not be taken within two hours of using an iron supplement. Some herbs also contain tannic acid, and should be avoided during treatment with iron supplements. These include allspice (*Pimenta dioica*) and bayberry (*Myrica cerifera*, also called wax myrtle).

Individuals considering treatment with homeopathic remedies should also consult their healthcare professional about possible interactions with certain foods, beverages, prescription medications, aromatic compounds, and other environmental elements—factors known in **homeopathy** as remedy antidotes—that could counteract the efficacy of treatment for iron deficiency.

Resources

BOOKS

Medical Economics Company. *PDR for Herbal Medicines.* Montvale, NJ: Medical Economics Company, 1998.

Medical Economics Company. *PDR 2000 Physicians' Desk Reference.* Montvale, NJ: Medical Economics Company, 1998.

Ody, Penelope. *The Complete Medicinal Herbal.* New York: DK Publishing, 1993.

PERIODICALS

de Valk, B. and J.J.M. Marx. "Iron, Atherosclerosis, and Ischemic Heart Disease." *Archives of Internal Medicine* 159, no. 14: 1542.

Paula Ford-Martin

Iron deficiency anemia

Definition

Anemia can be caused by **iron** deficiency, folate deficiency, **vitamin B$_{12}$** deficiency, and other causes. Iron deficiency anemia is due to a shortage of iron. It is characterized by the production of red **blood** cells that are smaller than normal (microcytic) and appear pale or light colored (hypochromic) when viewed under a **microscope**. For this reason, the anemia that occurs with iron deficiency is also called hypochromic microcytic anemia.

Description

Iron deficiency anemia is the most common type of anemia throughout the world. In the United States, iron deficiency anemia occurs to a lesser extent than in developing countries because of the higher consumption of red meat and the practice of food fortification (addition of iron to foods by manufacturers). In the United States, iron deficiency anemia is caused by a variety of factors, including excessive losses of iron in menstrual fluids and excessive bleeding into the gastrointestinal tract. In developing countries located in tropical climates, the most common cause of iron deficiency anemia is infestation with hookworm.

Causes and symptoms

Infancy is a period of increased risk for iron deficiency. A human infant is born with a built-in supply of iron, which can be tapped during periods of drinking low-iron milk or formula. Both human milk and cow milk contain rather low levels of iron (0.5-1.0 mg iron/liter). However, about 50% of the iron in human milk is absorbed by an infant, while only 10% of the iron in cow milk is absorbed. During the first six months of life, growth of an infant is made possible by milk in the diet and by the infant's built-in supply. **Premature infants** have a lower supply of iron. For this reason, it is recommended that pre-term infants (beginning at two months of age) be given oral supplements of 7 mg iron/day, in the form of ferrous sulfate. Iron deficiency can develop when infants are fed formulas that are based on cow milk that has not been fortified. For example, unfortified cow milk is given free of charge to mothers in Chile. This practice prevents general malnutrition, but results in the development of mild iron deficiency.

The normal rate of blood loss in the feces is 0.5-1.0 ml per day. About 60% of persons with **cancer** of the colon and rectum experience further blood loss in the range of 10 ml/day, which can lead to iron deficiency anemia. The **fecal occult blood test** is widely used to screen for the presence of cancer of the colon or rectum. In the absence of testing, **colorectal cancer** may be first detected because of the resulting iron deficiency anemia.

Infection with hookworm can also cause iron deficiency anemia. The hookworm is a parasite that thrives in warm climates, including in the southern United States. A hookworm enters the body through the skin, very commonly through bare feet. The hookworm then migrates to the small intestines where it attaches itself to the villi (small, finger-like structures found on the walls of the intestines, which are used for the absorption of nutrients). Hookworms damage the villi, resulting in blood loss. Further, they produce anticoagulants which promote continued bleeding. Each hookworm can cause the loss of up to 0.25 ml of blood per day.

Bleeding and blood loss through the gastrointestinal tract can also be caused by hemorrhoids, anal fissures, irritable bowel syndrome, aspirin-induced bleeding, blood clotting disorders, and diverticulosis (a condition caused by an abnormal opening from the intestine). Several genetic diseases are characterized by **bleeding disorders**. These include **hemophilia** A, hemophilia B, and von Willebrand's disease. Of these, only von Willebrand's disease leads to gastrointestinal bleeding.

The symptoms of iron deficiency anemia include weakness and fatigue. These symptoms result from the lack of function of red blood cells, and the reduced ability of red blood cells to carry iron to exercising muscles. Iron deficiency can also affect other tissues, including the tongue and fingernails. Prolonged iron deficiency can result in changes of the tongue, which may become smooth, shiny, and reddened, a condition known as glossitis. Fingernails may grow abnormally and acquire a spoon-shaped appearance.

Decreased iron intake is a contributing factor in iron deficiency and the resulting iron deficiency anemia. The iron content of some common foods is:

• whole wheat bread (43 mg/kg)

• spinach (33 mg/kg)

• beef (28 mg/kg)

• raisins (20 mg/kg)

• eggs (20 mg/kg)

• lima beans (15 mg/kg)

• potatoes (14 mg/kg)

• canned tuna (13 mg/kg)

• chicken (11 mg/kg)

• peanut butter (6.0 mg/kg)

• tomatoes (3.0 mg/kg)

• cabbage (1.6 mg/kg)

• apples (1.5 mg/kg)

• corn oil (0.6 mg/kg)

It is readily apparent that apples, tomatoes, and corn oil are relatively low in iron, while whole wheat bread, spinach, and beef are relatively high in iron. The assessment of whether a food is low or high in iron can also be made by comparing the amount of that food eaten per day with the recommended dietary allowance (RDA) for iron. The RDA for iron for an adult male is 10 mg/day, while that for an adult woman is 15 mg/day. The RDA during pregnancy is 30 mg/day. The RDA for infants of 0-0.5 years of age is 6 mg/day, while that for infants of 0.5-1.0 year of age is 10 mg/day. RDA values are based on the assumption that a person eats a mixture of plant and animal foods.

The above list of iron values alone may be deceptive, because bioavailability varies. Bioavailability means the percent of iron in the food that is absorbed via the gastrointestinal tract to the bloodstream. Non-absorbed iron is lost in the feces. The bioavailability of iron in fruits, vegetables, and grains is very low, but is much higher in meats. The bioavailability of iron in plants ranges from only 1-10%, while that in meat, fish, chicken, and liver is 20-30%. The most readily absorbable source of iron is human milk, which has a 50% bioavailability.

Interactions between various foods also influence the absorption of dietary iron. **Vitamin C**, for example, increases the absorption of dietary iron. Thus, if rice is consumed with a vitamin C-rich food such as orange juice, then the absorption of the rice's iron is enhanced. The increased use of formulas fortified with both iron and vitamin C has led to a marked reduction in anemia in infants and young children in the United States. In contrast, if rice is consumed with tea, certain chemicals (tannins) in the tea reduce the absorption of iron. Another potent inhibitor of iron absorption is phytic acid, a chemical that occurs naturally in legumes, cereals, and nuts.

Diagnosis

Iron deficiency anemia in infants is defined as a hemoglobin level below 109 mg/ml of whole blood, and a **hematocrit** of under 33%. Anemia in adult males is defined as hemoglobin under 130 mg/ml and a hematocrit of under 38%. Anemia in adult females is defined as hemoglobin under 120 mg/ml and a hematocrit of under 32%. Anemia in pregnant women is defined as hemoglobin of under 110 mg/ml and a hematocrit of under 31%.

When an abnormally high presence of blood is found in feces during a fecal occult blood test, a physician needs to examine the gastrointestinal tract to determine the cause or source of bleeding. For this, a sigmoidoscope may be used. This is an instrument that consists of a flexible tube with a light at the end and allows an examiner to directly visualize and examine the interior of the large bowel or colon to a distance of 60 cm from the anus. A **barium enema**, with an x ray, may also be used to detect abnormalities that can cause bleeding.

KEY TERMS

Barium—An element used in liquid suspension with radiography (x rays) due to its high contrast with human tissue.

Diverticulitis—A disease caused by abnormal outpocketings in the walls of the intestines.

Ferrous—A form of iron that has two electrons available for chemical reactions and is readily absorbed by humans; ferrous iron is also referred to as reduced.

Gastroenterology—The study of the structures of the gastrointestinal tract, commonly including the stomach, small intestines and large intestines.

Glossitis—A condition of the tongue in which the tongue becomes red, smooth, and shiny.

Hematocrit—The proportion of whole blood in the body, by volume, that is composed of red blood cells.

Heme—A protein comprising most of the mass of red blood cells that transports oxygen and carbon dioxide.

Hemoglobin—An iron-containing protein within red blood cells. Hemoglobin accounts for about 95% of the protein in the red blood cell.

Hypochromic—Having less than normal color.

Microcytic—Cells that are smaller than normal size.

Occult—Hidden or difficult to observe.

Protoporphyrin IX—A protein. Measuring proporphyrin IX is useful to assess iron status. Hemoglobin consists of a complex of a protein plus heme. Heme consists of iron plus protoporphyrin IX. Normally during the course of red blood cell formation, protoporphyrin IX acquires iron to generate heme. Protoporphyrin IX builds up to abnormally high levels when iron is deficient.

Recommended Dietary Allowance (RDA)—Quantities of nutrients in the diet that are required to maintain human health. RDAs are established by the Food and Nutrition Board of the National Academy of Sciences and may be revised every few years.

Villi—Small, finger-like structures found on the walls of the intestines that are used for the absorption of nutrients.

If evidence suggests that oral iron supplements are failng in treating anemia, a test for oral iron absorption is indicated. The oral iron absorption test is conducted by ingesting 64 mg iron (325 mg ferrous sulfate) in a single dose. Blood samples are then taken after two hours and four hours. The iron content of the person's serum is then measured. If iron absorption is normal, the concentration of iron should rise by an increment of about 22 micromoles. Smaller increases in concentration mean that iron absorption is abnormal, and that therapy should involve injections or infusions of iron.

Treatment

Oral iron supplements (pills) may contain various chemical compounds containing iron, often called iron salts. Iron salts include ferrous sulfate, ferrous gluconate, or ferrous fumarate. Injections and infusions of iron can be given using a preparation called iron dextran. In patients with poor gastrointestinal absorption of iron, therapy with injection or infusion is preferable over oral supplements. Treatment of iron deficiency anemia sometimes requires more than therapy with iron. If iron deficiency is due to bleeding from hemorrhoids, surgical correction of the hemorrhoids may be essential to prevent recurrent iron deficiency anemia. If iron deficiency is caused by bleeding due to aspirin treatment, aspirin should be discontinued. If iron deficiency is due to hookworm infestations, therapy for this parasite should be given in conjunction with protection of feet by wearing shoes whenever walking in areas that are potentially infested with hookworms.

Prognosis

The prognosis for treating and curing iron deficiency anemia is excellent. One important issue, however, is failure to take iron supplements. Pregnant women may be advised to take 100-200 mg iron/day, a dose that leads to nausea, **diarrhea**, or abdominal **pain** in 10-20% of women. Such a high dosage is recommended to rapidly cure the anemia during pregnancy. Before conception, problems associated with side effects and nonadherence may be avoided by taking iron doses (100-200 mg) only once a week. This can be continued throughout a woman's fertile period. The problem of adherence is not an issue when infusions are used, although a fraction of persons treated with iron infusions experience flushing, headache, nausea, seizures, or **anaphylaxis**.

A number of studies have shown that iron deficiency anemia in infancy can result in reduced intelligence in early childhood. It is not clear whether iron supplementation given to children with reduced intelligence due to iron-deficiency anemia in infancy has any influence in allowing a "catch-up" in intellectual development.

Health care team roles

Screening for iron deficiency anemia is commonly conducted by nurses and physicians. However, when professionally-trained personnel are not available, other people may be given specific training to administer the screening test. Laboratory technicians process blood samples collected by screening tests. Physicians and nurses administer iron injections or intravenous infusions. Surgeons or physicians trained in gastroentnerology perform gastroscopic examinations. Radiologists interpret the results of x rays taken after infusion of a barium enema.

Prevention

In a healthy population, all mineral deficiencies can be prevented by ingesting inorganic nutrients at levels defined by the RDA. Iron deficiency anemia in infants and young children can be prevented by consuming fortified foods. Cow milk-based infant formulas are generally supplemented with iron (12 mg/L). The iron in liquid formulas is added as ferrous sulfate or ferrous gluconate. Commercial infant cereals are also fortified with iron. In addition, small particles of elemental iron may be added to the cereal. The levels used are about 0.5 gram iron/kg dry cereal, an amount about 10-fold greater than what is naturally present.

Resources

BOOKS

Hazelwood, Loren F. *Can't Live Without It: The Story of Hemoglobin in Sickness and in Health.* Huntington, NY, Nova Science Publishers, 2001.

Hillman, Robert S. "Iron Deficiency and Other Hypoproliferative Anemias." In *Harrison's Principles of Internal Medicine*, edited by Anthony S. Fauci. New York: McGraw Hill, 1998.

Ramakrishnan, U. *Nutritional Anemias.* Boca Raton, FL: Lewis Publishers, 2000.

Uthman, Ed. *Understanding Anemias.* Jackson, MS: University Press of Mississippi, 1998.

PERIODICALS

Abelson, HT. "Complexities in recognizing and treating iron deficiency anemia." *Archives of Pediatric and Adolescent Medicine*, 155(3):332-333, 2001.

Anonymous. "Iron deficiency anemia: reexamining the nature and magnitude of the public health problem." *Journal of Nutrition* 131(2S-2):563S-703S, 2001.

Couper, R.T. and K.N. Simmer. "Iron deficiency in children: food for thought." *Medical Journal of Australia* 174(4):162-163, 2001.

Jolobe, O. "Guidelines for the management of iron deficiency anemia." *Gut* 48(2):283-284, 2001.

ORGANIZATIONS

American Academy of Family Physicians, 11400 Tomahawk Creek Parkway, Leawood, KS 66211-2672. (913) 906-6000. <http://www.aafp.org/>. fp@aafp.org.

American Academy of Pediatrics, 141 Northwest Point Boulevard, Elk Grove Village, IL 60007-1098. (847) 434-4000. Fax (847) 434-8000. <http://www.aap.org/default.htm>. kidsdoc@aap.org.

American Association for Clinical Chemistry, 2101 L Street, NW - Suite 202, Washington, D.C. 20037-1558. (800) 892-1400 or (202) 857-0717. Fax: (202) 887-5093. <http://www.aacc.org>. info@aacc.org.

American Society of Hematology, 1900 M Street NW, Suite 200, Washington, D.C. 20036. (202) 776-0544. Fax: (202) 776-0545. <http://www.hematology.org/>. ash@hematology.org.

OTHER

Centers for Disease Control and Prevention. <http://www.cdc.gov/epo/mmwr/preview/mmwrhtml/000 51880.htm>.

Columbia Presbyterian Medical Center. <http://cpmcnet.columbia.edu/texts/gcps/gcps0032.html>.

Oregon Health Sciences University. <http://www.ohsu.edu/som-hemonc/handouts/deloughery/fe.shtml>.

University of Virginia Health Sciences College. <http://hsc.virginia.edu/medicine/clinical/pathology/educ/innes/text/rcd/iron.html>.

L. Fleming Fallon, Jr., MD, PhD, DrPH

▌Iron tests

Definition

Iron tests consist of four assays performed on serum or plasma to aid in the diagnosis and treatment of iron deficiency or iron overload. These tests are serum iron, total iron binding capacity (TIBC), serum ferritin, and serum transferrin. Iron is an essential trace element needed for the production of hemoglobin as well as the function of cytochromes (compound molecules that are important in cell respiration) and certain enzymes. Iron in plasma is almost entirely bound to transport **proteins**. The total iron binding capacity (TIBC) is the maximum amount of iron that these proteins can bind. Transferrin, a beta globulin (molecular weight 75,000) is the principal transport protein for iron in plasma. Therefore, the TIBC is determined mainly by the concentration of serum transferrin. Iron is stored in the epithelial cells of the gastrointestinal tract and in the reticuloendothelial cells of the **liver**, spleen, and bone marrow. Ferritin is the principal form of storage iron. It consists of a protein (apoferritin) and iron in the form of ferric salts.

Purpose

Serum or plasma iron tests are used for the following purposes:

- To help in the differential diagnosis of **anemias**. **Iron deficiency anemia** is the most common form of anemia worldwide and is quite common in the United States—especially in multiparous females, young children, and persons with chronic intestinal bleeding.

- To assess the severity of anemia and monitor the treatment of patients with chronic anemia.

- To diagnose conditions of iron excess, including iron ingestion, thalassemia, hemosiderosis, and hemochromatosis. Hemosiderosis and hemochromatosis are conditions produced by excessive iron stores in the tissues. Hemosiderosis, which results from repeated **blood** transfusions, is not associated with tissue damage. Hemochromatosis, which is a disorder of iron absorption, can cause painful joints, skin bronzing, diabetes, and liver damage if the iron concentration in the body is not lowered. Hemachromatosis is still underdiagnosed because of its long latency period and lack of awareness on the part of medical professionals.

A serum iron test can be used without the others to evaluate cases of iron **poisoning**.

Precautions

Collection of blood samples

Patients should not have their blood tested for iron within four days of a blood transfusion or tests and treatments that use radioactive materials. Recent high **stress** levels or sleep deprivation are additional reasons for postponing iron tests. Clinicians should ask if patients are taking oral contraceptives or multivitamins, since these may alter results.

Blood samples for iron tests should be taken early in the morning because serum iron levels vary during the day, being higher in the morning and lower at night. This precaution is especially important in evaluating the results of iron replacement therapy.

Hemolysis must be avoided during collection of blood samples to prevent interference with test results from iron in the red blood cells.

Interpretation of test results

Some acute and chronic illnesses can increase the release of ferritin from the body stores, resulting in high serum levels. These disorders include infections, late-stage cancers, lymphomas, and severe inflammations. Alcoholics often have high ferritin levels owing to liver inflammation.

Medications and substances that can cause *increased* serum iron levels include chloramphenicol, estrogen preparations, dietary iron supplements, alcoholic beverages, methyldopa, and birth control pills. Medications that can cause *decreased* iron levels include aspirin, cholestyramine, cortisone, methicillin, and testosterone.

Medications and treatments that can cause *increased* ferritin levels include dietary iron supplements, oral contraceptives, theophylline, and x-ray therapy. Decreases in ferritin levels are seen with antithyroid therapy and high doses of ascorbic acid.

Medications that can cause *increased* transferrin levels include cortisone and cortisol. Those that can cause *decreased* transferrin levels include oral contraceptives and carbamazepine.

Description

Iron tests are performed on samples of the patient's blood, withdrawn from a vein into a vacuum tube. The amount of blood taken is between 6 mL and 10 mL (1/3 of a fluid ounce). The procedure, which is called a venipuncture, takes about five minutes.

Iron level test

The iron level test measures the amount of iron in the blood serum that is being carried by a protein (transferrin) in the blood plasma. Serum iron is most often measured by colorimetric analysis. Iron is deconjugated from the transferrin by adding dilute acid or guinidinium. The iron is reduced to Fe^{2+} by ascorbic acid. The reduced iron forms coordinate bonds with the nitrogen groups (a chromophore) forming a colored complex. The most common chromophore is FerroZine which reacts with Fe^{2+} to form a magenta-colored complex that is measured at 570 nm. Thiourea is added to prevent a reaction between FerroZine and **copper**.

Total iron-binding capacity (TIBC) test

The TIBC test measures the amount of iron that the blood would carry if the transferrin were fully saturated. Since transferrin is produced by the liver, the TIBC can be used to monitor liver function and **nutrition**.

Transferrin test

The transferrin test is a direct measurement of transferrin—which is also called siderophilin—levels in the blood. Transferrin is most often measured by rate immunophelometry. Some laboratories prefer this measurement to the TIBC. The saturation level of the transferrin can be calculated by dividing the serum iron level by the TIBC.

Ferritin test

The ferritin test measures the level of a protein in the blood that stores iron for later use by the body. Ferritin is most often measured by double antibody sandwich immunoassay. It is the most sensitive indicator of iron deficiency because a low serum level reflects depleted body stores. The body stores must be fully depleted before the serum iron becomes low or iron deficiency anemia develops. In persons with acute and chronic illness, however, ferritin levels may not reflect the status of the iron stores since more ferritin escapes into the circulation in these conditions.

Preparation

Iron absorption and **metabolism** are influenced by several factors. These should be identified prior to testing via a medical history that includes the following:

- prescription medications and multivitamins that affect iron levels, absorption, or storage
- blood transfusion within the last four days
- recent extreme stress or sleep deprivation
- recent eating habits

Blood collected for iron level or TIBC tests should be collected following a 12-hour fast. Fasting is not required for serum or plasma ferritin.

Aftercare

Aftercare consists of routine care of the area around the venipuncture.

Complications

The primary complication is the possibility of a bruise or swelling in the area of the venipuncture. The patient can apply moist warm compresses if there is any discomfort.

Results

Iron level test

Normal serum iron values are as follows:

- Adult males: 65-175 micrograms/dL.
- Adult females: 50-170 micrograms/dL.
- Children: 50-120 micrograms/dL.
- Infant: 40-100 micrograms/dL.
- Newborns: 100-250 micrograms/dL.

TIBC test

Normal TIBC values are as follows:

- Adult males: 300-400 micrograms/dL.
- Adult females: 300-450 micrograms/dL.

Transferrin test

Normal transferrin values are as follows:

- Adults: 200-400 mg/dL.
- Children: 203-360 mg/dL.
- Newborns: 130-275 mg/dL.

Normal transferrin saturation values are between 30% and 40%.

Ferritin test

Normal ferritin values are as follows:

- Adult males: 20-300 ng/mL.
- Adult females: 20-120 ng/mL.
- Children (one month): 200-600 ng/mL.
- Children (two to five months): 50-200 ng/mL.
- Children (six months to 15 years): 7-140 ng/mL.
- Newborns: 25-200 ng/mL.

Abnormal test results

Serum iron level is *increased* in thalassemia, hemochromatosis, severe hepatitis, liver disease, lead poisoning, acute leukemia, and kidney disease. It is also increased by multiple blood transfusions and intramuscular iron injections.

KEY TERMS

Anemia—A disorder marked by low hemoglobin levels in red blood cells, which leads to a decrease in the oxygen carrying capacity of the blood.

Chromophore—Any chemical group that produces color in a compound.

Cytochrome—A compound molecule consisting of a protein and a porphyrin ring. Cytochromes participate in cell respiration by electron transfer.

Ferritin—A protein found in the liver, spleen, and bone marrow that stores iron. Ferritin consists of a protein called apoferritin and iron in the form of ferric salts.

Hemochromatosis—A disorder of iron absorption characterized by increased iron absorption and excess deposition of iron in the tissues. It can cause painful joints, pancreatic, heart and liver damage if the iron concentration is not lowered.

Hemolysis—The breakdown of red blood cells with liberation of hemoglobin.

Hemosiderosis—An overload of iron in the body resulting from repeated blood transfusions. Hemosiderosis occurs most often in patients with thalassemia.

Iron poisoning—A potentially fatal condition caused by swallowing large amounts of iron dietary supplements. Most cases occur in children who have taken adult-strength iron formulas. The symptoms of iron poisoning include vomiting, bloody diarrhea, convulsions, low blood pressure, and turning blue.

Plasma—The liquid part of blood.

Siderophilin—Another name for transferrin.

Thalassemia—A hereditary form of anemia that occurs most frequently in people of Mediterranean origin.

Transferrin—A protein in the plasma that carries iron derived from food intake to the liver, spleen, and bone marrow.

Iron levels above 350-500 micrograms/dL are considered toxic; levels over 1000 micrograms/dL indicate severe iron poisoning.

Serum iron level is *decreased* in iron deficiency anemia, chronic blood loss, chronic diseases (lupus, rheumatoid arthritis), late **pregnancy**, chronically heavy menstrual periods, and thyroid deficiency.

Abnormal TIBC test

The TIBC is *increased* in iron deficiency anemia, polycythemia vera, pregnancy, blood loss, severe hepatitis, and the use of birth control pills.

The TIBC is *decreased* in malnutrition, severe **burns**, hemochromatosis, anemia caused by infections and chronic diseases, cirrhosis of the liver, and kidney disease.

Abnormal transferrin test

Transferrin is *increased* in iron deficiency anemia, pregnancy, hormone replacement therapy (HRT), and the use of birth control pills.

Transferrin is *decreased* in protein deficiency, liver damage, malnutrition, severe burns, kidney disease, chronic infections, and certain genetic disorders.

Abnormal ferritin test

Ferritin is *increased* in liver disease, iron overload from hemochromatosis, certain types of anemia, acute leukemia, Hodgkin's disease, **breast cancer**, thalassemia, infections, inflammatory diseases, and hemosiderosis. Ferritin levels may be normal or slightly above normal in patients with kidney disease.

Ferritin is *decreased* in chronic iron deficiency and severe protein depletion.

Health care team roles

Iron tests may be ordered by physicians or by nurse practitioners. Blood samples are usually drawn by nurses or phlebotomists. The samples are analyzed in the laboratory by medical laboratory technicians, with the results returned to the physician.

Patient education

Patients should be informed of any abnormal test results. Health care professionals may refer patients with iron deficiency to a dietitian to discuss nutrition therapy. With regard to excessive iron storage, all health care professionals should monitor patients for signs of hemochromatosis, which is easily treated but fatal if untreated.

Resources

BOOKS

Burtis, Carl A., and Edward R. Ashwood. *Teitz Textbook of Clinical Chemistry,* 3rd ed. Washington, DC: American Association of Clinical Chemistry (AACC) Press, 1999.

Fischbach, Frances Talaska. *A Manual of Laboratory and Diagnostic Tests.* Philadelphia and New York: Lippincott, 1996.

Mosby's Diagnostic and Laboratory Test Reference, 5th ed., edited by Kathleen Deska Pagana and Timothy James Pagana. St. Louis, MO: Mosby-Year Book, Inc., 2000.

Springhouse Corporation. *Everything You Need to Know About Medical Tests,* edited by Michael Shaw et al. Springhouse, PA: Springhouse Corporation, 1996.

PERIODICALS

Powell, Lawrie W., MD, et al. "Diagnosis of Hemachromatosis." *Annals of Internal Medicine* 129 (December 1, 1998): 925-931.

Jane E. Phillips

Irregular bite *see* **Malocclusion**

IV fluid regulation *see* **Intravenous fluid regulation**

IV medication administration *see* **Intravenous medication administration**

IV tubing and dressing change *see* **Intravenous tubing and dressing change**

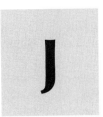

Jaundice

Definition

Jaundice is a condition in which the patient has a yellow hue because of high **blood** levels of bilirubin, a breakdown product of hemoglobin that is potentially toxic. The yellow discoloration is most noticeable in the skin, the sclera (whites of the eyes), and the inner surface of the eyelids.

Description

Jaundice is a physical sign or finding, not a disease. Many different diseases or conditions may cause a person's bilirubin level to be elevated. Most important to the understanding of causes of this sign is a good explanation of normal **liver** function with regard to the production and excretion of bile. Bile is a fluid excreted by the liver that aids in digestion and absorption of **fats**.

The liver is a large, solid organ in the right upper quadrant of the abdomen. It is the premier "chemical processing plant" in the body; most incoming and outgoing chemicals pass through it. It is the first stop for all nutrients, toxins, and drugs absorbed by the digestive tract. The liver also collects waste products from the blood for disposal. Many of these outward-bound chemicals (including bilirubin) are excreted into the bile.

Bile is made up of water; chemicals that act as detergents; and substances such as glycogen, bilirubin, cholesterol, and other byproducts of hepatic **metabolism**. It is formed by cellular metabolism and passes into the network of hepatic bile ducts, which join to form the common duct. A branch of this tube carries bile to the **gallbladder**, where it is stored and concentrated. When fats enter the **stomach**, the gallbladder secretes bile into the common bile duct. Before the common bile duct reaches the duodenum, it is joined by another duct from the **pancreas**. The bile and the pancreatic juice are triggered to enter the intestine through a valve called the ampulla of Vater by the presence of partially digested fats in the duodenum. After entering the intestine, the bile and pancreatic secretions together help to complete the process of digestion.

The liver removes toxins from the bloodstream, including bilirubin. Bilirubin is a potentially toxic waste product from the breakdown of hemoglobin, the oxygen-carrying molecule of red blood cells (RBCs). When bilirubin is first released from old RBCs or other sources, it cannot be dissolved in water. The liver changes it so that it is soluble in water. These two forms are called unconjugated (insoluble) and conjugated (soluble) bilirubin. Because of the type of laboratory test performed on the different forms of this molecule, unconjugated bilirubin is also called indirect bilirubin, and conjugated bilirubin is called direct bilirubin. Bilirubin is a bright yellow pigment and gives bile its characteristic color. If bilirubin cannot be cleared from the body in a timely fashion, it leaks into body tissues and stains them yellow temporarily, resulting in jaundice. The normal level of bilirubin in blood serum is between 0.2 mg/dL and 1.2 mg/dL. When it rises to 3 mg/dL or higher, jaundice becomes evident. "Icteric" is an adjective (based on the Greek word for jaundice) used to describe a jaundiced patient.

Causes and symptoms

There are many different causes of jaundice, but they can be divided into three categories: before, during, or after the liver has performed its task of making bilirubin soluble. These categories can also be called prehepatic, hepatic, and posthepatic causes of jaundice.

Prehepatic causes of jaundice

There are many different prehepatic causes of jaundice. When old RBCs die, hemoglobin is released into the bloodstream. When the rate of formation of new RBCs and the rate of loss of old RBCs are well balanced, the normal liver can keep pace with disposal of used hemoglobin. If the body is having difficulty making

RBCs (due to mineral or vitamin deficiencies), hemoglobin may leak into circulation and overwhelm the liver. Conversely, if RBCs are destroyed rapidly, the liver may also be overwhelmed. Disorders that cause RBCs to disintegrate prematurely are called hemolytic disorders.

One cause of hemolysis (or prematurely destroyed RBCs) to be aware of starts at the neonatal point, in babies born of Rh-negative mothers. Other causes include a long list of drugs, among them rifampin, methyldopa, certain **antibiotics**, quinine, and levodopa. Trauma can also destroy RBCs. Some common causes of trauma include surgery for mechanical **heart** valves, implants, and roughened surfaces of **blood vessels** such as occur in microangiopathic hemolytic anemia. The parasite that causes **malaria** develops inside red blood cells and ruptures the RBCs when it is mature. A number of hereditary defects affect red blood cells, including glucose-6-phosphate dehydrogenase (G6PD) deficiency (in which RBCs disintegrate under certain stresses, particularly when exposed to certain drugs), sickle-cell disease (in which the structure of hemoglobin is abnormal), and spherocytosis (in which a protein in the outer membrane of the RBC causes weakness in the membrane).

An enlarged spleen can also cause hemolysis. The spleen is the reservoir organ, located near the upper end of the stomach, that filters the blood. It is supposed to filter out and destroy only worn-out RBCs. If it becomes enlarged, it filters out normal cells as well. A wide variety of conditions, including many causes of hemolysis listed above, can enlarge the spleen to the point where it removes too many red blood cells. Also, in several types of **cancer** (such as chronic leukemia) and immune-system diseases, antibodies are produced that react with RBCs and destroy them. In addition, if a patient is given an incompatible blood type, it sets off an immune reaction, and hemolysis results.

In all causes of prehepatic jaundice, the predominant bilirubin is insoluble—that is, unconjugated. Hemolysis alone will rarely cause the total bilirubin level to rise above 7 mg/dL.

Hepatic causes of jaundice

Liver diseases of all kinds, whether temporary or life-long, threaten the organ's ability to keep up with bilirubin processing. Some of the more common causes of jaundice include infectious hepatitis (types A, B, C, D, and E, and various other **viruses**), alcoholic hepatitis, and cirrhosis (scarring of the liver, due to various diseases, to the degree that it can no longer function). Starvation, circulating infections, and certain medications (acetaminophen **overdose**, isoniazid, and others) can cause inefficiency in bilirubin disposal. Certain hereditary defects

also affect how the liver processes bilirubin (such as Gilbert's syndrome and Crigler-Najjar syndrome), causing elevated levels of unconjugated bilirubin. Also, there are several inherited conditions in which the liver cannot excrete bilirubin after it is made soluble (such as Dubin-Johnson syndrome and Rotor syndrome), resulting in direct (or conjugated) bilirubin being the predominant form of the molecule. Unlike hemolytic causes of jaundice, which always involve unconjugated bilirubin, the hepatic sources of jaundice often represent mixed results.

Posthepatic causes of jaundice

Posthepatic forms of jaundice include those caused when soluble bilirubin does not reach the intestines after it has left the liver, resulting in elevated direct bilirubin levels. These disorders are called obstructive jaundices. The most common cause of obstructive jaundice is the presence of gallstones in the ducts of the biliary system. Other causes include diseases where the bile ducts have been destroyed, such as the autoimmune disease primary biliary sclerosis, lesions (whether benign or malignant), and trauma. Some drugs (such as anabolic and contraceptive steroids), and occasionally pressures caused by a normal **pregnancy**, cause the bile in the ducts to stop flowing. This process is called cholestasis.

Neonatal jaundice

Several conditions can cause jaundice in a newborn baby. Erythroblastosis fetalis is a disease of newborns marked by the presence of too many immature red blood cells (erythroblasts) in the baby's blood. When a baby and mother have different Rh factors (positive-RH baby and negative-Rh mother), antibodies from the mother may leak into the baby's circulation through the placental exchange and destroy blood cells. This reaction may produce severe hemolysis and jaundice in the newborn. Rh-factor incompatibility is the most common cause. These births are usually induced a week or two early to keep third-trimester hemolysis to a minimum.

Even in the absence of Rh-factor incompatibility, the newborn's bilirubin level may reach threatening levels. Normal newborn jaundice is the result of two conditions occurring at the same time: a prehepatic and a hepatic source of excess bilirubin. During development, the fetal-type hemoglobin is important to extract oxygen from the mother's blood. At birth, the infant extracts oxygen directly from the **lungs** and no longer needs the fetal hemoglobin. So, fetal hemoglobin is removed from the system and replaced with mature hemoglobin. The resulting hemoglobin overload overwhelms the immature system, and bilirubin levels may rise until the third day of life, and then decline by day five to day 10. During that time, the baby is jaundiced.

These forms of jaundice in the newborn may result in high levels of unconjugated bilirubin. If conjugated bilirubin is found, it is usually due to serious causes, such as obstruction of the biliary system or overwhelming **infection**.

Symptoms

Certain chemicals in bile may cause itching in jaundiced patients. Fatigue is a very common symptom in people with liver disease. In more severe illness, nausea may occur. Poor appetite and weight loss can be a problem for some patients, usually those with acute infection or advanced scarring of the liver (cirrhosis). Depending on the cause of jaundice, patients may or may not have **pain** over the liver (upper right quadrant). Liver pain is common if there are gallstones, and may also occur in acute hepatitis. Patients whose bile does not drain into the **small intestine** adequately will have clay-colored stools. The conjugated form of bilirubin may be excreted by the **kidneys** and result in dark urine. Long-standing jaundice may upset the balance of chemicals in the bile and cause stones to form in the gallbladder or in the ducts.

In newborns, the concern about jaundice is that insoluble or unconjugated bilirubin may get into the **brain** and do permanent damage to the **central nervous system**. This serious condition is called kernicterus. It becomes a concern as bilirubin levels approach 20 mg/dL. Newborns are more likely to have problems with jaundice if they are premature, Asian or Native American, or bruised significantly during the birth process. Jaundice is also more common if a newborn was born after an induced labor, has lost too much weight during the first few days of life, was born at high altitude, or was born to a diabetic mother.

Diagnosis

In most cases, the sign of jaundice is identified based on the appearance of the patient's sclera and complexion. The liver and spleen are palpated to check for enlargement and to evaluate any abdominal pain. The location and severity of abdominal pain and the presence of masses in the abdomen, together with the presence of **fever**, help to distinguish among the causes for jaundice. The differential diagnosis of the cause of jaundice is primarily based on blood-test results.

Laboratory testing reveals the total bilirubin and its components. The capability to evaluate total bilirubin levels and the fractionation into direct (conjugated) and indirect (unconjugated) components is available in most laboratories. The jaundice may be determined to be of indirect (prehepatic sources, Gilbert's syndrome, or Crigler-Najjar syndrome) or direct (primarily obstructive posthepatic sources, and some hepatic diseases) origin. Liver enzymes, such as aspartate aminotransferase (AST) and alanine aminotransferase (ALT), should be evaluated; elevations would be signs of inflammation or destruction of liver cells. If the AST is at least twice the level of the ALT, this finding strongly supports the suggestion of alcohol abuse as a source of liver disease. If alkaline phosphatase is elevated, this suggests an obstructive (posthepatic) component in the cause of jaundice. Albumin levels and prothrombin times will be abnormal (elevated) if the liver is severely damaged. Microscopic analysis of blood smears for signs of hemolysis is performed.

Liver disease is usually assessed from blood studies and physical-examination findings, but a biopsy may be necessary to clarify less obvious disease. A **liver biopsy** may be performed at the bedside. A thin, cannulated needle is inserted to draw a core of tissue from the liver. The tissue sample is sent for patholic examination.

Diseases of the biliary system may be identified by imaging techniques, especially with the use of contrast dye. The most common and cost-effective method for beginning to assess the liver and bile ducts is ultrasound. Dilated bile ducts are very suggestive of obstruction, and abnormal amounts of fat or scar tissue may be noticed. Much more detailed information about the structure of the liver and biliary tree is gained with computed tomography (CT) or **magnetic resonance imaging** (MRI). Very detailed investigation of the bile ducts is achieved with endoscopic retrograde cholangiopancreatography (ERCP), for which a fiber-optic scope is put down the gastrointestinal tract via the mouth, all the way to the ampulla of Vater. Dye is injected to map the bile ducts and identify obstruction. A tiny brush-tipped device at the end of the scope light is used to scrape tissue from the duct lining for analysis. Treatment can also be achieved at the same time, as stones can be removed or stents placed to aid in passage of a stone or maintaining bile flow in spite of a tumor.

Treatment

Newborns are the one group of patients in whom the jaundice itself requires attention. Because the insoluble bilirubin can get into the brain, the amount in the blood must not go over certain levels. If there is reason to suspect increased hemolysis in the newborn, the bilirubin level must be measured repeatedly during the first few days of life. If the level of bilirubin shortly after birth

KEY TERMS

Ampulla of Vater—A valve at the distal end of the widened portion of the common bile duct, through which the bile and pancreatic juices enter the duodenum.

Anemia—A condition in which the blood does not contain enough hemoglobin. There are many causes of anemia, including hemolysis, bleeding, and problems producing red blood cells (RBCs).

Biliary system/bile ducts—The gallbladder and the system of tubes that carries bile from the liver into the intestines.

Bilirubin—A breakdown product of hemoglobin that is potentially toxic. The liver collects bilirubin from the bloodstream, alters it, and secretes it into bile.

Hemoglobin—The red pigment in red blood cells that carries oxygen.

Hemolysis—The premature destruction of red blood cells.

Hepatic jaundice—A cause of jaundice; jaundice that occurs while the liver is performing its task of making bilirubin soluble.

Icteric—An adjective, based on the Greek word for jaundice, used to describe a jaundiced patient.

Liver—A large, solid organ in the right upper quadrant of the abdomen that is the body's premier "chemical processing plant" of drugs, nutrients, and toxins.

Neonatal jaundice—Jaundice in a newborn baby, resulting from various conditions.

Pancreas—The organ adjacent to the stomach that produces digestive juices, insulin, and other hormones.

Posthepatic jaundice—A cause of jaundice; jaundice that occurs after the liver has performed its task of making bilirubin soluble.

Prehepatic jaundice—A cause of jaundice; jaundice that occurs before the liver has performed its task of making bilirubin soluble.

Rh incompatibility—When a baby and mother have different Rh factors; a common cause of jaundice in newborns.

Splenectomy—Surgical removal of the spleen, sometimes necessary to control certain types of hemolytic anemia.

threatens to go too high, treatment must begin immediately. Exchanging most of the baby's blood (an exchange transfusion) was the only way to reduce the amount of bilirubin until the late 1960s. Then it was discovered that bright blue light renders the bilirubin harmless. Now jaundiced babies are fitted with eye protection and placed under special lights, wearing only a diaper so that more skin surface can be exposed. The **phototherapy** alters the bilirubin in the blood as it passes through and close to the baby's skin. Under certain conditions, exchange transfusions are still done to rapidly gain control over bilirubin levels.

Most adult patients are treated based on the underlying cause of the jaundice. Surgical removal of the spleen (splenectomy) may arrest hemolytic anemia. Drugs that cause hemolysis or arrest the flow of bile are discontinued or replaced with alternate therapy. The abuse of alcohol or street drugs must stop if the liver is to begin to heal and the jaundice given a chance to subside. Obstructive jaundice frequently requires surgical repair. The gallbladder may need to be removed, or small stones removed from lower in the biliary tract. If there is neoplasm of the liver or biliary tree, partial or total removal is necessary. If the original biliary passageways cannot be restored, new ones are created in surgery.

Prognosis

Prognosis is based on the underlying cause of jaundice. The liver is a very resilient organ, and many patients do well after supportive therapy or surgical intervention for acute causes of jaundice. High bilirubin levels themselves are not dangerous to patients other than neonates, so all symptoms of high bilirubin levels are reversible if the underlying condition is treatable.

Health care team roles

Good supportive care of the jaundiced patient, regardless of the underlying disorder, is important. If alcohol abuse has been an acute or long-standing problem, nursing staff can contribute much in educating the patient about the importance of avoiding alcohol.

Prevention

Many of the numerous causes of jaundice cannot be anticipated or avoided. Alcohol abuse in patients should be identified and support provided to aid in recovery. Erythroblastosis fetalis can be prevented by giving an Rh-negative mother a gamma globulin solution called RhoGAM as a routine part of **prenatal care**. This will decrease the chances her antibody titer will rise against her baby's blood. Liver problems due to medications can be minimized with appropriate screening blood tests and cessation of the drug if necessary. One cause of liver failure not mentioned previously is anorexia nervosa, in which patients intentionally starve themselves, disabling the body's immune-defense system and overwhelming the liver's ability to detoxify the blood. Patients with this condition need specific psychiatric therapy in addition to adequate nutritional supplementation therapy to prevent liver failure. If it occurs, transplantation may be the only recourse. Malaria may be prevented by taking certain precautions when traveling in tropical or subtropical countries and climates.

Resources

BOOKS

Braunwald, E., et al. *Harrison's Principles of Internal Medicine,* 15th ed. New York: McGraw-Hill, 2001; pp. 255-259, 1715-1720.

Fischbach, F. *A Manual of Laboratory and Diagnostic Tests.* Philadelphia: Lippincott, 2000; pp. 385-389.

Tierney, L. M., S. J. McPhee, and M. A. Papadakis. *Current Medical Diagnosis and Treatment 2001;* New York: Lange Medical Books/McGraw-Hill, 2000; pp.662-667.

PERIODICALS

Furuta, S., et al. "Anorexia Nervosa with Severe Liver Dysfunction and Subsequent Critical Complications." *Internal Medicine* 38, no. 7 (July 1999): 575-579.

Himal, H. S. "Common Bile Duct Stones: The Role of Preoperative, Intraoperative, and Postoperative ERCP." *Seminars in Laparoscopic Surgery* 7, no. 4 (December 2000): 237-245.

Madlon-Kay, D. J. "Health Nurse Clinical Assessment of Neonatal Jaundice: Comparison of Three Methods." *Archives of Pediatric and Adolescent Medicine* 155, no. 5 (May 2001): 583-586.

Narang, A., P. Kumar, and R. Kumar. "Neonatal Jaundice in Very Low Birth Weight Babies." *Indian Journal of Pediatrics* 68, no. 4 (April 2001): 307-309.

Erika J. Norris

Jejunostomy *see* **Enterostomy**

Joint aspiration *see* **Joint fluid analysis**

Joint endoscopy *see* **Arthroscopy**

▌ Joint fluid analysis

Definition

Joint fluid analysis, also called synovial fluid analysis, or arthrocentesis, is a procedure used to assess joint-related abnormalities, such as occur in the knee or elbow. Synovial or joint fluid is an ultrafiltrate of plasma formed in the synovial membrane of movable joints. The fluid lubricates the bone and cartilage tissues of the joint.

Purpose

The purpose of joint fluid analysis is to diagnose arthritis, an inflammation of the joint, and identify its cause. In addition, removal of the fluid can decrease **pain** in the joint. Diseases which may cause joint swelling include rheumatoid arthritis, systemic lupus erythematosus, **gout**, gonococcal arthritis (caused by the **bacteria** that causes gonorrhea), other types of bacterial arthritis, and viral inflammation of the synovial lining.

Precautions

Universal precautions for the prevention of transmission of bloodborne pathogens should be observed when collecting synovial fluid. Arthrocentesis should not be performed on a patient who is uncooperative, especially if the patient cannot or will not keep the joint immobile throughout the procedure. Sampling of a joint may be contraindicated when there is evidence of **infection** in overlying skin or tissue. The joint space should be accessible. Therefore, a poorly accessible joint space, such as in hip aspiration in an obese patient, should not be subjected to this procedure.

Description

Arthrocentesis

The removal of synovial fluid, arthrocentesis, is also called a joint tap, or closed joint aspiration. The procedure is done by passing a needle into a joint space and aspirating synovial fluid using **aseptic technique**. The joint must be cleaned thoroughly with iodine before inserting the needle to prevent any infection. The size of the needle and volume of fluid withdrawn depends on the size of the joint. The patient is asked to lie on their back and remain relaxed. A local anesthetic, typically a **subcutaneous injection** of lidocaine, xylocaine, or ethyl chloride, is then administered. As the needle enters the joint, a "pop" may be felt or heard; this is normal. Correct placement of the needle in the joint space is normally painless. At this point, the clinician slowly drains some of the fluid into the syringe. The syringe may contain a small amount of sodium heparin. The needle is then withdrawn and an adhesive bandage is placed over the puncture site. The sample is transferred to one or more tubes containing liquid heparin or liquid EDTA anticoagulant.

The procedure takes about 10 minutes. The physician may need to prioritize the tests that he or she orders since fluid yields from this procedure may be very small. Only a drop of fluid is needed for culture and microscopic examination and these two procedures are given top priority because of their diagnostic importance. Some tests, such as glucose and total hemolytic complement must be evaluated with respect to **blood** levels. Therefore, a blood sample should be collected at the same time.

Causes of arthritis

Arthritis can be classified by cause into five categories. Noninflammatory or **osteoarthritis** is the most common form and results from loss of cartilage covering the bone. Inflammatory arthritis results from damage to the joint caused by immune complexes that deposit in the joint or autoantibodies that attach to and destroy the synovial membrane. The most common cause of inflammatory arthritis is rheumatoid arthritis. Septic arthritis is caused by bacterial infection of the joint, The most commonly implicated organism in sexually active persons is *Neisseria gonorrhoeae*. Gout is joint inflammation caused by deposition of uric acid crystals. When other crystals such as **calcium** pyrophosphate are the cause, the condition is called pseudogout. Hemorrhagic arthritis, bleeding into the joint, is caused by trauma, **hemophilia**, or other bleeding disorder such as thrombocytopenia (low platelet count).

Laboratory tests

Laboratory analysis of joint fluid should include determination of color, transparency, volume, and viscosity; red and white blood cell counts with a differential; examination of wet mounts for synovial crystals; microbiological culture; and tests for glucose, total protein, complement, rheumatoid factor, and mucin clot.

Physical characteristics

Normal joint fluid has a volume between 0.15-3.5 mL. An increased volume is common in all five classes of arthritis. The fluid should be clear and pale yellow. Observation of the color of the supernatant after centrifugation helps to discriminate between a hemorrhagic fluid (bleeding from injury to the joint) and a traumatic tap (puncture of a blood vessel during arthrocentesis). Deep yellow or pink fluid points to a hemorrhagic process whereas a normal color points to a traumatic tap. A clot in the fluid also points to a traumatic tap because large protein molecules such as fibrinogen are not found in the fluid. The specific gravity is normally the same as plasma, but the viscosity is much greater. The viscosity is measured by inserting a wooden applicator stick into the fluid and removing it. The fluid should form a thread of at least 1.6 in (4 cm) at the end of the applicator stick. Failure to do so indicates a low level of mucoprotein which is most common in inflammatory arthritis.

Microscopic analysis

The white blood cell (WBC) count is performed manually using a hemacytometer. The fluid is diluted in saline rather than a WBC counting fluid because the acetic acid will cause the formation of a mucin plug. The normal WBC count is very low, less than 200 per microliter. High counts are seen in septic arthritis, rheumatoid arthritis, and gout. Persons with osteoarthritis or hemorrhagic arthritis may or may not have a high WBC count. The highest counts with neutrophils predominating are associated with septic arthritis.

The normal differential shows 50-65% monocytes with neutrophils and lymphocytes each accounting for less than 25% of the WBCs. Neutrophils above 80% signal septic arthritis. A higher percentage of lymphocytes favors a diagnosis of rheumatoid arthritis. Neutrophils with dark staining cytoplasmic inclusions (ingested immunoglobulins) point to a diagnosis of rheumatoid arthritis. The red blood cell (RBC) count of synovial fluid is also performed manually. The count is normally less than 2000 per microliter. Higher counts especially in the presence of xanthochromia (abnormal color) indicate a synovial hemorrhage.

Microscopic examination of the fluid for crystals requires a polarizing **microscope** with a red compensating filter. This type of microscope transmits light in a single plane through the specimen. An analyzer filter is placed above the specimen before the ocular is aligned, so that it is out of phase with the polarizing filter. The analyzer filter blocks the light transmitted through the specimen, causing a dark background unless the light is rotated by the object on the slide. Uric acid and calcium pyrophosphate are the two most common crystals seen in joint fluid. They both rotate plane polarized light which causes them to be illuminated by the polarizing microscope. However, they can be differentiated using the red compensating filter. Uric acid crystals are seen as yellow needles when the long axis of the crystal is parallel to the slow vibrating light from the filter. Calcium pyrophosphate crystals are blue when the long axis of the crystal is parallel to the slow vibrating light.

Biochemical and immunological tests

Glucose in synovial fluid is normally within 10 mg/dL of the plasma level. Low glucose is seen in septic and rheumatoid arthritis. Very low levels (less than half of the plasma level) are seen in rheumatoid arthritis. The total protein of synovial fluid is normally below 2.0 g/dL. Increased total protein is seen in rheumatoid and hemorrhagic arthritis. In rheumatoid arthritis, complement will be low owing to chronic consumption and local immunoglobulin production will cause the ratio of synovial to serum IgG to be greater than 0.5. Rheumatoid factor in joint fluid is positive in about 60% of persons with rheumatoid arthritis and in a lesser number of persons with other autoimmune diseases.

The mucin clot test is used to measure the amount of mucin in the fluid. This substance consists of repeating subunits of hyaluronic acid that will cross link forming a mucin clot when acetic acid is added to the fluid. In infection bacterial hyaluronidase may destroy the mucoprotein causing no clot. In rheumatoid arthritis, damage to the synovial cells results in deficient production of mucoprotein and the mucin clot is either absent or easily broken apart.

Microbiological analysis

All samples of synovial fluid should be cultured and Gram-stained. The **Gram stain** results can be definitive for septic arthritis if neutrophils and bacteria are found, but is not always positive. The fluid should be inoculated on blood agar plates; on chocolate (heated blood) agar plates for gonococcus and *Haemophilus*; and in broth such as thioglycolate for the isolation of anaerobic bacteria. *N. gonorrhoeae* is responsible for about 75% of septic arthritis in young and middle aged adults. *Staphylococcus spp.* account for about 75% of septic arthritis in the elderly. *Staphylococcus, Streptococcus*, and *Haemophilus* are the most common genera isolated from children.

Preparation

Prior to the procedure, any risks that are involved should be explained to the patient. The patient will be given a local anesthetic but no pain medications or sedatives are required. If the clinician requests a glucose test, the patient will be asked to fast for six to 12 hours before the procedure. If not, there is no special preparation required for a joint fluid analysis.

Aftercare

Some post-procedural pain may be experienced. For this reason, the patient should arrange to be driven home by someone else. Aftercare of the joints will depend on the results of the analysis.

KEY TERMS

Aspirate—The removal by suction of a fluid from a body cavity using a needle.

Bursae—A closed sac lined with a synovial membrane and filled with fluid, usually found in areas subject to friction, such as where a tendon passes over a bone.

Gout—A painful joint disease characterized by the deposition of uric acid crystals in the joint. These crystals cause swelling and redness.

Hematoma—A localized mass of blood that is confined within an organ or tissue.

Hyaluronic acid—A high molecular weight made of carbohydrate and glucuronic acid that is found in high concentrations in the synovial fluid. This provides thickness to the fluid so it can cushion the joint.

Joint—A moveable portion of bone found between two bones.

Lupus erythematosus—A multisystem disease with an autoimmune etiology. Lupus causes problems with the skin, kidneys, joints and the serosal membranes.

Rheumatiod arthritis—A chronic and progressive inflammation of the joints whose cause is unknown.

Synovial fluid—A transparent lubricating fluid secreted in a sac to protect an area where a tendon passes over a bone.

Complications

While joint fluid analysis is generally a safe procedure, especially when performed on a large, easily accessible joint, such as the knee, some risks are possible. Some of the complications to the procedure, although rare, include infection at the site of the needle stick, an accumulation of blood (hematoma) formation, local pain, injury to cartilage, tendon rupture, and nerve damage.

Results

Normal values typical for synovial fluid are shown below:

- Volume: 0.15-3.5 mL.
- Transparency: clear.
- Color: straw or pale yellow.

- Viscosity: 1.6 in (4 cm) thread or greater.

- Mucin clot: firm.

- Glucose: different from plasma by 10 mg/dL or less.

- Total protein: less than or equal to 2.0 g/dL.

- White blood cell count: less than 200 per microliter.

- Differential: less than 25% granulocytes.

- Crystals: negative.

Health care team roles

The removal of synovial fluid from a joint should be done by a physician. Laboratory tests are performed by clinical laboratory scientists/medical technologists. Physicians interpret the results of laboratory tests.

Resources

BOOKS

Burtis, Carl A. and Edward R. Ashwood. *Tietz Textbook of Clinical Chemistry.* Philadelphia: W.B. Saunders Company, 1999.

Kaplan, Lawrence A. and Amadeo J. Pesce. *Clinical Chemistry, Theory, Analysis and Correlation.* St. Louis: Mosby Publishers, 1996.

Stobo, John D., David B. Hellman, Paul W. Ladenson,, Brent G. Petty and Thomas A. Traill. *Principles and Practice of Medicine, 23rd Edition.* Stamford, CT: Appleton and Lange, 1996.

Jane E. Phillips, PhD

Joint integrity and function

Definition

Joints serve as links between structures; in this case, bones in the human body. There are numerous joints in the body that act to stabilize and control bony segments. One example is the knee joint, which joins the femur and tibia. This joint allows the lower leg to swing freely, but also to be stable during the stance phase of gait. Some joints provide the body with stability, while others provide it with mobility. However, most joints provide both stability and mobility.

Description

There are two major types of joints: synarthroses and diarthroses. Synarthroses are joints connected by fibrous tissue. Diarthroses are synovial joints, where two bones are bound together by a joint capsule, forming a joint cavity. In synovial joints, there is a nourishing lubricating fluid called synovial fluid.

Function

Synarthoses

There are two types of synarthroses: fibrous joints and cartilaginous joints.

FIBROUS JOINTS. In fibrous joints, bones are united by fibrous tissue. There are three types of fibrous joints: gomphosis, suture, and syndesmosis. A gomphosis joint occurs where one bone fits into another bone. The articulating edges are bound together by connective tissue, and the bony surfaces in the articulation are close together. An example of a gomphosis joint is a tooth in the jawbone. An example of a suture is the fibrous joints between the bones of the **skull** of an infant. Before birth fibrous tissue forms soft spots on the skull, called fontanelles. As growth and development occurs the sutures ossify. A syndesmosis joint connects two bones through connective tissue and is found throughout the human body. An example is the tibio-fibular syndesmosis, the connective tissue that binds the distal ends of the fibula and tibia. A syndesmosis allows the fibula and tibia to work in unison as part of the lower leg. The limited motion available at this joint allows the tibia and fibula to move about each other, yet still function as a unit.

CARTILAGINOUS JOINTS. In cartilaginous joints, bones are connected by either fibrocartilage or hyaline cartilage. There are two types of cartilaginous joints: symphyses and synchondroses. A symphysis is a cartilaginous joint where the connecting entity is fibrocartilage. The symphysis is stable but it allows limited motion. An example of a symphysis joint is the attachment of one vertebra to another by an intervertebral disk, a fibrocartilage ring, in the **vertebral column**. In this symphysis joint only minimal motion occurs between vertebrae, thus maintaining stability. The combination of small movements between each successive vertebral attachment is what allows the vertebral column to flex and extend. A synchondrosis is a joint where the articulating surfaces are close together, yet are bound by hyaline cartilage. An example of a synchondrosis is the two distinct portions of long bone separated by a hyaline cartilaginous plate. This typically occurs at the ends of long bones, where a cartilaginous plate separates the diaphysis from the epiphysis. This plate allows the end of bones to grow throughout early human development. As growth and development continues, the hyaline cartilage ossifies and by adulthood the joint is gone. Another example of a synchondrosis in the human body is the articulation between the first rib and the manubrium, the upper portion of the sternum.

Diarthroses

A diarthroses has a synovial component. The bones are connected to a joint capsule that surrounds the bones and creates a joint cavity. Ligaments also attach bone-to-bone stabilizing the joint and making the diarthrotic joint stable, yet mobile. Again, the knee joint is a good example of a diarthroses; two bones (tibia and femur) that are attached by ligaments called the anterior and posterior cruciate ligaments. An extensive joint capsule also surrounds the knee joint. In synarthroses there are also disks or menisci that aid in maintaining congruency between bones, i.e., the medial and lateral menisci of the knee joint. Making the diarthroses even more unique from the synarthroses is the addition of synovial fluid. The synovial fluid provides lubrication within the joint. In summary, the diarthroses is complex, with ligaments and capsule providing stability, disks or menisci aiding in congruency, and synovial fluid providing lubrication.

Synovial-type joints can be further classified into three categories: uniaxial, biaxial, and triaxial.

UNIAXIAL JOINTS. Uniaxial joints can be further categorized into hinge and pivot joints. Examples of hinge joints are the joints of the fingers, i.e. interphalangeal joints. An example of a pivot-type joint is the articulation between the axis and atlas in the cervical region, allowing true rotation of the head. In a uniaxial joint the motion is in one plane or is said to have one degree of freedom.

BIAXIAL JOINTS. In a biaxial joint, motion occurs in two planes; thus, there are two degrees of freedom. There are two types of biaxial joints: saddle and condyloid. An example of a saddle joint is the carpmetocarpal joint of the thumb, where bones fit together like an individual riding a horse while sitting on a saddle. One bone is concave, the other is convex. Examples of condyloid joints are the metacarpophalangeal joints of the fingers.

TRIAXIAL JOINTS. Triaxial joints have three degrees of motion and can move in three planes. There are two types of triaxial joints: ball and socket, and plane joints. An example of a **ball and socket joint** is the hip. The attachment of the carpal bones in the hand are considered plane joints where gliding is permitted between bones.

Role in human health

Synarthrotic joints allow little or no movement. Their main function is to provide stability, and they also join bones to form a larger unit. Diarthrotic joints provide stability and mobility. Joints can be affected by injury,

increased demand, immobilization, or long-term bed rest, and diseases, such as **osteoarthritis**. Injury can occur if a large stress or load is placed on a joint. Constant excessive loading over time can also cause joint structure to break down. Immobilization or long-term bed rest causes muscles around joints to weaken. Furthermore, joints and articular surfaces need some load, such as gravity, to maintain proper integrity. Over time, if load is not present, articular surfaces will weaken and degenerate due to lack of stimulus. Disease processes such as osteoarthritis can also disrupt the integrity of the joint. All of the above problems can affect joint structure and eventually disrupt functions such as walking. Severe joint degradation can lead to disability.

Common diseases and disorders

Increased demand or trauma placed on a joint can cause tearing or even rupture of the ligaments, joint capsule, or hyaline cartilage. Furthermore, immobilization and disease can degrade the joint surfaces. Any one of these complications can disrupt the integrity of the joint. If the integrity of a joint is compromised, there could be decreased motion at the joint and possibly **pain**. Thus, pain and decreased joint mobility can lead to decreased function and eventual disability.

Other pathologies such as osteoarthritis, rheumatoid arthritis, trauma, and **gout** can all negatively affect joint integrity and function. In the acute phases of gout, joint effusion secondary to injury, and rheumatoid arthritis the joint capsule of diarthroidal joints becomes distended due to over production of synovial fluid. Because of this distention, joint receptors are impaired and may provide inaccurate information on position and movement. Furthermore, there is pain associated with these conditions. If treatment is not effective in reducing pain and inflammation, joint integrity and eventual function will be compromised. In situations where injury has occurred to a joint, such as ligament tear or rupture, the joint is unstable. This instability leads to further stresses placed on other structures within the joint. Eventually, if the ligament is not healed or repaired, further damage to the joint will occur because of the increased demand on other structures. An example is tearing of a ligament in the knee or ankle.

Osteoarthritis is a disease process that negatively affects the integrity and function of a joint. In this degenerative disease the articular surfaces of the joint are degrading. As time passes, the degradation of the joint continues. The most common joints affected by osteoarthritis are the knee and the hip. Conservative treatments such as medications and rehabilitation may be used to decrease pain and restore mobility. However,

KEY TERMS

Diathroses—Synovial joints.

Femur—The large upper bone, also known as the thigh bone.

Gait—Refers to walking, i.e. ambulation.

Gomphosis—A joint where a bony structure is implanted deep into another bony structure. An example would be the joint between a tooth and the mandible (jaw bone).

Immobilization—Keeping a joint from moving, i.e. when an individual breaks the lower leg; a cast may be used that covers the knee, thus preventing motion.

Knee joint—A lower limb joint connecting the tibia to the femur. It allows for straightening and bending of the knee.

Stance phase—The point where, when walking, one foot is in contact with the ground.

Suture—A joint where two bony structures are united by dense fibrous tissue. An example is the sutures of the skull.

Symphyses—Joints where bones are connected by a fibrocartilage disk. An example is the symphesis pubis.

Synchondroses—Joints that connect two bony structures by hyaline cartilage. Examples are the ends of long bones, where the bone growth is not yet complete. As the skeleton matures, the hyaline cartilage eventually ossifies.

Syndesmosis—A joint where two bones are joined by a ligament or membrane. An example is the membrane that joins the shaft of the tibia to the shaft of the fibula in the lower leg.

Tibia—The large lower leg bone between the knee and ankle.

there are instances where conservative treatments fail and joint replacement is a viable option, i.e. total knee arthroplasty.

Joint structures need optimum motion and stress to maintain proper function. Moreover, proper cartilage and joint **nutrition** are required for proper joint function. Therefore, it is important to have synovial fluid maintaining nourishment to the joint surfaces and cartilage in an effort to maintain the integrity of the joint. Since joints are not well supplied by **blood** flow it is important that

movement and weight-bearing are encouraged to promote fluid flow between joint surfaces and disks, i.e., menisci.

Resources

BOOKS

Hertling, D., and R.M. Kessler. *Management of Common Musculoskeletal Disorders.* Baltimore: Lippincott, Williams & Wilkins, 1996.

Lehmkuhl, L.D., and L.K. Smith. *Brunnstrom's Clinical Kinesiology.* Philadelphia: F.A. Davis Co., 1996.

Magee, D.J. *Orthopedic Physical Assessment.* Philadelphia: W.B. Saunders Co., 1997.

ORGANIZATIONS

American Physical Therapy Association, 1111 North Fairfax St., Alexandria, VA 22314-1488. Phone: (703) 684-APTA or (800) 999-APTA. TDD: (703) 683-6748. Fax: (703) 684-7343. <http://www.apta.org>.

OTHER

Sports Medicine and Orthopedic Center, University of Washington. <http://www.orthop.washington.edu>.

Mark Damian Rossi, Ph.D., P.T., C.S.C.S.

Joint mobilization and manipulation

Definition

Joint mobilization is a treatment technique used to manage musculoskeletal dysfunction. Most manipulative and mobilization techniques are performed by physical therapists, and fall under the category of manual therapy.

In most cases, at the end of a long bone there is a joint or articulation. The long bone is attached or joined to another bone by a joint. For example, the femur is attached to the tibia at the knee joint. The knee joint is made up of the surface of the tibia, femur, ligaments, and capsule. Thus, the knee joint is stable and yet mobile. When an individual is sitting in a chair and freely kicks his leg out (knee extension), the tibia moves, while the femur is stationary. However, at the surface of the articulating bones (tibia and femur), there is other movement. This movement is known as slide or glide; some have termed it "joint play." When an individual kicks his leg out, the lower leg or tibia is not only moving forward, but also gliding across the end of the femur. Mobilization is the treatment technique that involves the clinician applying a force to mimic the gliding that occurs between bones. It is a passive movement, the goal of which is to produce a slide or glide. Mobilizations are usually completed at slow speed, sometimes with oscillations, and even with a "hold" or stretch. Manipulations are more aggressive, high velocity techniques, or thrusts. They occur very fast, and at the end of available joint play.

Purpose

Mobilizations are used to restore joint play that has been lost due to injury or disease. In order for an individual to kick his leg out, there must be sufficient joint play, or freedom for the tibia to move on the femur. Thus, mobilizations are used when range of motion or mobility is lacking. Furthermore, gentle oscillations within the available joint play range is a technique used to decrease **pain**. Manipulations are quick movements that occur beyond the available joint play range. The purpose of manipulations, or joint thrusts, is to increase the available range if it is not full. Secondly, manipulations are done to break adhesions that disrupt joint movement.

Precautions

Mobilizations and manipulations should not be done in the following circumstances:

- to the spine if there is severe **osteoarthritis** or osteoporosis
- if there is any tumor or malignancy in the area
- to the cervical region if there is dysfunction with the flow of **blood** within the vertebral artery
- if there is bleeding in a joint
- if there is a loose body in the joint
- to total joint replacements
- to joints near a growth plate
- if the joint is degenerative
- until a full diagnosis is reached

Description

Peripheral joint mobilization means mobilizing the joints of the periphery or limbs. There is a grading system for completing mobilizations. The grading system is based on how much joint play is available. Thus, the clinician must know what the total range is by examination through passive movement. Furthermore, there are stretching mobilizations used for **pain management** and stretching. The first common mobilization techniques are sustained joint play movements that have three grades. These mobilizations aid in decreasing pain and increasing mobility.

Grade 1

The clinician applies passive movement in a very small range, approximately 15-25% of the available joint play range.

Grade 2

Bone is passively moved in a moderate range to 50% or half of the available joint play range.

Grade 3

Passive force by the clinician causes one bone to move on the other to the end of the available joint play range.

Within these three grades the stretch or "hold" is approximately five to seven seconds.

The other common mobilization technique is termed oscillatory mobilization. These mobilizations have five grades associated with them. Grades one to two are used to help decrease pain within a joint. Grades three to five are used to increase mobility of joint play. Interestingly, a grade five mobilization is really a manipulation. The following are grades for oscillatory mobilizations:

Grade 1

Slow oscillations within the first 20-25% of the available joint play range.

Grade 2

Slow oscillations within 45-55% of the available joint play range, or from the beginning to the middle of available joint play range.

Grade 3

Slow oscillations from the middle of the available joint play range to the end of available joint play range.

Grade 4

Slow oscillations at the end of the available joint play range.

Grade 5

Bone is passively moved to the end-range, and a fast thrust is performed. This is manipulation.

Preparation

The clinician should be aware of the following prior to performing manipulations:

KEY TERMS

Cryotherapy—Usually an ice or cold treatment after physical therapy treatment.

Femur—The long bone of the thigh which articulates with the hip bone and the tibia.

Knee extension—The act of straightening the knee or kicking the leg out, as in kicking a ball.

Ligaments—Fibrous structures that provide an attachment on bone to bone, and provide stability to joint structures.

Musculoskeletal—Pertains to the muscular and skeletal systems, and the relationship between the two.

Passive movement—Movement that occurs under the power of an outside source such as a clinician. There is no voluntary muscular contraction by the individual who is being passively moved.

Tibia—The larger, longer bone of the lower leg which articulates or joins with the ankle and knee.

• The clinician must use good body mechanics and be comfortable with the patient and the technique.

• The clinician must understand the patient's pain and not proceed if the patient has pain.

• The patient must be comfortable with the clinician, and the procedure must be explained fully to the patient.

• The patient must be relaxed.

Aftercare

Individuals with a chronic joint problem may have Grade 1 and Grade 2 techniques used at the beginning of treatment to decrease pain. Then, after treatment, the patient progresses to more aggressive rehabilitation such as **therapeutic exercise**. At the end of a rehabilitation session, Grades 3 and 4 can be used in conjunction with stretching to increase mobility. In an acute joint pathology, only Grades 1 and 2 should be used. Grades 1 and 2 mobilizations can be used at the beginning of therapy to reduce pain in an effort to increase performance during therapeutic **exercise**. Grades 1 and 2 mobilizations can be used again at the end of the treatment before cryotherapy to help alleviate pain.

Complications

Some complications associated with mobilizations, but more so with manipulations are:

• fracture

• dislocation

• joint capsule tearing

• ligamentous tearing

• muscle or tendon injury

• nerve damage

Results

If done appropriately, mobilizations can help reduce pain and restore joint play, which is critical for normal mobility. Manipulations are beneficial for releasing adhesions and are usually done under anesthesia by a medical physician. Chiropractic manipulations are not discussed here.

Health care team roles

It is important that nurses and other members of the allied health care team be aware of patients who undergo mobilization and monitor pain and any possible inflammation after treatment. Moreover, pain and inflammation may need to be more closely monitored in individuals having manipulation to restore joint mobility. An example of a patient requiring closer monitoring is an individual having manipulation after total knee replacement secondary to increased adhesions and limited range of motion. Today, most manual therapy is done by physical therapists. However, the education for physical therapists to conduct forceful or thrust manipulations continues to grow and is becoming more a part of **physical therapy** education and post education.

Resources

BOOKS

Hertling D., and R.M. Kessler. *Management of Common Musculoskeletal Disorders.* Baltimore: Lippincott, Williams & Wilkins, 1996.

Lehmkuhl L.D., and L. K. Smith. *Brunnstroms Clinical Kinesiology.* Philadelphia: F.A. Davis Co., 1996.

Magee D. J. *Orthopedic Physical Assessment.* Philadelphia: W.B. Saunders Co., 1997.

ORGANIZATIONS

American Physical Therapy Association. 1111 N. Fairfax Street, Alexandria, Va 22314. (703) 684-2782. <http://www.apta.org>.

Mark Damian Rossi Ph.D., P.T., C.S.C.S.

Joint sprain *see* **Sprains and strains**

Joint testing *see* **Joint integrity and function**

Joint x rays *see* **Arthrography**

Journal therapy

Definition

Journal therapy is the purposeful and intentional use of a written record of one's own thoughts or feelings to further psychological healing and personal growth. It is often used as an adjunct to many **psychotherapy** and recovery programs. Healthcare practitioners maintain that written expression fills a very important role in the therapeutic process by providing a mechanism of emotional expression in circumstances in which interpersonal expression is not possible or viable.

Origins

People have kept journals and diaries to record dreams, memories, and thoughts since ancient times. Emotional expression has also long held a central role in the study and practice of psychology. Throughout history, psychologists have advocated the expression of emotions as essential for good mental and physical health. Since the early 1980s, interest in this topic has resulted in numerous research studies investigating the health benefits of expressive writing.

Benefits

Journal writing produces a number of benefits in healthy people—among other things, it enhances creativity, helps cope with **stress**, and provides a written record of memorable life experiences. Likewise, some researchers have found that journal writing has a number of psychological and physical health benefits for people who are ill.

Aside from a reduction in physical symptoms of disease, the psychological benefits include reconciling emotional conflicts, fostering self-awareness, managing behavior, solving problems, reducing **anxiety**, aiding reality orientation, and increasing self-esteem. Writing therapy has been used as an effective treatment for the developmentally, medically, educationally, socially, or psychologically impaired and is practiced in mental health, rehabilitation, medical, educational, and forensic institutions. Populations of all ages, races, and ethnic backgrounds are served by writing therapy in individual, couple, family, and group therapy formats.

The therapeutic use of expressive writing allows individuals to confront upsetting topics, thus alleviating the constraints or inhibitions associated with not talking about the event. The psychological drain of the inhibition is believed to cause and/or exacerbate stress-related disease processes. Researchers have found that emotional expression facilitates cognitive processing of the traumatic **memory**, which leads to emotional and physiological change. Specifically, written emotional expression promotes integration and understanding of the event while reducing negative emotions associated with it.

Description

Journal writing and other forms of writing therapy are based on the premise that the mind and the body are inseparably joined in the healing process. Although there are many methods of conducting journal writing therapy depending on the therapeutic technique of the psychologist or psychiatrist, the therapist often instructs the participant to write about a distressing or traumatic event or thought in one or more sessions.

Although researchers are uncertain about exactly how writing about traumas produces improvements in psychological well-being, traumatic stress researchers have pointed out that ordinary memories are qualitatively different from traumatic memories. Traumatic memories are more emotional and perceptual in nature. The memory is stored as a sensory perception, obsessional thought, or behavioral reenactment. It is associated with persistent, intrusive, and distressing symptoms, avoidance, and intense anxiety that results in observed psychological and biological dysfunction. Thus, one goal in treating traumatic memories is to find a means of processing them.

A narrative that becomes more focused and coherent over a number of writing sessions is often associated with increased improvement, according to several research studies. The memories become deconditioned and restructured into a personal, integrated narrative. Changes in psychological well-being after writing therapy may result from cognitive shifts about the trauma either during or after the writing process.

Preparations

In a health care setting, the participant often prepares for journal writing by receiving (from the therapist) a set of instructions regarding the length and focus of the writing session or sessions. Other instructions may include writing in a stream-of-consciousness fashion, without censorship or concern about grammar or style.

Precautions

It is advisable that journal therapy be conducted only by a licensed health professional, such as a certified **art therapy** practitioner or trained psychologist or psychiatrist. While journal writing classes available to the general public may perform a variety of useful functions, these classes are not intended to provide medical therapy. In journal therapy, the participant may, for example, uncover potentially traumatic, repressed, or painful memories. Therefore, a trained health professional may be necessary to supervise the process and treat these symptoms as they arise.

Side effects

There are no known side effects of journal or writing therapy.

Research and general acceptance

Therapeutic writing became an increasingly popular topic in the final decades of the twentieth century, not only among trained health care professionals, but also among self-improvement speakers without medical training. Seminars, workshops, and Internet sites purportedly offering therapy through expressive writing sprang up around the nation and gained popular acceptance. Despite the large body of research indicating that writing confers benefits on healthy people, the topic of writing therapy's effects on diseased individuals has not received a great deal of research attention. Although increasingly used by health care professionals as an adjunct to various therapeutic approaches, the practice has been criticized by some members of the health care community. Some researchers are distrustful of the findings that so much measurable improvement in health status can occur in just a few brief writing sessions.

In the United Kingdom, the focus of journal therapy has been on descriptive accounts and psychodynamic explanations for subjective improvements in the health status of participants. In the United States, on the other hand, the focus is on formal scientific research aimed at validating the impact of brief, highly standardized writing exercises on physical measures of illness. The research demonstrates that although physical measures of illness may change, the reasons for the change are not always clear.

In the United States, one study on the effects of writing about stressful experiences on symptom reduction in patients with **asthma** or rheumatoid arthritis found that after four months of writing therapy—in conjunction with standard pharmacotherapy—nearly half the patients enrolled in the study experienced clinically relevant improvement. A growing number of studies have documented symptom improvement in patients with psychiatric disorders as well, suggesting that addressing patients' psychological needs produces both psychological and physical health benefits.

Training and certification

Although journal therapy is often provided by certified instructors who receive variable amounts of training in a number of programs around the country, journal therapy is best administered by a licensed psychologist (who may also be an art therapist) or psychiatrist.

Educational, professional, and ethical standards for art therapists who conduct writing therapy are regulated by The American Art Therapy Association, Inc. The American Art Therapy Credentials Board, Inc., an independent organization, grants postgraduate supervised experience. A registered art therapist who successfully completes the written examination administered by the Art Therapy Credentials Board qualifies as Board Certified (ATR-BC), a credential requiring maintenance through continuing education credits.

Resources

BOOKS

Adams, Kathleen. *Journal to the Self.* New York: Warner Books,1990.

PERIODICALS

Greenhalgh, Tricia. "Writing as Therapy." *British Medical Journal* (July 1999): 270-271.

Nye, Emily F. "Writing as Healing." *Qualitative Inquiry* (December 1997): 439-450.

Smyth, Joshua M. et al. "Effects of Writing About Stressful Experiences on Symptom Reduction in Patients With Asthma or Rheumatoid Arthritis." *Journal of the American Medical Association* (April 1999): 1304-1309.

Smyth, Joshua M. "Written Emotional Expression: Effect Sizes, Outcome Types, and Moderating Variables." *Journal of Consulting and Clinical Psychology* (1998): 174-184.

Spiegel, David. "Healing Words: Emotional Expression and Disease Outcome." *Journal of the American Medical Association* (April 1999): 1328-1329.

Walker, B. Lee, Lillian M. Nail, and Robert T. Croyle. "Does Emotional Expression Make a Difference in Reactions to Breast Cancer?" *Oncology Nursing Journal* (July 1999): 1025-1032.

ORGANIZATIONS

The American Art Therapy Association. 1202 Allanson Road. Mundelein, IL 60060-3808. <http://www.arttherapy.org>.

The Center for Journal Therapy. 12477 W. Cedar Drive, #102. Lakewood, CO 80228. <http://www.journaltherapy.com>.

Genevieve Slomski

Journal therapy

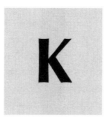

K

Ketone test *see* **Urinalysis**

Kidney dialysis *see* **Dialysis, kidney**

Kidney failure, acute *see* **Acute kidney failure**

Kidney failure, chronic *see* **Chronic kidney failure**

Kidney function tests

Definition

Kidney function tests are a cadre of tests that are used to screen for and manage renal disease. Tests commonly used for this purpose are plasma creatinine, **blood urea nitrogen (BUN)**, electrolytes, and routine **urinalysis**. Additional laboratory tests are performed to evaluate abnormal renal function and help differentiate between causes. The most commonly used follow-up tests are creatinine clearance, plasma and urine osmolality, and urine sodium.

Purpose

Renal function tests are used to screen for renal disease, to differentiate the cause of renal disease, and to determine the extent of renal dysfunction. These tests attempt to define the clinical state of renal dysfunction and not the process of injury. The latter is determined primarily by a combination of clinical data and biopsy to determine the histological pattern of injury.

Precautions

A complete history should be taken prior to kidney function tests to assess the patient's symptoms and food and drug intake. A wide variety of prescription and over-the-counter medications can affect blood and urine kidney function test results, as can some food and beverages. Renal function tests are performed on both blood and urine. Blood samples are collected by venipuncture from a vein in the crease of the arm. The nurse or phlebotomist performing the procedure should observe **universal precautions** for the prevention of transmission of blood-borne pathogens. The creatinine clearance test requires a timed urine sample. Explicit written instruction must accompany the explanation of how to collect this sample. It is imperative that the patient empty his or her bladder at the start of the test and not include this urine in the collection. It is equally important that all urine produced during the time of the test be saved and refrigerated, and that the bladder be emptied completely and this urine added to the collection at the end of the test.

Description

The **kidneys** are a pair of organs located in the back of the abdominal cavity on either side of the **vertebral column**. Their purpose is to filter the blood and remove wastes and excess water. They also selectively reabsorb compounds that have been filtered, thus conserving essential nutrients, electrolytes, amino acids and other biomolecules. Approximately one-quarter of the cardiac output, 1200 mL of blood per minute are received by the kidneys. Each kidney is made up of functional microscopic units called nephrons. Each nephron contains a capillary tuft, the glomerulus and a tubule. Blood flows into the kidneys, and engorges the capillary tufts. Water and small solutes pass through the vessel walls forming a filtrate of the plasma which enters the underlying space, Bowman's capsule. The walls of the capsule form a tubule that traverses the kidney. Blood leaves the glomerular capillaries through an efferent arteriole which forms a capillary network, the vasa recta, that follows the path of the tubules. The cells of the renal tubule modify the filtrate along its length ultimately forming urine that passes out of the body. The tubule is responsible for two processes, reabsorption and secretion. Reabsorption is the process of moving solutes from the tubular lumen into the interstitium that bathes the tubules, so that they can be absorbed by the vasa recta. Some substances such as glucose and sodium are one-hundred percent reabsorbed until the plasma level exceeds a certain concentration called the renal threshold. Secretion is the process of transporting solutes from the interstitium into the tubular lumen, so that they can be excreted in the urine. Secretion allows substances such as hydrogen ions to be eliminated at a rate that exceeds glomerular filtration. These processes are controlled by the selective permeability of different segments of the tubule to water, salt and urea, and the response of the distal collecting tubules to hormones such as aldosterone, antidiuretic hormone, and parathyroid hormone.

When kidney function becomes compromised by disease, the processes of glomerular filtration and tubular reabsorption and secretion become affected to different extents. This can result in retention of waste products that are incompletely filtered, loss of essential solutes that are not reabsorbed, and failure of the tubules to respond to hormonal control of electrolyte and water balance. Blood and urine biochemistry tests reflect the extent of this dysfunction and are used to characterize the clinical state of the patient. Fortunately, the kidneys have a large reserve capacity, and a significant amount of damage must be incurred before kidney function tests become significantly abnormal.

There are several renal states that can be categorized by renal function test results, but the two major ones are acute and chronic renal failure. Renal failure is a term used to describe a loss of renal function characterized by uremia, the retention of nitrogenous wastes in the blood. The acute form is rapid in onset and often reversible. It can occur as three different states, termed prerenal, renal (intrarenal), and postrenal failure. Prerenal failure results from decreased blood flow to the kidneys, and its most common cause is congestive **heart failure**. Renal failure results from injury to the glomerulus and the tubules. The most common causes are glomerulonephritis which is mediated by autoantibodies that damage the glomerulus and obstruct the tubules; pyelonephritis which is caused by a bacterial **infection** of the interstitium; and tubular damage caused by drugs, heavy metals, and viral infections. Post renal failure is caused by obstruction below the kidneys. This can result from urinary tract stones, tumors, or anatomic obstruction as in benign prostatic hypertrophy. The chronic form is characterized by slow onset without accompanying symptoms in its early stage. Chronic renal failure often follows episodes of acute renal failure, and it is not reversible. Chronic renal failure is most commonly a sequalae to acute glomerulonephritis or pyelonephritis which together account for

more than half the cases. Other causes of chronic renal failure are chronic diseases such as **diabetes mellitus**, renal vascular disease (e.g., atherosclerosis of the renal vessels), **hypertension**, polycystic kidney disease, drug damage, and **kidney stones**. Kidneys from patients with chronic renal failure will appear smaller than average and a biopsy of the kidney will demonstrate scarring of the tubules.

Laboratory tests

Regardless of the cause, most persons with acute renal failure are characterized by three common laboratory findings: reduced creatinine clearance, azotemia (excessive nitrogen compounds in the blood), and hyperkalemia (excessive potassium in the blood). Creatinine is a waste product of muscle **metabolism**. It is produced at a constant rate and filtered freely by the glomeruli without reabsorption. Therefore, creatinine levels in the blood are increased when there is reduced glomerular filtration. Although specific for glomerular disease, plasma creatinine is not a sensitive test, and about 60% of the renal capacity is usually lost before levels become abnormal. A more sensitive indicator of glomerular dysfunction is the creatinine clearance test. This test measures the ratio of urine to plasma creatinine. As plasma levels rise, urine levels fall causing the ratio to decrease before plasma creatinine becomes definitively abnormal.

CREATININE CLEARANCE TEST. The creatinine clearance is defined as the volume of plasma that contains the same amount of creatinine as is excreted in the urine in one minute. Because the tubules do not reabsorb creatinine, all of the creatinine filtered by the glomeruli in a given amount of time is excreted in the urine. This test is an estimate of the glomerular filtration rate. The test is performed by measuring creatinine in a timed urine specimen—a cumulative sample collected over a four, 12, or 24-hour hour period. Determination of the plasma creatinine is also required to calculate the urine clearance. The clearance formula is U/P x V x 1.73/A. "U" is the urine creatinine in gm/dL; "P" is the plasma creatinine in mg/dL; and "V" is the volume of urine produced per minute. This is usually calculated by dividing the volume of urine produced per day by 1440 minutes per day. "A" is the person's body surface area expressed in square meters, and 1.73 is the average body surface area in square meters. During the test, the patient must be well hydrated because under conditions of slow filtrate flow the tubules will secrete some creatinine causing an overestimate of clearance. Creatinine can be measured by a colormetric method called the Jaffe reaction or by a coupled enzymatic reaction. The Jaffe reaction is performed by mixing a plasma or diluted urine sample with a solution of sodium hydroxide and saturated picric acid. At an alkaline pH, the creatinine combines with picric acid to form creatinine picrate and the rate of absorbance change is measured over a precisely defined timed interval to eliminate interference from **proteins** and other reducing agents

Azotemia is the accumulation of nitrogenous (azo)waste products in the blood as a consequence of renal failure. The azo compounds routinely measured are creatinine, urea, and uric acid. While an increase of plasma urea or uric acid is not specific for renal disease, both compounds are retained whenever there is a reduction in the glomerular filtration rate. Of the two compounds, urea is the more sensitive, and urea levels can be used with creatinine to help differentiate prerenal and renal failure.

BLOOD UREA NITROGEN (BUN) TEST. Historically, urea concentration has been expressed as the concentration of nitrogen derived from urea, called the BUN. This test is performed by an enzymatic-ultraviolet photometric method using the enzyme urease. The enzyme catalyzes the hydrolysis of urea by water forming ammonia and carbon dioxide. A coupling enzyme, glutamate dehydrogenase, catalyzes the formation of glutamate from alpha-ketoglutamate and ammonia. In this reaction NADPH is converted to $NADP^+$ which causes a decrease in the absorbance of 340 nm light. The rate of absorbance decrease is proportional to the urea nitrogen concentration of the sample. Urea is freely filtered by the glomerulus but is reabsorbed by the tubules to a variable extent depending upon the movement of filtrate through the tubule. When filtrate flow is slow, 40% or more of the filtered urea can be reabsorbed. For this reason, BUN levels increase much more than creatinine in prerenal failure. In prerenal failure, the kidney is not damaged, but glomerular filtration is reduced because of insufficient blood flow to the glomeruli. This results in increased retention of all three azo compounds. However, poor renal blood flow is a stimulus for ADH secretion that promotes water and urea reabsorption. Since the tubules are undamaged, they reabsorb a maximal amount of urea. This causes the ratio of plasma BUN to creatinine to increase dramatically. The reabsorption of BUN is impaired in renal failure caused by renal damage because the tubules are impaired. Ratios in prerenal failure are approximately 20:1, twice that seen in renal failure caused by damaged kidneys.

Electolyte disturbances are common to all forms of renal failure. Potassium is filtered by the glomerulus and partly reabsorbed in the proximal tubule. A significant amount of potassium is secreted by the collecting tubule in response to aldosterone. Therefore, when the kidneys receive insufficient blood flow potassium is incompletely filtered. When the tubules are damaged, potassium levels rise further because the exchange of potassium for sodium is impaired.

Plasma potassium levels must be maintained within a very narrow range to avoid cardiac arrhythmia. Elevated plasma potassium is the single most important (life-threatening) consequence of renal failure. Plasma potassium is the criterion used to determine the need for dialysis and the frequency and duration of treatment. Urine sodium is very useful in helping to differentiate prerenal from renal failure. In prerenal failure, the daily excretion of sodium is lower than normal because the kidneys attempt to reabsorb sodium in order to restore blood flow. However, in renal failure, daily urine sodium loss is increased owing to tubular failure. Urinary sodium is about twofold higher in intrarenal failure than in prerenal failure.

Urinalysis

There are a variety of urine tests that assess kidney function. A simple, inexpensive screening test, routine urinalysis, is often the first test administered when kidney problems are suspected. A first-morning or randomly voided urine sample is examined visually for color and clarity, and a series of up to ten dry reagent strip biochemical tests are performed. Protein, blood, leukocytes, and specific gravity are four tests that are often abnormal in persons with renal failure. Glomerular damage causes albumin and red blood cells to pass through the basement membrane and enter the filtrate in Bowman's space. Leukocytes migrate to the site of injury and enter the filtrate through glomerular lesions and by passing between the tubular cells. Tubular failure disables the concentrating and diluting capacity of the kidneys and the urine produced is consistently of the same specific gravity as the plasma (1.010). Glucose and pH are also useful because a high percentage of diabetics develop renovascular disease, and renal failure results in acidosis (hydrogen ion retention) with concomitant failure to acidify the urine. While these findings can occur in severe lower urinary tract disease, the renal origin of the cells can often be confirmed by microscopic analysis of urinary sediment. In renal injury, stasis, protein, and obstruction of the tubules by cells cause the precipitation of mucoproteins in the tubules. When these are washed out by urine flow, they can be seen using the **microscope**, and are called casts. The finding of cellular casts in the urinary sediment, identifies the kidney as the source of the cells. Experienced technologists can often distinguish glomerular bleeding from bleeding below the kidney because the former causes characteristic abnormalities in red blood cell structure (dysmorphic cells). Furthermore, the presence of cells and casts signifies renal damage and

KEY TERMS

Blood urea nitrogen (BUN)—The nitrogen portion of urea in the bloodstream. Urea is a waste product of protein metabolism in the body.

Creatinine—The metabolized by-product of creatine, an organic compound that assists the body in producing muscle contractions. Creatinine is found in the bloodstream and in muscle tissue. It is removed from the blood by the kidneys and excreted in the urine.

Creatinine clearance rate—The clearance of creatinine from the plasma compared to its appearance in the urine. Since there is no reabsorption of creatinine, this measurement can estimate glomerular filtration rate.

Diuretic—A drug that increases the excretion of salt and water, increasing the output of urine.

Glomerular filtration rate—The rate in millimeters per minute at which plasma is filtered through the glomerular membrane.

Hematuria—The presence of blood in the urine.

Nephrologist—A doctor specializing in kidney disease.

Nephron—The functional unit of the kidney.

Oliguria—The formation of very small amounts of urine.

Osmolality—A measurement of urine concentration that depends on the number of particles dissolved in it. Values are expressed as milliosmols per kilogram (mOsm/kg) of water.

Polyuria—The formation of very large amounts of urine.

Proteinuria—The presence of protein in the urine often caused by damage to the glomerular membrane.

Renal—Pertaining to the kidney

Specific gravity—The ratio of the weight of a body fluid when compared to water.

Urea—A by-product of protein metabolism that is formed in the liver. Because urea contains ammonia, which is toxic to the body, it must be quickly filtered from the blood by the kidneys and excreted in the urine.

Uric acid—A product of purine breakdown that is excreted by the kidney. High levels of uric acid, caused by various diseases, can cause the formation of kidney stones.

Urine—A fluid containing water and dissolved substances excreted by the kidney.

rules out prerenal failure as the cause of abnormal biochemistry results.

Glomerulonephritis is the most common cause of intrarenal failure. Urinary sediment in this condition displays large numbers of both red and white blood cells, and usually a predominance of red blood cell casts. Pyleonephritis, the second most common renal disease is characterized by a predomonance of white blood cells and white blood cell casts. **Bacteria** are usually abundant in the sediment signaling the causative infection.

Postrenal failure may also result in abnormal sediment. The presence of large numbers of crystals in association with biochemical evidence of worsening renal function and hematuria may alert the clinician to the presence of a urinary tract stone. The presence of large numbers of abnormal (cancerous) transitional epithelial cells may be shed into the urine by a bladder tumor and seen in the urine microscopic exam. In such cases, an imaging test, the intravenous pyelogram, is often performed in order to identify the size, location, and possible cause of the obstruction.

OSMOLALITY. Urine osmolality is a measure of the number of dissolved particles in urine. It is a more precise measurement than specific gravity for evaluating the ability of the kidneys to concentrate or dilute the urine. Kidneys that are functioning normally will excrete water in relation to the amount consumed. Those with failing kidneys may not be able to concentrate urine. Solutes will equilibrate by passive diffusion in the tubule and the osmolality will be the same as plasma, approximately 290 mOsm/Kg water. The test may be done on a urine sample collected first thing in the morning as water deprivation overnight should concentrate the urine; multiple timed samples, or on a cumulative sample collected over a 24-hour period. In addition, the ratio of urine to plasma osmolality is another useful way to differentiate prerenal and intrarenal failure. In prerenal failure the kidneys attempt to restore blood volume by reabsorbing sodium. This raises the plasma osmolality causing release of antidiuretic hormone (ADH) from the posterior pituitary. Under the influence of ADH, the tubules reabsorb more water concentrating the urine. As mentioned, the plasma and urine osmolality are the same in intrarenal disease. The urine to plasma osmolality ratio in prerenal failure is usually twofold higher than in renal disease, in which the ratio is one.

The acute and chronic forms of renal failure display some distinguishing characteristics. In chronic renal failure, the tubules become scarred causing water loss. This results in polyruria (increased urine volume) as opposed to oliguria (low urine volume) seen in acute renal failure. Scarring also results in salt wasting causing the serum potassium to be lower than seen in acute renal failure. The urinary sediment shows heavy proteinuria, hematuria (red blood cells) and abundant casts. The casts are usually broad and waxy, which are unique characteristics of end-stage renal failure.

OTHER BLOOD TESTS. Measurement of the blood levels of other analytes regulated or affected in part by the kidneys can be useful in evaluating kidney function and in managing conditions such as osteomalacia and renal acidosis that are secondary to renal disease. These include bicarbonate, **calcium**, magnesium, **phosphorus**, **plasma renin activity**, and parathyroid hormone.

Preparation

Patients will be given specific instructions for collection of urine samples, depending on the test to be performed. During routine urinalysis, the patient will be given a sealed cup to urinate into. Nurses stress that the patient obtain a "clean catch" by initiating urination and placing the sample cup in the urine stream after a few seconds. This prevents the collection of the initial urine which may contain bacteria that are present in the lower urethra or on the skin. Some timed urine tests require an extended collection period of up to 24 hours, during which time the patient collects all urine voided and transfers it to a specimen container. Refrigeration and/or preservatives are typically required to maintain the integrity of such urine specimens. Certain dietary and/or medication restrictions may be imposed for some of the blood and urine tests. The patient may also be instructed to avoid **exercise** for a period of time before a test to prevent changes in creatinine.

Aftercare

If medication was discontinued prior to a kidney function test, it may be resumed once the test is completed.

Complications

Complications for these tests are minimal, but may include slight bleeding from a venipuncture site, hematoma (accumulation of blood under a puncture site), or fainting or feeling light-headed after venipuncture. In addition, suspension of medication or dietary changes imposed in preparation for some blood or urine tests may trigger side-effects in some individuals.

Results

Normal values for many tests are determined by the patient's age and sex. Reference values can also vary by laboratory, but are generally within the ranges that follow.

Urine tests

• Creatinine clearance. For a 24-hour urine collection, normal results are 90-139 mL/min for adult males less than 40 years old, and 80-125 mL/min for adult females less than 40 years old. For people over 40, values decrease by 6.5 mL/min for each decade of life.

• Urine osmolality. With restricted fluid intake (concentration testing), osmolality should be greater than 800 mOsm/kg of water. With increased fluid intake (dilution testing), osmolality should be less than 100 mOSm/kg in at least one of the specimens collected. A 24-hour urine osmolality should average 300-900 mOsm/Kg. A random urine osmolality should average 500-800 mOsm/Kg.

• Urine protein. A 24-hour urine collection should contain no more than 150 mg of protein.

• Urine sodium. A 24-hour urine sodium should be within 75-200 mmol/day.

Blood tests

• Blood urea nitrogen (BUN) should average 8-20 mg/dL.

• Creatinine should be 0.8-1.2 mg/dL for males, and 0.6-0.9 mg/dL for females.

• Uric acid levels for males should be 3.5-7.2 mg/dL and for females 2.6-6.0 mg/dL.

Low clearance values for creatinine indicate diminished ability of the kidneys to filter waste products from the blood and excrete them in the urine. As clearance levels decrease, blood levels of creatinine, urea, and uric acid increase. Since it can be affected by other factors, an elevated BUN, by itself, is suggestive, but not diagnostic, for kidney dysfunction. An abnormally elevated plasma creatinine is a more specific indicator of kidney disease than is BUN.

Inability of the kidneys to concentrate the urine in response to restricted fluid intake, or to dilute the urine in response to increased fluid intake during osmolality testing indicates decreased tubular function. Because the kidneys normally excrete almost no protein in the urine, its persistent presence, in amounts that exceed the normal 24-hour urine value, usually indicates glomerular or tubular injury. These can be distinguished by urine protein electrophoresis. This procedure separates proteins in an electric field based upon their charge. Albuminuria is characteristic of glomerular disease, while urinary excretion of alpha-1 and beta-2 microglobulins is characteristic of tubular damage. Proteinuria of tubular origin is caused by drugs, heavy metals, or viral infection of the kidneys. Urine protein electrophoresis also detects monoclonal immunoglobulin light chains (multiple myeloma and related conditions) and immunoglobulin fragments (systemic autoimmune diseases), which are nonrenal causes of proteinuria.

Health care team roles

Kidney function tests are ordered and interpreted by a physician. Blood samples are collected by a nurse or phlebotomist. Nurses should educate the patient on why the tests are being done and how to collect timed urine samples. In addition, patients with kidney disease may be advised to change their diets. A dietitian may be consulted.

Patient education

Some kidney problems are the result of another disease process such as diabetes or high **blood pressure**. Clinicians should take the time to inform patients about how their disease or its treatment will alter kidney function and the different measures they can take to help prevent these changes.

Resources

BOOKS

Brenner, Barry M. and Floyd C. Rector Jr., eds. *The Kidney, 6th Edition*. Philadelphia, PA: W.B. Saunders Company, 1999.

Burtis, Carl A. and Edward R. Ashwood. *Tietz Textbook of Clinical Chemistry*. Philadelphia, PA: W.B. Saunders Company, 1999.

Kaplan, Lawrence A. and Amadeo J. Pesce. *Clinical Chemistry Theory, Analysis and Correlation*. St. Louis: Mosby Publishers, 1996.

ORGANIZATIONS

National Kidney Foundation (NKF). 30 East 33rd Street, New York, NY 10016. (800)622-9020. <http://www.kidney.org>.

Jane E. Phillips, PhD

Kidney radionuclide scan

Definition

A kidney radionuclide scan, also called a kidney scan or renal scan, is a diagnostic imaging test that involves administering a small amount of radionuclide, also called a radioactive tracer, into the body and then imaging the **kidneys** with a gamma camera. The images obtained can help in the diagnosis and treatment of various kidney diseases and conditions.

Purpose

While many tests—such as x rays, ultrasounds, or computed tomography (CT scans)—can reveal the structure of the kidneys, the kidney radionuclide scan is unique in that it also reveals how the kidneys are functioning. Candidates for a kidney scan may include patients who have acute or chronic renal failure, obstruction in their **urinary system**, renal artery stenosis, kidney transplant, trauma to the kidney, reflux nephropathy, renal vascular disorders and/or **hypertension**, or congenital abnormalities.

Precautions

A kidney scan requires the use of a radioactive material; therefore, patients who are pregnant or suspect they may be pregnant are cautioned not to have the test unless the benefits outweigh the risks. Women should inform their doctor if they are breast feeding. The doctor will recommend the woman stop breast feeding for a specified period of time, depending on the particular tracer and dose used.

Description

Kidney scans are performed either in a hospital nuclear medicine department or in an outpatient radiology or nuclear medicine facility. The patient is positioned in front of, or under, a gamma camera—a special piece of equipment that detects the radiation emitted from the body and produces an image. An intravenous injection of the radionuclide is administered. Immediately after the injection imaging begins, and, in most studies, the flow of **blood** to each kidney is evaluated. Serial images of the kidneys are obtained over a specified period of time, depending upon the particular radiopharmaceutical used. Kidney scans may be performed to determine the rate at which the kidneys are filtering a patient's blood. These studies use a radiopharmaceutical called technetium DTPA (Tc99m DTPA). This radiopharmaceutical also can identify obstruction in the renal collecting system. To

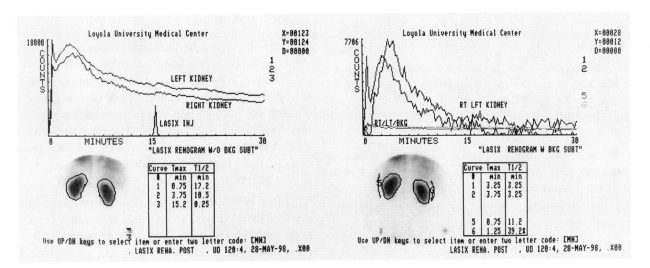

A computer-generated time activity curve generated from a renal scan. This time activity curve looks at the radiation count over a period of time. *(Photograph by Collette Placek. Reproduced by permission.)*

establish the function of the renal tubules, the radiopharmaceutical Technetium DMSA (Tc99m DMSA) is used.

A kidney scan ranges from 45 minutes to three hours in length, depending upon the goals of the test, but the test typically takes about an hour to an hour and a half. It is important to understand that kidney scans can reveal an abnormality, but they do not always identify the specific problem. They are very useful in providing information about how the various parts of the kidneys function, which, in turn, can assist in making a diagnosis.

Typically, posterior images are obtained but images are also obtained at oblique angles. If indicated, the patient may be positioned so that mobility of the kidney is demonstrated by sitting up or lying down for the images. If obstruction or renal function is being evaluated, a diuretic (drug to induce urination), such as Lasix, may be injected. If hypertension or renal artery sterosis is being evaluated, Captopril or Enalapril (ACE inhibitors) may be injected.

Preparation

No special preparation is necessary for a kidney scan. In some instances the patient may be required to drink additional liquids and to empty their bladder before the exam. If another nuclear medicine study was recently performed, the patient may have to wait for a specified period to avoid any interference from residual radioactivity in the body. The patient is instructed to remove metal items from the area to be scanned.

Aftercare

Patients can resume their normal daily activities immediately after the test. Most radioactive tracers are excreted through the urinary system, so drinking fluids after a kidney scan can help flush the tracer out of the body more quickly.

Complications

Nuclear medicine procedures are very safe. Unlike some of the dyes that may be used in x-ray studies, radioactive tracers rarely cause side effects. There are no long-lasting effects of the tracers themselves, because they have no functional effects on the body's tissues. If pharmaceuticals are injected these can temporarily raise or lower **blood pressure**, or cause one to urinate.

Results

The scan should reveal normal kidney function for the patient's age and medical status, as well as show normal relative position, size, configuration, and location of the kidneys. Initial blood flow images should reflect that blood circulation to both kidneys is equal. Patients whose images suggest a space-occupying lesion or obstruction may require other imaging procedures, such as CT or ultrasound, to provide more information. Also, if the kidneys appear to be abnormal in size, have an unusual contour, or are unusually positioned, other imaging procedures may be required.

Health care team roles

Kidney scans are performed by a nuclear medicine technologist trained in handling radioactive materials, operating the equipment, and processing data obtained during the procedure. The technologist is responsible for explaining the test to the patient, obtaining pertinent medical history, and administering injecting the radionuclide. All data collected is submitted either to a doctor who is a nuclear medicine specialist or a radiologist for interpretation. Patients obtain the results of the study from their primary care physician or the physician who ordered the study.

Resources

BOOKS

Henkin, Robert, et al. *Nuclear Medicine*. St. Louis: Mosby, 1996.

Klingensmith, Wm. C. III, Dennis Eshima, and John Goddard. *Nuclear Medicine Procedure Manual 2000-2002*.

Maisey, Michael. *Clinical Nuclear Medicine* 2nd ed. New York: Chapman and Hall, 1991.

ORGANIZATIONS

Society of Nuclear Medicine. 1850 Samuel Morse Drive, Reston, VA 20190-5316. (800) 633-2665.

OTHER

Interview with Robert H. Wagner, MD., Assistant Professor of Radiology, Section of Nuclear Medicine, Loyola University Medical Center. May 28, 1998, and June 5, 1998.

Renal Scan. <http://webmd.lycos.com/content/asset/adam_test_renogram>.

Christine Miner Minderovic, B.S., R.T., R.D.M.S.

Kidney stone analysis *see* **Stone analysis**

Kidney stones

Definition

Kidney stones are solid accumulations of material that form in the tubal system of the kidney. Kidney stones cause problems when they block the flow of urine through or out of the kidney. When the stones move along the ureter (the tube that connects the kidney and the urinary bladder), they cause severe **pain**.

Description

Urine is formed by the **kidneys**. **Blood** flows into the kidneys, and specialized tubes (nephrons) within the kidneys allow a certain amount of fluid from the blood, and certain substances dissolved in that fluid, to flow out of the body as urine. However, sometimes tiny crystals may form in the urine, meet, and cling together to create a larger solid mass called a kidney stone. A kidney stone is also called a nephrolith or urolith (nephro refers to the kidney, uro refers to urine, and lith means stone).

Many people do not ever find out that they have stones in their kidneys. These stones are small enough to allow the kidney to continue functioning normally, never causing any pain. These are called silent stones. Kidney stones cause problems when they interfere with the normal flow of urine. They can block (obstruct) the flow down the tube (the ureter) that carries urine from the kidney to the bladder. When pressure in the kidney builds from backed-up urine, the kidney may swell (hydronephrosis). If the kidney is subjected to this pressure for some time, it may cause damage to the delicate kidney structures. When the kidney stone is lodged further down the ureter, the backed-up urine may also cause the ureter to swell (hydroureter). Because the ureters are muscular tubes, the presence of a stone will make these muscular tubes spasm, causing severe pain.

About 10% of all people will have a kidney stone in their lifetime. Kidney stones are most common among:

- Caucasians
- males
- people over the age of 30
- people who previously have had kidney stones
- relatives of persons with kidney stones

Causes and symptoms

Kidney stones can be composed of a variety of substances. The most common types of kidney stones include:

- **Calcium** stones. About 80% of all kidney stones fall into this category. These stones are composed of either calcium and phosphate, or calcium and oxalate. People with calcium stones may have other diseases that cause them to have increased blood levels of calcium. These diseases include primary parathyroidism, sarcoidosis, hyperthyroidism, renal tubular acidosis, multiple myeloma, hyperoxaluria, and some types of **cancer**. A diet heavy in meat, fish, and poultry can cause calcium oxalate stones.

- Struvite stones. About 10% of all kidney stones fall into this category. This type of stone is composed of magnesium ammonium phosphate. These stones occur most often when persons have had repeated urinary tract infections with certain types of **bacteria**. These bacteria produce a substance called urease, which increases the pH of urine, making urine more alkaline and less acidic. This chemical environment allows struvite to precipitate in the urine, forming stones.

- Uric acid stones. About 5% of all kidney stones fall into this category. Uric acid stones occur when increased amounts of uric acid circulate in the bloodstream. When the uric acid content becomes very high, it can no longer remain dissolved. Molecules of uric acid precipitate out of the urine. A kidney stone is formed when these bits of uric acid begin to cling to each other within the kidney, slowly growing into a solid mass. About half of all persons with this type of stone also have deposits of uric acid elsewhere in their body, commonly in the joint of the big toe. This painful disorder is called **gout**. Other causes of uric acid stones include **chemotherapy** for cancer, certain bone marrow disorders where blood cells are over-produced, and an inherited disorder called Lesch-Nyhan syndrome.

- Cystine stones. About 2% of all kidney stones fall into this category. Cystine is a type of amino acid. People with this type of kidney stone have an abnormality in the way their bodies process amino acids in the diet.

People who have kidney stones usually do not have symptoms until the stones pass into the ureter. Prior to this, some individuals may notice blood in their urine. Once the stone is in the ureter, however, most people will experience bouts of very severe pain. The pain is crampy and spasmodic, and is referred to as colic. The pain usually begins in the flank region, the area between the lower ribs and the pelvis. As the stone moves closer to the bladder, a person will often feel the pain radiating along the inner thigh. In women, the pain may be felt in the vulva. In men, the pain may be felt in the testicles. Nausea, vomiting, extremely frequent and painful urination, and obvious blood in the urine are common. **Fever** and chills usually mean that the ureter has become obstructed, allowing bacteria to become trapped in the kidney causing a kidney **infection** (pyelonephritis).

Diagnosis

Diagnosing kidney stones is based on a person's history of the very severe, distinctive pain associated with the stones. Diagnosis includes laboratory examination of a urine sample and an x-ray examination. During the passage of a stone, examination of the urine almost always reveals blood. A number of x-ray tests are used to diag-

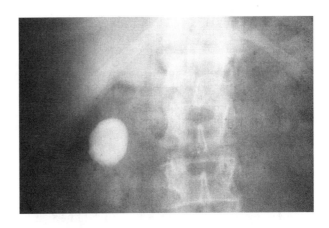

X ray of kidney stone. *(Custom Medical Stock Photo. Reproduced by permission.)*

nose kidney stones. A plain x ray of the kidneys, ureters, and bladder may or may not reveal the stone. A series of x rays taken after injecting iodine dye into a vein is usually a more reliable way of seeing a stone. This procedure is called an intravenous pyelogram (IVP). The dye highlights the **urinary system** as it travels through it. In the case of an obstruction, the dye will be stopped by the stone or will only be able to get past the stone at a slow trickle.

When a person is passing a kidney stone, it is important that all of the urine is strained through a special sieve. This is to ensure that the stone is caught. The stone can then be sent to a special laboratory for analysis so that the chemical composition of the stone can be determined. After the kidney stone has been passed, other tests will be required to understand the underlying condition that may have caused the stone to form. Collecting urine for 24 hours, followed by careful analysis of its chemical makeup, can often determine a number of reasons for stone formation.

Treatment

A person with a kidney stone will say that the most important aspect of treatment is adequate pain relief. Because the pain of passing a kidney stone is so severe, narcotic pain medications such as meperidine or morphine are often required. It is believed that stones may pass more quickly if a person is encouraged to drink large amounts of water (2–3 quarts, or 1.8–2.8 liters, per day). If an individual is vomiting or unable to drink because of the pain, it may be necessary to provide fluids through a vein. If symptoms and urine tests indicate the presence of infection, **antibiotics** will be required.

Although most kidney stones will pass on their own, some will not. Surgical removal of a stone may become necessary when a stone appears too large to pass. Surgery

KEY TERMS

Hydronephrosis—Swelling of a kidney due to elevated pressure from excess fluid accumulation.

Hydroureter—Swelling of a ureter due to elevated pressure from excess fluid accumulation.

Lithotripsy—Technique that uses focused sound waves to pulverize kidney stones, thus avoiding surgery.

Nephron—Tube within the kidney that processes filtrate from the blood, reclaiming some substances and creating urine.

Pyelonephritis—Infection of the kidney.

Ureter—Tube that connects the kidney and urinary bladder, whose function is to transport urine.

may also be required if the stone is causing serious obstructions, pain that cannot be treated, heavy bleeding, or infection. Several alternatives exist for removing stones. One method involves inserting a tube into the bladder and up into the ureter. A tiny basket is then passed through the tube, and an attempt is made to snare the stone and pull it out. Open surgery to remove an obstructing kidney stone was relatively common in the past, but current methods allow the stone to be crushed with shock waves (called **lithotripsy**). These shock waves may be aimed at the stone from outside of the body by passing the necessary equipment through the bladder and into the ureter. The shock waves may be aimed at the stone from inside the body by placing the instrument through a tiny incision located near the stone. The stone fragments may then pass naturally or may be removed through the incision. All of these methods reduce an individual's recovery time considerably when compared to the traditional open operation.

Alternative treatment

Alternative treatments for kidney stones include the use of herbal medicine, **homeopathy**, acupuncture, **acupressure**, hypnosis, or guided imagery to relieve pain. Starfruit (*Averrhoa carambola*) is recommended to increase the amount of urine a person passes and to relieve pain. Dietary changes can be made to reduce the risk of future stone formation and to facilitate the resorption of existing stones. Supplementation with magnesium, a smooth muscle relaxant, can help reduce pain and facilitate stone passing. Homeopathy and herbal medicine, both western and Chinese, recommend a number of remedies that may help prevent kidney stones.

Prognosis

A person's prognosis depends on the underlying disorder causing the development of kidney stones. In most cases, people with uncomplicated calcium stones will recover very well. About 60% of these individuals, however, will have other kidney stones. Struvite stones are particularly dangerous because they may grow extremely large, filling the tubes within the kidney. These are called staghorn stones and will not pass out in the urine. They will require surgical removal. Uric acid stones may also become staghorn stones.

Health care team roles

A physician makes an initial diagnosis of kidney stones. A radiologist confirms the diagnosis. A surgeon is needed to operatively remove a kidney stone. A technician performs a lithotripsy under the supervision of a physician.

Prevention

Prevention of kidney stones depends on the type of stone and the presence of an underlying disease. In almost all cases, increasing fluid intake so that a person consistently drinks several quarts of water a day is an important preventive measure. Persons with calcium stones may benefit from taking a medication called a diuretic, which has the effect of decreasing the amount of calcium passed in the urine. Eating less meat, fish, and chicken may be helpful for individuals with calcium oxalate stones. Other items in the diet that may encourage calcium oxalate stone formation include beer, black pepper, berries, broccoli, chocolate, spinach, and tea. Uric acid stones may require treatment with a medication called allopurinol. Struvite stones will require removal and an affected person should receive an antibiotic. When a disease is identified as the cause of stone formation, treatment specific to that disease may lessen the likelihood of repeated stones.

Resources

BOOKS

Asplin, John, Frederic L. Coe, and Murray Favus. "Nephrolithiasis." In *Harrison's Principles of Internal Medicine, 14th ed.*, edited by Anthony S. Fauci et al. New York: McGraw-Hill, 1998, 1569-74.

Gennari, F. John. *Medical Management of Kidney and Electrolyte Disorders.* New York: Marcel Dekker, 2001.

Hruska, Keith. "Renal Calculi (Nephrolithiasis)." In *Cecil Textbook of Medicine, 21st ed.*, edited by Lee Goldman and J. Claude Bennett. Philadelphia: W.B. Saunders, 2000, 622-27.

Massry, Shaul G., and Richard J. Glassock. *Massry & Glassock's Textbook of Nephrology, 4th ed*. Philadelphia: Lippincott Williams & Wilkins, 2001.

Savitz, Gail, Stephen W. Leslie, and Gail Golomb. *The Kidney Stones Handbook: A Patient's Guide to Hope, Cure, and Prevention*. Roseville, CA: Four Geez Press, 1999.

PERIODICALS

de Lorimier, A. A. "Alcohol, Wine, and Health." *American Journal of Surgery* 180(5) (2000): 357-61.

Grases, F., O. Sohnel, and A. Costa-Bauza. "Renal Stone Formation and Development." *International Journal of Urology and Nephrology* 31(5) (1999): 591-600.

Hulton, S. A. "Evaluation of Urinary Tract Calculi in Children." *Archives of Diseases of Children* 84(4) (April 2001): 320-23.

McConnell, E. A. "Myths & Facts... about Kidney Stones." *Nursing* 31(1) (January 2001): 73-7.

Portis, A. J., and C. P. Sundaram. "Diagnosis and Initial Management of Kidney Stones." *American Family Physician* 63(7) (April 2001): 1329-38.

Verkoelen, C. F., and M. S. Schepers. "Changing Concepts in the Aetiology of Renal Stones." *Current Opinion in Urology* 10(6) (2000): 539-44.

Young, J. "Action Stat. Kidney Stone." *Nursing* 30(7) (July 2000): 33-8.

ORGANIZATIONS

American Academy of Family Physicians. 11400 Tomahawk Creek Parkway, Leawood, KS 66211-2672. (913) 906-6000. <http://www.aafp.org>. fp@aafp.org.

American Association for Clinical Chemistry. 2101 L Street, NW, Suite 202, Washington, DC 20037-1558. (800) 892-1400. (202) 857-0717. Fax: (202) 887-5093. <http://www.aacc.org>. info@aacc.org.

American Foundation for Urologic Disease. 1128 North Charles Street, Baltimore, MD 21201. (800) 242-2383. (410) 468-1800. <http://www.afud.org>. admin@afud.org.

American Urological Association. 1120 North Charles Street, Baltimore, MD 21201. (410) 727-1100. Fax: (410) 223-4370. <http://www.auanet.org/index_hi.cfm>. aua@auanet.org.

National Kidney Foundation. 30 East 33rd Street, Suite 1100, New York, NY 10016. (800) 622-9010. (212) 889-2210. Fax: (212) 689-9261. <http://www.kidney.org/>. info@kidney.org.

OTHER

American Foundation for Urologic Disease. <http://www.afud.org/conditions/ksgloss.html>.

Kidney Stone Photographs. <http://www.herringlab.com/photos/>.

Lithotripsy. <http://pluto.apl.washington.edu/harlett2/artgwww/acoustic/medical/litho.html>.

Medical College of Georgia. <http://www.mcg.edu/news/96features/kidneystone.html>.

National Kidney and Urologic Diseases Information Clearinghouse. <http://www.niddk.nih.gov/health/kidney/pubs/stonadul/stonadul.htm>.

University of California Los Angeles. <http://www.radsci.ucla.edu:8000/gu/stones/kidneystone.html>.

L. Fleming Fallon, Jr., M.D., Dr.P.H.

Kidney, ureter, and bladder x-ray study

Definition

A kidney, ureter, and bladder (KUB) x ray is an AP (anteroposterior) abdominal x ray. Despite its name, KUB does not show the ureters and only sometimes shows the **kidneys** and bladder and, even then, with uncertainty.

Purpose

The KUB is used to detect **kidney stones, foreign bodies** in children, and to diagnose some gastrointestinal disorders. It is also used as a preliminary film for an intravenous pyelogram and **barium enema**, or as a follow-up x ray after the placement of devices such as ureteral stents and nasogastric or nasointestinal tubes (feeding tubes). It may also be requested in the operating room to detect sponges or clamps before the patient's incision is closed and would be done with the portable x-ray machine.

Precautions

Because of the risks of radiation exposure to the fetus, pregnant women are advised to avoid this x-ray procedure.

A KUB study is a preliminary screening test for kidney stones, and should be followed by a more sophisticated series of diagnostic tests [such as an **abdominal ultrasound, intravenous urography,** or computed tomography scan (CT scan)], if kidney stones are suspected.

Description

A KUB is typically a single x-ray procedure. The patient lies supine (face-up) on the x-ray table and may flex the knees if it is more comfortable. The x-ray technologist centers on the iliac crest, making sure the pubic

KEY TERMS

Pubic symphysis—The line of fusion between the pubic bones.

Ureteral stent—A surgical device implanted in patients with damaged ureters that holds the ureter open so that urine can flow freely from the kidneys to the bladder.

symphysis will be visualized. The collimation may be reduced to the ASIS (anterior superior iliac spine) for better detail of the kidney outline, ureter and bladder, especially during an intravenous pyelogram. The radiographic technique of the film should demonstrate peritoneal fat lines, psoas muscles, and both renal (kidney) outlines. The patient is asked to hold his or her breath on expiration. Sometimes a second film is obtained with the patient standing.

Preparation

A KUB study requires no special diet, fluid restrictions, medications, or other preparation. The patient is typically required to wear a hospital gown or similar attire. A lead apron can not be used since it will obstruct necessary structures of the abdomen.

Aftercare

No special aftercare treatment or regimen is required for a KUB study.

Complications

The KUB study is an x-ray procedure, so it does involve minor exposure to radiation.

Results

Normal KUB x-ray films show two kidneys of a similar size and shape, no renal calculi (stones), and a normal bowel gas pattern.

Abnormal KUB films may show calculi (kidney stones). If both kidneys are visible, it may be possible to diagnose renal size discrepancies. The film may also demonstrate an increase in bowel gas, indicating a possible bowel obstruction. In this case an additional film of the abdomen should be done either upright or in a lateral decubitus position. Soft tissue masses may also be visualized on a KUB.

Health care team roles

The x-ray technologist must confirm with the emergency physician that just a KUB is necessary to complete a diagnosis instead of a complete abdominal series. When a KUB is done with the mobile x-ray machine all staff remaining in the room must receive lead shielding. All radiographical technologists must be certified and registered with the A.S.R.T. and continue to upgrade and maintain their certification with ongoing education credits.

Patient education

The x-ray technologist must advise the patient to remain still and follow breathing instructions so that a detailed image of the abdomen may be taken.

Resources

BOOKS

Meschan, Isadore. *Radiographic Positioning and Related Anatomy.* 3rd ed. Philadelphia: W.B. Saunders and Co., 1996.

Pagana, Kathleen Deska, and Timothy James Pagana. *Mosby's Diagnostic and Laboratory Test Reference.* 4th ed. St. Louis, MO: Mosby, 1998.

Lorraine K. Ehresman

Kidneys

Definition

The kidneys maintain body fluid volumes and **blood pressure**, filter **blood**, and contribute to waste removal by producing urine.

Description

The kidneys are two bean-shaped organs that sit just below the rib cage on either side of the **spinal cord**. Each is about the size of a bar of soap. At any one time 20–25% of the body's blood flows through them, even though they comprise only 0.5% of the body's total weight. At this rate, the kidneys filter the entire blood supply 60 times per day.

Blood flows into the kidney through the renal artery and exits through the renal vein. Within the kidney are many small capillaries that perfuse it with blood, giving the organ its reddish-brown color.

The gross anatomy of the kidney can be divided into four parts:

- *Capsule:* A thin but tough outer membrane that protects the kidney against **infection** and trauma.

- *Cortex:* The outer layer of the kidney's interior, about 1 cm (0.4 inch) thick.

- *Medulla:* The inner layer of the kidney's interior, which contains triangular structures called renal pyramids. Between pyramids are sections of cortex called renal columns.

- *Renal pelvis:* A large funnel for collecting urine from all parts of the kidney, connected to the bladder by the ureter.

Each cortex and medulla together contain about a million nephrons, microscopic filtering systems that are the basic unit of each kidney. Each nephron has two main components. The first is a vascular system that includes 1) the glomerulus, 2) afferent and efferent arterioles, and 3) peritubular capillaries. The second, tubular component contains five main parts: Bowman's capsule, proximal tubule, loop of Henle, distal tubule, and the collecting duct.

Bowman's capsule forms one end of each nephron. It contains a bundle of tiny capillaries called the glomerulus, which receives its bloodflow from the afferent arteriole. The glomerulus filters **minerals**, nutrients, wastes, and water from the blood that flows through it, and passes them down into the proximal tubule. The glomerulus also returns large plasma **proteins** and red blood cells to the blood supply through the efferent arteriole. The efferent arteriole is connected to a second capillary bed called the peritubular capillaries. These two successive capillary beds create a pressure difference that forces fluid through the nephron.

Once filtrate enters the proximal tubule, specialized cells reabsorb sodium and other ions, water, glucose, and amino acids back into the blood. The fluid then goes into the loop of Henle, which helps concentrate the waste products to be excreted in urine. After the loop of Henle, fluid then flows into the highly coiled distal tubule, where potassium is secreted and more water and sodium are reabsorbed back into the blood. The fluid then flows into the last part of the nephron, the collecting duct, where final adjustments are made to the urine concentration. The collecting ducts respond to the antidiuretic hormone (ADH), which regulates the amount of water reabsorbed by the blood. The urine then flows through the renal pelvis to the ureter, which delivers urine to the bladder for excretion.

Function

By filtering the blood, the kidneys play a very important role in the body. They adjust the water volume, remove wastes such as urea, ammonia, and drugs, establish **acid-base balance**, determine the composition of blood, help maintain blood pressure, stimulate the production of red blood cells, and determine **calcium** levels.

The maintenance of water volume is a particularly important function. When the body sweats on a hot day or during **exercise**, it needs a way to sense water loss to avoid **dehydration**. Water volume is monitored by specialized osmoreceptors in the hypothalamus that measure sodium concentration in the blood. A high sodium concentration means there is insufficient water; this signals the hypothalamus to increase ADH secretion, which in turn prevents the kidneys from reabsorbing water from the blood in the collecting ducts. If the sodium concentration is low, there is too much water in the blood, so the hypothalamus reduces ADH secretion, which tells the kidneys to increase the water concentration of the urine.

The kidneys are also crucial in removing waste products such as urea, ammonia, and any chemical compounds such as medications from the blood. For this reason patients with damaged kidneys must be monitored closely when they take medications that are excreted in the urine. If the kidneys are not working properly, drug concentrations in the blood could rise to fatal levels.

In addition, the kidneys play a pivotal role in the body's acid-base balance. The blood's pH is maintained by a fixed ratio of hydrogen-to-bicarbonate ions in the blood. If the number of hydrogen ions increase, then the blood becomes acidic, a condition known as acidosis. Likewise, if the number of sodium bicarbonate ions rise, the blood becomes basic, a condition known as alkalosis. The kidneys help sustain this hydrogen-to-bicarbonate ratio by adjusting the amount of bicarbonate in the blood. If the blood is too basic the proximal and distal tubules of the kidney will decrease bicarbonate reabsorption and more bicarbonate will be excreted into the urine. If the blood is acidic, then the proximal tubule will allow reabsorption of bicarbonate back into the blood and excrete more hydrogen into the urine.

Another major task the kidneys perform is to help maintain blood pressure. Kidney cells can recognize when a drop in blood pressure occurs, because when this happens, blood flow to the kidney decreases. This means less sodium is present in the kidney cells, a condition that causes the kidney cells to release an enzyme called renin. Renin converts angiotensin I into angiotensin II, which in turn constricts **blood vessels** and causes sodium retention by the kidneys, thereby raising blood pressure. This is known as the renin-angiotensin system. Angiotensin II also causes the **adrenal glands** to release the hormone aldosterone, which tells the kidneys to allow more sodium and water to be reabsorbed back into the blood. This

KEY TERMS

Adrenal gland—Small gland on top of each kidney that produces and releases several different hormones that are involved in maintaining internal fluid and salt levels and also mediates stress responses.

Angiotensin I—Inactive form of angiotensin that circulates in the blood; it is a precursor of angiotensin II.

Angiotensin II—Active form of angiotensin that constricts blood vessels, thus raising blood pressure.

Capillary—Small blood vessel that is the point of connection for blood and veins and where exchanges occur between the blood and tissue.

Hydronephrosis—Distention of the renal pelvis that occurs when urine is trapped in the kidney and blocked from flowing into the bladder.

Ureter—Carries urine from the kidney to the bladder.

increase in water volume in the blood increases blood pressure. Many medications for high blood pressure act by working on the kidneys to decrease blood volume and therefore blood pressure. These blood pressure medications are collectively known as diuretics.

Role in human health

The kidneys play a crucial role in human health because they perform many vital functions. The kidneys work constantly, simultaneously, and influence each other. Individuals are born with two kidneys but can function with one. However, a person with kidney function at 10–15% of capacity will require dialysis or a kidney transplant to sustain life. Individuals with high blood pressure and diabetes have a significant risk of kidney disease.

Common diseases and disorders

Diabetic nephropathy

Diabetic patients cannot process blood glucose properly, and if their disease is untreated or poorly controlled, it can lead to high blood sugar levels. This can damage the nephrons, leading to diabetic neuropathy. This usually means that soft kidney tissue hardens and thickens, a process called sclerosis; this is especially true for the glomerulus. The American Diabetes Association esti-

mates that 35–45% of type 1 diabetics and 20–30% of type 2 diabetics have damaged kidneys. Because the symptoms of nephropathy may not appear until 80% of kidney function is gone, periodic tests of kidney function and strict compliance with diet and treatment regimens are important for patients with diabetes.

High blood pressure

The kidneys use small blood vessels called capillaries to filter blood and to help create a pressure gradient to move fluid through the nephron. Continuous high blood pressure can damage the fragile walls of these vessels. When this happens, blood may not filter properly, allowing waste products and/or drug levels to build up, sometimes to dangerous or fatal levels.

Kidney stones

Kidneys stones occur when crystals form in the lumen of the tubules or in the ureters. The stones are most commonly made of calcium and oxalate or phosphate. The basis of stone formation is not clear but certain foods in certain people can cause them to accrete. **Kidney stones** can be extremely painful, and can also cause hydronephrosis. Patients with kidney stones are encouraged to drink plenty of water in effort to have the stone excreted in the urine. In some cases, kidney stones must be surgically removed.

Polycystic kidney disease

Polycystic kidney disease (PKD) is an inherited disease in which cysts form in the kidney. These fluid-filled cysts can take over a significant amount of space in the kidney, eventually reducing kidney function and causing kidney failure. Most cases of PKD show no symptoms until the patient is well into adulthood. PKD that appears in children is often more virulent, frequently leading to kidney failure and death. **Nutrition** and dietary modification play a major role in controlling the progression of PKD.

Wilms' tumor

Wilms' tumor, or nephroblastoma, is a **cancer** of the kidney that appears during childhood. Both sporadic cases and a few rare inherited cases have been linked to mutations in the Wilm's tumor gene (WT1) on chromsome 11. Many cases of Wilms' tumor are curable if caught early enough.

Resources

BOOKS

Cohen, Barbara, and Dena Wood. *Structure and Function of the Human Body,* 7th ed. Philadelphia, PA: Lippincott Williams and Wilkins, 2000.

Johnson, R.J., and J. Feehally. *Comprehensive Clinical Nephrology.* London: Harcourt Publishers, 2000.

ORGANIZATIONS

National Kidney Foundation. 30 East 33rd St. Suite 1100, New York, NY 10016. (800) 622-9010. <http://www.kidney.org>.

Polycystic Kidney Disease Foundation. 4901 Main St. Suite 200, Kansas City, MO 64112. (800) PKD-CURE. <http://www.pkdcure.org>.

Susan M. Mockus, Ph.D.

Kleihauer-Betke test *see* **Fetal cell screen**

KOH test

Definition

The KOH (potassium hydroxide) test is the microscopic examination of a skin, nail, or hair sample for the presence of a fungus that infects these structures. The test takes its name from the chemical formula for potassium hydroxide (KOH), the substance used in the test to clear skin cells, protein, and cellular debris, making the **fungi** easier to observe. A sample from the infected area is analyzed under a **microscope** following the addition of a few drops of potassium hydroxide. A stain may be added to make the fungi more easily visible.

Purpose

The KOH test is used for the rapid, differential diagnosis of infections produced by dermatophytes from skin disorders such as eczema and psoriasis which may appear similar. Dermatophytes are a type of fungus that invade the skin, hair, or nails, and produce an **infection** commonly called ringworm (tinea). There are three genera of fungi commonly implicated in human skin, nail, and hair infections. These are *Trichophyton spp.*(found in skin, nail, and hair infections), *Epidermophyton spp.* (skin and nail infections), and *Microsporum spp.* (skin and hair infections). The KOH test may also be used on scrapings from the mouth or vagina for the rapid identification of *Candida spp.*, the cause of yeast infections of the mouth (thrush) and the vagina (vaginitis). If a dermatophyte or yeast infection is found, antibiotic treatment can be started immediately, and further testing is not usually required. The KOH prep cannot identify the specific causative organism. When fungus is found, the specimen can be submitted for **fungal culture** to identify the causative agent(s).

Precautions

There are no specific precautions for patients who require this test. Health care professionals who perform this test should be properly trained in skin scraping, nail, and hair follicle removal procedures, the identification of fungi and yeasts by microscopy, and the safe handling of specimens.

Description

Ringworm of the skin produces red or gray, scaly patches of itchy skin. Hair infection results in brittle hair shafts that fall out easily. Deeper infections may be ulcerative, discolored, and purulent. The health care provider selects an infected area from which to collect the sample. A scalpel or edge of a glass slide is used to gently scrape skin scales from the infected area. For hair samples, a forceps is used to remove hair shafts and follicles from the infected site. If the test is to be performed immediately, the scrapings are placed directly onto a microscope slide and are covered with 10% or 20% potassium hydroxide. If the test will be sent to a laboratory, the scrapings are placed in a sterile covered container for later testing.

After adding KOH, the slide should be allowed to stand for five minutes in order to dissolve skin cells, hair, and debris. If the sample remains unclear after five minutes, it may be left for an additional five to 10 minutes. Dimethyl sulfoxide can be added to the KOH to enhance clearing, and lactophenol cotton blue stain can be added to make the fungi easier to see. The slide may be gently heated to enhance the digestive action of the KOH. If a fluorescent microscope is available, calcofluor white stain may be added to the KOH preparation. This will cause the fungi to become fluorescent, making them easier to identify.

Dermatophytes are easily recognized under the microscope by their long branch-like tubular structures called hyphae. Fungi causing ringworm infections produce septate (segmented) hyphae. Some show the presence of spores formed directly from the hyphae (arthroconidia). Yeast infections of the skin can also be identified by the KOH test. Yeast cells appear round or oval and budding forms may be seen.

Fungal infections of the skin are described by the site of infection. Tinea cruris is a fungal infection occurring in the groin or inner thigh, tinea pedis on the feet, tinea capitis on the scalp and hair, and tinea unguium on the nails. Tinea versicolor refers to a fungal infection of the skin caused by *Malassezia furfur*. This organism cannot be cultured, and is recognized by characteristic yellowish skin patches and the microscopic appearance of the organism. The fungus produces curved hyphae and round yeast forms that give it a spaghetti-and-meatball appearance under the microscope.

Preparation

There is no special preparation for the patient prior to sample collection.

Aftercare

The patient will experience slight discomfort from sample collection. The skin site or area exposed when the nail is removed may need to be covered by a guaze bandage.

Complications

There are usually no complications for the patient associated with this test.

Results

A normal, or negative, KOH test shows no fungi (no dermatophytes or yeast). Dermatophytes or yeast seen on a KOH test indicate the patient's symptoms are caused by a fungal infection. Follow-up tests are usually unnecessary.

Health care team roles

Physicians, nurses, or physician assistants usually collect the skin, nail, or hair samples from the patient. The KOH test procedure may be performed by the physician or by a clinical laboratory scientist/medical technologist. If fungal cultures are required, they are performed by a clinical laboratory scientist/medical technologist who specializes in microbiology.

Patient education

The health care professional who collects the sample also explains the testing procedure to the patient, and explains why the test is required. The physician or nurse will also explain the treatment regimen, as well as the importance of adhering to the treatment as required, if a fungal infection is diagnosed.

Resources

BOOKS

Fischbach, Frances. "Diagnosis of Fungal Disease." In *A Manual of Laboratory & Diagnostic Tests*. 6th ed. Philadelphia: Lippincott Williams & Wilkins, 2000, pp.521-525.

Forbes, Betty A., Daniel F. Sahm, and Alice S. Weissfeld. "Laboratory Methods in Basic Mycology." In *Bailey & Scott's Diagnostic Microbiology*. 10th ed. St. Louis: Mosby, 1998, pp.870-961.

Sacher, Ronald A., Richard A. McPherson, with Joseph M. Campos. "Direct Visualization of Infectious Agents." In *Widmann's Clinical Interpretation of Laboratory Tests*. 11th ed. Philadelphia: F. A. Davis Company, 2000, pp.613-618.

ORGANIZATIONS

The American Society for Clinical Laboratory Science. 7910 Woodmont Ave., Suite 523, Bethesda, MD 20814. (301) 657-2768. <http://www.ascls.org>.

The American Society for Microbiology. 1752 N St. N.W., Washington, DC 20036. (202) 737-3600. <http://www.asmusa.org>.

OTHER

"Dermatologic Disorders: Fungal Skin Infections." In *The Merck Manual of Diagnosis and Therapy*. 17th ed., internet edition, <http://www.merck.com/pubs/mmanual>, 2001.

"Dermatologic Disorders: Special Diagnostic Methods." In *The Merck Manual of Diagnosis and Therapy*. 17th ed., internet edition, <http://www.merck.com/pubs/mmanual>, 2001.

Linda D. Jones, B.A., PBT (ASCP)

KUB *see* **Kidney, ureter, and bladder x-ray study**

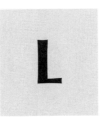

Labor and delivery *see* **Childbirth**

Lacerations *see* **Wounds**

Lactate dehydrogenase isoenzymes test *see*
   Liver function tests

Lactation

Definition

Lactation is the medical term used for breastfeeding. It also specifically refers to the synthesis and secretion of milk.

Purpose

Breastfeeding provides a baby with **nutrition** in the form of breast milk. Not only does breast milk contain all the nutrients needed by a rapidly developing newborn, but it also contains antibodies that provide the baby with additional protection from common early childhood diseases.

Precautions

Most common illnesses can not be transmitted via breast milk. However, some **viruses**, including HIV (the virus that causes **AIDS**) can be passed in breast milk; for this reason, women who are HIV-positive should not breastfeed.

Many medications have not been tested in nursing women, so it is not known if these drugs can affect a breast-fed child. A nursing woman should always check with her doctor before taking any medications, including over-the-counter drugs.

These drugs are not safe to take while nursing:

- radioactive drugs for some diagnostic tests

- chemotherapy drugs for **cancer**

- bromocriptine

- ergotamine

- lithium

- methotrexate

- street drugs (including **marijuana**, heroin, amphetamines)

- tobacco

Description

Early in a woman's **pregnancy** her milk-producing glands, called mammary glands, begin to prepare for the baby's arrival and by the sixteenth week of pregnancy the breasts are ready to produce milk. Shortly after the baby is born, the expulsion of the placenta triggers hormone shifts in the woman's body to activate lactation. The levels of the hormones estrogen and progesterone fall abruptly while the level of the hormone prolactin—the main hormone involved in the biosynthesis of milk—increases. The anterior **pituitary gland** secretes prolactin during lactation in very large quantities so that by 36 to 96 hours postpartum the woman's milk volume has dramatically increased. Subsequently, the volume of milk the mother produces levels off and the removal of milk becomes the predominant factor in regulating milk production.

Another hormone called oxytocin controls the release of milk from the breasts. The baby's sucking stimulates nerve endings in the nipple, which signal the mother's pituitary gland to release the oxytocin. This is called the "let-down reflex." While the baby's sucking is the primary stimulus for the reflex, a baby's cry, thoughts of the baby, or the sound of running water also may trigger the response.

Breast milk cannot be duplicated by artificial milk, although both contain protein, fat, and **carbohydrates**. Breast milk changes to meet the specific needs of a baby.

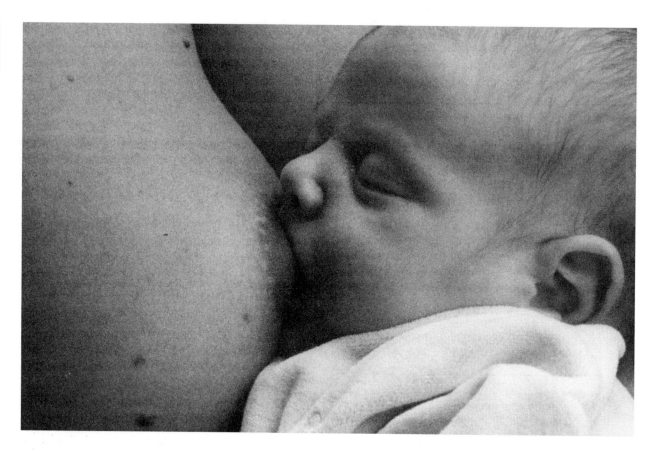

Breastfeeding is healthy for both mother and baby. *(Photograph by J.M. Trois. Science Source/Photo Researchers. Reproduced by permission.)*

In particular, the mother produces milk called colostrum at the end of pregnancy and in the initial postpartum period. Colostrum is called "first milk" and is thicker than mature milk. It is yellowish in color and is rich in **proteins**, many of which are immunoglobulins that can protect the child against illness and **allergies**. Immunoglobuoins are part of the body's natural defense system against infections and other agents that can cause disease. Breast milk also helps a baby's own **immune system** mature faster. As a result, breast-fed babies have fewer ear infections, bouts of **diarrhea**, rashes, allergies, and other medical problems than bottle-fed babies do.

There are many other benefits to breast milk. Because it is easily digested, babies do not get constipated. Breast-fed babies have fewer speech impediments due to good cheekbone development and jaw alignment.

Breastfeeding is also good for the mother. It releases hormones that stimulate the uterus to contract, helping the uterus to return to normal size after delivery and reducing the risk of bleeding. The act of producing milk burns calories, which helps the mother to lose excess weight gained during pregnancy. Breastfeeding also may be related to a lower risk of **breast cancer**, ovarian cancer, and cervical cancer.

Breast milk is free, and saves money by eliminating the need to buy artificial milk (formula), bottles, and nipples. Because breast-fed babies overall have fewer illnesses, their health care costs may be lower.

Breastfeeding should begin as soon as possible after birth and should continue every two to three hours. However, all babies are different; some need to nurse very frequently at first, while others can go much longer between feedings. A baby should be fed at least eight to 12 times in 24 hours. Because breast milk is easily digested, a baby may be hungry again as soon as one and one-half hours after the last meal. Frequent nursing will also help in increasing milk production.

Some babies have no trouble breastfeeding, while others may need some assistance. Once the baby begins to suck, the mother should make sure that most of the areola is in the baby's mouth. Proper latching-on will help stimulate milk flow and will prevent nipple soreness.

Breastfeeding mothers should offer the baby both breasts at each feeding. Breastfeeding takes about 15-20 minutes on each side. After stopping the feeding on one side, the mother should burp the baby before beginning the feeding on the other breast. The next feeding should begin with the breast that the baby nursed on last.

Mothers can tell if the baby is getting enough milk by checking diapers; a baby who is wetting between four to six disposable diapers (six to eight cloth) and who has three or four bowel movements in 24 hours is getting enough milk.

Preparation

Loose, front-opening clothes and a good nursing bra are recommended. Mothers should find a comfortable chair with lots of pillows, supporting the arm and back, to nurse in. Feet should rest on a low footstool with knees raised slightly. The baby should be level with the breast. The new mother may have to experiment with different ways of holding the baby before finding one that is comfortable for both the mother and baby.

Complications

Breastfeeding problems

New mothers may experience breastfeeding problems, including:

- Engorged breasts. Breasts that are too full can prevent the baby from sucking. Expressing milk manually or with a breast pump can help, as can warm showers and compresses.

- Sore nipples. In the early weeks nipples may become sore and even cracked. Treatments include changing the position that the baby nurses in, ensuring that the baby has latched on to most of the areola, and using lanolin-based lotion on the nipples. Nipple shields are sometimes effective as a short-term remedy but their use may reduce milk supply, further irritate the breast, and change the baby's sucking pattern.

- Inverted nipples: A mother with inverted nipples may still breastfeed in most instances. The baby should be enticed to open the mouth widely before latching on. The mother can use various techniques to evert the nipple such as wearing a breast shell between feedings, rolling the nipple, pulling the nipple out, and applying a breast pump on the breast for a few seconds before starting the breastfeeding session.

- **Infection**. Soreness and inflammation on the breast surface or a **fever** in the mother, may be an indication of a breast infection called **mastitis**. **Antibiotics** and

---

Suggestions for breastfeeding women who work outside the home

Stay at home as long as possible, and work part-time, if possible.

Try taking a few hours away from the baby to anticipate problems.

Have an extra set of towels, an extra bra, and a change of clothes at the work site.

Take a quart of liquid to work and remember to drink it frequently.

When choosing a pump, consider portability as well as cost and comfort.

Practice with a pump ahead of time to get used to it and so that the milk will let-down quickly.

If working full-time and manual expression or a manual pump is objectionable or does not work well, rent a dual hook-up electric pump to keep at work.

Find a place at work to feel comfortable and have some privacy while pumping, and have a backup place in mind as well.

If the baby will be in day care, be certain the day care provider is supportive of breastfeeding.

Arrange to nurse the baby during the day if possible.

Arrive early at the day care provider's site to nurse the baby right before going to work to help the baby settle down and allow time for talking with the provider.

SOURCE: Wheeler, L. *Nurse-Midwifery Handbook: A Practical Guide to Prenatal and Postpartum Care*. Philadelphia: Lippincott-Raven Pub., 1997.

---

continued nursing on the affected side may solve the problem.

Results

There are no rules about when to stop breastfeeding. A baby needs breast milk or artificial milk for at least the first year of life. As long as a baby eats age-appropriate solid food, the mother may nurse for several years.

Health care team roles

Several members of the health care team, including obstetricians, nurses, midwives, and lactation consultants, are equipped to provide guidance and support to mothers who wish to breastfeed their babies. By meeting specific eligibility requirements and passing an independent examination, lactation consultants may be certified by the International Board of Lactation Consultants. Such certification demonstrates that these consultants possess the necessary skills, knowledge, and attitudes to provide quality breastfeeding assistance. It is important for new mothers to understand that breastfeeding is something that mothers and babies must learn to do together. The development of a satisfying breastfeeding relationship requires patience on the mother's part and the mother may benefit from the support and guidance of a lactation consultant or other qualified member of her health care team.

KEY TERMS

Areola—The pigmented, circular area surrounding the nipple of each breast.

Bromocriptine—A drug used to treat Parkinson's disease that can decrease a woman's milk supply.

Ergotamine—A drug used to prevent or treat migraine headaches. This can cause vomiting, diarrhea, and convulsions in infants.

Immunoglobulin—A protein produced by plasma cells; a component of the immune system. Transferred in utero and through breast milk providing passive immunity to the baby.

Lactation—Secretion of milk from the breasts; the act of breastfeeding.

Latch-on—The process whereby the baby opens the mouth widely and first exerts negative pressure on the mother's nipple and then positive pressure. Good latch-on will result in adequate transfer of milk into the baby's mouth and prevent sore nipples from occurring.

Lithium—A drug used to treat manic depression (bipolar disorder) that can be transmitted in breast milk.

Methotrexate—An anticancer drug also used to treat arthritis that can suppress an infant's immune system when taken by a nursing mother.

Postpartum—Refers to the six-week period after childbirth.

Resources

BOOKS

Biancuzzo, Marie. *Breastfeeding the Newborn*. St. Louis: Mosby, 1999.

Cunningham, F. Gary, et al. *Williams Obstetrics*. 20th ed. Stamford, CT: Appleton & Lange, 1997.

Riordan, Jan, and Kathleen G. Auerbach. *Breastfeeding and Human Lactation*. 2nd ed. Boston: Jones & Bartlett, 1999.

ORGANIZATIONS

The International Board of Lactation Consultant Examiners (IBLCE). 7309 Arlington Blvd., Suite 300, Falls Church, VA 22042-3215. (703) 560-7330. <http://www.iblce.org/>.

The International Lactation Consultant Association (ILCA). 1500 Sunday Dr., Suite 102, Raleigh, NC 27607. (919) 787-4916. <http://users.erols.com/ilca/index.html>.

Nadine M. Jacobson

Lactation consulting

Definition

Lactation consultants assist lactating mothers in self-care and management techniques related to breast-feeding.

Description

Lactation consulting has emerged as a new field over the past twenty years. Because scientific inquiry has consistently shown breastfeeding to be the recommended source of **nutrition** for infants through the first year of life, more mothers are opting to nurse their infants. Lactation consultants try to meet the educational needs of these mothers and sometimes of other health care providers who have an interest in their patients' breastfeeding needs.

Lactation consulting is the only specialty within health care that places the advocation of the woman who wishes to breastfeed her baby as its primary responsibility. The mother and her baby are described as a nursing couple or a nursing dyad—two separate people forming one unit. If other members of the health care team choose a plan of care that could be detrimental to the nursing dyad relationship, then the lactation consultant may need to suggest an alternate course if one is available.

Caring for the mother and baby

The primary function of the lactation consultant is to gently guide the mother's breastfeeding in a manner that involves the least intrusion and generates a minimal amount of complications. The consultant's skills are based on scientific information and familiarity with breastfeeding.

A useful approach for the consultant is to make suggestions to the mother while explaining the rationale behind these recommendations. The mother can then determine how to adapt these recommendations to best promote her needs and the needs of her baby. Potential problems that a lactation consultant would assist a client with are nipple soreness, breast engorgement, and milk production. A lactation consultant should be knowledgeable in the various components of science of lactation: milk production, normal breastfeeding behaviors, and factors that may impact the breastfeeding relationship.

Work settings

Lactation consulting can occur in a variety of settings—within the hospital, in the home, in a clinic or physician's office, in prenatal classes, as part of routine **postpartum care**, by operating a telephone help line, or through referrals to peer support groups. The location of practice is frequently determined by what other credentials the individual had prior to becoming a lactation consultant. In the hospital setting, the lactation consultant often is a **registered nurse** on the maternity unit. In a clinic such as the Special Supplemental Food Program for Women, Infants and Children (WIC), the consultant may be a registered dietician.

Hospital setting

Every postpartum mother who is breastfeeding should ideally be observed feeding her newborn at least one time prior to being discharged home. In the hospital setting, the role of the lactation consultant is to observe every mother breastfeeding and to ensure that maternity staff receive training in basic breastfeeding management and common problems and are capable of making such observations. The maternity staff can then refer complicated problems to the lactation consultant.

Lactation consultants in the hospital setting also act as an advisor in the development of breastfeeding policies and procedures for the facility. The consultant may compile handouts and other reading resource materials for breastfeeding mothers, as well as design forms for documentation of breastfeeding activities. If the nursing mother needs to use a breast pump or other breastfeeding device, the consultant may be the one responsible for assisting the mother in obtaining the equipment and training the client in its use.

Outpatient settings

There are several outpatient facilities that the lactation consultant might practice in. Some of these are **public health** clinics, health care provider offices, home health care, or as a consultant in private practice.

PUBLIC HEALTH CLINIC. Working in a public health clinic, such as Women, Infants, and Children (WIC), the lactation consultant will be an active advocate for breastfeeding because WIC, through the U.S. Department of Agriculture (USDA) has undertaken a breastfeeding promotion program. WIC participants represent a significant proportion of the low income and at-risk population of women and infants. The WIC program is having an impact on meeting the Healthy People 2010 breastfeeding goals for the United States. Women who are breastfeeding in the WIC program receive priority treatment and additional services. The breastfeeding mother will receive an enhanced food package including additional fruit juice, dairy products, legumes, carrots, and canned tuna fish.

In the WIC program, the lactation consultant may be responsible for the training of peer counselors. Peer counselors are individuals of a similar background as other WIC clients who have breastfed or are breastfeeding a child and have an interest in supporting other mothers to do the same. WIC clients come from ethnically diverse backgrounds, and peer counselors are particularly useful in expressing sensitivity to the different cultures, socioeconomic backgrounds, and value systems. WIC uses peer counselors to promote breastfeeding and lactation consultants to manage breastfeeding problems.

HEALTH CARE PROVIDER OFFICES. In the clinic/ office setting the consultant will conduct prenatal education in breastfeeding, will make rounds in the hospital on patients who have delivered and will provide follow-up after discharge through home visits and a telephone help line sometimes referred to as a "warm line." The lactation consultant in a health care provider's office will serve as a resource person for doctors and nurses by providing updates on breastfeeding research and information on medications that are contraindicated for the mother to take while breastfeeding.

HOME HEALTH CARE. If a mother is discharged prior to 48 hours after delivery, the home health visit is particularly important for assessing proper initiation of breastfeeding. The lactation consultant making such a visit may also be a registered nurse and will be checking the mother and baby for recovery and transition, in addition to breastfeeding. As part of such an assessment conducted by a registered nurse, certain phenomena should be observed. The infant should be having at least six wet diapers and four stools a day after the milk is "in." The mother's bleeding should be decreasing, she should not have a temperature—be afebrile—and any incisional discomfort should be under control with proper medications. The home assessment may involve taking **vital signs** on the mother and the infant.

Relatives and siblings may make for a hectic environment as compared with another setting, but the home environment allows for a more realistic environment in which to observe breastfeeding, and the consultant also gets a view of the client's support system. Involving family members in breastfeeding education will help relatives to understand the benefit of breastfeeding and may prompt a more supportive environment for the mother. The lactation consultant may wish to encourage the mother to make use of a telephone help line if she has any problems and concerns that were not addressed during the home visit.

PRIVATE PRACTICE. A private practice affords the lactation consultant the greatest flexibility but simultaneously constrains the consultant with more administrative

KEY TERMS

Consulting—Providing advice or an opinion.

Lactation—Secretion of milk from the breasts; the act of breastfeeding.

responsibilities. The independent lactation consultant may operate out of a home office or maintain a regular office, possibly sharing it with other consultants or heath care providers. The source of referrals for the independent lactation consultant is from clients themselves, from other lactation consultants, from other health care providers, and from hospitals.

Education and training

The field of lactation consulting attracts people from a varied background. Some hold advanced degrees in medicine, nursing and nutrition and have been working in maternal child health. Others are lay counselors who obtained the necessary education to become lactation consultants after having had a positive breastfeeding experience of their own.

Professional education for lactation consultants was first offered in the early 1980s. The International Board of Lactation Consultant Examiners (IBLCE) started to offer a certification exam for lactation consulting in 1985. Shortly thereafter, the International Lactation Consultant Association (ILCA) became the professional association for lactation consultants.

Resources

BOOKS

Kutner, Linda., Barger, Jan., and Peterson, Carole. "The Lactation Consulting Profession." In *Counseling the Nursing Mother: A Lactation Consultant's Guide*, edited by Lauwers, Judith., Shinskie, Debbie., and Breck, Sandra. Boston: Jones and Bartlett, 2000, pp.7-23.

ORGANIZATIONS

The International Board of Lactation Consultant Examiners(IBLCE). 7309 Arlington Blvd., Suite 300, Falls Church, VA 22042-3215. (703) 560-7330. <http://www.iblce.org>.

The International Lactation Consultant Association (ILCA). 1500 Sunday Dr., Suite 102, Raleigh, NC 27607. (919) 787-4916. <http://www.users.erols.com/ilca/index.html>.

Nadine M. Jacobson, R.N.

Language acquisition

Definition

Language acquisition is defined as a natural progression or development in the use of language, typified by infants and young children learning to talk. It is an unconscious process that occurs when language is used in ordinary conversation. Language acquisition is distinguished from intentional study of a language by its informality.

Description

Theories of language acquisition

Developmental psychologists are not agreed as to how humans acquire the ability to speak their first language. It was only in the 1950s that the availability of portable tape recorders made it possible for researchers to record children's speech patterns for later analysis in the laboratory. One early theory of language acquisition was based on imitation, which is the notion that children learn to speak by imitating adults and older children. The difficulty with the imitation theory is that it fails to account for the ability of even small children to form new sentences from words they know. A second theory, associated with the behavioral school of psychology, maintains that language acquisition is explained by reinforcement. Children learn to speak because their parents give them positive reinforcement when they speak correctly and negative reinforcement (correction or criticism) when they speak ungrammatically. This theory does not hold up under the findings of recent research that parents reinforce the *meaning* of what children say rather than its grammatical correctness. In addition, children often chatter to themselves or to no one in particular for the sheer pleasure of talking. This activity is hard to explain in terms of the reinforcement theory.

A third theory of language acquisition is called nativism. This theory holds that humans are neurologically "programmed" from birth with the capacity to acquire language as soon as their nervous system reaches a certain point of maturation. Noam Chomsky maintained that the human **brain** has a built-in language acquisition device, or LAD, that analyzes the parts of speech in the language that a child hears. The phases of language acquisition and the age at which children begin to acquire language are similar enough across different cultures and different languages to give some support to the nativist view.

Biological and neuroanatomical features of language acquisition

EVOLUTION AND DEVELOPMENT OF THE HUMAN VOCAL TRACT AND NERVOUS SYSTEM. Language is, as far as we know, unique to humans. Chimpanzees are able to learn a rudimentary sign language, but they cannot combine vocalized sounds into meaningful structured combinations as humans do. The human mouth and throat appear to have been modified over the course of evolutionary history for speech. The human larynx is situated low in the throat, and the sharp right-angle bend at the back of the mouth divides the human vocal tract into two resonant cavities (the mouth and the throat) that allow for the production of a large range of vowel sounds.

The maturation of certain neural circuits in a child's brain may explain why language development proceeds most rapidly in young children after the first year of life. Although babies are born with most of their nerve cells already formed, their head size, brain weight, and junctions between nerve cells (synapses) continue to increase in the first year after birth. The long-distance connections in the child's nervous system are not complete until nine months of age, and the rate of **metabolism** in the child's brain reaches adult levels by ten months. There appears to be a neurologically determined critical period for language acquisition. Children acquire language easily until age four, or six at the latest. After **puberty**, it is rare for humans to learn to speak if they have not done so earlier.

AREAS OF THE BRAIN ASSOCIATED WITH LANGUAGE. The areas of the brain that govern the interpretation and production of language were discovered in the nineteenth century by physicians studying patients with **speech disorders**. In 1861, Pierre Paul Broca, a French physician, was able to demonstrate from post-mortems of patients who had lost the ability to speak, that the loss of this ability is associated with damage to an area of the brain toward the front of the left hemisphere. In 1876, a German physician named Karl Wernicke found that damage to an area in the posterior part of the left temporal lobe of the brain is also associated with **language disorders**. This area, now called Wernicke's area, is connected to Broca's area by a group of nerve fibers called the arcuate fasciculus.

When a person reads aloud, information from the eyes travels along the optic nerve to the primary visual cortex of the brain. From the primary visual cortex, the information is transmitted to Wernicke's area, where it is interpreted. From Wernicke's area, it is carried by the arcuate fasciculus to Broca's area, then to the primary motor cortex. When a person repeats a word that is spoken, the information is carried from the nerves in the ear to the primary auditory cortex in the brain. It is then transmitted from the primary auditory cortex to Wernicke's area, then to Broca's area via the arcuate fasciculus, then to the primary motor cortex.

Stages of language acquisition

A young human's acquisition of language takes place in a series of six stages:

- Prelinguistic stage (birth to six months): The baby cries, coos, laughs, and makes other sounds.

- Babbling (six to 12 months): The baby makes nonspecific sounds from all human languages.

- One-word (holophrastic) stage (1–2 years): The child speaks single words in isolation, in his or her first language.

- Two-word stage (24–30 months): The child forms two-word phrases or strings that reflect the language being acquired. The vocabulary increases; the child begins to learn words at the rate of one word every two waking hours.

- Telegraphic speech (30–36 months): Children begin to utter short phrases like telegraph messages, without formal grammatical structure.

- Fluent speech (three years +): The child learns grammar and syntax (patterns of sentence formation) with surprising rapidity and accuracy; sentences increase in length and complexity.

Function

Human language functions as a means of interpersonal communication, to convey thoughts, feelings, and many other forms of information. It is necessary to human social life as well as to intellectual development. Language also stimulates the expression of human creativity: poetry, drama, novels, short stories, vocal music, and similar forms of art are based on language.

Role in human health

The fact that language is unique to humans implies that language acquisition is necessary to full psychosocial as well as intellectual development. People who lose the ability to speak normally in later life because of a stroke or a condition known as primary progressive **aphasia** often become depressed because they feel cut off from others. Children and adolescents with dyslexia (a learning disability that affects reading and is sometimes related to problems understanding spoken language) often have additional difficulties learning to inter-

KEY TERMS

Aphasia—The loss of previously held ability to speak or to understand written or spoken language, caused by disease or injury to the brain.

Arcuate fasciculus—A group of nerve fibers in the brain that connects Wernicke's area with Broca's area.

Broca's area—An area in the left hemisphere of the brain associated with the motor impulses necessary for speech. It is named for Pierre Paul Broca (1824-1880), a French physician.

Dyslexia—A reading disorder associated with impairment of the ability to integrate auditory and visual information, or to process sounds accurately.

Holophrastic—An early stage in language acquisition in which a single word serves the function of a phrase or sentence.

Nativism—The theory that humans have neural circuits that are genetically programmed to acquire language.

Specific language impairment (SLI)—A developmental disorder of childhood characterized by significant delays in language development in the absence of deafness, autism, mental retardation, or similar handicaps.

Wernicke's area—An area in the left hemisphere of the brain that is important in the reception and interpretation of speech. Wernicke's area is connected to Broca's area by the arcuate fasciculus.

Williams syndrome—A rare congenital disorder caused by a deletion of the elastin gene on chromosome 7. Children with Williams syndrome have normal language skills even though they are usually mildly retarded.

act with others and feeling comfortable in social situations.

Studies of "wild" children and children reared by emotionally disturbed parents who did not talk to them indicate that children who do not learn to speak by age eight never achieve normal fluency. This feature of language acquisition implies that language is an important component of the social dimension of human nature. Humans who have never acquired the ability to communicate with others cannot be completely socialized.

Common diseases and disorders

Aphasia

Aphasia refers to the loss of a previously held ability to speak or to understand written or spoken language. Aphasia is most often the result of a stroke or head trauma, but it can occur in relation to other neurological disorders. Primary progressive aphasia is a disorder of the nervous system in which the person's ability to speak gradually deteriorates. In Broca's aphasia, caused by damage to Broca's area, the person can understand what words mean, but has trouble with speech output. Broca's aphasia is sometimes called motor or expressive aphasia. In Wernicke's aphasia, caused by damage to Wernicke's area, the person cannot understand spoken language. They can speak, but their speech is ungrammatical and incoherent. Wernicke's aphasia is sometimes called fluent or receptive aphasia.

Dyslexia

Dyslexia is a disorder that affects the ability to read. Its symptoms may include problems with spelling, difficulty recognizing the sounds in words, problems processing visual information, and difficulty saying words quickly when asked to do so. Present dyslexia research is focused on studying the parts of the brain that process speech sounds and relate them to **vision** and other language areas in the brain.

Williams syndrome

Williams syndrome is a rare congenital disorder that occurs once in every 20,000 births. It results from a deletion of the genetic material on human chromosome 7 that makes a protein called elastin. Although children with Williams are usually mildly retarded, they often have normal language abilities. The dissociation of language acquisition from general intelligence in Williams syndrome suggests that human speech is not simply a byproduct of intelligence as such.

Specific language impairment (SLI)

Specific language impairment, or SLI, refers to a group of inherited syndromes in which children with normal intelligence and **hearing** are slow to acquire and use language. SLI is thought to affect 5–7% of children starting school. A cross-cultural study done in 1999 suggests that SLI may differ from other language disorders in that the number and specific types of problems the children had were related to their specific first language. The study showed that children learning Italian or Hebrew had fewer difficulties with verbs, for example, than children learning English.

Resources

BOOKS

Fletcher, P., and B. MacWhinney. *The Handbook of Child Language*. Cambridge, MA: Blackwell Publishers, 1995.

Martin, John H., PhD. *Neuroanatomy: Text and Atlas*, second edition. Norwalk, CT: Appleton & Lange, 1996.

Pinker, Steven. *The Language Instinct*. New York: Morrow, 1994.

PERIODICALS

Toppelberg, Claudio O. "Several developmental disorders and bilingualism." *Journal of the American Academy of Child and Adolescent Psychiatry* 38, no. 9 (September, 1999).

ORGANIZATIONS

American Speech Language Hearing Association (ASHA). 10801 Rockville Pike, Rockville, MD 20852-3279. (301) 897-5700 or (800) 638-8255. Fax: (301) 571-0457. <http://www.asha.org>.

International Dyslexia Association. 8600 LaSalle Road, Chester Building, Suite 382, Baltimore, MD 21286-2044. (410) 296-0232. Fax: (410) 321-5069. <http://www.interdys.org>.

National Aphasia Foundation. 156 Fifth Avenue, Suite 707, New York, NY 10010. (800) 922-4622. <http://www.aphasia.org>.

National Institute of Child Health and Human Development (NICHD). National Institutes of Health, Bldg. 31, Room 2A32, Bethesda, MD 20892-2425. (301) 496-5133 or (800) 370-2943. <http://www.nichd.nih.gov>.

National Institute on Deafness and Other Communication Disorders (NIDCD). National Institutes of Health, Bldg. 31, Room 3C35, Bethesda, MD 20892-2320. (301) 496-7243. <http://www.nidcd.nih.gov>.

National Institute of Neurological Disorders and Stroke (NINDS). Building 31, Room 8A06, 9000 Rockville Pike, Bethesda, MD 20892. (301) 496-5751. <http://www.ninds.nih.gov>.

National Organization for Rare Disorders, Inc. (NORD) P. O. Box 8923, New Fairfield, CT 06812-8923. (203) 746-6518 or (800) 999-NORD. Fax: (203) 746-648. <http://www.rarediseases.org>.

Williams Syndrome Association. P.O. Box 297, Clawson, MI 48017-0297. (248) 541-3630. Fax: (248) 541-3631. <http://www.williams-syndrome.org>.

Rene Jackson, R.N.
Rebecca Frey

Language development *see* **Language acquisition**

Language disorders

Definition

A language disorder is a communication disorder characterized by an impaired ability to understand and/or use words in their proper context, whether verbal or nonverbal.

Description

Language disorders belong to a broad category of disorders called *communication disorders* that also include speech and **hearing** disorders. As of 1998, communication disorders were affecting one person out of every 10 in the United States. Language disorders are characterized by one or more of the following features: sound substitutions in words, difficulty in processing sounds into syllables and words, improper use of words, confusion about their meaning, difficulty in expressing ideas and thoughts, inappropriate use of grammatical forms, limited vocabulary development and inability to follow directions, remember questions or numbers and letters in sequence. Language disorders can be classified as either developmental or acquired.

Developmental language disorders

Developmental language disorders occur in children who do not develop functional language skills. Clinically, they are diagnosed as language-delayed or language-disordered. Language-delayed children can have receptive language impairments, expressive language impairments or both.

Receptive language impairments refer to a difficulty understanding language at the level of meaning. The vocabulary range is usually very limited. The purpose of simple grammatical constructions is also not properly understood. For example, that adding an "-s" to a noun makes it plural, or that "'s" is a possessive form, or that a verb with an "-ed" ending means that the action occurred in the past. There is also difficulty in understanding nonverbal signals, such as body language, or difficulty understanding sarcasm and irony, or indirect requests and sentences.

Expressive language impairments refer to the use of defective language patterns, for example using too few words in sentences. Or the sentences may be truncated, or contain words that lack proper endings, or miss the verbs "is" and "are." Limited or ambiguous vocabulary is also a feature. Affected individuals have difficulty using language properly, and as a result, they often seem rude or blunt. There is also a distinct pattern of changing topics very abruptly.

Acquired language disorders

Acquired language disorders, also called *aphasias*, are language impairments caused by damage to the areas of the **brain** responsible for language function. Various aspects of language may be affected depending on the location and extent of the brain damage. Language function is believed to be associated with the left hemisphere of the brain and some aphasias are accordingly classified with respect to the affected brain area:

- Broca's **aphasia**. This type of aphasia is an expressive aphasia and it is associated with damage to Broca's area, a region located in the frontal lobe of the left hemisphere of the brain. It is characterized by an impaired ability to produce language.

- Wernicke's aphasia. This type of aphasia is a receptive aphasia and it is associated with damage to Wernicke's area, a region located in the left temporal lobe of the brain. It is characterized by an impaired ability to understand language.

- Dyslexia. Dyslexia is a neurological learning difficulty that also affects the learning of language skills. It is characterized by an impaired ability to manage verbal codes in **memory** and difficulties with writing, spelling, and reading. Other symbolic functions, such as mathematics and musical notation, can also be affected.

Causes and symptoms

Developmental language disorders have been associated with a wide variety of causes, such as hearing impairment, cognitive impairment, autism, or a physical handicap that prevents the child from interacting normally with his environment, such as mental retardation, or a cleft lip or palate. Emotional/psychological problems may also be a cause, and lack of intellectual stimulation as well. Often, there is no identifiable cause for a developmental language disorder.

Acquired language disorders or aphasias resulting from brain damage can be caused by **cerebral palsy**, stroke, tumor or **head injury** affecting the left hemisphere of the brain. It should be noted that individual differences do exist in brain function and when coupled with differences in the extent of the brain damage, the degree of impairment caused by aphasia is then unique to the affected individual.

Although the symptoms of language disorders vary from one individual to the next, and also depend on whether they are developmental or acquired, they do present a range of characteristic symptoms. Generally speaking, in the case of developmental disorders, a child's language skills are considered delayed when the child is noticeably behind his or her peers in the acquisition of basic language skills. Sometimes a child will have a greater receptive (understanding) impairment than an expressive (speaking) impairment, but the overall result is the same as both functions are required for the full development of language skills.

Some general symptoms are typical of an aphasic language disorder. Most affected individuals experience *anomia*, or difficulty finding words and some aphasic people try to cope with this difficulty by providing descriptions or definitions for the missing words. This is called circumlocution. Another symptom is paraphasia, meaning the use of an incorrect or unrecognizable word in place of the desired word. There are three types of paraphasias. Phonemic or literal paraphasias are faulty words that sound very close to the intended word (for example, using "bait" instead of "bake"). Verbal or semantic paraphasias are faulty words that are close in meaning to the target word (for example, using "apple" instead of "orange"). The third type of paraphasias are neologisms, or invented words that do not exist in the speaker's language. Another symptom is perseveration, meaning the repetition of a word or sentence when it is not required. The aphasic person gets stuck in a pattern of repetitive sentences without being able to break out of it.

Diagnosis

The early diagnosis of language disorders is important because they are first and foremost a communication disorder that always leads to social and educational isolation. Evaluation procedures, usually performed by a speech-language pathologist, are used to diagnose the disorders and any child whose language is not similar to that of other children of the same age should be evaluated. While faulty language patterns are considered normal "baby talk" during early childhood, they become indicative of a language disorder if they are not outgrown as expected. Because of brain development patterns, it is easier to learn language and communication skills before the age of five, thus the importance of timely diagnosis. One or a combination of typical features usually occur in a child affected by a language disorder or developmental language delay. The child may hear or see a word but be incapable of understanding its meaning. He may have trouble getting others to understand what he wants to communicate or display a high level of inattention or lack of organizational skills. These are all pointers that are used to establish diagnosis.

Treatment

The treatment of language disorders belongs to speech pathology, the specialty concerned with disorders of speech and language. Language therapy with preschoolers is centered on working with parents and other family members to create an optimal environment for learning language. For example, when speaking with a child who has aphasia, it helps to minimize distractions, and to speak slowly and clearly. If the child has difficulty understanding, the use of short and simple sentences is beneficial. Pairing gestures with speech to help comprehension also helps. So does allowing the child ample time to respond and the formulation of questions that can be answered easily with a yes or no or other single word. Speech pathologists can recommend strategies to help families of children with language disorders. School-age children with developmental language disorders can benefit from special education programs, usually monitored by a speech pathologist.

Prognosis

Prognosis is dependent on the cause of the language disorder. If the cause is brain damage, the acquired disorder usually remains. In the case of developmental language disorders, many affected children are able to catch up with their peers, but many also continue to have difficulty with the gap between their skill level and that of their peers, which may increase over time. Since many factors influence outcome, it is not possible to predict which individuals are most likely to recover or how significant the progress will be. Developmental language disorders also have different stages that follow the overall development of children. At different ages, different demands are made on the language system. For example, language-disordered children in the preschool years may appear to catch up to peers by age five or six years, but in later years, as language demands evolve, (e.g., the stage of learning how to read), new impairments usually become apparent.

Health care team roles

Language disorders are usually treated by a speech pathologist working with a collaborative team consisting of the family, physicians, educational professionals as well as special educators. The team usually includes:

- Speech-language pathologists. These specialists have several responsibilities, including: providing individual therapy to the language-impaired; informing teachers and health care professionals on how to identify children who are at risk; performing the evaluation of spoken and written language skills; interviewing family members and teachers; observing the child in the classroom setting so as to evaluate language skills; assessing reading, spelling and writing levels for older children and adolescents.

- Audiologists. Audiologists are specialists of hearing disorders and their expertise may be required in cases where the language disorder is associated with a hearing deficiency.

- Reading specialists. These specialists are special educators who design remedial reading and language skill acquisition therapies.

- Teachers of the language handicapped. These specialized teachers are trained to teach language-delayed children.

Prevention

There are no specific preventive measures for language disorders, but their early detection will often improve the chances of a successful special education therapy. Thus, identifying children that are at risk of developing a language disorder is important. The following conditions are considered to represent high-risk factors and children exposed to them should be tested early and regularly:

- diagnosed medical conditions, such as chronic ear infections

- biological factors, such as fetal alcohol syndrome

- genetic defects, such as Down syndrome

- neurological defects, such as cerebral palsy

- family history, such as family incidence of literacy difficulties

Resources

BOOKS

Gunning, T. G. *Assessing and Correcting Reading and Writing Difficulties.* Boston: Allyn & Bacon, 1997.

Kamhi, A. G., Catts, H. W., ed. *Language and Reading Disabilities.* Boston: Allyn & Bacon, 1998.

Leonard, L. B. *Children With Specific Language Impairment.* Cambridge: MIT Press, 2000.

Paul, R. *Language Disorders From Infancy Through Adolescence: Assessment & Intervention.* St Louis: Mosby, 2001.

Ratner, V. and L. Harris. *Understanding Language Disorders: The Impact on Learning.* Eau Claire: Thinking Publications, 2001.

Smiley, L. R. and P. A. Goldstein. *Language Delays and Disorders: From Research to Practice.* San Diego: Singular Publishing Group, 1998.

KEY TERMS

Anomia—Difficulty finding words.

Aphasia—Acquired language disorder caused by damage to the areas of the brain responsible for language function.

Broca's aphasia—Language disorder associated with damage to Broca's area, a region in the frontal lobe of the left hemisphere of the brain. It is characterized by an impaired ability to produce language.

Communication disorder—Disorder characterized by an impaired ability to communicate. Communication disorders include language, speech and hearing disorders. They are associated with a wide variety of physical and psychological causes.

Dyslexia—Dyslexia is a specific learning difficulty that hinders the learning of literacy skills. This problem with managing verbal codes in memory is neurological and tends to run in families. Other symbolic systems, such as mathematics and musical notation, can also be affected.

Language disorder—Communication disorder characterized by an impaired ability to understand and/or use words in their proper context, whether verbal or nonverbal. The disorder can be either developmental or acquired.

Paraphasia—Use of an incorrect or unrecognizable word.

Speech disorder—Communication disorder characterized by an impaired ability to produce speech sounds or by problems with voice quality.

Speech pathology—The field of speech pathology, formerly known as speech therapy, is concerned with disorders of speech and language. A speech pathologist is a professional trained to diagnose and treat language and speech disorders.

Wernicke's aphasia—Language disorder associated with damage to Wernicke's area, a region in the left temporal lobe of the brain. It is characterized by an impaired ability to understand language.

PERIODICALS

Anderson, S. R., Lightfoot, D. W., "The human language faculty as an organ." *Annual Reviews of Physiology* 62 (2000): 697-722.

Coslett, H. B., "Acquired dyslexia." *Seminars in Neurology* 20 (2000): 419-426

Friederici, A. D., "The developmental cognitive neuroscience of language: a new research domain." *Brain and Language* 71 (January 2000): 65-68.

Grigorenko. E. L., "Developmental dyslexia: an update on genes, brains, and environments." *Journal of Child Psychology and Psychiatry* 42 (January 2001): 91-125

Martins I. P., "Childhood aphasias." *Clinical Neuroscience* 4 (1997): 73-77.

Pinker, S., "Acquiring language." *Science* 276 (May 1997): 1178-1181.

ORGANIZATIONS

American Speech-Language-Hearing Association (ASHA) 10801 Rockville Pike, Rockville, MD 20852. (800)638-8255. <http://www.asha.org/>.

The International Dyslexia Association 8600 LaSalle Road, Chester Building, Suite 382, Baltimore, MD 21286-2044. (410) 296-0232. <http://www.interdys.org/>.

It Takes Two To Talk—The Hanen Program for Parents of Children with Language Delays. The Hanen Center, Suite 403 - 1075 Bay Street, Toronto ON M5S 2B1, Canada. (416) 921-1073. <http://www.hanen.org/>.

National Institute on Deafness and Other Communication Disorders (NIDCD), National Institutes of Health, 31 Center Drive, MSC 2320, Bethesda, MD 20892-2320. <http://www.nidcd.nih.gov/>.

OTHER

Net Connections for Communication Disorders and Sciences. "A guide to communication disorders and science sources on the Internet." <http://www.mankato.msus.edu/dept/comdis/kuster2/welcome.html>.

The SLP Homepage. "Internet Searches and Resources on Speech Language Pathology." <http://members.tripod.com/Caroline_Bowen/slp-eureka.htm>.

Monique Laberge, PhD

Laparoscope

Definition

A laparoscope is a telescope-like **endoscope** used to view the abdominal cavity for diagnosis and treatment during a minimally invasive surgical procedure called **laparoscopy**.

Purpose

A laparoscope is used to directly examine the abdominal and pelvic organs to diagnose certain conditions and—depending upon the condition—to perform therapeutic surgery. Laparoscopes are commonly used in gynecologic laparoscopy to examine the outside of the uterus, the Fallopian tubes, and the ovaries—particularly in pelvic **pain** cases where the underlying cause of pain could not be determined using diagnostic imaging (e.g., ultrasound; computed tomography). Gynecologic conditions diagnosed using laparoscopy include endometriosis, ectopic **pregnancy**, ovarian cysts or tumors, pelvic inflammatory disease, pelvic **abscess**, **infertility**, uterine fibroids, and **cancer**. Laparascopes are used in general surgery to examine abdominal organs such as the **gallbladder**, bile ducts, **liver**, appendix, and intestines (external surface). Laparoscopy can identify **appendicitis**, cholecystitis, cirrhosis, hernias, ascites, and abdominal cancers.

During the laparoscopic procedure, certain conditions can be treated surgically using special laparoscopic instruments and devices designed to be used with laparoscopes. For example, appendectomy, cholecystectomy, biopsy of the ovary or liver, hernia repair, and removal of endometriotic tissue or cysts, can all be performed laparoscopically. Medical devices that can be used in conjunction with laparoscopy include surgical lasers and electrosurgical units. Other procedures that can be performed laparoscopically include hysterectomy, oophorectomy, tubal ligation, and lymphadenectomy. Laparoscopic surgery is now preferred over open surgery for several types of procedures due to its minimally invasive nature and associated lower complication rate.

A relatively new type of laparoscope is the microlaparoscope—a smaller laparoscope used to perform microlaparoscopy in the physician's office. Common clinical applications of microlaparoscopy in gynecology include pain mapping (e.g., endometriosis), and sterilization and fertility procedures. Common applications in general surgery include evaluation of chronic and acute abdominal pain (e.g., appendix), basic trauma evaluation, biopsies, and evaluation of abdominal masses.

Laparoscopes are most commonly used by gynecologists, urologists, and general surgeons for abdominal and pelvic applications. In addition to expanding applications in these areas, orthopedic surgeons are now using laparoscopes for spinal applications, and cardiac surgeons for minimally invasive **heart** surgery.

Description

Laparoscopes are rigid, telescope-like endoscopes used during laparoscopic procedures for either viewing or operating. Viewing laparoscopes typically range from 5 to 10 mm in diameter, and operating laparoscopes usually range from 8 to 12 mm in diameter. Operating laparoscopes have a separate instrument channel in their shaft where laparoscopic **surgical instruments** can be inserted to perform therapeutic procedures. Viewing laparoscopes do not have an instrument channel and are used primarily for diagnosis. Microlaparoscopes of approximately 2 mm in diameter are available for diagnostic procedures performed in the physician's office. Although most laparoscopes are rigid, some manufacturers supply semi-flexible or flexible laparoscopes to increase the viewing range. The size and type of laparoscope chosen depends upon the type of procedure being performed, the patient's size and age, and the patient's medical condition.

Laparoscopes have an optical system of lenses, prisms, and mirrors to provide magnification of tissue and organs, a wide field of view, and high image resolution. A bundle of illuminating fibers are located in the laparoscope's shaft surrounding the lenses and are connected to a separate fiber-optic light source that provides light during the procedure. Most laparoscopes have integral cameras or allow connection of a camera for transmitting images during the procedure. The images from the laparoscope are transmitted to one or more viewing monitors, which the surgeon uses to visualize the internal anatomy and guide any surgical procedures. Video and photographic equipment are used to document the procedure.

Operation

Laparoscopy is typically performed in the hospital under **general anesthesia**, although some laparoscopic procedures can be performed using **local anesthesia** and conscious sedation. Once the patient is under anesthesia, a urinary catheter is inserted to collect urine during the procedure. As the procedure begins, a small incision is made just below the navel and a cannula or trocar is inserted into the incision to accommodate the insertion of the laparoscope. Other incisions (one or two) may be made in other areas of the abdomen to allow for insertion of other laparoscopic instrumentation. A laparoscopic insufflation device is used to inflate the abdomen with carbon dioxide gas to create a space in which the laparoscopic surgeon can maneuver the instruments.

Once the laparoscope is inserted, the surgeon manipulates it to view the anatomical areas of interest. Depending on the surgeon's preference and the type of

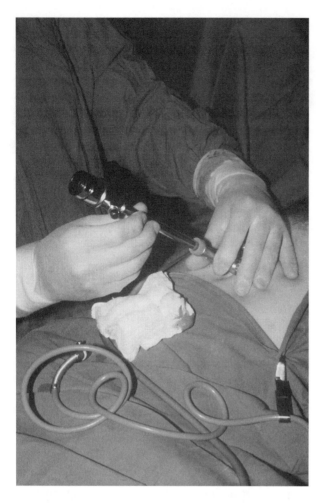

A laparoscope can be used for internal examination and minor surgery through only a small incision. *(Photograph by John Watney. Science Source/Photo Researchers. Reproduced by permission.)*

procedure, an eyepiece can be attached to the scope for direct viewing, or television/video cameras can be attached for viewing on a monitor. Instruments such as forceps, graspers, and manipulators can be used in conjunction with operating laparoscopes. For example, a uterine manipulator would be used in gynecologic procedures involving the uterus (e.g., hysterectomy).

After laparoscopic diagnosis and treatment are completed, the laparoscope, cannula, and other instrumentation are removed, and the incision is sutured and bandaged.

Complications related to the use of a laparoscope can occur during laparoscopy. The most serious complication is laceration of a major abdominal **blood** vessel resulting from improper positioning, inadequate insufflation (inflation) of the abdomen, abnormal pelvic anatomy, or too much force during scope insertion. Thin patients with well-developed abdominal muscles are at higher risk, since the aorta may only be an inch (2-3 cm) or so below the skin. Obese patients are also at higher risk because more forceful and deeper needle and scope penetration is required. There is also a risk of bleeding from vessels, and adhesions that may require repair by open surgery if bleeding cannot be stopped using laparoscopic instrumentation. In laparoscopic procedures that use electrosurgical devices, **burns** to the incision site are possible due to conduction of electrical current through the laparoscope due to a fault or malfunction in the equipment.

Any abdominal surgery, including laparoscopy, carries the risk of unintentional organ injury (punctures and perforations). For example, the bowel, bladder, ureters, or fallopian tubes may be injured during the procedure by the laparoscope itself. These injuries are often unavoidable due to the patient's anatomy or medical condition. Patients at higher risk for bowel injury include those with chronic bowel disease, pelvic inflammatory disease, a history of pervious abdominal surgery, or severe endometriosis. Some types of laparoscopic procedures have a higher risk of organ injury. For instance, during laparoscopic removal of endometriosis adhesions or ovaries, the ureters may be injured due to its proximity to each other.

Several clinical studies have shown that the complication rate during laparoscopy is associated with surgeon experience. Surgeons experienced in laparoscopic procedures have fewer complications than surgeons performing their first 100 cases.

Maintenance

The success of the laparoscopic procedure is highly dependent upon the condition of the laparoscope and its associated accessories. Improper disinfection, sterilization, and handling of laparoscopic equipment can result in equipment damage, unnecessary wear, and ultimately surgical errors. All clinical staff using laparoscopes and related equipment should be well-trained and familiar with disassembling and assembling scopes and accessory parts (e.g., couplers; adapters; instrumentation) so that defects in equipment can be recognized before a complication occurs or equipment malfunctions. Manufacturers of laparoscopic equipment usually provide maintenance guidelines, including cleaning techniques, for their scopes and accessories. The hospital **biomedical engineering** department and/or the scope manufacturer will implement actual repairs to equipment. The introduction of disposable accessories (e.g., trocars; couplers) has simplified preparation for procedures and minimized maintenance needs.

Health care team roles

Laparoscopy may be performed by a gynecologist, general surgeon, gastroenterologist, or other physician, depending upon the patient's condition. An anesthesiologist is required during the procedure to administer general and/or local anesthesia and to perform patient monitoring. Nurses and surgical technicians/assistants aid with scope positioning, video system adjustments and image recording, and laparoscopic instrumentation. Clinical staff trained in the daily maintenance, disinfection, and sterilization of laparoscopes are required to sterilize equipment between procedures and make sure all scopes are in working order.

Training

Physicians and surgeons using laparoscopes should be well-trained in laparoscopic techniques. A surgeon skilled and experienced in open surgical techniques cannot necessarily transfer those skills to laparoscopic techniques because a different skill set is involved in minimally invasive surgery. Organizations focused on laparoscopy, and laparoscope manufacturers, offer clinical training in laparoscopic surgery.

Resources

BOOKS

Soderstrom, Richard M. "Laparoscopic Equipment." In *Operative Laparoscopy* 2nd ed. Ed. Richard M. Soderstrom. Philadelphia: Lippincott-Raven, 1998, 1-9.

Soderstrom, Richard M., ed. *Operative Laparoscopy,* 2nd ed. Philadelphia: Lippincott-Raven, 1998.

Soderstrom, Richard M., Carl J. Levinson, Barbara S. Levy. "Complications of Operative Laparoscopy." In *Operative Laparoscopy,* 2nd ed. Ed. Richard M. Soderstrom. Philadelphia: Lippincott-Raven, 1998, 257-267.

PERIODICALS

Boike, Guy M., and Brian Dobbins. "New Equipment for Operative Laparoscopy." *Contemporary OB/GYN* no. 2 (April 1998). <http://consumer.pdr.net/consumer/psrecord.htm>.

Pritts, Elizabeth A., David L. Olive, Tracey Gilhuly, and Steven F. Palter. "The Role of Microlaparoscopy in the New Era of Gynecology." *Contemporary OB/GYN* (April 15, 1999). <http://consumer.pdr.net/consumer/psrecord.htm>.

ORGANIZATIONS

American College of Obstetricians and Gynecologists. 409 12th Street SW, P.O. Box 96920, Washington, DC 20090-6920. <http://www.acog.org>.

Society of American Gastrointestinal Endoscopic Surgeons (SAGES). 2716 Ocean Park Boulevard, Suite 3000, Santa Monica, CA 90405. (310) 314-2404. <http://www.endoscopy-sages.com>.

Society of Laparoendoscopic Surgeons. 7330 SW 62nd Place, Suite 410, Miami, FL 33143-4825. (305) 665-9959. <http://www.sls.org>.

KEY TERMS

Ascites—Accumulation of fluid in the abdominal cavity; Laparoscopy may be used to determine its cause.

Cannula—A small tube inserted into the incision site through which laparoscopes and instruments are inserted; used in conjunction with a trocar.

Cholecystitis—Inflammation of the gallbladder; often diagnosed using laparoscopy.

Electrosurgical device—A medical device that uses electrical current to cauterize or coagulate tissue during surgical procedures; often used in conjunction with laparoscopy.

Endometriosis—A disease involving occurrence of endometrial tissue (lining of the uterus) outside the uterus in the abdominal cavity; often diagnosed and treated using laparoscopy.

Hysterectomy—Surgical removal of the uterus; often performed laparoscopically.

Insufflation—Inflation of the abdominal cavity using carbon dioxide; performed prior to laparoscopy to give the surgeon space to maneuver surgical equipment.

Oophorectomy—Surgical removal of the ovaries; often performed laparoscopically.

Trocar—A small sharp instrument used to puncture the abdomen at the beginning of the laparoscopic procedure.

OTHER

"Diagnostic Laparoscopy." Society of Gastrointestinal Endoscopic Surgeons. <http://www.sages.org/pi_diaglap.html>.

Jennifer E. Sisk, M.A.

Laparoscopy

Definition

Laparoscopy is a minimally invasive surgical procedure performed to examine the abdominal and pelvic organs.

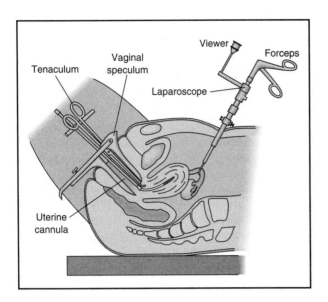

Viewer
Forceps
Vaginal
speculum
Tenaculum
Laparoscope
Uterine
cannula

A laparoscopy procedure. *(Delmar Publishers, Inc. Reproduced by permission.)*

Purpose

Laparoscopy is performed to directly examine the abdominal and pelvic organs to diagnose certain conditions and—depending upon the condition—to perform surgery. Laparoscopy is commonly used in gynecology to examine the outside of the uterus, the Fallopian tubes, and the ovaries—particularly in pelvic **pain** cases where the underlying cause of pain cannot be determined using diagnostic imaging (e.g., ultrasound; computed tomography). Gynecologic conditions diagnosed using laparoscopy include endometriosis, ectopic **pregnancy**, ovarian cysts or tumors, pelvic inflammatory disease, pelvic **abscess**, **infertility**, uterine fibroids, and **cancer**. Laparoscopy is used in general surgery to examine abdominal organs such as the **gallbladder**, bile ducts, **liver**, appendix, and intestines (external surface). Laparoscopy can identify **appendicitis**, cholecystitis, cirrhosis, hernias, ascites, and abdominal cancers.

During the laparoscopic procedure, certain conditions can be treated surgically using special laparoscopic instruments and devices designed to be used with laparoscopes. For example, appendectomy, cholecystectomy, biopsy of the ovary or liver, hernia repair, and removal of endometriotic tissue or cysts can all be performed laparoscopically. Medical devices that can be used in conjunction with laparoscopy include surgical lasers and electrosurgical units. Other procedures that can be performed laparoscopically include hysterectomy, oophorectomy, tubal ligation, and lymphadenectomy. Laparoscopic surgery is now preferred over open surgery for several types of procedures due to its minimally invasive nature and associated lower complication rate.

A relatively new development is microlaparoscopy performed in the physician's office using smaller laparoscopes. Common clinical applications in gynecology include pain mapping (e.g., endometriosis), and sterilization and fertility procedures. Common applications in general surgery include evaluation of chronic and acute abdominal pain (e.g., appendix), basic trauma evaluation, biopsies, and evaluation of abdominal masses.

Laparoscopy has been most commonly used by gynecologists, urologists, and general surgeons for abdominal and pelvic applications. In addition to expanding applications in these areas, laparoscopy is now being used by orthopedic surgeons for spinal applications and by cardiac surgeons for minimally invasive **heart** surgery.

Precautions

Patients should be carefully screened for **allergies** to anesthetic agents used for laparoscopy. Obese patients, very thin patients, and patients with abnormal anatomy have a higher risk of complications, and laparoscopy should be performed with caution in these patients. Preoperative imaging examinations may be helpful to visualize any anatomical abnormalities. Some daily medications, such as **blood** thinners or arthritis medications, may need to be stopped for a certain time period prior to the procedure. Any medications taken on a regular basis, including over-the-counter medicines, should be discussed with the physician and anesthesiologist. Patients who have had prior abdominal surgical procedures may have resulting scar tissue that would interfere with laparoscopy; thus, these patients are usually not considered good candidates for laparoscopic procedures.

Description

Laparoscopy is typically performed in the hospital under **general anesthesia**, although some laparoscopic procedures can be performed using **local anesthesia**. Once the patient is under anesthesia, a urinary catheter is inserted to collect urine during the procedure. To begin the procedure, a small incision is made just below the navel and a cannula or trocar is inserted into the incision to accommodate the insertion of the **laparoscope**. Other incisions (one or two) may be made in other areas of the abdomen to allow for insertion of other laparoscopic instrumentation. A laparoscopic insufflation device is used to inflate the abdomen with carbon dioxide gas to create a space in which the laparoscopic surgeon can maneuver the instruments.

Laparoscopes, which have integral cameras for transmitting images during the procedure, are available in various sizes depending upon the type of procedure being performed. The images from the laparoscope are transmitted to a viewing monitor, which the surgeon uses to visualize the internal anatomy and guide any surgical procedure. Video and photographic equipment are used to document the procedure.

After laparoscopic diagnosis and treatment are completed, the laparoscope, cannula, and other instrumentation are removed, and the incision is sutured and bandaged.

Robotic systems are available to assist with laparoscopy. A robotic arm attached to the operating table may be used to hold and position the laparoscope in order to reduce unintentional camera movement that is common when a surgical assistant holds the laparoscope. The surgeon controls the robotic arm movement by foot pedal, voice-activated command, or handheld control panel.

Microlaparoscopy has become more common over the past few years. This procedure involves the use of smaller laparoscopes (e.g., 2 mm compared to 5 to 10 mm for hospital laparoscopy) with the patient undergoing local anesthesia with conscious sedation in a physician's office. Video and photographic equipment used are similar to that used for general laparoscopy.

Preparation

Because laparoscopy requires general anesthesia in most cases, the patient is required to fast for several hours before the procedure. Sometimes bowel cleansing is also required. The patient is screened by anesthesiology staff regarding allergies to medication and previous experiences (e.g., allergic reaction) with anesthesia.

Aftercare

Following laparoscopy, patients are required to remain in a recovery area until the immediate effects of anesthesia wear off and until normal voiding is accomplished after urinary catheter removal. **Vital signs** are monitored to ensure that no reactions to anesthesia have occurred and no internal injuries are present. For healthy patients undergoing elective procedures such as tubal ligation, diagnostic laparoscopy, or hernia repair, laparoscopy is usually an outpatient procedure and patients are discharged from the recovery area within a few hours after the laparoscopy. Due to the aftereffects of anesthesia, patients should not drive themselves home. Patients with more serious medical conditions, or patients undergoing emergency laparoscopy, may be kept in the hospital overnight or for a few days.

Discharged patients receive instructions regarding activity level, medications, and side effects of the proce-

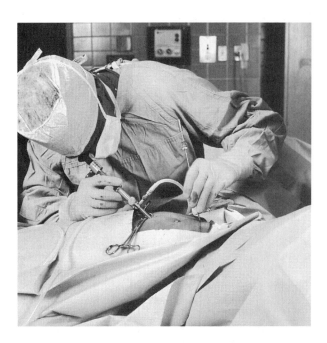

This surgeon is performing a laparoscopic procedure on a patient. *(Photo Researchers, Inc. Reproduced by permission.)*

dure. Depending upon the nature of the laparoscopic procedure and the patient's medical condition, daily activity may be restricted for a few days and strenuous activity restricted for several days to weeks. Pain-relieving medications are usually prescribed for several days following the procedure. In addition, **antibiotics** to prevent **infection** may also be prescribed. Patients are instructed to watch for signs of a urinary tract infection or unusual pain, which may indicate organ injury.

Complications

The most serious complication that can occur during laparoscopy is laceration of a major abdominal blood vessel resulting from improper positioning, inadequate insufflation (inflation) of the abdomen, abnormal pelvic anatomy, and too much force exerted during scope insertion. Thin patients with well-developed abdominal muscles are at higher risk, since the aorta may only be an inch or so below the skin. Obese patients are also at higher risk because more forceful and deeper needle and scope penetration is required. During laparoscopy, there is also a risk of bleeding from vessels, and adhesions that may require repair by open surgery if bleeding cannot be stopped using laparoscopic instrumentation. In laparoscopic procedures that use electrosurgical devices, **burns** to the incision site are possible due to conduction of electrical current through the laparoscope caused by a fault or malfunction in the equipment.

KEY TERMS

Ascites—Accumulation of fluid in the abdominal cavity; Laparoscopy may be used to determine its cause.

Cholecystitis—Inflammation of the gallbladder, often diagnosed using laparoscopy.

Electrosurgical device—A medical device that uses electrical current to cauterize or coagulate tissue during surgical procedures; often used in conjunction with laparoscopy.

Embolism—Blockage of an artery by a clot, air or gas, or foreign material. Gas embolism may occur as a result of insufflation of the abdominal cavity during laparoscopy.

Endometriosis—A disease involving occurrence of endometrial tissue (lining of the uterus) outside the uterus in the abdominal cavity; often diagnosed and treated using laparoscopy.

Hysterectomy—Surgical removal of the uterus; often performed laparoscopically.

Insufflation—Inflation of the abdominal cavity using carbon dioxide; performed prior to laparoscopy to give the surgeon space to maneuver surgical equipment.

Oophorectomy—Surgical removal of the ovaries; often performed laparoscopically.

Pneumothorax—Air or gas in the pleural space (lung area) that may occur as a complication of laparoscopy and insufflation.

Subcutaneous emphysema—A pathologic accumulation of air underneath the skin resulting from improper insufflation technique.

Trocar—A small sharp instrument used to puncture the abdomen at the beginning of the laparoscopic procedure.

Complications related to insufflation of the abdominal cavity include gas inadvertently entering a blood vessel and causing an embolism, pneumothorax, and subcutaneous **emphysema**. One common, but not serious, side effect of insufflation is pain in the shoulder and upper chest area for a day or two following the procedure.

Any abdominal surgery, including laparoscopy, carries the risk of unintentional organ injury (punctures and perforations). For example, the bowel, bladder, ureters, or fallopian tubes may be injured during the laparoscop-

ic procedure. Many times these injuries are unavoidable due to the patient's anatomy or medical condition. Patients at higher risk for bowel injury include those with chronic bowel disease, pelvic inflammatory disease, a history of pervious abdominal surgery, or severe endometriosis. Some types of laparoscopic procedures have a higher risk of organ injury. For instance, during laparoscopic removal of endometriosis adhesions or ovaries, the ureters may be injured due to their proximity to each other.

During the recovery period following laparoscopy, complications may also occur. An organ injury may be overlooked, so patients should be monitored for any unusual pain, particularly in association with the bowel, as bowel injuries may not be apparent during the procedure. Other complications include urinary tract infection (resulting from catheterization) and minor infection of the incision site.

Several clinical studies have shown that the complication rate during laparoscopy is associated with surgeon experience. Surgeons experienced in laparoscopic procedures have fewer complications than surgeons performing their first 100 cases.

Results

In diagnostic laparoscopy, the surgeon will be able to see signs of a disease or condition (e.g., endometriosis adhesions; ovarian cysts; diseased gallbladder) immediately, and can either treat the condition surgically or proceed with appropriate medical management. In diagnostic laparoscopy, biopsies may be taken of questionable areas, and laboratory results will govern medical treatment. In therapeutic laparoscopy, the surgeon performs a procedure that rectifies a known medical problem, such as hernia repair or appendix removal. Because laparoscopy is minimally invasive in comparison to open surgery, patients experience less trauma and postoperative discomfort, have fewer procedural complications, can return to daily activities sooner, and have a shorter hospital stay.

Health care team roles

Laparoscopy may be performed by a gynecologist, general surgeon, gastroenterologist, or other physician—depending upon the patient's condition. An anesthesiologist is required during the procedure to administer general and/or local anesthesia and to perform patient monitoring. Nurses and surgical technicians/assistants are needed during the procedure to assist with scope positioning, video system adjustments and image recording, and laparoscopic instrumentation.

Resources

BOOKS

Soderstrom, Richard M., ed. *Operative Laparoscopy,* 2nd ed. Philadelphia: Lippincott-Raven, 1998.

Soderstrom, Richard M., Carl J. Levinson, Barbara S. Levy. "Complications of Operative Laparoscopy." In *Operative Laparoscopy,* 2nd ed. Ed. Richard M. Soderstrom. Philadelphia: Lippincott-Raven, 1998, 257-267.

PERIODICALS

Boike, Guy M., and Brian Dobbins. "New Equipment for Operative Laparoscopy." *Contemporary OB/GYN* no. 2 (April 1998). <http://consumer.pdr.net/consumer/psrecord.htm>.

Pritts, Elizabeth A., David L. Olive, Tracey Gilhuly, and Steven F. Palter. "The Role of Microlaparoscopy in the New Era of Gynecology." *Contemporary OB/GYN* (April 15, 1999). <http://consumer.pdr.net/consumer/psrecord.htm>.

ORGANIZATIONS

American College of Obstetricians and Gynecologists. 409 12th Street SW, P.O. Box 96920, Washington, DC 20090-6920. <http://www.acog.org>.

Society of American Gastrointestinal Endoscopic Surgeons(SAGES). 2716 Ocean Park Boulevard, Suite 3000, Santa Monica, CA 90405. (310) 314-2404. <http://www.endoscopy-sages.com>.

Society of Laparoendoscopic Surgeons. 7330 SW 62nd Place, Suite 410, Miami, FL 33143-4825. (305) 665-9959. <http://www.sls.org>.

OTHER

"Diagnostic Laparoscopy." Society of Gastrointestinal Endoscopic Surgeons. <http://www.sages.org/pi_diaglap.html>.

Jennifer E. Sisk, M.A.

Large intestine *see* **Intestine, large**

Laryngeal cancer *see* **Head and neck cancer**

Laryngitis *see* **Sore throat**

Laryngoscopy

Definition

Laryngoscopy is a procedure used to view the inside of the larynx (the voice box).

Purpose

The purpose of seeing inside the larynx is to assess the vocal cords and to detect tumors, **foreign bodies**, nerve or structural injury, or other abnormalities.

Precautions

A patient undergoing a laryngoscopy should be assessed for **allergies** to local anesthetics or other pharmacologic agents in order to prevent possible allergic reactions.

Patients may have fears concerning this procedure. Prior to laryngoscopy, the physician should explain the procedure in detail and assure the patient that he or she will be closely monitored for respiratory or other problems.

Description

Two methods of laryngoscopy allow the examiner to view the structures of the larynx and the surrounding areas. A light and lens affixed to a surgical viewing instrument called an **endoscope** are used in both methods.

Indirect laryngoscopy

Indirect laryngoscopy, the simplest form of laryngeal examination, involves the placement of a small, angled mirror at the back of the throat, allowing the examiner to reflect light onto the larynx and view its major structures. However, since the mirror must remain in the back of the throat, examination of the larynx during normal speech is hindered. Also, a strong gag reflex in some patients may limit the usefulness of this procedure.

A rigid endoscope may also be used to perform an indirect laryngoscopy. An examination using a rigid scope involves placement of the tip of the instrument through the mouth and into the back of the throat. A prism at the tip allows the examiner to view the larynx. This type of exam provides clear and highly magnified images of the vocal cords and allows better examination of the larynx during phonation (the production of vocal sounds). Another advantage to these instruments is that photographic or video recordings can be made through the endoscope for future review, also allowing more than one person to observe the laryngeal area.

Direct laryngoscopy

In direct laryngoscopy, a flexible, fiber-optic endoscope is threaded through the nasal passage and down into the throat. This procedure is used to detect or remove

KEY TERMS

Aspirate—To draw by suction.

Biopsy—The removal of a sample of tissue for study under the microscope.

Endoscope—An instrument used for visualizing the interior of a hollow organ such as the larynx.

Epiglottis—The lid-like appendage that covers the glottis during swallowing.

False cords—The protective valves of the larynx that prevent food from entering the trachea.

Laryngectomy—The surgical removal of the larynx.

Larynx—The organ of sound production, sometimes called the voice box. The larynx is made of cartilage and muscle.

Phonation—The production of vocal sounds. Examination of the larynx may be facilitated by asking the patient to produce a high-pitched "e-e-e" sound, since this lifts the epiglottis.

True cords—Also called vocal cords, these are two small shelves of muscular tissue within the larynx. They supplement the protective valves of the larynx that prevent food from entering the trachea. Their main function is to vibrate against each other and generate a sound tone.

lesions or foreign bodies in the larynx, or to diagnose **cancer** by removing tissue for biopsy or samples for culture. Once the instrument is inserted, flexible glass fibers illuminate the laryngeal area and transmit the image to the external part of the scope. From this position, an image of the larynx and vocal folds (including their movement and position during respiration and speech) can be clearly obtained.

Bronchoscopy is a similar, but more extensive procedure in which the tube is continued through the larynx and down into the trachea and bronchi.

Preparation

Patients should not eat for several hours before the examination.

Patients undergoing indirect laryngoscopy should sit in an upright position and breathe normally. The patient should be leaning slightly forward, with the head lifted. This facilitates the passage of the laryngeal mirror into the mouth and facilitates the procedure.

Topical anesthetics, such as lidocaine or dyclonine, may be used during laryngoscopy to suppress the gag reflex. The patient should be warned that the agent may **taste** bad and that the effects may be unpleasant. Anesthetized patients may feel as if their swallowing mechanism is impaired, and many experience an ill-defined sense of insecurity. Patients who are receiving anesthesia should be warned about these side effects and reassured throughout the procedure.

The gag reflex can also be reduced in the adult by the intravenous injection of diazepam (Valium). The typical dose is 10 mg. Diazepam may be used as an alternative for patients who are allergic to local anesthetics or who require both agents to allow adequate examination. Diazepam should be injected slowly into a large vein, and is only appropriate for healthy adults.

Complications

This procedure carries no serious risks, although the patient may experience soreness of the throat or cough up small amounts of **blood** until the irritation subsides. After the procedure, the patient should ingest nothing by mouth until the gag reflex returns. Once the reflex returns, fluid intake should be encouraged because it promotes the expectoration of secretions, and lozenges or gargles may be used relieve a **sore throat**.

Vital signs should be assessed frequently for 24 hours to detect bleeding or complications such as difficult or labored respiration (dyspnea).

Results

A normal result would be the absence of signs of disease or damage.

An abnormal finding, such as a tumor or an object lodged in the tissue, would either be removed or examined for further medical attention.

Health care team roles

A nurse plays an important role in explaining the procedure to the patient, preparing the patient for the procedure, and assisting the physician in conducting the procedure. A nurse also assists patient recovery after the procedure, administering fluids and lozenges once the gag reflex returns, and monitoring vital signs.

Resources

BOOKS

Clinical ENT: An Illustrated Textbook, 2nd ed. O'Donoghue, G.M., A.A. Narula, and G.J. Bates, eds. Albany, NY: Singular Publishing Group, Thomson Learning, 2000.

Essentials of Otolaryngology, 4th ed. Lucente, F.E. and G. Har-El, eds. Philadelphia: Lippincott Williams & Wilkins, 1999.

Foundations of Nursing: Caring for the Whole Person. White, Lois, ed. Albany, NY: Delmar Thomson Learning, 2001.

Medical-Surgical Nursing across the Health Care Continuum, 3rd ed. Ignatavicius, D.D., M.L. Workman, and M.A. Mishler, eds. Philadelphia: W.B. Saunders, 1999.

PERIODICALS

Altman, L.K. "New Direction for Transplants Raises Hopes and Questions." *New York Times* 148, no. 51510 (2 May 1999): 1.

Monaco, A.P. "Transplantation of the Larynx—A Case Report that Speaks for Itself." *New England Journal of Medicine* 344, no. 22 (31 May 2001): 1712.

Sabin, S.L. and R.M. Rosenfeld. "The Impact of Comorbidity and Age on Survival with Laryngeal Cancer." *ENT: Ear, Nose & Throat Journal* 78, no. 8 (August 1999): 578.

ORGANIZATIONS

American Board of Otolaryngology, 3050 Post Oak Blvd., Suite 1700, Houston, TX 77056. (713) 850-0399. <http://www.aboto.org>.

National Institute on Deafness and Other Communication Disorders, 31 Center Dr., MSC 2320, Bethesda, MD 20892-2320. <http://www.nidcd.nih.gov>.

Jennifer F. Wilson

Laser-assisted in-situ keratomileusis *see*
Refractive eye surgeries

Laser surgery

Definition

Laser is an acronym that stands for Light Amplification by Stimulated Emission of Radiation. Laser surgery uses an intensely hot, precisely focused beam of light to remove or vaporize tissue and control bleeding in a wide variety of noninvasive and minimally invasive procedures.

Purpose

Laser surgery may be used to:

- cut or destroy tissue that is abnormal or diseased without harming healthy, normal tissue

- shrink or destroy tumors and lesions

- cauterize (seal) **blood vessels** to prevent excessive bleeding

Precautions

Although many laser surgeries can be performed in the physician's office rather than in a hospital, practitioners must be at least as thoroughly trained and highly skilled their counterparts in a hospital setting. The American Society for Laser Medicine and Surgery, Inc. recommends that:

- All operative areas be equipped with oxygen and other drugs and equipment required for **cardiopulmonary resuscitation** (CPR).

- Nonphysicians performing laser procedures be properly trained, licensed, and insured.

- A qualified and experienced supervising physician be able to respond to and manage unanticipated events or other emergencies within five minutes of the time they occur.

- Emergency transportation to a hospital or other acute-care facility be available whenever laser surgery is performed in a nonhospital setting.

All patients who are considering laser surgery should be fully informed about the procedure's relative risks and benefits, as well as any alternatives that may exist. Some types of laser surgery, for example, should not be performed on pregnant women or on patients with severe cardiopulmonary disease or other serious health problems. The patient should understand why laser surgery a better choice than traditional surgery (in this instance), and how much experience the physician has in performing the laser procedure the patient is considering. Generally, surgical nurses will inform patients about the planned procedure and, if hospital policy permits nurses to do so, obtain their **informed consent** to proceed; some hospitals require doctors to do this.

Description

The first working lasers were introduced in 1960. They were initially used to treat diseases and disorders of the eye, where transparent tissues gave ophthalmic surgeons a clear view of how the narrow, concentrated beam was being directed. Dermatologic surgeons helped further pioneer laser surgery, developing and improving many early techniques and refining surgical procedures.

Lasers are medically useful because they can be directed with pinpoint accuracy to cut, vaporize, or weld tissue while cauterizing **blood** vessels and nerves to reduce or eliminate surgical bleeding and postoperative **pain**. This reduces postoperative swelling and scarring as well as the length of the recovery period. A laser's heat often destroys **bacteria** and **viruses** in the surgical field, creating a more sterile environment that is less prone to

infection. Because a smaller incision is required, laser procedures often take less time than traditional surgery. Lasers can also be tailored to particular applications.

All lasers operate on the principle of selective photothermolysis, meaning that the laser's wavelength, energy density, power, and exposure time determine what types of tissue will be affected and the effects that will be produced. Lasers can be further adapted to different medical procedures with special delivery (such as fiberoptic cables) that help apply the laser beam.

Laser applications

Sometimes described as "scalpels of light," lasers are used alone or with conventional **surgical instruments** and can be tailored with seemingly infinite precision for a vast number of surgical procedures. For these reasons laser surgery is often standard operating procedure for specialists in cardiology, dentistry, dermatology, gastroenterology, gynecology, neurosurgery, oncology, ophthalmology, orthopedics, otolaryngology, pulmonology, and urology.

Lasers are used to erase birthmarks, skin discolorations, and skin changes due to aging; to remove benign, precancerous, or cancerous tissues or tumors; to stop snoring; remove tonsils; remove or transplant hair; and relieve pain and restore function in patients too weak to undergo more invasive surgery. Lasers are also used to treat angina; cancerous or noncancerous tumors that cannot be removed or destroyed; cold and canker sores, gum disease and tooth sensitivity or decay; ectopic **pregnancy**, endometriosis, and fibroid tumors; gallstones; **glaucoma**, mild-to-moderate nearsightedness, **astigmatism**, and other conditions that impair **vision**; migraine headaches; noncancerous enlargement of the prostate gland; nosebleeds; ovarian cysts; ulcers; **varicose veins**; warts; and numerous other conditions, diseases, and disorders.

Types of lasers

CARBON DIOXIDE LASER. Carbon dioxide (CO_2) lasers were the first to find surgical applications, and they remain the most used of all **medical lasers**. CO_2 laser light is absorbed readily by water in the cells, allowing tissue to be cut precisely with minimal bleeding. The laser beams can be concentrated into a fine beam that slices like a scalpel, or diffused to shave or vaporize tissue. This versatility makes them valuable in many types of procedures from wart removal to **brain** surgery.

NEODYMIUM:YTTRIUM-ALUMINUM-GARNET LASER. Neodymium:yttrium-aluminum-garnet laser (Nd:YAG) lasers can penetrate tissue more deeply than other lasers, allowing surgeons to operate on parts of the body that could previously be reached only through invasive surgery. Nd:YAG lasers are the most frequently used laser in dental procedures, and are also well suited for respiratory surgery because they cauterize and seal the tiny vessels of the lung. They are also used to excise tumors with minimal damage to healthy tissue, and may even eliminate micrometastases before they can spread to another region.

Other types of YAG lasers are:

- The KTP laser, produced when Nd:YAG laser light is passed through a potassium-titanyl-phosphate (KTP) crystal. This green laser is used frequently for vascular lesions (such as leg veins) and to remove certain tattoo colors.

- The erbium (Er:YAG) laser, which penetrates less deeply into tissue; it is used in dental and hair removal procedures.

- The holmium (Ho:YAG) laser, used in orthopedic surgery to eliminate extraneous bone and cartilage, to destroy **kidney stones**, in endoscopic sinus procedures, and for prostate removal.

ARGON LASER. Another laser to find early medical application, the argon laser produces a blue-green light that is selectively absorbed by hemoglobin and melanin. This means that argon laser light is drawn to areas that are heavily pigmented or rich in blood vessels. Argon lasers are most often used for opthalmic surgery and surface skin blemishes (birthmarks, enlarged blood vessels) because they vaporize and seal blood vessels on contact. In a special procedure known as photodynamic therapy (PDT), this laser is also used in conjunction with light-sensitive dyes to shrink or dissolve tumors.

Preparation

Because laser surgery is used to treat such a wide variety of conditions, patients should be given specific, detailed instructions about how to prepare for their procedure. Diet, activities, and medications may or may not have to be limited prior to surgery, so it's important that nurses offer written and/or verbal preoperative **patient education** and instructions. Many procedures require a preoperative **physical examination** to determine the patient's general health and current medical status, especially if **general anesthesia** will be used. Patients should also be given a realistic expectation of the procedure's outcome and the duration of recovery.

Aftercare

Many laser surgeries are be performed on an outpatient basis, and patients are usually permitted to leave the

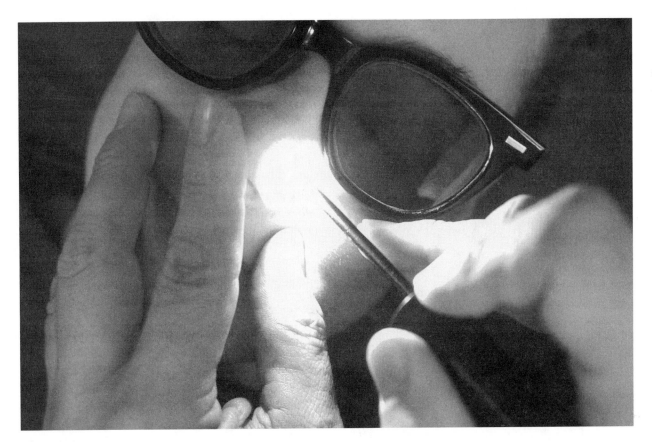

Cosmetic laser surgery in progress. The wavelengths of the laser's light can be matched to a specific target, enabling the physician to destroy the capillaries near the skin's surface without damaging the surrounding tissue. *(Photograph by Will & Deni McIntyre, Photo Researchers, Inc. Reproduced by permission.)*

hospital, medical office, or surgical center once their **vital signs** have stabilized. Patients who have been sedated should not be discharged until they have completely recovered from the anesthesia and they are oriented and alert. Most practitioners require discharged patients to be accompanied by a responsible adult. Patients should not drive themselves to or from the facility.

The physician may prescribe analgesic medication for postoperative pain, and should provide easy-to-understand written instructions that describe how the patient's recovery should progress, the actions to take in the event of complications, and how to recognize complications requiring emergency medical treatment.

Complications

The risks and complications associated with laser surgery are comparable to those for other surgical procedures. Treated areas can become infected following laser surgery; this should be suspected if burning, crusting of the skin, itching, pain, scarring, severe redness, and swelling appear at the treatment site. Other risks are associated with anesthesia and complications such as hemor-

rhage, perforation, or infection. Fortunately, errors of this sort tend to occur when a physician is poorly supervised while learning a new skill. Serious complications are rare with experienced doctors.

Some complications may be cosmetic: lighter or darker skin may appear when a laser is used to remove sun damage or age spots from an olive- or dark-skinned individual. This abnormal pigmentation may or may not disappear in time. Black, Asian, Hispanic, or dark-skinned patients should make sure that their surgeon has performed laser procedures successfully on people of color.

Laser surgery also involves unique risks: Imprecisely aimed lasers can burn or destroy healthy tissue, cause injuries that are painful and sometimes permanent, and even compound the problems they are supposed to solve. Errors or inaccuracies in laser eye surgery can damage or worsen a patient's vision, for example. Scarring or rupturing of the cornea is uncommon, but laser surgery on one or both eyes can increase sensitivity to light or glare, reduce night vision, permanently cloud vision, or cause sharpness of vision to decline throughout

KEY TERMS

Argon—A colorless, odorless gas, which, when used in a laser, emits a blue-green beam.

Astigmatism—A condition in which one or both eyes cannot filter light properly because the corneal surface is irregular. This results in blurred, indistinct images unless corrected by glasses, contact lenses, or laser surgery.

Carbon dioxide—A heavy, colorless gas that dissolves in water.

Cauterize—The use of heat or chemicals to stop bleeding, prevent the spread of infection, or destroy tissue.

Cornea—The outer, transparent lens that covers the pupil of the eye and admits light.

Endometriosis—An often painful gynecologic condition in which endometrial tissue migrates from the inside of the uterus to other organs inside and beyond the abdominal cavity.

Glaucoma—A disease of the eye in which increased pressure within the eyeball can cause gradual loss of vision. Iridectomy is the laser surgical procedure that helps relieve the pressure.

Invasive surgery—Surgery that involves making an incision in the patient's body and inserting instruments or other medical devices into it.

Nearsightedness—A condition in which one or both eyes cannot focus normally, causing objects at a distance to appear blurred and indistinct. Also called myopia.

Ovarian cyst—A benign or malignant growth on an ovary. An ovarian cyst can disappear without treatment or become extremely painful and have to be surgically removed.

Papillomavirus—A group of viruses that cause several types of warts, some of which can cause cancer.

Vaporize—To dissolve solid material or convert it into smoke or gas with a laser.

Varicose veins—Peripheral veins, usually in the legs, that have valvular insufficiency. This allows blood to pool in the vessels of the lower extremities, permanently dilating the veins.

the day. To guard against some of these risks, patients must wear protective eye shields while undergoing laser

surgery on any part of the face near the eyes or eyelids, and a United States Food and Drug Administration (FDA) mandate requires both health care personnel and patients to use special protective eyewear whenever a CO_2 laser is used.

An unexpected risk associated with laser surgery is the "plume" or smoke that is emitted when lasers vaporize tissue. Studies have shown that although the particles in the smoke are very small ($0.5–5.0\mu m$), they are small enough to pass through a surgical mask. This is a concern for both patient and health care personnel because viral DNA has been shown to survive in the smoke produced when warts are removed by a laser, and some forms of papillomavirus are infectious. To guard against any possible contagion, a vacuum system with a multistage filter is recommend to suction the smoke produced during laser procedures; it must be held very close (about 1 cm) from the target to be effective.

Results

The nature and severity of the problem addressed by the laser procedure, the skill of the surgeon performing the procedure, as well as the patient's general health and realistic expectations about the result of the procedure are among the factors that influence the outcome of laser surgery.

Patients considering any type of laser surgery should be fully apprised of the risks, benefits and potential complications of the procedure as well as any alternative treatment that might be feasible in place of laser surgery. It is especially important for patients undergoing cosmetic procedures to have realistic expectations about the outcomes of these procedures.

Health care team roles

Laser surgery may be performed by a general surgeon, cardiologist, dentist, oral surgeon, dermatologist, gynecologist, ophthalmologist, otolaryngologist, plastic surgeon, urologist or other physician specialist, assisted by specially trained surgical nurses. Preoperative blood work is performed by laboratory technologists, and when necessary, imaging studies may be performed by radiologic technicians.

Patient education

Nurses have a vital role in delivering pre- and postoperative patient education. There is considerable evidence that well-informed patients achieve better clinical outcomes and experience higher levels of satisfaction with treatment. Patients considering laser surgery should be provided with detailed information about the anticipated outcomes of the surgery and the duration of recovery process.

Resources

BOOKS

Dover, J.S., et al., ed. *Illustrated Cutaneous and Aesthetic Laser Surgery.* New York: McGraw-Hill. 2000.

Lask, G.P., and N.J. Lowe. *Lasers in Cutaneous and Cosmetic Surgery.* Philadelphia PA: Churchill Livingstone. 2000.

PERIODICALS

"High-Power Potassium-Titanyl_Phosphate Laser Vaporization Prostatectomy." *Journal of Urology* (June 2000):1730–1733.

"Laser-Assisted Uvulopalatoplasty for Snoring." *Archives of Otolaryngology: Head & Neck Surgery* (April 2001): 412–417.

"Percutaneous Myocardial Laser Revascularization." *Heart* (March 1, 2000): 253–254.

Stratigos, Alexander J., Jeffrey S. Dover, and Kenneth A. Arndt. "Laser Treatment of Pigmented Lesions—2000: How Far Have We Gone?" *Archives of Dermatology* (July 2000): 915–921.

ORGANIZATIONS

American Society for Dermatologic Surgery. 930 North Meacham Road, Schaumburg, IL 60173-6016. (847) 330-9830. <http://www.asds-net.org>.

American Society for Laser Medicine and Surgery, Inc. 2404 Stewart Square, Wausau, WI 54401. (715) 845-9283 <http://www.aslms.org/index.html>.

OTHER

Arieli, Rami. "Lasers and Their Applications." <http://www.phys.ksu.edu/perg/vqm/laserweb/Preface/Toc.htm> (22 July 2001).

Facts About Laser Surgery. <http://www.glaucoma.org/fs-laser-sur.html> (22 July 2001).

Shore Laser Center. "Medical Lasers." <http://www.shorelaser.com/AboutLasersMed.html>. (22 July 2001).

U.S. Department of Health. Occupational Health and Safety Administration. " Hazard of Laser Surgery Smoke." <http://www.osha-slc.gov/dts/hib/hib_data/hib19880411.html>. (22 July 2001).

Barbara Wexler

Lasers in medicine *see* **Medical lasers**

LASIK *see* **Refractive eye surgeries**

Laughing gas *see* **Nitrous oxide**

Laxatives

Definition

Laxatives are products that promote bowel movements.

Purpose

Laxatives are used to treat constipation—the passage of small amounts of hard, dry stools, usually fewer than three times a week. Before recommending use of laxatives, differential diagnosis should be performed. Prolonged constipation may be evidence of a significant problem, such as localized peritonitis or diverticulitis. Complaints of constipation may be associated with obsessive-compulsive disorder. Use of laxatives should be avoided in these cases. Patients should be aware that patterns of defecation are highly variable, and may vary from two to three times daily to two to three times weekly.

Laxatives may also be used prophylacticly for patients, such as those recovering from a **myocardial infarction** or those who have had recent surgery, who should not strain during defecation.

Description

Laxatives may be grouped by mechanism of action.

Saline cathartics include dibasic sodium phosphate (Phospo-Soda), magnesium citrate, magnesium hydroxide (milk of magnesia), magnesium sulfate (Epsom salts), sodium biphosphate, and others. They act by attracting and holding water in the intestinal lumen, and may produce a watery stool. Magnesium sulfate is the most potent of the laxatives in this group.

Stimulant and irritant laxatives increase the peristaltic movement of the intestine. Examples include cascara and bisadocyl (Dulcolax). Castor oil works in a similar fashion.

Bulk producing laxatives increase the volume of the stool, and will both soften the stool and stimulate intestinal motility. Psyllium (Metamucil, Konsil) and methylcellulose (Citrucel) are examples of this type. The overall effect is similar to that of eating high-fiber foods, and this class of laxative is most suitable for regular use.

Docusate (Colace) is the only representative example of the stool softener class. It holds water within the fecal mass, providing a larger, softer stool. Docusate has no effect on acute constipation, since it must be present before the fecal mass forms to have any effect, but may be useful for prevention of constipation in patients with

KEY TERMS

Carbohydrates—Compounds, such as cellulose, sugar, and starch, that contain only carbon, hydrogen, and oxygen, and are a major part of the diets of people and other animals.

Cathartic colon—A poorly functioning colon, resulting from the chronic abuse of stimulant cathartics.

Colon—The large intestine.

Diverticulitis—Inflammation of the part of the intestine known as the diverticulum.

Fiber—Carbohydrate material in food that cannot be digested.

Hyperosmetic—Hypertonic, containing a higher concentration of salts or other dissolved materials than normal tissues.

Osteomalacia—A disease of adults, characterized by softening of the bone. Similar to Rickets which is seen in children.

Pregnancy category—A system of classifying drugs according to their established risks for use during pregnancy. Category A: Controlled human studies have demonstrated no fetal risk. Category B: Animal studies indicate no fetal risk, but no human studies, or adverse effects in animals, but not in well-controlled human studies. Category C: No adequate human or animal studies, or adverse fetal effects in animal studies, but no available human data. Category D: Evidence of fetal risk, but benefits outweigh risks. Category X: Evidence of fetal risk. Risks outweigh any benefits.

Steatorrhea—An excess of fat in the stool.

Stool—The solid waste that is left after food is digested. Stool forms in the intestines and passes out of the body through the anus.

recurrent problems, or those who are about to take a constipating drug, such as narcotic **analgesics**.

Mineral oil is an emollient laxative. It acts by retarding intestinal absorption of fecal water, thereby softening the stool.

The hyperosmotic laxatives are glycerin and lactulose (Chronulac, Duphalac), both of which act by holding water within the intestine. Lactulose may also increase peristaltic action of the intestine.

Precautions

Short term use of laxatives is generally safe except in **appendicitis**, fecal impaction, or intestinal obstruction. Lactulose is composed of two sugar molecules; galactose and fructose, and should not be administered to patients who require a low galactose diet.

Chronic use of laxatives may result in fluid and electrolyte imbalances, steatorrhea, osteomalacia, **diarrhea**, cathartic colon, and **liver** disease. Excessive intake of mineral oil may cause impaired absorption of oil soluble **vitamins**, particularly A and D. Excessive use of magnesium salts may cause hypermanesemia.

Lactulose and magnesium sulfate are **pregnancy** category B. Casanthranol, cascara sagrada, danthron, docusate sodium, docusate **calcium**, docusate potassium, mineral oil and senna are category C. Casanthranol, cascara sagrada and danthron are excreted in breast milk, resulting in a potential increased incidence of diarrhea in the nursing infant.

Interactions

Mineral oil and docusate should not be used in combination. Docusate is an emulsifying agent which will increase the absorption of mineral oil.

Bisacodyl tablets are enteric coated, and so should not be used in combination with **antacids**. The antacids will cause premature rupture of the enteric coating.

Recommended dosage

See specific resources.

Resources

PERIODICALS

"Constipation, Laxatives and Dietary Fiber." *HealthTips* (April 1993): 9.

"Overuse Hazardous: Laxatives Rarely Needed." (Includes related article on types of laxatives.) *FDA Consumer* (April 1991): 33.

ORGANIZATIONS

National Digestive Diseases Information Clearinghouse. 2 Information Way, Bethesda, MD 20892-3570. nddic@aerie.com. <http://www.niddk.nih.gov/Brochures/NDDIC.htm>.

Samuel D. Uretsky, PharmD

Lead poisoning *see* **Trace metal tests**

Learning theory

Definition

Learning is defined as a relatively permanent change in behavior as a result of experience. This definition excludes changes that might occur solely as a result of maturation, injury, or disease. To learn is to adapt. A child might stick his or her finger in a light socket, but not more than once. Sea lions in an aquarium will learn to bark and slap the water if these behaviors prompt people to toss them food. Changes that occur as a result of learning are not always positive. We may acquire bad (maladaptive) habits, as well as good ones. Three basic kinds of learning have been studied extensively by psychologists. These are: classical conditioning, operant conditioning, and observational learning.

Description

Classical conditioning

The pioneer of the study of classical conditioning was Ivan Pavlov. While studying salivation in dogs as part of his research on digestion, Pavlov discovered an interesting phenomenon. Dogs that had been repeatedly given meat in order to induce salivation began to salivate before the presentation of the meat. The sight of the pan containing the meat, or the sound of the experimenter's footsteps coming toward the laboratory was enough to initiate salivation. This was curious. Dogs do not normally salivate to the sound of footsteps, thus they must have acquired this response as a result of experience. In other words, learning had taken place.

Pavlov recognized the potential importance of the dogs' behavior, and subsequently turned his attention to the study of what we now know as conditioned **reflexes**. By carefully scrutinizing the dogs' behaviors under controlled laboratory conditions, Pavlov discovered and described the principles of classical conditioning. In order to understand its operation, there are a few key terms that need to be explained. An unconditional stimulus refers to a thing or event that triggers a response (change) reflexively or automatically. This response is referred to as an unconditional response. It is automatically produced; no learning is needed for it to occur. A neutral stimulus is a stimulus that elicits no response (or at least not the response being studied). When a neutral stimulus is repeatedly paired with an unconditional stimulus it will produce an effect similar to that of the unconditional stimulus. This mutated neutral stimulus, if you will, is referred to as a conditioned stimulus and the response it produces is called a conditioned response. The conditioned response, unlike the unconditioned

response, is learned. Each pairing of an unconditional stimulus with a conditional stimulus is referred to as reinforcement. The pairing strengthens or reinforces the conditioned response. In classical conditioning it is important to remember that the initial stimulus and its response (i.e., the unconditioned stimulus and response) occur naturally; they are instinctual, so to speak.

HOW CLASSICAL CONDITIONING WORKS. In the first stage, the unconditioned (natural) response to an unconditioned stimulus occurs automatically. It is a natural, reflexive reaction. For example, eating meat will make a dog salivate to aid in digestion. In the second stage, a neutral stimulus is paired with the natural or unconditioned stimulus. Using our example of the dog and meat, suppose we ring a bell just before the meat is given to the dog. If we do this repeatedly the bell alone will cause the dog to salivate and this represents the third stage of classical conditioning. In other words the conditioned stimulus now produces a conditioned response. This response was not present before the conditioning process (or learning) took place. Conditioning occurs most quickly and effectively when the conditioned stimulus immediately precedes the unconditioned stimulus.

Because of classical conditioning, certain events can produce unwanted distress for reasons that are largely unrelated to the event itself. Young children, for example, often become fearful during their first visit to a barber. Barbers often wear white smocks, similar to those worn by doctors. There are also numerous metallic instruments (scissors, razors) in plain sight in the barbershop. Unpleasant experiences at the doctor's office (e.g., an injection) could become associated with accompanying stimuli (the doctor's white coat, silver instruments) in such a way that similar stimuli (in other settings) could trigger an **anxiety** response. Some children's barbers make a point of wearing colored (as opposed to white) jackets, and take pains to reduce any similarities between their work areas and doctors' examining rooms.

Viewpoints

On the basis of his research, Pavlov assumed that the basic associations established through classical conditioning were universal. In other words, he believed that all animals would show conditioning, and that any natural response could be conditioned to any and all neutral stimuli. More recent research has shown that there are restrictions on the kinds of associations that are amenable to conditioning. For example when tastes, sounds, and visual stimuli were used as conditioned stimuli prior to being given a nausea-inducing drink, rats very quickly learned to associate **taste** with illness, and forever after avoided similar tasting food. This happened even if the nausea occurred several hours after the ingestion. Moreover, neither the visual nor the auditory stimuli created aversion responses. Apparently all animals, including humans, are biologically prepared to learn some associations rather than others. It is as if nature prepares each species to learn what is best suited to its survival.

Operant conditioning

If the sole mechanism of learning were classical conditioning only a very limited number of responses could be learned. A dog may learn to salivate at the sound of a bell but how are new, voluntary responses learned? How does the animal learn to operate on its environment?

Operant conditioning provides some insight. In classical conditioning the animal is relatively passive. In operant conditioning the animal is an active part of its environment. It operates on the environment. Two pioneers of this approach are Edward L. Thorndike (1874-1949) and B. F. Skinner (1904-1990). At about the same time that Pavlov was performing his experiments with dogs, Thorndike began experimenting with cats. He devised a box from which a cat could escape only if it performed a particular action. For example, the cat would have to press a lever, which would, in turn, cause a rope to pull a bolt from the door and thus allow it to escape. Through trial-and-error the cat would eventually escape from the box. Thorndike noticed that over successive trials, it took progressively less and less time for the cat to solve its problem. Thorndike reasoned that the gratifying experience of being released from the box caused the correct response (pressing the lever) to occur more rapidly on the subsequent trials.

Skinner's research extended and elaborated this simple fact of life: behavior that is rewarded is more likely to recur.

Much of Skinner's research utilized laboratory rats and pigeons. He designed the now famous Skinner Box—a soundproof chamber with a bar or key, which, if pressed or pecked, would dispense a reward of food or water. Once the rat was placed into the box, the experimenter had total control over its environment. The equipment could be programmed to deliver positive or negative reinforcement. For example, the box could be rigged with a lever that, when pressed, turned off a mild electric shock (negative reinforcement). A negative reinforcer is one that strengthens a response by removing an aversive or unpleasant stimulus.

Before a response can be reinforced, it must first occur. Suppose you wanted to teach a dog to climb a ladder. Because this action has no probability of occurring spontaneously, you would wait forever for it to occur so that it could be reinforced. What to do? The solution is to use a procedure known as shaping. When we shape a behavior, we define some ultimate target behavior and then reinforce all actions that are even remotely related to the target behavior. Thus the dog might receive a reward for placing a paw on the bottom rung of the ladder. The trainer then requires responses that are more and more similar to the final, desired response. These responses that are rewarded on the way to the final target behavior are called successive approximations. With shaping (and patience) various animals can be taught to produce extraordinary sequences of behaviors. There are bears in the Russian circus that drive motorcycles. Seeing eye dogs act as the "eyes" for the blind, and can also be taught to assist people with **spinal cord** injuries by turning on light switches or opening doors. The basic principles of operant conditioning have important practical implications. These principles are at the **heart** of behavior modification therapy—a treatment approach that has demonstrated some impressive successes in schools, prisons, mental hospitals, and rehabilitation wards.

Observational learning

While classical conditioning and reinforcement principles are powerful and ubiquitous determinants of behavior, they do not tell the whole story, especially when it comes to human learning. We do not always learn through direct experience. Indeed, we wouldn't survive for very long if we could not learn from watching others. Observational learning plays a role in almost every aspect of our activities, from learning how to hold a fork, drive a car, smoke a cigarette, or have sex. Observational learning occurs in fish, birds, and mammals too. For example, if given a choice, rats will prefer to eat food that they have seen other rats choose. Research has demonstrated that children imitate their parents' food aversions. After the first few months of *The Simpsons* television show, many young girls across the country began expressing an interest in playing the baritone saxophone—Lisa Simpson's instrument of choice.

The observational learning perspective emphasizes that what is learned is 'knowledge' about behavior, in addition to the behavior itself. Role models can be quite influential. If you want to encourage a child to read, read to them, surround him or her with books and with people who read them. Not surprisingly, modeling effects cut both ways. Antisocial role models can cultivate negative patterns of behavior in the observer. Children who grow up in households where wife abuse is common are "learning" that physical assaults and intimidation are effective ways of controlling others. Models are most likely to be imitated when they have status, when their actions are rewarded, when the modeled behaviors are in the observer's repertoire, and when the observer is motivated to emulate the model. While it is disheartening to realize how easily antisocial behaviors can be acquired, the overall legacy from learning theories is one of hope. What is learnable is also (potentially) teachable. This fact inspires parents, teachers and therapists. And what is learned can also be unlearned. No matter how distressed we may feel, we are not stuck forever with our current state. Humans are remarkably capable of change through learning.

Resources

BOOKS

Barone, D., Maddux, J., & Snyder, C. R. *Social cognitive psychology: History and current domains.* New York: Plenum Press, 1997.

Chance, Paul. *Learning and Behavior.* Pacific Grove: Brooks/Cole, 1999.

Geller, E. S. *The psychology of safety: How to improve behaviors and attitudes on the job.* Radnor, PA: Chilton Book Co., 1996.

PERIODICALS

Steinmetz, J. E. "A renewed interest in human classical conditioning." *Psychological Science* 10 (1999): 24-25.

Timothy E. Moore

Leg veins x ray *see* **Phlebography**

Leukemias, acute

Definition

Acute leukemia is a type of **cancer** in which excessive quantities of abnormal white **blood** cells are produced.

Description

Medical science further classifies acute leukemia by the type of white blood cell that undergoes mutation. The most common of these are:

• Acute lymphoblastic leukemia (ALL), in which excessive quantities of lymphoblasts, or immature lymphocyte white blood cells, are produced.

• Acute myeloblastic leukemia (AML), also known as acute nonlymphocytic leukemia (ANLL), in which excessive quantities of other types of immature white blood cells are produced.

Acute leukemias progress rapidly, while the **chronic leukemias** progress more slowly. The vast majority of the childhood leukemias are of the acute form.

The cells that make up blood are produced in the bone marrow and the **lymphatic system**. Bone marrow is the spongy tissue found in the large bones of the body. The lymphatic system includes the spleen (an organ in the upper abdomen), the thymus (a small gland beneath the breastbone), and the tonsils (a mass of lymphatic tissue located in the throat). In addition, the lymphatic vessels (tiny tubes that branch like **blood vessels** into all parts of the body) and lymph nodes (pea-shaped organs that are found along the network of lymphatic vessels) are also part of the lymphatic system. Lymph is a milky fluid that contains cells. Clusters of lymph nodes are found in the neck, underarm, pelvis, abdomen, and chest.

The cells found in the blood include red blood cells (RBCs) that carry oxygen and other materials to all tissues of the body; white blood cells (WBCs) that fight **infection**; and platelets, which play an important role in the clotting of the blood. White blood cells can be further subdivided into three main types: granulocytes, monocytes, and lymphocytes.

The granulocytes, as their name suggests, have particles (granules) inside them. These granules contain special **proteins** (enzymes) and several other substances that can break down chemicals and destroy microorganisms, such as **bacteria**. Monocytes are the second type of white blood cell. They are also important in defending the body against pathogens.

Lymphocytes are the third type of white blood cell. There are two primary types of lymphocytes—T lymphocytes and B lymphocytes—with different functions in the **immune system**. B cells protect the body by making antibodies. Antibodies are proteins that can attach to the surfaces of bacteria and **viruses**. This "attachment" sends signals to many other cell types to come and destroy the antibody-coated organism. T cells protect the body against viruses. When a virus enters a cell, it produces certain proteins that are projected onto the surface of the infected cell. T cells recognize these proteins and make certain chemicals that are capable of destroying the virus-infected cells. In addition, T cells can destroy some types of cancer cells.

Bone marrow makes stem cells, which are the precursors of the different blood cells. These stem cells mature through stages into either RBCs, WBCs, or platelets. In acute leukemias, the maturation process of the white blood cells is interrupted. The immature cells (or "blasts") proliferate rapidly and begin to accumulate in various organs and tissues, thereby affecting their normal function. This uncontrolled proliferation of the immature cells in the bone marrow affects the production of the normal red blood cells and platelets as well.

As noted, there are two types of acute leukemias—acute lymphocytic leukemia and acute myelogenous leukemia. Different types of white blood cells are involved in the two leukemias. In acute lymphocytic leukemia (ALL), it is the T or the B lymphocytes that are involved. The B cell leukemias are more common than T cell leukemias. Acute myelogenous leukemia, also known as acute nonlymphocytic leukemia (ANLL), is a cancer of the monocytes and/or granulocytes.

Leukemias account for 2% of all cancers. Because leukemia is the most common form of childhood cancer, it is often regarded as a disease of childhood. However, leukemias affect far more adults than children. Half of the cases occur in people who are 60 years of age or older. The incidence of acute and chronic leukemias is about the same. According to the estimates of the American Cancer Society (ACS), approximately 29,000 new cases of leukemia are diagnosed each year in the United States. Of these, 27,000 will be diagnosed in adults, 2,000 in children.

Causes and symptoms

Leukemia strikes both sexes and all ages. The human T-cell leukemia virus (HTLV-I), a virus with similarities to the human **immunodeficiency** virus (HIV), is believed to be the causative agent for some kinds of leukemias, but this has not yet been proven, and the cause of most leukemias is not known. Acute lymphoid leukemia (ALL) is more common among Caucasians than among African-Americans, while acute myeloid leukemia (AML) affects both races equally. The incidence of acute leukemia is slightly higher among men than women. People with Jewish ancestry have a higher likelihood of getting leukemia. A higher incidence of leukemia has also been observed among persons with **Down syndrome** and some other genetic abnormalities.

Reports in *Science News* cited studies that found a gene that regulates folic acid **metabolism** in the body to be more prevalent in acute lymphocytic leukemia (ALL) patients. **Folic acid** is known to be involved in the process of DNA maintenance and repair, and this gene diverts folic acid from this function. It is therefore hypothesized that this gene plays a role in the development of ALL, and that folic acid supplementation could lower the risk for developing ALL. This gene has not been found to play a part in other leukemias, such as AML.

Exposure to ionizing radiation, such as occurred in Japan after the atomic bomb explosions, has been shown to increase the risk of getting leukemia. Electromagnetic fields are suspected of being a possible cause, as are certain organic chemicals, such as benzene. Having a history of diseases that damage the bone marrow, such as aplastic anemia, or a history of cancers of the lymphatic system puts people at a high risk for developing acute leukemias. Similarly, the use of anticancer medications, immunosuppressants, and the antibiotic chloramphenicol are also considered risk factors for developing acute leukemias.

The symptoms of leukemia are generally vague and non-specific. A patient may experience all or some of the following symptoms:

- weakness or chronic fatigue
- fever of unknown origin, chills and flu-like symptoms
- weight loss that is not due to dieting or **exercise**
- frequent bacterial or viral infections
- headaches
- skin rash
- non-specific bone **pain**
- easy bruising
- bleeding from gums or nose
- blood in urine or stools
- swollen and tender lymph nodes and/or spleen
- abdominal fullness
- night sweats
- petechiae, or tiny red spots under the skin
- more rarely, sores in the eyes or on the skin

Diagnosis

For a successful outcome, treatment for acute leukemia must begin as soon as possible, but there are no screening tests available. If the doctor has reason to suspect leukemia, he or she will conduct a very thorough **physical examination** to look for enlarged lymph nodes in the neck, underarm, and pelvic region. Swollen gums, enlarged **liver** or spleen, bruises, or pinpoint red rashes all over the body are some of the signs of leukemia. Urine and blood tests may be ordered to check for microscopic amounts of blood in the urine and to obtain a complete differential blood count. This count will give the numbers and percentages of the different cells found in the blood. An abnormal blood test might suggest leukemia; however, the diagnosis must be confirmed by more specific tests.

The doctor may perform a bone marrow biopsy to confirm the diagnosis of leukemia. During the biopsy, a cylindrical piece of bone and marrow is removed. The tissue is generally taken out of the hipbone. These samples are sent to the laboratory where they are examined under a **microscope** by a hematologist, oncologist, or pathologist. In addition to the diagnostic biopsy, another biopsy will also be performed during the treatment phase of the disease to see if the leukemia is responding to therapy.

A spinal tap (lumbar puncture) is another procedure that the doctor may order to diagnose leukemia. In this procedure, a small needle is inserted into the spinal cavity in the lower back to withdraw some cerebrospinal fluid and to look for leukemic cells.

Standard imaging tests, such as x rays, computed tomography scans (**CT scans**), and **magnetic resonance imaging** (MRI) may be used to check whether the leukemic cells have invaded other areas of the body, such as the bones, chest, **kidneys**, abdomen, or **brain**. A gallium scan or bone scan is a test in which a radioactive chemical is injected into the body. This chemical accumulates in the areas of cancer or infection, allowing them to be viewed with a special camera.

Treatment

As noted, treatment must be begun as soon as possible. The goal of treatment is remission, or an arresting of the disease process of the leukemia. There are two phases of treatment for leukemia. The first phase is called induction therapy. As the name suggests, during this phase, the primary aim of the treatment is to reduce the number of leukemic cells as much as possible and induce a remission in the patient. Once the patient shows no obvious signs of leukemia (no leukemic cells are detected in blood tests and bone marrow biopsies), the patient is said to be in remission.

The second phase of treatment is then initiated. This is called continuation or maintenance therapy, and the goal is to kill any remaining cancer cells and to maintain the remission for as long as possible.

Chemotherapy

Chemotherapy is the use of drugs to kill cancer cells. It is usually the treatment of choice in leukemia, and is used to relieve symptoms and achieve long-term remission of the disease. Generally, combination chemotherapy, in which multiple drugs are used, is more efficient than using a single drug for the treatment. Some drugs may be administered intravenously through a vein in the arm; others may be given by mouth in the form of pills. If the cancer cells have invaded the brain, then chemotherapeutic drugs may be put into the fluid that surrounds the brain through a needle in the brain or back.

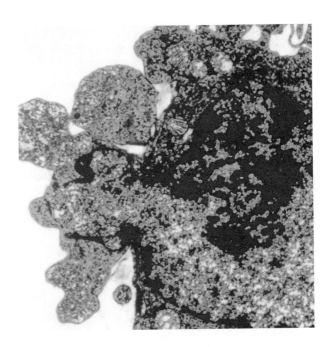

An enhanced transmission electron microscopy (TEM) of acute myelogenous leukemia cells. *(Photograph by Robert Becker, Ph.D., Custom Medical Stock Photo. Reproduced by permission.)*

This is known as intrathecal chemotherapy. Because leukemia cells can spread to all the organs via the blood stream and the lymphatic vessels, surgery is not considered an option for treating leukemias.

Radiation

Radiation therapy, which involves the use of x rays or other high-energy rays to kill cancer cells and shrink tumors, may be used in some cases. For acute leukemias, the source of radiation is usually outside the body (external radiation therapy). If the leukemic cells have spread to the brain, radiation therapy can be given to the brain.

Bone marrow transplantation

Bone marrow transplantation is a process in which the patient's diseased bone marrow is replaced with healthy marrow. There are two ways of doing a bone marrow transplant. In an *allogeneic* bone marrow transplant, healthy marrow is taken from a donor whose tissue is either the same as or very closely resembles the patient's tissues. The donor may be a twin, a brother or sister (sibling), or a person who is not related at all. First, the patient's bone marrow is destroyed with very high doses of chemotherapy and radiation therapy. Healthy marrow from the donor is then given to the patient through a needle in a vein to replace the destroyed marrow.

KEY TERMS

Antibodies—Proteins made by the B lymphocytes in response to the presence in the body of infectious agents, such as bacteria or viruses.

Biopsy—The surgical removal and microscopic examination of living tissue for diagnostic purposes.

Chemotherapy—Treatment with drugs that act against cancer.

Computerized tomography (CT) scan—A series of x rays put together by a computer in order to form detailed pictures of areas inside the body.

Cytokines—Chemicals made by the cells that act on other cells to stimulate or inhibit their function. Cytokines that stimulate growth are called growth factors.

Immunotherapy—Treatment of cancer by stimulating the body's immune defense system.

Lumbar puncture—A procedure in which the doctor inserts a small needle into the spinal cavity in the lower back to withdraw some spinal fluid for testing. Also known as a spinal tap.

Magnetic resonance imaging (MRI)—A medical procedure using a magnet linked to a computer to picture areas inside the body.

Maturation—The process by which stem cells transform from immature cells without a specific function into a particular type of blood cell with defined functions.

Radiation therapy—Treatment using high-energy radiation from x-ray machines, cobalt, radium, or other sources.

Remission—A disappearance of a disease as a result of treatment. Complete remission means that all disease is gone. Partial remission means that the disease is significantly improved by treatment, but residual traces of the disease are still present.

In the second type of bone marrow transplant, called an autologous bone marrow transplant, some of the patient's own marrow is taken out and treated with a combination of **anticancer drugs** to kill all the abnormal cells. This marrow is then frozen to preserve it. The marrow remaining in the patient's body is destroyed with high-dose chemotherapy and radiation therapy. The marrow that was frozen is then thawed and given back to the patient through a needle in a vein. This type of bone marrow transplant is currently being investigated in clinical trials.

Biological therapy or immunotherapy is a mode of treatment in which the body's own immune system is harnessed to fight the cancer. Interferon is a biological therapy that is increasingly being used. Substances that are routinely made by the immune system (such as growth factors, hormones, and disease-fighting proteins) are either synthetically made in a laboratory or their effectiveness is boosted and they are then put back into the patient's body. This treatment mode is also being investigated in clinical trials all over the country at major cancer centers.

Prognosis

Like all cancers, the prognosis for leukemia depends on the patient's age and general health. According to statistics, more than 60% of the patients with leukemia survive for at least a year after diagnosis. Acute myelocytic leukemia (AML) has a poorer prognosis rate than acute lymphocytic leukemias (ALL) and the chronic leukemias. In the last 15 to 20 years, the five-year survival rate for patients with ALL has increased from 38% to 57%.

Interestingly enough, since most childhood leukemias are of the ALL type, chemotherapy has been highly successful in their treatment. This is because chemotherapeutic drugs are most effective against actively growing cells. Due to the new combinations of anticancer drugs being used, the survival rates among children with ALL have improved dramatically. Ninety-five percent of all childhood ALL patients will enter remission, and 60–75% will remain in remission after five years, depending upon the type. T-cell ALL is considered cureable in half of all cases, while B-cell ALL is rarely, if ever cureable. The worst prognosis is for non-typable ALL, whose victims are usually below one year of age.

Health care team roles

In most cases, a diagnosis of leukemia is made in a physician's office, a general medical clinic, or emergency room by a primary care practitioner. Children and adolescents with leukemia are likely to be diagnosed by their primary care physician, or pediatrician. However, oncologists, or physicians that specialize in the diagnosis and treatment of cancer are also often involved. Hematologists, physicians that specialize in the diagnosis and treatment of disorders of the blood and the organs that produce blood cells, may become involved through consultation. A pathologist, or physician who specializes in studying tissue and cell samples, often to assist other physicians in reaching the correct diagnosis, also may be consulted.

Both registered nurses and licensed practical nurses provide direct care to leukemia patients in general hospitals, homes, or other healthcare facilities. Good supportive nursing care and observation are necessary to:

- Prevent or monitor for the infections to which leukemia patients are so susceptible.

- Monitor for anemia and bleeding.

- Assist in treatments such as chemotherapy, radiation, bone-marrow transplantation, or in giving blood transfusions.

- Monitor vital signs.

- Provide teaching regarding the prevention of infection, the normal course of leukemia, including the fatigue so many patients feel, the signs and symptoms of anemia, and good dental care (both leukemia and chemotherapy are apt to cause sensitivity in the mouth, vulnerability to infection and bleeding).

Clinical laboratory scientists draw blood samples that are ordered by the physician to monitor the leukemia from the outset, during treatment, and also during remission. Radiologic technologists take x rays to visualize and monitor parts of the body that may be affected by the leukemia.

Prevention

Most cancers can be prevented by changes in lifestyle or diet, which will reduce the risk factors. However, in leukemias, there are no such known risk factors. Therefore, at the present time, no way is known to prevent leukemias from developing. People who are at an increased risk for developing leukemia because of proven exposure to ionizing radiation or exposure to the toxic liquid benzene, and people with Down syndrome, should undergo periodic medical checkups.

Resources

BOOKS

Beers, Mark H., et al., eds. *Merck Manual of Diagnosis and Therapy.* 17th ed. Rahway, NJ: Merck & Co., 1999.

Keene, Nancy, and Linda Lamb, eds. *Childhood Leukemia: A Guide for Families, Friends and Caregivers.* Cambridge, MA: O'Reilly & Associates, 1999.

Lackritz, Barbara. *Adult Leukemia: A Comprehensive Guide for Patients and Families.* Cambridge, MA: O'Reilly & Associates, 2001.

Murphy, Gerald P. *Informed Decisions: The Complete Book of Cancer Diagnosis, Treatment and Recovery.* Atlanta, GA: American Cancer Society, 1997.

PERIODICALS

Seppa, N. "Genetic Variants May Ease Leukemia Risk." *Science News* 156 (November 6,1999): 293.

ORGANIZATIONS

American Cancer Society. 1599 Clifton Road, N.E., Atlanta, Georgia 30329. (800) 227-2345. <http://www.cancer.org>.

Cancer Research Institute. 681 Fifth Avenue, New York, N.Y. 10022. (800) 992-2623. <http://www.cancerresearch.org>.

National Cancer Institute. 9000 Rockville Pike, Building 31, Room 10A16, Bethesda, Maryland, 20892. (800) 422-6237. <http://wwwicic.nci.nih.gov>.

Leukemia Society of America, Inc. 600 Third Avenue, New York, NY 10016. (800) 955-4572. <http://www.leukemia.org>.

OTHER

University of Pennsylvania Cancer Center. Oncolink. <http://cancer.med.upenn.edu>.

Joan M. Schonbeck

Leukemias, chronic

Definition

Chronic leukemia is a type of **cancer** in which excessive quantities of abnormal white **blood** cells are produced, usually slowly, often over a period of years.

Description

Medical science further classifies chronic leukemia by the type of white blood cell that undergoes mutation. The most common of these are:

- Chronic lymphocytic leukemia (CLL), in which mature-appearing white blood cells called lymphocytes are produced.

- Chronic myeloid (or myelogenous) leukemia (CML), also known as chronic granulocytic leukemia (CGL), is the result of uncontrolled proliferation of white blood cells called granulocytes.

Chronic leukemias are much less rapid-growing than acute leukemia, and affect adults far more often than children. In fact, nearly all the people who develop CLL are over 50 years of age. CML is also a disease primarily of middle-aged to elderly people, but 3% of all childhood leukemias are classified as CML, and the average age for developing CML is between ages 10 and 12.

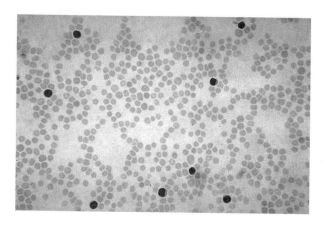

A magnified stain of chronic lymphocytic leukemia cells.
(Custom Medical Stock Photo. Reproduced by permission.)

The cells that make up blood are produced in the bone marrow and the lymph system. The bone marrow is the spongy tissue found in the large bones of the body. The lymph system includes the spleen (an organ in the upper abdomen), the thymus (a small organ beneath the breastbone), and the tonsils (an organ in the throat). The lymph vessels (tiny tubes that branch like **blood vessels** into all parts of the body) and lymph nodes (small pea-shaped organs that are found along the network of lymph vessels) are also part of the lymph system. The lymph itself is a milky fluid that contains cells. Clusters of lymph nodes are found in the neck, underarm, pelvis, abdomen, and chest.

The cells found in the blood are the red blood cells (RBCs), which carry oxygen and other materials to all tissues of the body; white blood cells (WBCs), which fight **infection**; and the platelets, which play an important role in the clotting of the blood. The white blood cells can be further subdivided into three main types: granulocytes, monocytes, and lymphocytes.

The granulocytes have particles (granules) inside them that contain special **proteins** (enzymes) and several other substances that can break down chemicals and destroy microorganisms such as **bacteria**. Monocytes are the second type of white blood cell. They are also important in defending the body against pathogens.

The lymphocytes form the third type of white blood cell. The two primary types of lymphocytes, T lymphocytes and B lymphocytes, have different functions within the **immune system**. The B cells protect the body by making antibodies, which are proteins that can attach to the surfaces of bacteria and **viruses**. This attachment sends signals to many other cell types to destroy the antibody-coated organism. The T cells protect the body against viruses. When a virus enters a cell, it produces certain proteins that are projected onto the surface of the

infected cell. The T cells recognize these proteins and make certain chemicals that are capable of destroying the virus-infected cells. In addition, the T cells can destroy some types of cancer cells.

The bone marrow makes stem cells, which are the precursors of the different blood cells. Stem cells mature into RBCs, WBCs, or platelets. In chronic leukemias, blood cells suddenly begin to proliferate rapidly and begin to accumulate in various organs and tissues, thereby affecting their normal function. This uncontrolled proliferation of the immature cells in the bone marrow affects the production of the normal red blood cells and platelets as well.

Different types of white blood cells are involved in chronic lymphocytic leukemia and chronic myeloid leukemia. Although some blasts, or immature cells (the hallmark of acute leukemia), are also present in chronic leukemia, it is the T or B lymphocytes that gradually mutate and become cancerous. The scenario is similar for chronic myelogenous leukemia, also known as chronic granulocytic leukemia (CGL), which occurs when unusually large numbers of granulocytes begin to appear in the bloodstream.

Leukemias account for 2% of all cancers. According to the estimates of the American Cancer Society (ACS), approximately 29,000 new cases of leukemia are diagnosed each year in the United States. Of these, 27,000 will be diagnosed in adults, 2000 in children. Leukemia is the most common form of childhood cancer, and it is often regarded as a disease of childhood However, leukemias, especially chronic leukemia, affect far more adults than children. Half of all leukemia cases occur in people who are 60 years of age or older, and the overwhelming majority of chronic leukemias occur in adults. The incidence of both acute and chronic leukemias is about the same.

Causes and symptoms

Leukemia strikes both sexes and all ages. The human T-cell leukemia virus (HTLV-I), a virus with similarities to the human immunovirus (HIV), is believed to be the causative agent for some kinds of leukemias, but this has not yet been proven. To date, the cause of most leukemias is not known. Lymphoid leukemias are more common among Caucasians than among African-Americans, while myeloid leukemias affects both races equally. The incidence of leukemia is slightly higher among men than women. People with Jewish ancestry have a higher likelihood of getting leukemia. A higher incidence of leukemia has also been observed among persons with **Down syndrome** and some other genetic abnormalities. Patients with chronic myeloid leukemia often show a chromosome abnormality called the Philadelphia chromosome, that occurs when one chromosome attaches to another.

Exposure to ionizing radiation, such as occurred in Japan after the atomic bomb explosions, has been shown to increase the risk of getting leukemia. Electromagnetic fields are suspected of being a possible cause, as are certain organic chemicals such as benzene. Having a history of diseases that damage the bone marrow, such as aplastic anemia, or a history of cancers of the **lymphatic system** puts people at a high risk for developing leukemias. Similarly, the use of anticancer medications, immunosuppressants, and the antibiotic chloramphenicol are also considered risk factors for developing leukemias.

The symptoms of chronic leukemia are generally vague and non-specific, and are frequently overlooked until they are noticed on routine **physical examination**, especially when a routine blood test such as a **complete blood count** (CBC) is performed. A CBC may show unusually large numbers of a certain type of lymphocyte in the blood. Chronic leukemias may go for years without manifesting any symptoms at all, but also can develop symptoms similar to **acute leukemias**. Chronic myeloid leukemia, in particular, has two phases, a chronic one that can last for several years, and a malignant phase in which immature granulocytes are suddenly generated in huge numbers, producing similar symptoms to acute leukemia. In such cases, a patient may experience all or some of the following symptoms:

- weakness or chronic fatigue
- fever of unknown origin, chills, and flu-like symptoms
- unexplained weight loss
- frequent bacterial or viral infections
- viscous (sticky) blood (which slows down the supply to various organs)
- headache
- non-specific bone pain
- easy bruising
- bleeding from gums or nose
- blood in urine or stools
- swollen and tender lymph nodes and/or spleen
- abdominal fullness
- night sweats
- petechiae, or tiny red spots under the skin
- priapism, or persistent, painful erection of the penis
- rarely, sores in the eyes or on the skin

Diagnosis

As noted, there are often no symptoms present for chronic leukemia, and there are no screening tests available. If the physician has reason to suspect leukemia, a very thorough physical examination will be conducted to look for enlarged lymph nodes in the neck, underarm, and pelvic region. Swollen gums, enlarged **liver** or spleen, bruises, or pinpoint red rashes all over the body are some of the signs of leukemia. Urine and blood tests may be ordered to check for microscopic amounts of blood in the urine and to obtain a complete differential blood count, which gives the numbers and percentages of the different cells found in the blood. An abnormal blood test might suggest leukemia. However, the diagnosis has to be confirmed by more specific tests.

The physician may perform a bone marrow biopsy, during which a cylindrical piece of bone and marrow is removed, generally taken from hipbone. A spinal tap (lumbar puncture) is another procedure that may be ordered. In this procedure, a small needle is inserted into the spinal cavity in the lower back to withdraw some cerebrospinal fluid and to look for leukemic cells.

Standard imaging tests such as x rays, computed tomography (CT) scans, and **magnetic resonance imaging** (MRI) may be used to check whether the leukemic cells have invaded other areas of the body, such as the bones, chest, **kidneys**, abdomen, or **brain**. A gallium scan, or bone scan, is a test in which a radioactive chemical is injected into the body. The chemical accumulates in the areas of cancer or infection, allowing them to be viewed with a special camera.

Treatment

The need for treatment is assessed according to the degree of enlargement of the liver and spleen, a serious decline in the number of platelets in the blood, and whether or not anemia is present, and if present, how severe. Once begun, the goal of treatment is the same as for acute leukemia: remission, or an arresting of the disease process. There are two phases of treatment for leukemia. The first phase is called induction therapy, in which the main aim is to reduce the number of leukemic cells as much as possible and induce a remission in the patient. Once no leukemic cells are detected in blood tests and bone marrow biopsies, the patient is said to be in remission.

The second phase of treatment is then initiated. This is called continuation, or maintenance therapy, and the aim in this case is to kill any remaining cells and to maintain the remission for as long as possible.

KEY TERMS

Antibodies—Proteins made by the B lymphocytes in response to the presence of infectious agents in the body, such as bacteria or viruses.

Biopsy—The surgical removal and microscopic examination of living tissue for diagnostic purposes.

Chemotherapy—Treatment with anticancer drugs.

Computerized tomography (CT) scan—A series of x rays put together by a computer in order to form detailed pictures of areas inside the body.

Immunotherapy—Treatment of cancer by stimulating the body's immune defense system.

Lumbar puncture—A procedure in which the doctor inserts a small needle into the spinal cavity in the lower back to withdraw some spinal fluid for testing; also known as a spinal tap.

Magnetic resonance imaging (MRI)—A medical procedure using a magnet linked to a computer to picture areas inside the body.

Maturation—The process by which stem cells transform from immature cells without a specific function into a particular type of blood cell with defined functions.

Radiation therapy—Treatment using high-energy radiation from x-ray machines, cobalt, radium, or other sources.

Remission—A disappearance of a disease as a result of treatment. Complete remission means that all disease is gone; partial remission means that the disease is significantly improved by treatment, but residual traces are still present.

Chemotherapy

Chemotherapy is usually the treatment of choice in leukemia, and is used to relieve symptoms and achieve long-term remission of the disease. Generally, combination chemotherapy, in which multiple drugs are used, is more efficient than using a single drug for the treatment. Some drugs may be administered intravenously (through a vein), while others may be given by mouth in the form of pills. If the cancer cells have invaded the brain, then chemotherapeutic drugs may be put into the fluid that surrounds the brain through a needle in the brain or back. This is known as intrathecal chemotherapy.

Radiation

Radiation therapy, which involves the use of x rays or other high-energy rays to kill cancer cells and shrink tumors, may be used in some cases. For leukemias, the source of radiation is usually outside the body (external radiation therapy). If the leukemic cells have spread to the brain, radiation therapy can be given to the brain.

Bone marrow transplantation

Bone marrow transplantation is a process in which the patient's diseased bone marrow is replaced with healthy marrow. There are two ways of doing a bone marrow transplant. In an allogeneic bone marrow transplant, healthy marrow is taken from a donor whose tissue is either the same as or very closely resembles the patient's tissues. The donor may be a twin, a sibling, or a person who is not related at all. First, the patient's bone marrow is destroyed with very high doses of chemotherapy and radiation therapy. Healthy marrow from the donor is then administered to the patient through a needle in a vein to replace the destroyed marrow.

In the second type of bone marrow transplant, called an autologous bone marrow transplant, some of the patient's own marrow is taken out and treated with a combination of **anticancer drugs** to kill all the abnormal cells. This marrow is then frozen to save it. The marrow remaining in the patient's body is destroyed with high-dose chemotherapy and radiation therapy. The thawed marrow is returned to the patient intravenously. This mode of bone marrow transplant is currently being investigated in clinical trials.

Biological therapy, or immunotherapy, is a mode of treatment in which the body's own immune system is harnessed to fight the cancer. Interferon is a biological therapy that is increasingly being used. Substances that are routinely made by the immune system, such as growth factors, hormones, and disease-fighting proteins, are either synthetically made in a laboratory or their effectiveness is boosted, and they are then put back into the patient's body. This treatment mode is also being investigated in clinical trials all over the country at major cancer centers.

Because leukemia cells can spread to all the organs via the bloodstream and the lymph vessels, surgery is not considered an option for treating leukemias.

Prognosis

Like all cancers, the prognosis for leukemia depends on the patient's age and general health. According to statistics, more than 60% of the patients with leukemia survive for at least a year after diagnosis. More than half the patients diagnosed with chronic lymphocytic leukemia survive for at least five years due to the slowness of the disease process. Eventual death for CLL patients usually is the result of repeated and overwhelming infections. The outlook for chronic myeloid leukemia is generally less optimistic. Overall, average survival time for CML patients from the time of diagnosis is three years. However, 20% of all CML patients survive for at least 10 years, and bone marrow transplantation is improving the outcome.

Health care team roles

In most cases, a diagnosis of leukemia is made in a physician's office, a general medical clinic, or an emergency room by a primary care practitioner. Children and adolescents with leukemia are likely to be diagnosed by their primary care physician, pediatrician, or pediatric nurse practitioner. Oncologists, specialists in the diagnosis and treatment of cancer, are also often involved.

Hematologists, specialists in the diagnosis and treatment of disorders of the blood and the organs that produce blood cells, may be consulted. A pathologist, a specialist in studying tissue and cell samples, may also assist in diagnosis.

Both registered Nurses (RNs) and licensed practical nurses (LPNs) are often the people who deal the most with leukemia patients both in general hospitals, homes, or other health care facilities. Good supportive nursing care and observation are necessary to:

• Prevent or monitor for infections.

• Monitor for anemia and bleeding.

• Assist in treatments such as chemotherapy, radiation, bone-marrow transplantation, or blood transfusions.

• Monitor vital signs.

• Provide teaching regarding the prevention of infection, the normal course of leukemia, including fatigue, the signs and symptoms of anemia, and good dental care (both leukemia and chemotherapy can cause sensitivity in the mouth, and vulnerability to infection and bleeding).

Clinical laboratory scientists draw blood samples to monitor the leukemia from the outset, during treatment, and also during remission. Radiologic technologists chest x rays to visualize and monitor parts of the body that may be affected.

Prevention

There is no known way to prevent leukemias. People who are at an increased risk for developing leukemia because of proven exposure to ionizing radiation or exposure to the toxic liquid benzene, and people with Down syndrome, should undergo periodic medical checkups.

Resources

BOOKS

Behrman, Richard E. *Nelson Textbook of Pediatrics.* Philadephia: W. B. Saunders, 1995.

Berkow, Robert, and Mark H. Beers, eds. *Merck Manual of Diagnosis and Therapy, 17th ed.* Whitehouse Station, NJ: Merck Research Laboratories, 1999.

Murphy, Gerald P. *Informed Decisions: The Complete Book of Cancer Diagnosis, Treatment and Recovery.* Atlanta, GA: American Cancer Society, 1997.

ORGANIZATIONS

American Cancer Society. 1599 Clifton Road, N.E., Atlanta, Georgia 30329. (800) 227-2345. <http://www.cancer.org>.

Cancer Research Institute. 681 Fifth Avenue, New York, N.Y. 10022. (800) 992-2623. <http://www.cancerresearch.org>.

Leukemia Society of America, Inc. 600 Third Avenue, New York, NY 10016. (800) 955 4572. <http://www.leukemia.org>.

National Cancer Institute. 9000 Rockville Pike, Building 31, Room 10A16, Bethesda, Maryland, 20892. (800) 422-6237. <http://wwwicic.nci.nih.gov>.

Oncolink. University of Pennsylvania Cancer Center. <http://cancer.med.upenn.edu>.

Joan M. Schonbeck

Levodopa *see* **Antiparkinson drugs**

LGI *see* **Barium enema**

Licensed practical nurse

Definition

Licensed practical nurses (L.P.N.s) work under the direction of physicians and registered nurses to provide wellness, preventive, and other health care services to people of all walks of life, including those who are sick, injured, convalescent, and disabled.

Description

L.P.N.s, or licensed vocational nurses (L.V.N.s), as they are called in Texas and California, provide basic bedside care. They work under the supervision of an **registered nurse**, physician, or other health care provider.

Licensed practical nurse

L.P.N.s work as part of the health care team taking **vital signs**, including temperature, pulse, **blood pressure**, and respiration. They record patients' progress, including patients' food and beverage intake and output. L.P.N.s help hospitalized, bedridden, and other patients with personal hygiene, assisting with bathing and dressing, as well as caring for patients' comfort and emotional well-being.

L.P.N.s can be scrub nurses. Scrub nurses directly assist surgeons in the operating room. They are responsible for setting up sterile instruments and supplies and handing them to the operating surgeon or surgical assistant during the procedure. L.P.N.s prepare and give injections and **enemas**. They treat bedsores, apply dressings, give alcohol rubs and massages, care for tracheostomies, apply ice packs and hot water bottles, and insert catheters. Often, L.P.N.s observe patients so that the nurses can report adverse reactions to treatments or medications. They help to prepare patients for testing by feeding them or giving them necessary liquids. L.P.N.s also collect patient samples for testing and perform some routine laboratory tests. In some states, L.P.N.s are allowed to administer prescribed medications or start intravenous fluids. L.P.N.s also help deliver babies, and care for and feed infants.

In some cases, experienced L.P.N.s supervise other health care professionals, including nursing assistants and aides. In addition to clinical tasks, L.P.N.s provide a variety of clerical or administrative services. Especially when they work in doctors' offices and clinics, L.P.N.s often assist the administrative staff by making appointments, keeping records and answering phones. As other types of nurses, L.P.N.s take part in educating patients about health care, preventive health maintenance, and at-home treatment. They help to promote preventive measures in community health and act to safeguard health and life. L.P.N.s who work in private homes, caring for people who are unable to care for themselves full-time, often help with daily tasks, such as cooking and running errands.

L.P.N.s often assume broad responsibilities when working in **nursing homes**. In addition to providing general bedside services, L.P.N.s employed in nursing homes might assist the health care team, which general includes registered nurses and physicians, with evaluating residents' needs, initiating care plans and overseeing the activities of nurse aides.

In 1998, L.P.N.s held about 692,000 jobs. It is important that anyone considering a career as a L.P.N. is caring and sympathetic in nature. The job can be emotionally stressful because these nurses often work with the critically or chronically ill. It requires that the nurse exhibit emotional stability and be able to take direction from other types of nurses, doctors and other supervisory staff.

L.P.N.s enjoy flexible work schedules, especially in the hospital setting, where they can work nights and weekends. Most who work full time work a 40-hour week. One in four L.P.N.s worked part time in 1998. Some of the drawbacks of the job are the **stress** levels, which can be exacerbated by heavy workloads and patients who are confused or irrational due to their illnesses. Most L.P.N.s spend much of their working hours on their feet, and the job can often require heavy lifting. At times, because of the nature of their work, L.P.N.s can be at risk for exposure to caustic chemicals, radiation and infectious diseases, including hepatitis. It is important that L.P.N.s always observe health guidelines.

L.P.N.s earned median annual earnings of $26,940 in 1998. The highest area of reported median annual earnings was in personnel supply services, which was at $30,200 a year. The lowest annual earnings were reported by L.P.N.s working in doctors' offices and clinics, which was $24,500. L.P.N.s who work hourly are reported to make from $12 to $18 an hour.

Work settings

L.P.N.s work in all types of health care settings, including hospitals, clinics, **public health** environments, home health care agencies, assisted living facilities, rehabilitation facilities and nursing homes. Thirty-two percent of L.P.N.s worked in acute care hospitals in 1998, while 28% worked in nursing homes and 14% worked in doctors' offices and health care clinics. Many others work for temporary help agencies, residential care facilities, schools and government agencies.

Education and training

L.P.N.s must pass a licensing examination once they complete a state-approved practical nursing program. While most state-approved programs require a high school diploma, some do not and will allow someone with a high school diploma or specific GED score to participate in the program. Many programs require that potential students pass an entrance exam and interview with the program's director.

About 1,100 state-approved programs provided practical nursing training in 1998. Nearly six in every 10 of these students went to technical or vocational schools. Three in 10 of these students attended programs in community and junior colleges; while the remaining students graduated from programs in high schools, hospitals, colleges, and universities.

Practical nursing programs prepare students to qualify and pass the National Council Licensure Examination. After their scholastic training, L.P.N.s should be able to utilize the nursing process to care for patients. They learn to teach patients about health maintenance and prevention of disease. Essentially, L.P.N.s learn to function as generalists in practical nursing in a variety of health care settings. Practical nursing programs usually require that students go through about a year of learning in the classroom and supervised clinical practice. In the classroom, these nurses discover basic nursing concepts and patient care. These nurses take classes in such subjects as: anatomy, physiology, medical-surgical nursing, **medical terminology**, pediatrics, **pharmacology**, obstetrics, psychiatric nursing, advanced nursing procedures, geriatrics, administration of drugs, **nutrition**, health and wellness, and **first aid**. Clinical practice might be in the hospitals in addition to other health care settings, including community health care clinics, schools, nursing homes and rehabilitation settings.

Advanced education and training

L.P.N.s can continue their educations to become registered nurses, or RNs. RNs have expanded roles, working collaboratively with physicians and other health care providers. They often oversee the work of L.P.N.s. RNs must graduate from a nursing program and pass a national licensing examination to become licensed. They must periodically renew their licenses and, depending on which state they work, must also take continued education courses for license renewal. There were more than 2,200 entry-level RN programs in the United States in 1998. RNs can pursue one of three educational options. They can achieve an associate degree in nursing, which is usually offered at community and junior colleges and is about two years long; a bachelor of science degree in nursing, taken at colleges and universities and usually taking from four to five years; or a diploma program, which is given in hospitals and lasts about two to three years. Licensed graduates of any of these levels usually qualify to start work at the staff nurse level. Most RNs graduate with either an associate's or bachelor's degree. There has been talk of the requirement for an RN changing to a bachelor's degree or higher; however, this would not affect current associate degree RNs and would probably take place on a state-by-state basis. Most agree that there are more opportunities for advancement for RNs with bachelor's degrees in nursing. A bachelor's often is necessary for administrative positions and is required for admission to graduate nursing programs of all types, including research, consulting, teaching and clinical specialization. Today an increasing number of nurse executives are saying that they want a majority of their hospi-

---

KEY TERMS

Registered nurse—A nurse who has graduated from a nursing program, including an associate degree, bachelor of science degree or diploma program, and passed a national licensing examination.

Scrub nurse—Scrub nurses directly assist surgeons in the operating room. They are responsible for setting up sterile instruments and supplies and handing them to the operating surgeon or surgical assistant during the procedure.

---

tal staff nurses to have bachelor's degrees because of the more complex demands of patient care. In 1996, 27 percent of RNs reported having a diploma, 31% had a bachelor's degree and 32% held an associate's degree.

Students in R.N. programs take courses in anatomy, physiology, microbiology, nutrition, psychology, chemistry, nursing, and other behavioral sciences. In addition to classroom instruction, nursing students receive supervised clinical experience in hospitals and other health care facilities. Nursing students received a variety of clinical experience in settings such as hospital maternity, psychiatric, pediatric, and surgical wards. They also gain experience in public health departments, home health agencies and ambulatory clinics.

Once they become RNs, nurses can go on to become **advanced practice nurses**, which include nurse practitioners, clinical nurse specialists, certified registered nurse anesthetists and certified nurse-midwives. Advanced practice nurses generally have master's degrees or certificates. Nurse practitioners deliver front-line primary and acute care. They can prescribe medications and diagnose and treat common acute illnesses and injuries. Nurse practitioners provide immunizations, conduct physical exams and provide care to manage chronic diseases, such as diabetes. Certified nurse-midwives are trained to provide prenatal and gynecological care to healthy women. They also deliver babies in all types of settings, including at the patient's home, and provide **postpartum care**. Clinical nurse specialists specialize in areas such as cardiology, oncology and pediatrics. Certified registered nurse anesthetists administer anesthetics to patients in in-patient, outpatient and in-office settings. They are often the sole providers of anesthesia.

RNs can also go on to careers in teaching, research or administration. These areas require master's in nursing degrees or Ph.D. or other doctorate level degrees.

Doctorally-prepared RNs tend to go into education or research.

Future outlook

The future looks good for L.P.N.s. Job growth in this area of nursing is expected to grow as fast as the average for all occupations through 2008. The job growth can be attributed to a rapidly aging population, which will require long-term care. The area that appears to be not as promising for L.P.N.s is in the acute care hospital setting, where the number of openings for L.P.N.s is expected to decline. This is due to an expected decrease in the number of admitted patients. Nursing home employment for L.P.N.s is expected to grow; in fact, geriatric care is where L.P.N.s will find the most opportunity. The growth is nursing home employment of L.P.N.s is not only attributed to the growth in the aging population but also to an expected increase in the number of patients who are released early from hospitals but cannot yet take care of themselves at home.

Home health care looks promising for L.P.N.s. Many of the aged and ill will prefer to stay at home rather than be admitted to a nursing home. Technological advances will make it possible for more people to live out much of their remaining years at home.

Employment also is expected to grow much faster than average in settings that will benefit from advances in health care technology, including outpatient surgery centers, emergency medical centers and some physicians' offices and clinics. Here, too, L.P.N.s will find more opportunity in the future.

Resources

ORGANIZATIONS

Central School of Practicing Nursing, 4600 Carnegie Avenue, Cleveland, OH 44103. <www.cspnohio.org>.

OTHER

Occupational Outlook Handbook, U.S. Department of Labor, Bureau of Labor Statistics, Division of Information Services, 2 Massachusetts Ave. NE, Room 2860, Washington, DC 20212. (202) 691-5200. <http://stats.bls.gov>.

Lisette Hilton

Ligament sprain *see* **Sprains and strains**

Ligament tests *see* **Orthopedic tests**

Light therapy *see* **Phototherapy**

Lipase tests *see* **Amylase and lipase tests**

Lipid tests

Definition

Lipid tests routinely performed on plasma include measurement of total cholesterol, triglycerides, high-density lipoprotein (HDL) cholesterol, and low-density lipoprotein (LDL) cholesterol. Lipid tests may also be performed on amniotic fluid and include tests for lecithin and other pulmonary surfactants.

Purpose

The purpose of **blood** lipid testing is to determine whether abnormally high or low concentrations of a specific lipid are present. Low levels of cholesterol are associated with **liver** failure and inherited disorders of cholesterol production. Cholesterol is a primary component of the plaques that form in atherosclerosis and is therefore the major risk factor for the rapid progression of **coronary artery disease**. High blood cholesterol may be inherited, or result from other conditions such as biliary obstruction, **diabetes mellitus**, hypothyroidism, and nephrotic syndrome. In addition, cholesterol may be increased in persons who have a diet rich in saturated **fats** and cholesterol and who lead a sedentary lifestyle. Low levels of triglyceride are seen in persons who have malnutrition or malabsorption. Increased levels are associated with diabetes mellitus, hypothyroidism, **pancreatitis**, glycogen storage diseases, and estrogens. Diets rich in either **carbohydrates** or fats may cause elevated triglycerides in some persons. Although not a component of the atherosclerotic plaque, triglycerides increase blood viscosity and promote **obesity** that can contribute to coronary disease. The majority of cholesterol and triglyceride testing is performed to screen persons for increased risk of coronary artery disease.

Lipid tests are performed on amniotic fluid to determine the maturity of the fetal **lungs**. Tests are performed prior to delivery to ensure that there is sufficient pulmonary surfactant to prevent collapse of the lungs during exhalation.

Description

Cholesterol screening can be performed with or without fasting and should include total and HDL cholesterol tests. The frequency of cholesterol testing depends on the patient's risk for CAD. Adults over 20 with total cholesterol levels below 200 mg/dL need to be tested once every five years. People with higher levels should be tested for LDL cholesterol and tested at least once per year thereafter, if the LDL cholesterol is 130 mg/dL or higher. The National Cholesterol Education Program (NCEP) suggests further evaluation when the patient has any of the symptoms of CAD or if she or he has two or more of the following risk factors for CAD:

- high **blood pressure**
- cigarette smoking
- diabetes
- low HDL levels
- family history of CAD
- age, men over 45 years and women over 55 years

Measurements of cholesterol and triglycerides are routinely performed using enzymatic methods. For cholesterol, the cholesterol oxidase method is used. Plasma or serum is mixed with a reagent containing cholesterol ester hydrolyase, cholesterol oxidase, peroxidase, and a chromogen. The cholesterol ester hydrolyase converts cholesterol esters (cholesterol coupled to a fatty acid) to free cholesterol. This reacts with cholesterol oxidase forming an oxidation product and hydrogen peroxide. The peroxidase enzyme catalyzes the oxidation of the chromogen by the hydrogen peroxide. This forms a red colored product that can be measured with a spectrophotometer. The amount of light absorbed at 500 nm is directly proportional to cholesterol concentration. HDL cholesterol is usually measured by the same reaction except that the enzymes are coupled to polyethylene glycol (PEG). In the presence of sulfated cyclodextrin, these enzymes will not react with the cholesterol in LDL, VLDL, or chylomicrons. LDL cholesterol is measured by first precipitating the other lipoproteins using a mixture of antibodies to apolipoprotein C and apolipoprotein E. The LDL cholesterol can be separated by centrifugation and then measured using the cholesterol oxidase reaction. Alternatively, LDL cholesterol can be calculated using the Friedewald formula. LDL cholesterol = total cholesterol minus (HDL cholesterol + triglyceride/5). This formula will underestimate LDL cholesterol when triglycerides are above 400 mg/dL.

Triglycerides are routinely measured using the glycerol kinase reaction. The reagent contains the enzymes lipase, glycerol kinase, glycerol phosphate oxidase, and peroxidase. It also contains adenosine triphosphate (ATP) and a chromogen. Triglycerides are composed of glycerol that is bound (esterified) to three long chain fatty acids. The lipase sequentially splits the fatty acids from the molecule forming glycerol and free fatty acids. The glycerol kinase catalyzes the transfer of **phosphorus** from ATP to the glycerol forming glycerol-phosphate. The glycerol phosphate oxidase is used to oxidize this to dihydroxyacetone phosphate. This reaction generates hydrogen peroxide. In the final step, the peroxidase enzyme catalyzes the oxidation of the chromogen by the hydrogen peroxide. This forms a red-colored product that can be measured with a spectrophotometer. The amount of light absorbed at 500 nm is directly proportional to triglyceride concentration. An important potential interfering substance in this reaction is glycerol, which is a common additive to many medications. If the Friedewald formula is used to calculate LDL cholesterol, the triglyceride measurement must be corrected by subtracting the plasma glycerol concentration from the triglyceride result.

Measurement of pulmonary surfactants

During the first half of gestation, lecithin and sphingomyelin levels in amniotic fluid are approximately equal. During the second half of **pregnancy**, lecithin production increases, but the sphingomyelin remains constant. Lecithin is the principal pulmonary surfactant secreted by the alveolar cells (type II granular pneumocytes) of the lung. Lecithin and the other surfactants prevent collapse of the air sacs during expiration. Infants born prematurely may suffer from **respiratory distress syndrome** (RDS) because levels of pulmonary surfactant are insufficient to prevent collapse of the air sacs. Tests for RDS are called fetal lung maturity (FLM) tests. The reference method for determining fetal lung maturity is the amniotic fluid L/S ratio. This is measured by thin layer chromatography in which lecithin and sphingomyelin in the amniotic fluid are separated and stained to determine their relative concentrations. An L/S ratio of 2:1 or higher is consistent with fetal lung maturity. Amniotic fluid levels of other surfactants such as phosphatidyl glycerol (PG), phosphatidyl glycerol, phosphatidyl inositol, and phosphatidyl ethanolamine may be measured by high performance liquid chromatography (HPLC). PG in amniotic fluid can be detected by a latex-coated antibody (latex agglutination) test. PG is an important marker for fetal lung maturity because a falsely positive test for lecithin may occur when the fluid is contaminated with blood or meconium. Since PG is not present in blood or meconium, and is only present when lecithin is adequate, a positive test is conclusive evidence of lung maturity. Measurement of lecithin which comprises about three quarters of the total surfactant composition at birth is most often measured by fluorescence polarization. This assay has replaced the L/S ratio as the FLM test in most labs. Most of the pulmonary surfactants are present in the form of lamellar bodies. These can be counted in the amniotic fluid using an electronic cell counter at the platelet threshold. The number of lamellar bodies is proportional to the quantity of surfactant.

KEY TERMS

Amniocentesis—A procedure to remove amniotic fluid from the womb using a fine needle.

Atherosclerosis—A disease of the coronary arteries in which cholesterol is deposited in plaques on the arterial walls. The plaque narrows or blocks blood flow to the heart. Atherosclerosis is sometimes called coronary artery disease, or CAD.

High-density lipoprotein (HDL)—A type of lipoprotein that protects against CAD by removing cholesterol deposits from arteries or preventing their formation.

Hypercholesterolemia—The presence of excessively high levels of cholesterol in the blood.

Hypertriglyceridemia—The presence of excessively high levels of TAG in the blood.

Lecithin—A phospholipid found in high concentrations in surfactant.

Lipid—Any organic compound that is greasy, insoluble in water, but soluble in alcohol. Fats, waxes, and oils are examples of lipids.

Lipoprotein—A complex molecule that consists of a protein membrane surrounding a core of lipids. Lipoproteins carry cholesterol and other lipids from the digestive tract to the liver and other body tissues. There are five major types of lipoproteins.

Low-density lipoprotein (LDL)—A type of lipoprotein that consists of about 50% cholesterol and is associated with an increased risk of CAD.

Plaque—An abnormal deposit of cholesterol, TAG, dead cells, lipoproteins and calcium on the wall of an artery.

Surfactant—A compound made of fats and proteins that is found in a thin film along the walls of the air sacs of the lungs. Surfactant keeps the surface pressure low so that the sacs can inflate easily and not collapse.

Tocolytic drug—A compound given to women to stop the progression of labor.

Triacylglyceride—A chemical compound that forms about 95% of the fats and oils stored in animal and vegetable cells. TAG levels are sometimes measured as well as cholesterol when a patient is screened for heart disease.

Precautions

Tests for triglycerides and LDL cholesterol must be performed following a 12-hour fast. The nurse or phlebotomist collecting the blood sample should observe **universal precautions** for the prevention of transmission of bloodborne pathogens. Acute illness, high **fever**, starvation, or recent surgery lowers blood cholesterol and triglyceride levels. If possible, patients should also stop taking any medications that may affect the accuracy of the test.

Amniotic fluid is collected by a process called **amniocentesis**. This procedure is usually performed between the after the 33rd week of gestation to evaluate lung maturity. Spontaneous abortion can occur as a consequence of this procedure. Its overall incidence following amniocentesis is approximately 1%. Complications include premature labor and placental bleeding. The fluid may be contaminated with blood or meconium (intestinal contents of the fetus), which can interfere with some fetal lung maturity tests.

Preparation

Patients who are scheduled for a lipid profile test should fast (except for water) for 12-14 hours before the blood sample is drawn. If the patient's LDL cholesterol is to be measured, he or she should also avoid alcohol for 24 hours before the test. When possible, patients should also stop taking any medications that may affect the accuracy of the test results. These include **corticosteroids**, estrogen or androgens, oral contraceptives, some diuretics, haloperidol, some **antibiotics**, and **niacin**. Antilipemics are drugs that lower the concentration of fatty substances in the blood. When these are taken by the patient, blood testing may be done frequently to evaluate liver function as well as lipid levels.

Aftercare

Aftercare with the blood lipid tests includes routine care of the skin around the needle puncture. Most patients have no aftereffects, but some may have a small bruise or swelling. A washcloth soaked in warm water usually relieves any discomfort. In addition, the patient should resume taking any prescription medications that were discontinued before the test.

Care after amniocentesis requires that the clinician watch the patient for any signs of **infection** or possible injury to the fetus. Some things to look for are fever, vaginal bleeding, or vaginal discharge. The patient may feel sick and there may be some cramping. She should be advised to rest and to avoid strenuous activity. If labor is impending, supportive care should be provided to the patient and tocolytic agents may be necessary to prevent the premature birth of the baby.

Complications

The primary risk to the patient with the lipid blood tests is a mild stinging or burning sensation during the venipuncture, with minor swelling or bruising afterward.

Amniocentesis, while much safer in the third trimester, and much safer now that it is done with the guidance of ultrasound technology does present a risk of **miscarriage** and fetal injury. The patient should be watched for any signs of bleeding, infection, or impending labor.

Results

The normal values for serum **lipids** depend on the patient's age, sex, and race. Normal values for people in Western countries are usually given as 140-220 mg/dL for total cholesterol in adults, although as many as 5% of the population have a total cholesterol higher than 300 mg/dL. Among Asians, the figures are about 20% lower. As a rule, both total and LDL cholesterol levels rise as people get older. Normal values for HDL cholesterol are also age and sex dependent. The range for males between 20-29 years is approximately 30-63 mg/dL and for females of the same age group it is 33-83 mg/dL. Normal values for fasting triglycerides are also age and sex dependent. The reference range for adult males 20-29 years is 45-200 mg/dL and for females of the same age group it is 37-144 mg/dL. As with cholesterol, the normal range increases with age.

Since diet and lifestyle affect normal values, which are determined by the interval between the 5th and 95th percentile of the group, it is more helpful to evaluate cholesterol and triglycerides from the perspective of desirable plasma levels. Desirable values defined by the Nation Cholesterol Education Program (NCEP) in 2001 are as follows:

• Total cholesterol: Less than 200 mg/dL; 200-239 mg/dL is borderline high and greater than 240 mg/dL is high.

• HDL cholesterol: Less than 40mg/dL is low.

• LDL cholesterol: Less than 100 mg/dL is optimal; near optimal is 100-129 mg/dL; borderline high is 130-159 mg/dL; high is 160-189 mg/dL; and very high is anything over 190 mg/dL.

• Total cholesterol: HDL ratio: Under 4.0 in males; 3.8 in females.

FLM tests

Low levels of surfactant in amniotic fluid are denoted by an L/S ratio less than 2.0 or a lecithin level less than or equal to 0.10 mg/dL. Lung development can be delayed in premature births and in babies whose mothers have diabetes.

Health care team roles

Physicians will order the blood lipid tests on patients who have risk factors for **heart** disease or who have not been tested within the past five years. A dietician may be consulted if test results are abnormal. FLM tests are ordered by a physician, usually an obstetrician. Lipid tests are performed by clinical laboratory scientists/medical technologists or clinical laboratory technicians/medical laboratory technicians.

Patient education

Nurses should explain the results of abnormal blood lipid tests to patients and advise them on lifestyle changes. **Patient education** is important in fetal lung maturity testing. The situation faced by the expectant parents may be very critical, and the more information they can be given, the better choices they can make.

Resources

BOOKS

Baron, Robert B. and Warren S. Browner. "Lipid Abnormalities." In *Current Medical Diagnosis & Treatment 1998.* edited by Lawrence M. Tierney et al. Stamford, CT: Appleton & Lange, 1997.

Kaplan, Lawrence A. and Amadeo J. Pesce. *Clinical Chemistry, Theory, Analysis and Correlation.* St. Louis: Mosby Publishers, 1996.

OTHER

National Cholesterol Education Program. The National Heart, Lung, and Blood Institute. National Institutes of Health. PO Box 30105, Bethesda, MD, 20824-0105. 301-251-1222. <http://www.nhlbi.nih.gov/guidelines/cholesterol/atglance.pdf>. (May 2001).

Jane E. Phillips

Lipids

Definition

Lipids are a wide-ranging group of organic compounds found in all living organisms, including humans,

KEY TERMS

Hypercholesterolemia—An excess of cholesterol in the blood.

Hyperlipidemia—A group of disorders characterized by an excess of fatty substances, such as cholesterol, triglycerides, and lipoproteins, in the blood.

Protoplasmic—Relating to protoplasm, a colorless jellylike substance that is the main constituent of all human cells and tissue.

plants, and animals. Lipids are the body's reserve supply of energy. Unlike other organic compounds, lipids are soluble in alcohol, ether, and other organic substances but not in water.

Description

Lipid comes from the Greek word *lipos*, meaning fat. Cells make lipids in the human body and, along with **carbohydrates** and **proteins**, are components of all life. Among the major classes of lipids in humans are acids, glycerol-derived lipids (including **fats** and oils), and steroids. The two major lipids found in the **blood** are cholesterol and triglycerides.

Cholesterol

Cholesterol is a lipid that is essential for repairing **cell membranes**, manufacturing **vitamin D** on the skin's surface, and creating hormones, especially testosterone and estrogen. To circulate in the bloodstream, cholesterol must attach to proteins. The combination of cholesterol and protein is called lipoprotein.

The two major lipoprotein groups are high-density lipoprotein (HDL), commonly referred to as "good" cholesterol, and low-density lipoprotein (LDL), also known as "bad" cholesterol. HDL helps prevent fat buildup throughout the body by carrying cholesterol from the arteries to the **liver**, where it is disposed of. LDL carries most of the cholesterol in the body, so an excess of LDL can clog the arteries with cholesterol buildup.

High levels of LDL are 100 milligrams or more per deciliter (mg/dL) of blood for people with **heart** or vascular disease or diabetes, 160 mg/dL for people with two risk factors, and 190 mg/dL or more for people with no risk factors. A high LDL level is a primary cause of coronary heart disease (CHD) and stroke. This is because when LDL accumulates in the body, it forms a plaque

that sticks to the walls of arteries, slowing or restricting blood flow and oxygen delivery to the heart and other vital organs. This causes atherosclerosis, commonly referred to as hardening of the arteries. The buildup of plaque usually occurs over a few years and without cholesterol tests the patient may not know about the problem until angina (chest pains) or an acute **myocardial infarction** (heart attack) occurs.

Among the key risk factors for high LDL are age, gender, smoking, diabetes, and a family history of the disorder. About 25% of people with high LDL can control the disorder with a diet low in saturated fats and cholesterol, weight control, and regular **exercise**. About 75% of people with high LDL require lipid-lowering medications in addition to the weight, diet, and exercise guidelines. First-line drugs recommended by the National Cholesterol Education Program to treat high LDL are bile acid sequestrants such as cholestyramine (Questran) and colestipol (Colestid), **niacin** (either over-the-counter or time-released prescription drugs such as Niaspan, Slo-Niacin, and Nicobid), and HMG-CoA reductase inhibitors, including fluvastatin (Lescol), pravastatin (Pravachol), cervistatin (Baycol), lovastatin (Mevacor), simvastatin (Zocor), and atorvastatin (Lipitor). The second-line drug choice are fibric acid derivatives such as gemfibrozil, clofibrate, and fenofibrate (Tricor.) Estrogen replacement therapy should also be considered as complementary therapy in postmenopausal women.

Levels of HDL between 30 and 75 mg/dL are associated with decreased risk of CHD and stroke. But HDL levels under 30 mg/dL are associated with a greater risk for CHD and stroke.

Triglycerides

Triglycerides are another form of fat that comes from foods and is carried through the bloodstream to the tissues. High levels of triglycerides in the blood can mean that there is too much fat in the diet. Hypertriglyceridemia (high levels of triglycerides) is associated with coronary heart disease, especially since elevated triglycerides levels are usually associated with unhealthy low levels of HDL, which is necessary for good health.

High triglyceride levels (more than 150 mg/dL) can be caused by excessive intake of alcohol or high-calorie foods. Other risk factors include a family history of high triglycerides, **obesity**, **hypertension** (high **blood pressure**), and diabetes. Treatment generally includes controlling other disorders such as diabetes and high blood pressure, proper diet and regular exercise, and fibric acid derivatives such as gemfibrozil, clofibrate, or fenofibrate.

Other lipids

Lipoprotein(a) is a cholesterol-carrying molecule similar in structure to LDL and is believed to carry a protein that interferes with the body's ability to dissolve blood clots. Elevated levels may contribute to heart attacks. Apolipoprotein A-1 is a molecule associated with healthy hearts and may lower the risk of heart disease due to high HDL. Apolipoprotein B is associated with high LDL and may be more effective in predicting heart disease in women. Remnant lipoproteins are byproducts of chylomicrons, lipid particles common in the blood during fat digestion and assimilation, and/or very low density lipoproteins. Initial research suggest they may be a risk factor for CHD.

Function

Lipids manufactured by cells in the body form part of the protoplasmic structure of cells. Lipids act as a reserve source of energy. When broken down to be used as energy, lipids are converted to an energy-rich compound called adenosine triphosphate by a process known as fatty acid oxidation or beta oxidation.

Role in human health

Lipids are important to the human body since they helps produce hormones, and builds cell membranes and other needed tissue. Lipids, both lipoproteins and triglycerides, are made and stored in the body and are used as energy sources. Lipids also play a major role in cardiovascular health.

Common diseases and disorders

The two primary conditions associated with lipids are hyperlipidemia and hypercholesterolemia. These conditions have no overt symptoms but can lead to several serious disorders, primarily:

- Angina, which is chest **pain** that occurs when the heart does not get enough oxygen. When angina is not caused by **stress** or physical exertion and becomes frequent and more severe, it is called unstable angina, and may indicate an impending heart attack.

- Atherosclerosis, also called hardening of the arteries, a condition in which fatty deposits called plaque build up inside the arteries, restricting blood flow.

- Coronary heart disease, in which the arteries narrow, restricting the flow of blood and oxygen to the heart. Lack of sufficient oxygen to the heart can lead to angina or a heart attack. Most cases of CHD are due to atherosclerosis.

- Stroke, a group of **brain** disorders involving loss of brain functions that occur when the blood supply to any part of the brain is interrupted. Strokes are most commonly caused by atherosclerosis.

Resources

BOOKS

Gotto, Antonio M. and Pownall, Henry J. *Manual of Lipid Disorders: Reducing the Risk for Coronary Heart Disease.* New York: Lippincott Williams & Wilkins Publishers, 1999.

Gurr, M. I., et al. *Lipid Biochemistry.* Malden, MA: Blackwell Science Inc., 2001.

Pond, Caroline M. *The Fats of Life.* New York: Cambridge University Press, 1998.

Tyman, J. H. P. *Lipids in Health and Nutrition.* London: Royal Society of Chemistry, 1999.

PERIODICALS

Barnard, N., et al. "Does a Low-Fat Vegetarian Diet Alter Serum Lipids?" *Nutrition Research Letter* (Sept. 2000): 15.

Bell, Stacey J., et al. "The New Dietary Fats in Health and Disease." *Journal of the American Dietary Association* (March 1997): 280–286.

Franklin, Deborah. "What This CEO Didn't Know About His Cholesterol Almost Killed Him: Half of all Heart Attacks Happen to People Whose Blood Tests are Normal. New Screening May Help Reveal Who is Really at Risk." *Fortune* (March 19, 2001): 154+.

Mormando, Robert M. "Lipid Levels: Applying the Second National Cholesterol Education Program Report to Geriatric Medicine." *Geriatrics* (Aug. 2000): 48+.

Raloff, Janet. "Sphinx of Fats: Some Lipids, Wallflowers for a Century, Show Therapeutic Promise." *Science News* (May 31, 1997): 342–343.

Steiner, George. "The Diabetes Atherosclerosis Intervention Study (DAIS): Interim Lipid Results." *Diabetes* (May 1999): SA2.

Yu, Harry H., et al. "Dyslipidemia in Patients with CAD: Rational Use of Diets and Drugs." *Consultant* (Sept. 2000): 1740.

ORGANIZATIONS

American Heart Association. National Center, 7272 Greenville Ave., Dallas, TX 75231. (800) 242-8721. <http://www.americanheart.org>.

National Cholesterol Education Program. National Heart, Lung and Blood Institute, P.O. Box 30105, Bethesda, MD 20824. (301) 592-8573. <http://www.nhlbi.nih.gov>.

Ken R. Wells

Lipoproteins test

Definition

Lipids are water insoluble molecules and must be transported in the plasma as macromolecular complexes containing protein called lipoproteins. The lipoproteins are large aggregates (micelles) composed of cholesterol, triglycerides, phospholipids, **proteins**, and small amounts of **carbohydrates**. Generally, the core of the lipoprotein contains hydrophobic lipids surrounded by a sheath of protein and lipids arranged with the hydrophilic ends directed outward. Carbohydrates and enzymes are present in the outer sheath. The proteins that become part of the lipoprotein are called apoproteins. Lipoproteins are grouped into four main classes depending upon their density. In order from least to greatest density these are: chylomicrons, very low density lipoprotein (VLDL), low density lipoprotein (LDL), and high density lipoprotein (HDL).

Purpose

Lipoproteins are measured to classify persons with severe hyperlipoproteinemia or hypolipoproteinemia. The hyperlipoproteinemias result from increased production or decreased clearance of lipoproteins from the **blood** and may be inherited or secondary to other diseases or conditions. Some common causes of secondary hyperlipoproteinemia include **diabetes mellitus**, hypothyroidism, biliary cirrhosis, estrogens and **pancreatitis**. The cholesterol content of the LDL (LDL cholesterol) and HDL (HDL cholesterol) are measured, along with total cholesterol and triglycerides, to evaluate the patient's risk for coronary **heart** disease. In addition, a subclass of LDL called lipoprotein(a) or Lp(a) may be measured in persons who have a family history of **coronary artery disease** (CAD) or predisposing risk factors for CAD.

Description

Measurement

Measurement of lipoproteins may be performed by ultracentrifugation of the plasma. When plasma is subjected to very high centrifugal force, the lipoproteins can be separated in a gradient salt solution on the basis of their density. Since the density is directly related to protein content, the lipoproteins can also be separated by electrophoresis.

Electrophoresis is the separation of charged particles in an electrical field and is dependent on the amount and nature of the apoproteins within the lipoprotein. The electrophoretic positions of the lipoproteins are often used to describe them. Thus, HDL is also called alpha-1 lipoprotein, VLDL is called prebeta lipoprotein, and LDL is called beta lipoprotein. Chylomicrons do not migrate and are not given any designation. When one or more plasma lipid levels are extremely elevated or reduced, either of these methods may be used to determine which lipoproteins are abnormal. On the basis of these findings, abnormal lipoproteins are classified into patterns. Since severe disorders of lipoprotein **metabolism** are often inherited, the abnormal patterns are called phenotypes. There are five abnormal lipoprotein phenotypes (Type I through Type V), each characterized by the presence of an extremely high quantity of one or two lipoproteins. Persons with severe hyperlipoproteinemia often have skin and tissue infiltration of fat deposits, and persons with Type II and Type III are predisposed to premature atherosclerosis owing to high levels of plasma cholesterol. Lipoprotein phenotyping is not performed as a screening test to evaluate risk of coronary artery disease.

Immunological methods are used to measure the quantity of specific apoproteins present in the plasma. Testing for apoA-I and apoB-100 the principal apoproteins of HDL and LDL, respectively is often performed in persons with elevated lipids who have risk factors associated with coronary artery disease. Measurement of a form of LDL, called Lp(a) is performed on these persons as well as on those who have normal lipid levels, but a family history of CAD.

HDL cholesterol is routinely measured along with total cholesterol and triglycerides as a screening test for coronary artery disease. If the total cholesterol is 200 mg/dL or higher the LDL cholesterol is measured. The measurement of HDL cholesterol is based upon the measurement of cholesterol (see entry on **lipid tests**) under conditions that inhibit the reaction with all lipoproteins except HDL. The measurement of LDL cholesterol involves precipitating the HDL, VLDL, and cholymicrons using antibodies to apoproteins A, and E, followed by measurement of the LDL cholesterol in the supernatant. When the triglyceride concentration is below 400 mg/dL, the LDL cholesterol is often estimated using the Friedewald formula [LDL cholesterol = total cholesterol minus (HDL cholesterol + triglyceride/5)]. It should be noted that this formula will underestimate LDL cholesterol when triglycerides are above 400 mg/dL.

Chylomicrons

Chylomicrons are made in the intestines mainly from dietary triglycerides. They are approximately 95% triglyceride and only 2% protein by weight. The major apoproteins of chylomicrons are apoC, B, and A.

Chylomicrons are degraded in the plasma by the enzyme lipoprotein lipase, which splits the triglycerides into glycerides, and fatty acids, which are mainly absorbed by cells. Smaller chylomicron remnants are returned to the **liver**, where they are degraded by hepatic lipase. In the blood, some of the apoprotein A and C from chylomicrons are transferred to HDL. The chylomicrons are lighter than water and will float to the top of the plasma when it is stored overnight in the refrigerator. Since plasma from a fasting specimen should not contain chylomicrons, the observation of this floating layer is significant and indicates a deficiency of peripheral lipase activity. Chylomicrons are found in the fasting plasma of persons with Type I and Type V hyperlipoproteinemia.

Very low-density lipoproteins (VLDL)

VLDL are formed in the liver using apoproteins partly recycled from chylomicron remnants. VLDLs are about 10% protein and 60-70% triglycerides by weight; consequently they account for only 10-15% of the plasma cholesterol. The triglycerides carried by the VLDL are derived from carbohydrate metabolism. VLDL is released into the circulation, where it is partly degraded. Excessively elevated VLDL is responsible for Type IV hyperlipoproteinemia and is most often caused by hyperinsulinemia, which promotes triglyceride production. When both chylomicrons and VLDL are greatly increased, the abnormality is defined as Type V hyperlipoproteinemia.

Some free cholesterol, triglycerides, and apoproteins from VLDL are transferred to HDL in the circulation. This forms a lipoprotein of greater density and roughly equal cholesterol and triglyceride content called intermediate density lipoprotein (IDL). The IDL is converted to LDL by enzymatic removal of triglycerides and apoC. IDL is not found in significant amounts in the circulation unless there is a defect in conversion of VLDL to LDL. Such cases are caused by a deficiency of apo E-III or apo C-III activated lipase. This results in the accumulation of IDL in the plasma. This is responsible for Type III hyperlipoporteinemia.

Low-density lipoprotein (LDL)

The LDL is composed of about 25% protein and 45-55% cholesterol by weight. LDL carries cholesterol to the cells and is then degraded by lysosomal hydrolysis. Since LDL contains the majority of the plasma cholesterol and is responsible for cholesterol transport to cells, it is positively correlated with the risk of coronary artery disease. LDL accumulates in the plasma when there is a deficiency of the apoB-100 receptor on cells. This is responsible for the Type II hyperlipoprotienimia. Low

levels of LDL occur in two inherited conditions. Abetalipoproteinemia results from a complete deficiency of apoB. This is an autosomal recessive condition associated with severe metabolic problems including intestinal malabsorption, motor nerve dysfunction, fat soluble vitamin deficiency and anemia. Hypobetalipoproteinemia is an autosomal dominant condition in which LDL levels are about 10% of normal. This condition may be associated with fat soluble vitamin deficiency that is treated by vitamin supplementation and with a very low risk for coronary artery disease.

High-density lipoproteins (HDL)

HDL is approximately 50% protein by weight. Phospholipids account for 25-30% of its mass and cholesterol for 15-20%. HDL is made in the liver partly from VLDL and chylomicrons. It binds to and esterifies cellular cholesterol and transports it to the liver, where it is used to make bile salts and acids. HDL provides the main route for cellular cholesterol clearance and its level is inversely related to coronary artery disease. Absent or nearly absent HDL occurs in an autosomal recessive hypolipoproteinemia called Tangier disease. This is caused by a deficiency of both apoA-I and apoA-II, the principal lipoproteins of HDL. Persons with this disease develop premature CAD.

Lipoprotein a or Lp(a)

Lp(a) contains apoB bound to another apoprotein that is designated apo(a). Like LDL it is about 27% protein and 65% lipid by weight and has prebata mobility on electropohoresis. The amount of Lp(a) in plasma is normally below 150 mg/dL. Elevated levels are considered to be an independent risk factor for developing coronary artery disease. High levels are inherited as an autosomal dominant trait and are not influenced by diet or **exercise**. It is speculated that the link betweeen Lp(a) and atherosclerosis is related to the similarity between apo(a) and plasminogen. Plasminogen is the precuror of plasmin which initiates the lysis of blood clots.

Measurement guidelines

The Expert Panel of the National Cholesterol Education Program (NCEP) sponsored by the National Institutes of Health has published guidelines for the detection of high cholesterol in adults which are listed below. The NCEP panel recommends that adults over the age of 20 be tested for cholesterol and HDL every five years. If the cholesterol is high, the HDL is low (below 40 mg/dl), or other risk factors are present, a complete lipoprotein profile that includes total cholesterol, triglycerides, HDL cholesterol, and LDL cholesterol should be performed.

Preparation

Initial screening for total cholesterol and HDL cholesterol may be performed on nonfasting persons. The tests require a blood specimen usually collected by venipuncture or fingerstick. The nurse or phlebotomist performing the test should observe **universal precautions** for the prevention of transmission of bloodborne pathogens. If results require follow-up testing, the patient must fast for 12 hours before the test, eating nothing and drinking only water. The person should not have alcohol for 24 hours before the test. There should be a stable diet and no illnesses occurring in the preceding two weeks. A test for lipoprotein electrophoresis requires a 12-hour fast and a blood sample collected in EDTA.

Complications

Discomfort or bruising may occur at the puncture site or the person may feel dizzy or faint. Pressure to the puncture site until the bleeding stops reduces bruising. Warm packs to the puncture site relieve discomfort.

Results

In April 2001, the NIH released new NCEP guidelines to assist doctors and nurses in identifying who is at risk for CAD.

Total cholesterol guidelines are:

- desirable: < 200 mg/dL
- borderline high: 200-239 mg/dL
- high: > 240 mg/dL

High density lipoprotein guidelines reflect the fact that this lipoprotein is inversely related to risk for CAD.

LDL cholesterol guidelines are:

- low: < 40 mg/dL
- desirable: < 130 mg/dL (deciliter)
- optimal: < 100 mg/dL
- near optimal: 100-129 mg/dL
- borderline high: 130-159 mg/dL
- high: 160-189 mg/dL
- very high: > 190 mg/dL

The NCEP also identified factors that patients may have that make the risk of heart disease higher. Health care professionals are advised to help the patient lower their cholesterol as much as possible, if they have two or more of these risk factors:

- Cigarette smoking.
- High **blood pressure**, with a measurement of > 140/90 mm Hg (millimeters of mercury). In addition, it is considered a risk factor if the patient is on blood pressure lowering medications, even if they have achieved a normal blood pressure.
- Age, over 45 years in men and over 55 years in women. Estrogen, a sex hormone in women protects against heart disease. The levels of estrogen are lower after a woman goes through **menopause**, roughly after the age of 55.
- Low HDL cholesterol (less than 35 mg/dL). Note that HDL > 60 mg/dL is a negative risk factor for CAD.
- Family history of premature heart disease. Premature heart disease is defined as heart disease seen before age 55 in a male relative or before age 65 in a female relative.
- Diabetes mellitus.

Some people have normal variations in their lipoprotein and total cholesterol levels. Repeat testing may be necessary, especially if a value is at a borderline risk category point.

Health care team roles

Lipoprotein testing is ordered by a physician. A nurse or phlebotomist usually collects the blood sample for the tests. Testing is most often performed by clinical laboratory scientists/medical technologists or clinical laboratory technicians/medical laboratory technicians. All clinicians should be well versed in the NCEP guidelines and treatment recommendations including both dietary and drug interventions. Patient's with high cholesterol levels may be requested to consult a dietician in order to evaluate their meal plans, and learn how to follow the Step 1 or 2 diets that may be needed to lower the LDL cholesterol.

Resources

BOOKS

Burtix, Carl A. and Edward R. Ashwood. *Tietz Textbook of Clinical Chemistry,* Third ed., Philadelphia, W.B. Saunders Company, 1999.

Rifai, Nader, G. Russell Warnick, and Marek H. Dominiczak. *Handbook of Lipoprotein Testing.* Washington, D.C.: American Association of Clinical Chemistry (AACC) Press, 1997.

ORGANIZATIONS

American Heart Association. 7272 Greenville Avenue, Dallas, TX, 75231-4596. 214-706-1220. <http://www.american-heart.org/>.

National Cholesterol Education Program. The National Heart, Lung, and Blood Institute. National Institutes of Health. PO Box 30105, Bethesda, MD, 20824-0105. 301-251-1222. <http://www.nhlbi.nih.gov/guidelines/cholesterol/atglance.pdf> May 2001.

Jane E. Phillips

Liquid diets *see* **Fad diets**

Lithotripsy

Definition

Lithotripsy is a therapeutic medical procedure used to disintegrate stones (calculi) in the urinary tract and **kidneys**. Extracorporeal shock wave lithotripsy (ESWL) uses shock waves generated outside the body and is noninvasive. Intracorporeal shock wave lithotripsy (ISWL) delivers shock waves through a specially designed scope used for the urinary tract (ureteroscope) and kidneys (nephroscope) and is a minimally invasive procedure. Ultrasound lithotripsy also uses a scope to deliver ultrasonic waves (mechanical vibrations) and is minimally invasive.

Purpose

Lithotripsy is used when a kidney stone is too large to pass on its own, or when a stone becomes stuck in a ureter (a tube which carries urine from the kidney to the bladder) and will not pass. **Kidney stones** are extremely painful and can cause serious medical complications,

such as kidney damage, if not removed. Usually, stones smaller than 5 mm in diameter can pass without intervention, while stones larger than 7 mm in diameter require lithotripsy or the placement of a urethral or ureteral stent to help them pass. Stones larger than 10 mm require lithotripsy or surgery.

ESWL is a noninvasive alternative to open surgery (which is only very rarely performed for stones now) or percutaneous nephrolithotomy. ESWL is used in patients with stones less than or equal to 1 cm located in the kidneys or ureters. ISWL is a minimally invasive endoscopic technique that is used in patients with stones over 1 cm, with stones in the lower urinary tract, with impacted stones, and when ESWL is unsuccessful. Both ESWL and ISWL can also be used to fragment **gallbladder** and bile duct stones.

Precautions

ESWL should not be considered for patients with severe skeletal deformities, patients weighing over 300 lbs (136 kg), patients with abdominal aortic aneurysms, or patients with uncontrollable **bleeding disorders**. Patients who are pregnant should not be treated with ESWL. Patients with cardiac **pacemakers** should be evaluated by a cardiologist familiar with lithotripsy. Lithotripsy may temporarily inhibit the pacemaker or cause circuit damage leading to erratic functioning or cessation of the pacemaker. The cardiologist should be present during the lithotripsy procedure in the event there are problems with the pacemaker.

Description

Lithotripsy uses focused shock waves to fragment a stone in the kidney or the ureter. In ESWL, the patient is placed on a table in contact with a water-filled cushion; and a shock wave is generated, travels through the water, and shatters and fragments the stone. Older ESWL systems involved immersing the patient in a tub of water; but this space-consuming, awkward method has been replaced by water-filled cushions. Once the stone is fragmented, the resulting gravel is left to pass on its own; the patient may have been stented prior to the procedure to widen the urethra and or ureters to allow the fragments to pass easily and with less **pain**. In ISWL, a ureteroscope is inserted through the urethra and bladder and into the ureters, or a nephroscope is inserted, usually through an incision in the patient's back. Once the stone is located using the **endoscope**, an electrohydraulic, laser, or ultrasound lithotripter can be used to fragment the stone. In ISWL using an electrohydraulic lithotripter, a probe is inserted through the endoscope and against the stone, and shock waves are delivered by a generator. In laser ISWL,

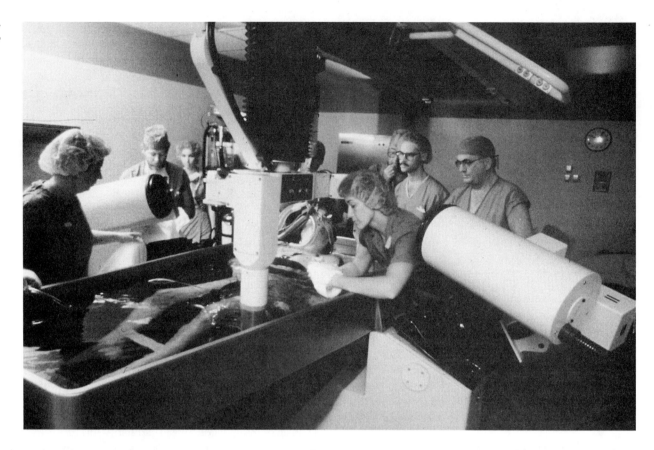

A lithotriptor in use by patient in tub. This noninvasive method crushes kidney stones through shock waves. *(Photo Researchers, Inc. Reproduced by permission.)*

a pulsed-dye laser is used to deliver laser energy through a fiber inserted through the endoscope and into the stone. Ultrasound ISWL uses a generator to produce mechanical vibrations delivered to the stone via a probe tip inserted through the generator. In ISWL, after the stone is fragmented, the pieces can be removed using a grasper or basket or left to pass on their own if they are small enough.

Preparation

Prior to the lithotripsy procedure, a complete **physical examination** is done, including a urine analysis, followed by imaging tests to determine the number, location, and size of the stone or stones. A test called an intravenous pyelogram, or IVP, is often used to locate the stones and determine the degree of obstruction (blockage). An IVP involves injecting a dye (contrast medium) into a vein in the arm. This dye, which shows up on x ray, travels through the bloodstream and is excreted by the kidneys. The dye then flows down the ureters and into the bladder. The dye surrounds the stones, and x rays are then used to evaluate the stones and the anatomy of the **urinary system**. For those patients who are allergic to the dye, ultrasound, which uses focused sound waves, or

computed tomography without contrast dye is performed. **Blood** tests are done to determine if any potential bleeding problems exist. For women of childbearing age, a **pregnancy test** is done to make sure the patient isn't pregnant; and elderly patients have an elctrocardiogram (ECG) done to make sure no potential **heart** problems exist. Some patients may have a stent placed prior to the lithotripsy procedure. A stent is a plastic tube placed in the ureter which allows the passage of gravel and urine after the procedure is completed.

Aftercare

Most patients have a lot of blood in their urine after the lithotripsy procedure. This is normal and should clear after several days to a week or so. Lots of fluids should be taken to encourage the flushing of any gravel remaining in the urinary system. The patient may be asked to urinate through a strainer and collect any stone fragments that pass for examination by the physician. Patients with stents may experience some discomfort during urination or during certain movements; this is normal. The patient should follow up with the urologist in about two weeks to make sure that everything is going as planned. If a stent

KEY TERMS

Aneurysm—A dilation of the wall of an artery which causes a weak area prone to rupturing.

Bladder—Organ in which urine is stored prior to urination.

Bleeding disorder—Problems with the clotting mechanism of the blood.

Cardiologist—A physician who specializes in problems with the heart and its vessels.

Computed tomography—An imaging examination that uses x-rays to produce a cross-sectional image of the anatomical area of interest; used to image the urinary tract and kidneys to detect kidney stones.

ECG—Electrocardiogram; a tracing of the electrical activity of the heart.

Gravel—The debris which is formed from a fragmented kidney stone.

IVP (Intravenous pyelogram)—The use of a dye, injected into the veins, used to locate kidney stones. Also used to determine the anatomy of the urinary system.

Kidney stones—Also called calculi; hard masses that form in the urinary tract and which can cause pain, bleeding, obstruction, or infection. Stones are primarily made up of calcium and can vary in size from a few millimeters to over a centimeter and more in diameter.

Nephroscope—An endoscope, a thin flexible tube with optics, used to examine the kidneys and through which intracorporeal lithotripsy can be performed.

Percutaneous nephrolithotomy—A minimally invasive endoscopic procedure involving a small incision in the back through which a nephroscope is inserted to remove stones from the kidney; used in conjunction with ISWL and after unsuccessful ESWL.

Stent—A small, short plastic tubular device placed in the urethra or ureters to widen them in order for stones and stone fragments to pass easily.

Ultrasound—Sound waves used to determine the internal structures of the body.

Ureter—A tube which carries urine from the kidney to the bladder.

Ureteroscope—An endoscope, a thin flexible tube with optics, used to examine the ureters and through which intracorporeal lithotripsy can be performed.

Urethra—A tube through which urine passes during urination.

Urologist—A physician who specializes in problems of the urinary system.

has been inserted, it is normally removed at this time. Patients may return to work whenever they feel able.

Occasionally, the ESWL procedure does not break stones into pieces small enough to pass. In these cases, an endoscope may be used to remove the pieces after the ESWL procedure.

Complications

Abdominal pain is not uncommon after lithotripsy, but it is usually not cause to worry. However, persistent or severe abdominal pain may imply unexpected internal injury. Colicky renal pain is very common as gravel is still passing. Other problems may include perirenal hematomas (blood clots around the kidneys); hemorrhage; **pancreatitis** (inflammation of the **pancreas**); damage to nearby organs and tissues (during ISWL); and obstruction by stone fragments. The most common complication is urinary tract **infection**, sometimes present

prior to the procedure due to obstruction by stones. Prophylactic **antibiotics** are administered to treat infection. Other postprocedural complications sometimes associated with the administration of anesthetics include nausea, vomiting, and allergic reaction.

Health care team roles

Lithotripsy is performed by a urologist or urologic surgeon, sometimes in conjunction with a radiologist, and with assistance from nursing staff for patient monitoring and medication administration during the procedure. The procedure may also be performed by a uroradiologist. If ISWL requires **general anesthesia** or conscious sedation, an anesthesiologist and/or **nurse anesthetist** may need to be present for the procedure. Because ESWL uses x rays to locate the stones, a radiologic technologist may be required to assist with operating the x-ray equipment.

Lithotripsy

GALE ENCYCLOPEDIA OF NURSING AND ALLIED HEALTH

1415

Resources

BOOKS

Tanagho, Emil, and Jack McAninch, eds. *Smith's General Urology.* 14th ed. Norwalk, CT: Appleton and Lange Publishers, 1995.

PERIODICALS

Portis, Andrew J. and Chandru P. Sundaram. "Diagnosis and Initial Management of Kidney Stones." *American Family Physician* 63, no. 7 (April 1, 2001): 1329-1338.

Shagam, Janet Yagoda. "Extracorporeal Shock Wave Lithotripsy." *Radiologic Technology* 72, no. 2 (November-December 2000): 145-163.

ORGANIZATIONS

American Urological Association. 1120 North Charles Street, Baltimore, MD 21201. 410-727-1100. <http://www.auanet.org>.

National Kidney Foundation. 30 East 33rd Street, Suite 1100, New York, NY 10016. (800) 622-9010. <http://www.kidney.org>.

Society of Urologic Nurses and Associates. East Holly Avenue, Box 56, Pitman, NJ 08071-0056. 609-256-2335. <http://suna.inurse.com/>.

Jennifer E. Sisk, M.A.

Liver-spleen scan *see* **Liver radionuclide scan**

Liver

Definition

The liver is the largest gland and largest internal organ in the human body (the skin is the largest organ overall).

Description

Weighing 3-3.5 lbs (1.4-1.6 kg), the liver is a dark red, wedge-shaped gland approximately eight and a half inches long (roughly the size of a football). It is located in the right side of the abdominal area just below the diaphragm and above the **stomach**.

Approximately 1.5 qts (1.5 L) of **blood** flow through the liver each minute. The liver holds about 13% of the body's blood supply. It is furnished with blood from two large vessels, the portal vein and the hepatic artery (hepatic means liver). Blood that has circulated through the stomach, spleen, and intestine enters the liver through the portal vein as part of the portal circulation system.

The liver extracts nutrients and toxins from this blood, which is then returned through the hepatic vein to the right side of the **heart**. The hepatic artery supplies oxygenated blood directly from the heart to the liver.

Function

Some of the liver's many important functions include:

- Production of bile which is stored in the gall bladder and used to digest **fats**. If the excretion of bile is blocked, the stools become pale and retain fat. As a result, fat-soluble **vitamins** (vitamins A,D, E, and K) are not properly absorbed and levels of bilirubin, the main component of bile, rises in the blood. Once bilirubin levels reach a certain level, **jaundice** or yellowing of the skin and eyes occurs.

- Synthesis of **proteins**, including albumin. Albumin is the predominant protein in blood plasma and helps to retain fluid within the **blood vessels**. The loss of albumin results in fluid shifting from blood vessels to the surrounding tissue. The result is swelling of tissue, a condition called edema.

- Production of blood-clotting factors that control bleeding. Loss of clotting factors leads to increased chance of hemorrhage.

- **Metabolism** of hormones and medications, such as estrogen and acetaminophen (Tylenol). When the liver is damaged, its ability to metabolize hormones decreases. This can result in changes to estrogen and testosterone levels in the body. Symptoms of these changes include loss of pubic hair and the development of spider angiomas, small clusters of red blood vessels on the skin of the upper body, in both males and females. Men sometimes experience a decrease of testicular size and development of breast tissue (a condition called *gynecomastia*). A decline in the body's ability to metabolize medications means that normal doses can turn into toxic levels. Therefore, doses of medicines are often reduced for people who have liver disease.

- Regulation of glucose levels. Loss of liver cells leads to poorly controlled glucose levels. Glucose levels may soar after eating (hyperglycemia) or fall dangerously low between meals (hypoglycemia). This poor regulation of blood sugar is due to a different mechanism than the mechanisms that lead to diabetes types I and II.

- Conversion of ammonia, a by-product of metabolism, into a less toxic form called urea. Inability to convert ammonia to urea results in elevated ammonia levels in the blood. This can result in a condition called hepatic encephalopathy, which is a neurological syndrome characterized by alterations in mental status and behavior. Although acute episodes can be reversible, severe cases of hepatic encephalopathy can lead to **coma** and death.

Role in human health

A healthy liver enables the human body to:

- produce energy when needed
- manufacture new proteins
- store certain vitamins, **minerals**, and sugars
- regulate transport of fat stores
- regulate blood clotting
- facilitate the digestive process by producing bile
- control the production and excretion of cholesterol
- neutralize and destroy toxic substances
- metabolize alcohol
- monitor proper chemical and drug blood levels
- cleanse the blood and discharging waste products into the bile
- maintain hormone balance
- serve as the main fetal blood forming organ
- resist infection
- regenerate its damaged tissue
- store **iron**

Common diseases and disorders

Symptoms and signs of liver disease:

- jaundice, or abnormal yellowing of the skin and eyes (often the first, and may be the only, sign of liver disease)
- dark urine
- gray, yellow, or light colored stools
- nausea, vomiting, and/or loss of appetite
- intestinal bleeding due to liver diseases obstructing blood flow. (Bleeding may result in vomiting of blood, and bloody or black stools.)
- abdominal swelling (Liver disease may cause ascites, an accumulation of fluid in the abdominal cavity.)
- prolonged generalized itching
- an increase or decrease of more than 5% body weight in two months
- abdominal **pain**

- sleep disturbances, mental confusion, and coma that may result from an accumulation of toxic substances that impair **brain** function
- fatigue or loss of stamina
- loss of sexual drive or diminished performance

The most common liver diseases are as follows:

Viral hepatitis

- Hepatitis A spreads through contaminated water and food.
- Hepatitis B may be transmitted through transfusions, cuts, kissing, tooth brushing, ear piercing, tattooing, dental work, or during sexual contact.
- Hepatitis C primarily spreads through infected blood.

The liver often becomes tender and enlarged, and the patient usually experiences **fever**, weakness, nausea, vomiting, jaundice, and aversion to food. The virus may be present in the bloodstream, intestines, feces, saliva, and other body secretions. Hepatitis is common in the United States and some forms of it can be extremely infectious. Most people recover from viral forms of the disease without treatment, but some die and others may develop a chronic, disabling illness. In the United States there are more than four million hepatitis carriers.

Alcohol-related liver disorders

Liver disorders related to alcohol include fatty liver, alcoholic hepatitis, and alcoholic cirrhosis.

Fatty liver, the most common alcohol-related liver disorder, causes liver enlargement and abdominal discomfort. Swollen livers are often tender or painful, and may cause jaundice and liver function abnormalities.

Alcoholic hepatitis often results in nausea, vomiting, abdominal pain, fever, jaundice, liver enlargement and tenderness, and white blood cell count elevation. At times alcoholic hepatitis may be asymptomatic.

Cirrhosis

Over 25,000 Americans die from cirrhosis each year. It is the seventh leading cause of death. Among those 25-44, it is the fourth disease-related cause of death. Cirrhosis of the liver occurs when damaged liver cells are replaced by scar tissue causing diminished blood flow, which causes additional liver cell death. Loss of liver function results in gastrointestinal disturbances, emaciation, liver and spleen enlargement, jaundice, fluid accumulation in the abdomen and other tissues. Obstructed circulation often causes massive vomiting of blood.

Any severe liver injury may cause cirrhosis. Over half of the deaths from cirrhosis result from alcohol abuse, hepatitis, and other **viruses**. Toxins, chemicals, excessive iron or **copper**, severe drug reactions, and bile duct obstruction may also cause cirrhosis.

Gallstones

Gallstones form when cholesterol and/or pigment in bile crystallize into gall stones. Gall stones vary in size from small pebbles to golf balls. Occasionally gallstones become lodged in the bile ducts leading from the **gallbladder** to the duodenum (first part of the **small intestine**). This may cause extreme abdominal pain. When gall stones block bile ducts, bile cannot flow into the intestines, and backs up into the bloodstream causing jaundice.

Gallstones are more common in people over 40, especially among women and the obese. Each year in the United States, 400-500,000 gallbladders are surgically removed.

Children's liver disorders

Tens of thousands of American children contract liver diseases causing hundreds of deaths each year. The most common of these diseases are:

Biliary atresia is caused by the lack, or inadequate size, of bile ducts connecting the liver to the intestine. Unable to excrete bile, death results from cirrhosis and bleeding by two years of age.

Chronic active hepatitis destroys liver cells replacing them with scar tissue. It is caused by an unknown process that resembles an allergy to the child's own liver tissue.

Galactosemia, an inherited disease, is caused by the lack of an enzyme needed to digest milk sugar. As a result, milk sugar accumulates in the liver and other organs, leading to cirrhosis of the liver, **cataracts**, and brain damage.

Wilson's disease occurs when copper accumulates in the liver due to an inherited abnormality, causing cirrhosis and brain damage.

Reyes syndrome is a fatal disorder in which fat accumulates in the liver.

Cirrhosis may result from extensive liver injury.

Liver cancer

Most **liver cancer** results from the spread of **cancer** from other organs to the liver (metastasis).

Resources

BOOKS

Cotran, Ramzi, S. *Robbins Pathologic Basis of Disease. 6th ed.* Philadelphia: W.B. Saunders Company, 1999.

Guyton, Arthur C. *Textbook of Medical Physiology. 10th ed.* Philadelphia: W.B. Saunders Company, 2000.

PERIODICALS

Smales, Caroline. "Hepatitis: Symptoms, Treatments, and Prevention." *Nursing Times* (4 November 1998): 58-60.

ORGANIZATIONS

American Liver Foundation. 75 Maiden Lane, Suite 603, New York, NY 10038. 1-800-GOLIVER (1-800) 465-4837) <http://www.liverfoundation.org/>.

Bill Asenjo, MS, CRC

Liver biopsy

Definition

A **liver** biopsy is a medical procedure performed to obtain a small piece of liver tissue for diagnostic testing. The sample is examined under a **microscope** by a doctor who specializes in the effects of disease on body tissues (a pathologist) to detect abnormalities of the liver. Liver biopsies are sometimes called percutaneous liver biopsies, because the tissue sample is obtained by going through the patient's skin. This is a useful diagnostic procedure with very low risk and little discomfort to the patient.

Purpose

A liver biopsy is usually done to evaluate the extent of damage that has occurred to the liver because of chronic and acute disease processes or toxic injury. Biopsies are often performed to identify abnormalities in liver tissues after imaging studies and radiopharmaceutical scans have failed to yield clear results.

A liver biopsy may be ordered to diagnose or stage any of the following conditions or disorders:

- jaundice

- cirrhosis

- repeated abnormal results from liver function tests

- alcoholic liver disease

- unexplained swelling or enlargement of the liver (hepatomegaly)

- suspected drug-related liver damage such as acetaminophen poisoning

- hemochromatosis, a condition of excess **iron** in the liver

- intrahepatic cholestasis, the build up of bile in the liver

- hepatitis

- primary cancers of the liver, such as hepatomas, cholangiocarcinomas, and angiosarcomas

- metastatic cancers of the liver (These are over 20 times as common in the United States as primary cancers.)

- post liver transplant to measure graft rejection

- fever of unknown origin

- suspected **tuberculosis**, sarcoidosis, or amyloidosis

Precautions

When performing the liver biopsy and **blood** collection that precedes it, the physician and other health care providers should follow **universal precautions** for the prevention of transmission of bloodborne pathogens. Some patients should not have percutaneous liver biopsies. They include those with any of the following conditions:

- a platelet count below 100,000

- a prothrombin test time greater than three seconds over the reference interval

- a liver tumor with a large number of veins

- a large amount of abdominal fluid (ascites)

- **infection** anywhere in the **lungs**, the lining of the chest or abdominal wall, the biliary tract, or the liver

- benign tumors (angiomas) of the liver (These tumors consist mostly of enlarged or newly formed **blood vessels** and may bleed heavily.)

- biliary obstruction

Description

Percutaneous liver biopsy is sometimes called aspiration biopsy or fine needle aspiration (FNA) because it is done with a hollow needle attached to a suction syringe. The special needles that are used to perform a

liver biopsy are called Menghini or Jamshedi needles. The amount of specimen collected should be about 1-2 cc. In many cases the biopsy is done by a doctor who specializes in x rays and imaging studies (a radiologist). The radiologist will use computed tomography scan (CT scan) or ultrasound to guide the needle to the target site for the biopsy. Some ultrasound guided biopsies are performed using a biopsy gun which has a spring mechanism which contains a cutting sheath. This type of procedure gives a greater yield of tissue.

An hour or so before the biopsy, the patient will be given a sedative to aid in **relaxation**. The patient is then asked to lie on the back with the right elbow to the side and the right hand under the head. The patient is instructed to lie as still as possible during the procedure. He or she is warned to expect a sensation resembling a punch in the right shoulder when the needle passes a certain nerve (the phrenic nerve) but to hold still in spite of the momentary feeling.

Following these instructions to the patient, the doctor marks a spot on the skin where the needle will be inserted. The right side of the upper abdomen is thoroughly cleansed with an antiseptic solution, generally iodine. The patient is then given a local anesthetic at the biopsy site.

The doctor prepares the needle by drawing sterile saline solution into a syringe. The syringe is then attached to the biopsy needle, which is inserted into the patient's chest wall. The doctor then draws the plunger of the syringe back to create a vacuum. At this point the patient is asked to take a deep breath and hold it. The needle is inserted into the liver and withdrawn quickly, usually within two seconds or less. The negative pressure in the syringe draws or pulls a sample of liver tissue into the biopsy needle. As soon as the needle is withdrawn, the patient can breathe normally. This step takes only a few seconds. Pressure is applied at the biopsy site to stop any bleeding and a bandage is placed over it. The liver tissue sample is placed in a cup with a 10% formalin solution and sent to the laboratory immediately. The entire procedure takes 10 to 15 minutes. Test results are usually available within a day.

Most patients experience minor discomfort during the procedure, but not severe **pain**. Mild medications of a non-aspirin type can be given after the biopsy if the pain lasts for several hours.

Preparation

Liver biopsies require some preparation of the patient. Since aspirin and ibuprofen (Advil, Motrin) are known to inhibit platelets and lessen clotting function, it is best to avoid these medications for at least a week

KEY TERMS

Aspiration—The technique of removing a tissue sample for biopsy through a hollow needle attached to a suction syringe.

Bile—Liquid produced by the liver that is excreted into the intestine to aid in the digestion of fats.

Biliary—Relating to bile.

Biopsy—The surgical removal and microscopic examination of living tissue for diagnostic purposes.

Cholestasis—A blockage in the flow of bile.

Cirrhosis—A progressive disease of the liver characterized by the death of liver cells and their replacement with fibrous tissue.

Formalin—A clear solution of diluted formaldehyde that is used to preserve liver biopsy specimens until they can be examined in the laboratory.

Gross inspection—A visual examination of the tissue with the unaided eye performed by a pathologist.

Hepatitis—Inflammation of the liver, caused by infection or toxic injury.

Jaundice—Also termed icterus. An increase in blood bile pigments that are deposited in the skin, eyes, deeper tissue and excretions. The skin and whites of the eye will appear yellow.

Menghini needle/Jamshedi needle—Special needles used to obtain a sample of liver tissue by aspiration.

Percutaneous biopsy—A biopsy in which the needle is inserted and the sample removed through the skin.

Prothrombin test—A common test to measure the amount of time it takes for a patient's blood to clot. Units are in seconds.

Vital signs—A person's essential body functions, usually defined as the pulse, body temperature, and breathing rate. Vital signs are checked periodically during procedures like liver biopsies to make sure that the patient is not having physical problems as a result of the procedure.

(or **complete blood count**) and prothrombin time are performed prior to the biopsy. These tests determine whether there is an abnormally high risk of uncontrolled bleeding from the biopsy site which may contraindicate the procedure. The patient should limit food or drink for a period of four to eight hours before the biopsy.

Before the procedure, the patient or family member should sign a consent form. The patient will be questioned for any history of allergy to the local anesthetic and asked to empty the bladder so that he or she will be more comfortable during the procedure. His or her pulse rate, temperature, and breathing rate (**vital signs**) will be noted so that the doctor can tell during the procedure if he or she is having any physical problems.

Aftercare

Liver biopsies are now considered outpatient procedures in most hospitals. Patients are asked to lie on their right sides for one hour and then to rest quietly for three more. At regular intervals, a nurse checks the patient's vital signs. If there are no complications, the patient is sent home but is asked to stay within an hour from the hospital since delayed bleeding may occur.

Patients should arrange to have a friend or relative take them home after discharge. Bed rest for a day is recommended, followed by a week of avoiding heavy work or strenuous **exercise**. The patient can resume eating a normal diet.

Some mild soreness in the area of the biopsy is normal after the anesthetic wears off. Irritation of the muscle that lies over the liver can also cause mild discomfort in the shoulder for some patients. Acetaminophen can be taken for minor soreness, but aspirin and ibuprofen products are best avoided. The patient should, however, call the doctor if there is severe pain in the abdomen, chest, or shoulder; difficulty breathing; or persistent bleeding. These signs may indicate that there has been leakage of bile into the abdominal cavity, or that air has been introduced into the cavity around the lungs.

Complications

The complications associated with a liver biopsy are usually very small. The most significant risk is prolonged internal bleeding. In about 0.4% of cases, a patient with **liver cancer** will develop a fatal hemorrhage from a percutaneous biopsy. These fatalities result because some liver tumors are supplied with a large number of blood vessels and bleed very easily. Other complications from percutaneous liver biopsies include the leakage of bile or the introduction of air into the chest cavity (pneumothorax). There is also a small chance that an infection may

before the biopsy. The doctor should check the patient's records to see whether he or she is taking any other medications that may affect blood clotting. A platelet count occur, or an internal organ such as the lung, gall bladder, or kidney could be punctured. This risk is decreased when using the ultrasound or CT guided procedure.

Results

After the biopsy, the liver sample is sent to the pathology laboratory and examined. A normal (negative) result would find no evidence of pathology in the tissue sample. It should be noted that many diseases of the liver are focal and not diffuse; an abnormality may not be detected, if the sample was taken from an unaffected site. If symptoms persist, the patient may need to undergo a repeat biopsy.

The pathologist will perform a gross inspection of the sample to note any changes in appearance. In cirrhosis, the sample will be fragmented and hard. Fatty liver, seen in heavy drinkers, will float in the formalin solution and will be yellow. Carcinomas are white. The pathologist will also look for deposition of bile pigments (green) indicating cholestasis (obstruction of bile flow). In preparation for microscopic examination, the tissue will be frozen and cut into thin sections. These will be mounted on glass slides and stained with various dyes to aid in identifying microscopic structures. Using the microscope, the pathologist will examine the tissue samples, and identify abnormal cells or microarchitecture and any deposited substances such as iron or **copper**. In liver **cancer**, small dark malignant cells will be visible within the liver tissue. An infiltration of white blood cells may signal infection. The pathologist also checks for the number of bile ducts and whether they are dilated. He or she also looks at the health of the small arteries and portal veins. Fibrosis will appear as scar tissue and fatty changes are diagnosed by the presence of lipid droplets. Many different findings may be noted and a differential diagnosis (one out of many possibilities) can often be made. In difficult cases, other laboratory tests such as liver function enzymes, will aid the clinician in determining the final diagnosis.

Health care team roles

The liver biopsy requires the skill of many clinicians including the radiologist, hepatologist and pathologist in order to make the diagnosis. Nurses will assist the physician during the biopsy procedure and in caring for the patient after the procedure. Tissues are prepared for microscopic evaluation by a histologic technician.

Patient education

Patients should be told what to expect in the way of discomfort pre- and post-procedure. In addition, they should be advised about what medications they should not take before or after the biopsy. It is important for the clinician to reassure the patient concerning the safety of the procedure.

Resources

BOOKS

"Hepatobiliary Disorders: Introduction." In *Professional Guide to Diseases,* edited by Stanley Loeb, et al. Springhouse, PA: Springhouse Corporation, 2001.

Kanel, Gary C. and Jacob Korula. *Liver Biopsy Evaluation, Histologic Diagnosis and Clinical Correlations.* Philadelphia, PA: W.B. Saunders Company, 2000.

"Screening and Diagnostic Evaluation." In *The Merck Manual of Diagnosis and Therapy, 17th Edition,* edited by Robert Berkow, et al. Whitehouse Station, NJ: Merck Research Laboratories, 1999.

ORGANIZATIONS

American Liver Foundation. 1425 Pompton Avenue, Cedar Grove, NJ 07009. (800) 465-4837. <http://www.liverfoundation.org>.

Jane E. Phillips, PhD

Liver cancer

Definition

Liver cancer is a form of cancer with a high mortality rate. Liver cancers are classified into two types. They are either primary, when the cancer starts in the liver itself; or metastatic, when the cancer has metastasized (spread) to the liver from some other part of the body.

Description

Primary liver cancer

Primary liver cancer is a relatively rare disease in the United States, representing about 2% of all malignancies. It is much more common in other parts of the world, representing from 10-50% of malignancies in Africa and parts of Asia. According to the American Cancer Society, in the United States during 1998, more than 14,000 new cases of primary liver cancer were diagnosed, and approximately 13,000 deaths were attributable to it.

TYPES OF PRIMARY LIVER CANCER. In adults, most primary liver cancers belong to one of two types: hepatomas, also known as hepatocellular carcinomas, which start in the liver tissue itself; and cholangiocarcinomas, which are cancers that develop in the bile ducts

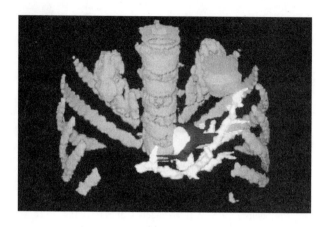

A three-dimensional computed tomography (CAT) scan of a patient's abdomen showing a malignant tumor (upper right) in the liver. *(Photo Researchers, Inc. Reproduced by permission.)*

inside the liver. About 90% of primary liver cancers are hepatomas. In the United States, about one person in every 40,000 will develop a hepatoma; in Africa and Asia, over 8 persons in 40,000 will develop this form of cancer. Two rare types of primary liver cancer are mixed-cell tumors and Kupffer cell **sarcomas.**

There is one type of primary liver cancer that usually occurs in children younger than four years of age and between the ages of 12-15. This type of childhood liver cancer is called a hepatoblastoma. Unlike liver cancers in adults, hepatoblastomas have a good chance of being treated successfully. Approximately 70% of children with hepatoblastomas experience complete cures. When the tumor is detected early, the survival rate is over 90%.

Metastatic liver cancer

The second major category of liver cancer, metastatic liver cancer, is about 20 times as common in the United States as primary liver cancer. Because **blood** from all parts of the body must pass through the liver for filtration, cancer cells from other organs and tissues easily reach the liver, where they can lodge and grow into secondary tumors. Primary cancers in the colon, **stomach**, **pancreas**, rectum, esophagus, breast, lung, or skin are the most likely to metastasize to the liver. It is not unusual for the metastatic cancer in the liver to be the first noticeable sign of a cancer that started in another organ. Second only to cirrhosis, metastatic liver cancer is the most common cause of fatal liver disease.

Causes and symptoms

Risk factors for primary liver cancer

The exact cause of primary liver cancer is still unknown. In adults, however, certain factors are known to place some individuals at higher risk of developing liver cancer. These factors include:

- Gender. The male/female ratio for hepatoma is 4:1.

- Age over 60 years.

- Environmental exposure to carcinogens (cancer causing substances). Examples of environmental carcinogens are aflatoxin, substance produced by a mold that grows on rice and peanuts; thorium dioxide, used at one time as a contrast dye for x rays of the liver; and vinyl chloride, used in manufacturing plastics.

- Use of oral estrogens for **contraception** (birth control).

- Hereditary hemochromatosis. Hemochromatosis is a disorder characterized by abnormally high levels of **iron** storage in the body. It often progresses to cirrhosis.

- Cirrhosis. Hepatomas appear to be a frequent complication of cirrhosis of the liver. Between 30-70% of hepatoma patients also have cirrhosis. It is estimated that a patient with cirrhosis has 40 times the chance of developing a hepatoma than a person with a healthy liver. Cirrhosis usually results from alcohol abuse or chronic viral hepatitis.

- Exposure to hepatitis B (HBV) or hepatitis C (HBC) **viruses.** In Africa and most of Asia, exposure to hepatitis B is an important factor; in Japan and some Western countries, exposure to hepatitis C is associated with a higher risk of developing liver cancer. In the United States, nearly 25% of patients with liver cancer have evidence of HBV **infection.** Hepatitis B and C are commonly found among intravenous drug abusers.

Symptoms of liver cancer

The early symptoms of primary, as well as metastatic, liver cancer are often vague and not specific to liver disorders. The long delay between the beginning of the tumor's growth and signs of illness is the major reason the disease has such a high mortality rate. At the time of diagnosis, patients are often tired, with **fever**, abdominal **pain**, and loss of appetite. They may look emaciated and generally ill. As the tumor grows bigger, it stretches the membrane surrounding the liver (the capsule), causing pain in the upper abdomen on the right side. The pain may extend into the back and shoulder. Some patients develop ascites (a collection of fluid) in the abdominal cavity. Others may have gastrointestinal bleeding. In addition, the tumor may block the ducts of the liver or the gall bladder, leading to **jaundice.** In patients with jaundice, the whites of the eyes and the skin may turn yellow, and the urine becomes dark-colored.

Diagnosis

Physical examination

When a diagnosis of primary liver cancer is suspected, the physician will scrutinize the patient's history for risk factors and pay close attention to the condition of the abdomen during the **physical examination**. Masses or lumps in the liver and ascites can often be felt while the patient is lying flat on the examination table. The liver is usually swollen and hard in patients with liver cancer; it may be sore when the physician presses on it. In some cases, the patient's spleen is also enlarged. The physician may be able to hear a bruit (an abnormal sound) or friction rub when a **stethoscope** is used to listen to the **blood vessels** that lie near the liver. These abnormal sounds are caused by the pressure of the tumor on the blood vessels.

Laboratory tests

Blood tests, performed by a laboratory technologist or technician, may be used to evaluate liver function or to confirm risk factors, such as hepatitis B or C infection. About 75% of patients with liver cancer show evidence of hepatitis infection. Between 50-75% of primary liver cancer patients have abnormally high blood serum levels of alpha-fetoprotein (AFP). The AFP test, however, cannot be used by itself to confirm a diagnosis of liver cancer, because cirrhosis or chronic hepatitis can also produce high alpha-fetoprotein levels. Tests for alkaline phosphatase, bilirubin, lactic dehydrogenase, and other chemicals indicate that the liver is not functioning normally. Though useful, abnormal liver function test results can not alone establish the diagnosis of liver cancer.

Imaging studies

Imaging studies are used to locate specific areas of abnormal tissue in the liver. Liver tumors as small as an inch across can be detected by ultrasound or computed tomography scan (CT scan). Imaging studies, however, cannot tell the difference between a hepatoma and other abnormal masses or nodules in the liver. A sample of liver tissue for biopsy is needed to make the definitive diagnosis of a primary liver cancer. CT or ultrasound may be used to guide the physician in selecting the best location for obtaining the biopsy sample.

Chest x rays may be used to see whether the liver tumor is primary or has metastasized from a primary tumor in the **lungs**. Imaging studies, including chest x rays, are usually performed by a radiology technician.

Liver biopsy

Liver biopsy provides the definite diagnosis of liver cancer. A sample of the liver or tissue fluid is removed with a fine needle and is examined by a pathologist, under a **microscope**, for the presence of cancer cells. In about 70% of cases, the biopsy is positive for cancer. In most cases, there is little risk to the patient from the biopsy procedure. In about 0.4% of cases, however, the patient develops a fatal hemorrhage from the biopsy because some tumors are supplied with a large number of blood vessels and bleed very easily.

Laparoscopy

The physician also may perform a **laparoscopy** to assist in the diagnosis of liver cancer. A **laparoscope** is a small tube-shaped instrument with a light at one end that is inserted into the patient's abdomen. A small piece of liver tissue is removed and sent for biopsy (microscopic examination for the presence of cancer cells).

Treatment

Treatment of liver cancer is based on several factors, including the type of cancer (primary or metastatic); stage (early or advanced); the location of other primary cancers or metastases; the patient's age; and other coexisting diseases, including cirrhosis. For many patients, treatment of liver cancer is primarily intended to relieve the pain caused by the cancer; it aims to relieve symptoms but not to cure the disease.

Surgery

Few liver cancers in adults can be cured surgically because they are usually too advanced by the time they are discovered. If the cancer is contained within one lobe of the liver, and if the patient does not have cirrhosis, jaundice, or ascites, then surgery is the best treatment option. Patients who can have their entire tumors removed have the best chances for survival. Unfortunately, only about 5% of patients with metastatic cancer (from primary tumors in the colon or rectum) fall into this group. If the entire visible tumor can be removed, about 25% of patients will be cured. The surgical procedure that is performed is called a partial hepatectomy, or partial removal of the liver. The surgeon will remove either an entire lobe of the liver (a lobectomy) or cut out the area around the tumor (a wedge resection).

Chemotherapy

Some patients with metastatic cancer of the liver may have their lives prolonged for a few months by **chemotherapy**, although cure is not possible. If the

KEY TERMS

Aflatoxin—A substance produced by molds that grow on rice and peanuts. Exposure to aflatoxin is thought to explain the high rates of primary liver cancer in Africa and parts of Asia.

Alpha-fetoprotein—A protein in blood serum that is found in abnormally high concentrations in most patients with primary liver cancer.

Cirrhosis—A chronic degenerative disease of the liver, in which normal cells are replaced by fibrous tissue. Cirrhosis is a major risk factor for the later development of liver cancer.

Hepatitis—A viral disease characterized by inflammation of the liver cells (hepatocytes). People infected with hepatitis B or hepatitis C virus are at an increased risk for developing liver cancer.

tumor cannot be removed by surgery, then a catheter may be placed in the main artery (hepatic artery) of the liver and an implantable infusion pump can be installed. The pump allows much higher concentrations of the anticancer drug to be carried to the tumor than is possible with chemotherapy carried through the bloodstream. The drug used for infusion pump therapy is usually floxuridine (FUDR), given for 14-day periods alternating with 14-day rests.

Systemic chemotherapy, given through a peripheral vein, can also be used to treat liver cancer. The drugs usually used are 5-fluorouracil (Adrucil, Efudex) or methotrexate (MTX, Mexate). Systemic chemotherapy does not, however, significantly increase survival time.

Radiation therapy

Radiation therapy may be used to relieve some symptoms of the disease. In general, radiation therapy will not prolong survival. Radioimmunotherapy is an experimental form of radiation therapy used to treat some types of liver cancer. A radioactive isotope is given intravenously and concentrates in the liver, where it radiates the tumor internally.

Liver transplantation

Since 1998, removal of the entire liver (total hepatectomy) and liver transplantation have very rarely been used to treat liver cancer. This is because very few patients are eligible for this procedure, either because the cancer has spread beyond the liver or because there are

no suitable donors. Further research in the field of transplant immunology may make liver transplantation a viable treatment modality.

Prognosis

Liver cancer has a very poor prognosis because it is often not diagnosed until it has metastasized. Fewer than 10% of patients survive three years after the initial diagnosis; the overall five-year survival rate for patients with hepatomas is around 4%. Most patients with primary liver cancer die within several months of diagnosis. Patients with liver cancers that metastasized from cancers in the colon live slightly longer than those whose cancers spread from cancers in the stomach or pancreas.

Health care team roles

Like other cancer patients, patients with liver cancer are usually cared for by a multidisciplinary team of health professionals. The patient's family physician or primary care physician collaborates with other physician specialists, such as surgeons and oncologists. Radiologic technicians perform x ray, CT and MRI scans and nurses and laboratory technicians may obtain samples of blood, urine and other laboratory tests. Nurses also perform patient and family education.

Before and after any surgical procedures, including biopsies, nurses explain the procedures and help to prepare patients and families. Patients may also benefit from counseling from social workers, other mental health professionals or pastoral counselors.

Prevention

Presently, there are no useful strategies for preventing metastatic cancers of the liver. Primary liver cancers, however, are 75-80% preventable. Current strategies focus on widespread **vaccination** for hepatitis B; early treatment of hereditary hemochromatosis; and screening of high-risk patients with alpha-fetoprotein testing and ultrasound examinations.

Lifestyle factors that may be modified in order to prevent liver cancer include avoidance of exposure to environmental carcinogens, toxic chemicals, and foods harboring molds that produce aflatoxin. Most important, however, is avoidance of alcohol and drug abuse. Alcohol abuse is responsible for 60-75% of cases of cirrhosis, which is a major risk factor for eventual development of primary liver cancer. Hepatitis is a widespread disease among persons who abuse intravenous drugs.

Resources

BOOKS

Friedman, Lawrence S. "Liver, Biliary Tract, & Pancreas." In *Current Medical Diagnosis & Treatment 1998,* edited by Lawrence M. Tierney, Jr., et al. Stamford, CT: Appleton & Lange, 1997.

Murphy, Gerald P. et al. *American Cancer Society Textbook of Clinical Oncology Second Edition* Atlanta, GA: The American Cancer Society, Inc. 1995.

Rudolph, Rebecca E., and Kris V. Kowdley. "Cirrhosis of the Liver." In *Current Diagnosis 9,* edited by Rex B. Conn, et al. Philadelphia: W. B. Saunders Company, 1997.

Way, Lawrence W. "Liver." In *Current Surgical Diagnosis & Treatment,* edited by Lawrence W. Way. Stamford, CT: Appleton & Lange, 1994.

ORGANIZATIONS

American Cancer Society. 1599 Clifton Road, N.E., Atlanta, GA 30329. (800)227-2345.

American Liver Foundation. 1425 Pompton Avenue, Cedar Grove, NJ 07009. (800)465-4837.

Cancer Research Institute. 681 Fifth Avenue, New York, NY 10022. (800)992-2623.

National Cancer Institute (National Institutes of Health). 9000 Rockville Pike, Bethesda, MD 20892. (800)422-6237.

Barbara Wexler

Liver function tests

Definition

Liver function tests, or LFTs, include tests that are routinely measured in all clinical laboratories. LFTs include bilirubin, a compound formed by the catabolism of hemoglobin; ammonia, a product of protein catabolism that is normally converted into urea by the liver before being excreted by the **kidneys; proteins** that are made by the liver including total protein, albumin, prothrombin, and fibrinogen; cholesterol and triglycerides, which are made and excreted via the liver; and the enzymes alanine aminotransferase (ALT), aspartate aminotransferase (AST), alkaline phosphatase (ALP), gamma-glutamyl transferase (GGT), and lactate dehydrogenase (LDH). Other liver function tests include serological (tests to demonstrate antibodies) and DNA tests for hepatitis and other **viruses**, tests for antimitochondrial and smooth muscle antibodies, transthyretin (prealbumin), protein electrophoresis, bile acids, alpha-fetoprotein, and a constellation of other enzymes that help differentiate necrotic versus obstructive liver disease.

Purpose

Liver function tests done individually do not give the physician very much information, but used in combination along with a careful history, **physical examination**, and imaging studies they contribute to making an accurate diagnosis of the specific liver disorder. Different tests will show abnormalities in response to liver inflammation, liver injury due to drugs, alcohol, toxins or viruses, liver malfunction due to blockage of the flow of bile, and liver cancers.

Precautions

Blood for LFTs is collected by venipuncture. The nurse or phlebotomist performing the procedure must be careful to observe **universal precautions** for the prevention of transmission of bloodborne pathogens. Blood for ammonia testing should be iced immediately after collection, stored anaerobically until measured, and assayed within 30 minutes to prevent an increase in ammonia caused by deamination of amino acids in the blood. Hemolysis will falsely increase tests for LD, AST, and ALT.

Bilirubin: Drugs that may cause increased blood levels of total bilirubin include anabolic steroids, **antibiotics**, antimalarials, ascorbic acid, Diabinese, codeine, diuretics, epinephrine, oral contraceptives, and **vitamin A**.

Ammonia: Muscular exertion can increase ammonia levels, while cigarette smoking produces significant increases within one hour of inhalation. Drugs that may cause increased levels include alcohol, barbiturates, narcotics, and diuretics. Drugs that may decrease levels include broad-spectrum antibiotics, levodopa, lactobacillus, and potassium salts.

ALT: Drugs that may increase ALT levels include acetaminophen, ampicillin, codeine, dicumarol, indomethacin, methotrexate, oral contraceptives, tetracyclines, and verapamil. Previous intramuscular injections may cause elevated levels.

GGT: Drugs that may cause increased GGT levels include alcohol, phenytoin, and phenobarbital. Drugs that may cause decreased levels include oral contraceptives.

LD: Strenous activity may raise levels of LDH. Alcohol, anesthetics, aspirin, narcotics, procainamide, and fluoride may also raise levels. Ascorbic acid (**vitamin C**) can lower levels of LDH.

Description

The liver is the largest and one of the most important organs in the body. As the body's "chemical factory," it regulates the levels of most of the biomolecules found in the blood, and acts with the kidneys to clear the blood of drugs and toxic substances. The liver metabolizes these products, alters their chemical structure, makes them water soluble, and excretes them in bile. Laboratory tests for total protein, albumin, ammonia, transthyretin, and cholesterol are markers for the synthetic function of the liver. Tests for cholesterol, bilirubin, ALP, and bile salts are measures of the secretory (excretory) function of the liver. The enzymes ALT, AST, GGT, LD, and tests for viruses are markers for liver injury.

Some liver function tests are used to determine if the liver has been damaged or its function impaired. Elevations of these markers for liver injury or disease tell the physician that something is wrong with the liver. ALT and bilirubin are the two primary tests used largely used for this purpose. Bilirubin is measured by two tests, called total and direct bilirubin. The total bilirubin measures both conjugated and unconjugated bilirubin while direct bilirubin measures only the conjugated bilirubin fraction in the blood. Unconjugated bilirubin is formed from heme in the reticuloendothelial cells in the spleen that remove old red blood cells from the circulation. The RE cells release the bilirubin into the blood where it is bound by albumin and transported to the liver. The bilirubin is taken up by liver cells and conjugated to glucuronic acid, which makes the bilirubin water soluble. This form will react directly with a Ehrlich's diazo reagent, hence the name direct bilirubin. While total bilirubin is elevated in various liver diseases, it is also increased in certain (hemolytic) **anemias** caused by increased red blood cell turnover. Neonatal hyperbilirubinemia is a condition caused by an immature liver than cannot conjugate the bilirubin. The level of total bilirubin in the blood becomes elevated, and must be monitored closely in order to prevent damage to the **brain** caused by unconjugated bilirubin, which has a high affinity for brain tissue. Bilirubin levels can be decreased by exposing the baby to UV light. Direct bilirubin is formed only by the liver, and therefore, it is specific for hepatic or biliary disease. Its concentration in the blood is very low (0-0.2 mg/dL) and therefore, even slight increases are significant. Highest levels of direct bilirubin are seen in obstructive liver diseases. However, direct biliruibn is not sensitive to all forms of liver disease (e.g., focal intrahepatic obstruction) and is not always elevated in the earliest stages of disease, and therefore, ALT is needed to exclude a diagnosis.

ALT is an enzyme that transfers an amino group from the amino acid alanine to a ketoacid acceptor (oxaloacetate). The enzyme was formerly called serum glutamic pyruvic transaminase (SGPT) after the products formed by this reaction. Although ALT is present in other tissues besides liver, its concentration in liver is far greater than any other tissue, and blood levels in nonhepatic conditions rarely produce levels of a magnitude seen in liver disease. The enzyme is very sensitive to necrotic or inflammatory liver injury. Consequently, if ALT or direct bilirubin are increased, then some form of liver disease is likely. If both are normal, then liver disease is unlikely.

These two tests along with others are used to help determine what is wrong. The most useful tests for this purpose are the liver function enzymes and the ratio of direct to total bilirubin. These tests are used to differentiate diseases characterized primarily by hepatocellular damage (necrosis) from those characterized by obstructive damage (cholestasis or blockage of bile flow). In hepatocellular damage, the transaminases, ALT and AST, are increased to a greater extent than alkaline phosphatase. This includes viral hepatitis, which gives the greatest increase in transaminases (10-50 fold normal), hepatitis induced by drugs or poisons (toxic hepatitis), alcoholic hepatitis, hypoxic necrosis (a consequence of congestive **heart failure**), chronic hepatitis, and cirrhosis of the liver. In obstructive liver diseases, the alkaline phosphatase is increased to a greater extent than the transaminases (ALP>ALT). This includes diffuse intrahepatic obstructive disease which may be caused by some drugs or biliary cirrhosis, focal obstruction that may be caused by malignancy, granuloma, or stones in the intrahepatic bile ducts, or extrahepatic obstruction such as gall bladder or common bile duct stones, or pancreatic or bile duct **cancer**. In both diffuse intrahepatic obstruction and extrahepatic obstruction, the direct bilirubin is often greatly elevated because the liver can conjugate the bilirubin, but this direct bilirubin cannot be excreted via the bile. In such cases the ratio of direct to total bilirubin is greater than 0.4.

Aspartate aminotransferase, formerly called serum glutamic oxaloacetic transaminase (SGOT), is not as specific for liver disease as is ALT, which is increased in **myocardial infarction**, **pancreatitis**, muscle wasting diseases, and many other conditions. However, differentiation of acute and chronic forms of hepatocellular injury are aided by examining the ratio of ALT to AST, called the DeRitis ratio. In acute hepatitis, Reye's syndrome, and infectious mononucleosis the ALT predominates. However, in alcoholic liver disease, chronic hepatitis, and cirrhosis the AST predominates.

Alkaline phosphatase is increased in obstructive liver diseases, but it is not specific for the liver. Increases of a similar magnitude (three- to five-fold normal) are commonly seen in bone diseases, late **pregnancy**, leukemia, and some other malignancies. The enzyme gamma-glutamyl transferase (GGT) is used to help differentiate the source of an elevated ALP. GGT is greatly increased in obstructive **jaundice**, alcoholic liver disease, and hepatic cancer. When the increase in GGT is two or more times greater than the increase in ALP, the source of the ALP is considered to be from the liver. When the increase in GGT is five or more times the increase in ALP, this points to a diagnosis of alcoholic hepatitis. GGT, but not AST and ALT, is elevated in the first stages of liver inflammation due to alcohol consumption, and GGT is useful as a marker for excessive drinking. GGT has been shown to rise after acute persistent alcohol ingestion and then fall when alcohol is avoided.

Lactate dehydrogenase (LD) is found in almost all cells in the body. Different forms of the enzyme (isoenzymes) exist in different tissues, especially in **heart**, liver, red blood cells, brain, kidney and muscles. LD is increased in megaloblastic and hemolytic anemias, leukemias and lymphomas, myocardial infarction, infectious mononucleosis, muscle wasting diseases, and both necrotic and obstructive jaundice. While LD is not specific for any one disorder, the enzyme is elevated (two- to five-fold normal) along with liver function enzymes in both necrotic and obstructive liver diseases. LD is markedly increased in most cases of **liver cancer**. An enzyme pattern showing a marked increase in LD and to a lesser degree ALP with only slightly increased transaminases (AST and ALT) is seen in cancer of the liver (space occupying disease). Such findings should be followed-up with imaging studies and measurement of alpha-fetoprotein and carcinoembryonic antigen, two tumor markers prevalent in hepatic cancers.

Some liver function tests are not sensitive enough to be used for diagnostic purposes, but are elevated in severe or chronic liver diseases. These tests are used primarily to indicate the extent of damage to the liver. Tests falling into this category are ammonia, total protein, albumin, cholesterol, transthyretin, fibrinogen, and the prothrombin time.

Analysis of blood ammonia aids in the diagnosis of severe liver diseases and helps to monitor the course of these diseases. Together with the AST and the ALT, ammonia levels are used to confirm a diagnosis of Reye's syndrome, a rare disorder usually seen in children and associated with **infection** and aspirin intake. Reye's syndrome is characterized by brain and liver damage following an upper respiratory tract infection, chickenpox, or **influenza**. Ammonia levels are also helpful in the diagnosis and treatment of hepatic encephalopathy, a serious brain condition caused by the accumulated toxins that result from liver disease and liver failure. Ammonia levels in the blood are normally very low. Ammonia produced by the breakdown of amino acids is converted by the liver to urea. When liver disease becomes severe, failure of the urea cycle results in elevated blood ammonia

and decreased urea (or blood urea nitrogen, BUN). Increasing ammonia signals end-stage liver disease and a high risk of hepatic **coma**.

Albumin is the protein found in the highest concentration in blood, making up over half of the protein mass. Albumin has a half-life in blood of about three weeks and decreased levels are not seen in the early stages of liver disease. A persistently low albumin in liver disease signals reduced synthetic capacity of the liver and is a sign of progressive liver failure. In the acute stages of liver disease, proteins such as transthyretin (prealbumin) with a shorter half-life may be measured to give an indication of the severity of the disease.

Cholesterol is synthesized by the liver and cholesterol balance is maintained by the liver's ability to remove cholesterol from lipoproteins, and use it to produce bile acids and salts that it excretes into the bile ducts. In obstructive jaundice caused by stones, biliary tract scarring, or cancer, the bile cannot be eliminated and cholesterol and triglycerides may accumulate in the blood as low-density lipoprotein cholesterol. In acute necrotic liver diseases triglycerides may be elevated due to hepatic lipase deficiency. In liver failure caused by necrosis, the liver's ability to synthesize cholesterol is reduced and blood levels may be low.

The liver is responsible for production of the **vitamin K** clotting factors. In obstructive liver diseases a deficiency of vitamin K-derived clotting factors results from failure to absorb vitamin K. In obstructive jaundice, **intramuscular injection** of vitamin K will correct the prolonged prothrombin time. In severe necrotic disease, the liver cannot synthesize factors I (fibrinogen) or factors II, VII, IX, and X from vitamin K. When attributable to hepatic necrosis, an increase in the prothrombin time by more than two seconds indicates severe liver disease.

Serum protein electrophoresis patterns will be abnormal in both necrotic and obstructive liver diseases. In the acute stages of hepatitis, the albumin will be low and the gamma globulin fraction will be elevated owing to a large increase in the production of antibodies. The alpha-1 globulin and alpha-2 globulin fractions will be elevated owing to production of acute phase proteins. In biliary cirrhosis the beta globulin may be elevated owing to an increase in beta lipoprotein. In hepatic cirrhosis the albumin will be greatly decreased, and the pattern will show bridging between the beta and gamma globulins owing to production of IgA. The albumin to globulin ratio (A/G) ratio will fall below one.

The most prevalent liver disease is viral hepatitis. Tests for this condition include a variety of antigen and antibody markers and nucleic acid tests that are discussed in detail elsewhere (see entry on hepatitis tests). Acute

KEY TERMS

Bile acid—A detergent that is made in the liver and excreted into the intestine to aid in the absorption of fats.

Biliary—Relating to bile.

Cirrhosis—A liver disease where there is a loss of normal liver tissues, replaced by scar tissue. This is usually caused by chronic alcohol abuse but can be caused by blockage of the bile ducts.

Detoxification—A process of altering the chemical struction of a compound to make it less toxic.

Hepatitis—Inflammation of the liver.

Hepatocyte—Liver cell.

Isoenzyme—One of a group of enzymes that brings about the same reactions on the same chemicals, but are different in their physical properties.

Jaundice—Hyperbilirubinemia or too much bilirubin in the blood. Bilirubin will be deposited in the skin and the mucosal membranes. The whites of the eyes and the skin appear yellow.

Neonatal jaundice—A disorder in newborns where the liver is too premature to conjugate bilirubin which builds up in the blood.

viral hepatitis is associated initially with 20 to 100 fold increases in transaminases and is followed shortly afterward by jaundice. Such patients should be tested for hepatitis B surface antigen (HbsAg) and IgM antibodies to hepatitis B core antigen (anti-HBc IgM), and anti-hepatitis C virus (anti-HVC) to identify these causes. In addition to hepatitis A-G, viral hepatitis may be caused by Epstein-Barr virus (EBV) and cytomegalovirus (CMV) infections of the liver. Tests for these viruses such as the infectious mononucleosis antibody test, anti- viral capsid antigen test (anti-VCA), and anti-CMV test are useful in diagnosing these infections.

Liver disease may be caused by autoimmune mechanisms in which autoantibodies destroy liver cells. Autoimmune necrosis is associated with systemic lupus erythematosus and chronic viral hepatitis usually caused by hepatitis B and hepatitis C virus infections. These conditions give rise to anti-smooth muscle antibodies and anti-nuclear antibodies, and tests for these are useful markers for chronic hepatitis. Antibodies to mitochondrial antigens (antimitochondrial antibodies) are found in the blood of more than 90% of persons with primary bil-

iary cirrhosis, and those with M2 specificity are considered specific for this disease.

Preparation

Patients are asked to fast and to inform clinicians of all drugs, even over the counter drugs, that they are taking. Many times liver function tests are done on an emergency basis and fasting and obtaining a medical history are not possible.

Aftercare

Patients will have blood drawn into a vacuum tube and may experience some **pain** and burning at the site of injection. A gauze bandage may be placed over the site to prevent further bleeding. If the person is suffering from severe liver disease, they may lack clotting factors. The nurse should be careful to monitor bleeding in these patients after obtaining blood.

Results

Reference ranges vary from laboratory to laboratory and also depend upon the method used. However, normal values are generally framed by the ranges shown below. Values for enzymes are based upon measurement at 37°C.

- ALT: 5-35 IU/L (values for the elderly may be slightly higher, and values also may be higher in men and in African-Americans).

- AST: 0-35 IU/L.

- ALP: 30-120 IU/LALP is higher in children, older adults and pregnant females.

- GGT: males 2-30 U/L; females 1-24 U/L.

- LD: 0-4 days old: 290-775 U/L; 4-10 days: 545-2000 U/L; 10 days-24 months:180-430 U/L; 24 months-12 years:110-295 U/L; 12-60 years:100-190 U/L; 60 years: >110-210 U/L.

- Bilirubin: (Adult, elderly, and child) Total bilirubin: 0.1-1.0 mg/dL; indirect bilirubin: 0.2-0.8 mg/dL; direct bilirubin: 0.0-0.3 mg/dL. (Newborn) Total bilirubin: 1-12 mg/dL. Note: critical values for adult: greater than 1.2 mg/dL. Critical values for newborn (requiring immediate treatment): greater than 15 mg/dL.

- Ammonia: 10-70 micrograms per dL (heparinized plasma). Normal values for this test vary widely, depending upon the age of the patient and the type of specimen.

- Albumin: 3.2-5.4 g/L.

Abnormal results

ALT: Values are significantly increased in cases of hepatitis, and moderately increased in cirrhosis, liver tumor, obstructive jaundice, and severe **burns**. Values are mildly increased in pancreatitis, heart attack, infectious mononucleosis, and **shock**. Most useful when compared with ALP levels.

AST: High levels may indicate liver cell damage, hepatitis, heart attack, heart failure, or gall stones.

ALP: Elevated levels occur in diseases that impair bile formation (cholestasis). ALP may also be elevated in many other liver disorders, as well as some lung cancers (bronchogenic carcinoma) and Hodgkin's lymphoma. However, elevated ALP levels may also occur in otherwise healthy people, especially among older people.

GGT: Increased levels are diagnostic of hepatitis, cirrhosis, liver tumor or metastasis, as well as injury from drugs toxic to the liver. GGT levels may increase with alcohol ingestion, heart attack, pancreatitis, infectious mononucleosis, and Reye's syndrome.

LD: Elevated LD is seen with heart attack, kidney disease, hemolysis, viral hepatitis, infectious mononucleosis, Hodgkin's disease, abdominal and lung cancers, germ cell tumors, progressive **muscular dystrophy** and pulmonary embolism. LD is not normally elevated in cirrhosis.

Bilirubin: Increased indirect or total bilirubin levels can indicate various serious anemias, including hemolytic disease of the newborn and transfusion reaction. Increased direct bilirubin levels can be diagnostic of bile duct obstruction, gallstones, cirrhosis, or hepatitis. It is important to note that if total bilirubin levels in the newborn reach or exceed critical levels, exchange transfusion is necessary to avoid kernicterus, a condition that causes brain damage.

Ammonia: Increased levels are seen in primary liver cell disease, Reye's syndrome, severe heart failure, hemolytic disease of the newborn, and hepatic encephalopathy.

Albumin: Albumin levels are increased due to **dehydration**. They are decreased due to a decrease in synthesis of the protein which is seen in severe liver failure and in conditions such as burns or renal disease that cause loss of albumin from the blood.

Health care team roles

A physician will order the liver function tests that he or she feels are necessary, and the nurse or phlebotomist will draw the blood. Patients will probably be referred to an internist or hepatologist if results are abnormal. LFTs are performed by clinical laboratory scientists/medical technologists or clinical laboratory technicians/medical laboratory technicians.

Patient education

Health care providers should inform the patient of any abnormal results and explain how these values reflect the status of their liver disease. It is important to guide the patient in ways to stop behaviors such as taking drugs or drinking alcohol, if these are the causes of the illness.

Resources

BOOKS

Burtis, Carl A., and Edward R. Ashwood. *Tietz Textbook of Clinical Chemistry.* Philadelphia: W.B. Saunders, 1999.

Cahill, Matthew. *Handbook of Diagnostic Tests, 2nd ed.* Springhouse, PA: Springhouse Corporation, 1999.

Pagana, Kathleen Deska, and Timothy James Pagana. *Mosby's Manual of Diagnostic and Laboratory Tests.* Philadelphia: Mosby, Inc., 1998.

Jane E. Phillips, PhD

Liver radionuclide scan

Definition

A **liver** scan, also known as a liver-spleen scan, is a diagnostic imaging procedure to evaluate the liver and spleen for suspected disease.

Purpose

A liver scan is performed to determine the size, configuration, relative function of the liver and spleen, and to detect space occupying lesions such as, cysts, an **abscess**, and tumors. Liver scans are indicated if a patient has abdominal **pain**, if a patient's liver enzymes (determined by **blood** tests) are abnormal, if the patient is jaundiced, and to detect and monitor metastatic disease. A liver scan may also be helpful in diagnosing specific disorders, by detecting features which are characteristic of a disorder, such as cirrhosis of the liver. This study may also be part of the battery of tests used to evaluate potential candidates for liver transplant.

Precautions

Women who are pregnant are cautioned against having this test unless the benefit of having the test outweighs the risks. If a woman is breast feeding, she will be required to stop for a specified period of time, depending on the dose given.

Description

This test is be performed in an out-patient facility or a hospital x-ray or nuclear medicine department. The patient is injected intravenously with a radioactive tracer, or radionuclide, that accumulates in certain cells of the liver, spleen, and bone marrow. Approximately 15 minutes after the injection, the patient is asked to lie down on a bed. A gamma camera or scintillation camera is positioned above the upper abdomen and may lightly touch the patient. It is important for the patient to lie quietly. Position changes and brief periods of breath holding may be required. The test usually takes approximately 30 minutes. Occasionally, a SPECT (Single Photon Emission Computed Tomography) study is indicated to further pinpoint an area of abnormality. The SPECT procedure is the same, but the camera will circle around the patient, in order to provide a cross sectional image of the liver.

Preparation

No physical preparation is required. The patient will be asked to remove metal objects from the area to be imaged. If the patient has had other recent nuclear scans, a waiting period may be necessary so that any residual radiation in the body will not interfere. The patients should understand that there is no danger of significant radioactive exposure to themselves or others. Only small amounts of radionuclide are used. The total amount of radiation absorbed is often less than the dose received from ordinary x rays.

Aftercare

No special aftercare is necessary.

Results

A normal scan will show a liver of normal size, shape, and position. It is expected that the liver will accumulate the radioactive tracer in a uniform fashion. Areas that appear absent may represent a cyst, abscess, or a

tumor and therefore other imaging tests such as ultrasound or CT may be required to assess the nature of the abnormality. Too much radioisotope in the spleen and bones compared to the liver, known as "colloid shift," can indicate portal **hypertension** or cirrhosis. Liver diseases such as hepatitis may also cause an abnormal scan, but is rarely diagnosed from the information revealed by this study alone. Again, other diagnostic tests are performed along with a liver scan to evaluate specific abnormalities and to arrive at a diagnosis.

Health care team roles

The injection and scan are performed by a nuclear medicine technologist, who will also obtain pertinent medical history from the patient and explain the test. The technologist is trained to handle radioactive materials, operate the scanner, and to process the data. The images are interpreted by a medical doctor who is a radiologist or nuclear medicine specialist. The patient received the results of the scan from their personal physician or doctor who ordered the test.

Resources

BOOKS

Klingensmith III, M.D., Wm. C., Dennis Eshima, Ph.D., John Goddard, Ph.D. *Nuclear Medicine Procedure Manual 2000-2001.*

Vitti, Richard A., and Leon S. Malmud. "Gastrointestinal System." In *Nuclear Medicine,* edited by Donald R. Bernier, et al. St. Louis: Mosby, 1997.

PERIODICALS

Drane, Walter E. "Scintigraphic Techniques for Hepatic Imaging." *Radiologic Clinics of North America,* 36 (March 1998): 309-318.

Christine Miner Minderovic, B.S., R.T., R.D.M.S.

Local anesthetic *see* **Anesthesia, local**

Long-term insurance

Definition

Long-term insurance provides for a person's care in cases of chronic illness or disability. Policies are available with a wide range of coverage options.

Long-term insurance refers to coverage of health services, which may include community health care, nursing **home care,** and home support. Long-term health insurance is normally for the elderly, but is sometimes also applicable to younger individuals with disabilities.

Description

A major health care challenge looms over America as the population ages and people live longer. The country lacks a comprehensive health system that serves the needs of millions of older persons and individuals with long-term disabilities.

Long-term care options are often fragmented, uncoordinated, and costly for patients, their families and, in some instances, public coffers. Millions of Americans, according to the American Association of Retired Persons (AARP), are denied access to long-term care services because they cannot pay for services, do not qualify for public funding or cannot access the types of services that they need and can afford.

People of all ages usually prefer to receive long-term care in their own homes, or in home-like assisted-living facilities. More than three-quarters of older Americans in need of long-term care live in the community, with most receiving no paid services. The majority of long-term care is provided by unpaid, informal caregivers, such as family and friends. In 1996, more than 22 million households in the United States included a caregiver who was age 50 or older. About 73% of unpaid caregivers were women, nearly one-third of whom were over age 65. Many caregivers, especially women, balance multiple caregiving roles by providing for both their parents and their children.

Medicare does not cover most long-term care services. In 1997, 68% of nursing home residents were dependent on **Medicaid** to finance at least some of their care. For many, long-term insurance is unaffordable, and many cannot qualify because of pre-existing conditions.

Long-term insurance policies are often complex. People who purchase them may not read the fine print, then are forced to cancel the policy later because it does not fit their needs. Increasing rates factored into some long-term policies, known as "climbing premiums," may also become prohibitively expensive.

Long-term care insurance can benefit the consumer, provided that such items as affordability, coverage gaps, and timing of purchase are carefully considered. It may be advisable to check the financial stability and the claims ratio of the insurance company. Long-term insurance is a serious financial investment and should be considered a part of estate planning. A qualified, independent professional should be consulted to review the policy before purchase. The state health insurance assistance program (SHIP) is also available to answer questions.

The type of care that a client seeks is another important consideration before purchasing a policy. There is as yet no universal standard for defining long-term care facilities. A placement that is covered under one company's policy may not be covered under another's. Physicians can also play a part in denial of a placement by stating that the facility of choice is either not adequate or too advanced for the patient's needs.

When to buy a policy is another important consideration. Individuals with a pre-existing diagnosis for a debilitating condition or illness may not be eligible for coverage. This clause is common in most insurance policies of any type. But purchasing a policy too far in advance of an anticipated need can work against a buyer. The health care industry is currently in a state of flux, and technological advances are rapid. The benefits provided in a policy that is purchased at one point in time may not match the care available in the distant future, giving the company reason to deny benefits.

Generally, long-term insurance operates as an indemnity program for potential nursing home and/or home health-care costs. Additionally, many policies provide coverage for adult daycare, for care delivered in an assisted-living facility, and for hospice care. Rarely are all costs covered.

Some long-term care policies are pure indemnity programs which pay the insured a daily benefit contracted for by the insured. The pure indemnity program pays the full daily benefit regardless of the amount of care that the insured receives per diem.

Other long-term care policies pay for covered losses, or the cost of care actually received each day, up to the selected daily benefit level. This type of policy is also referred to as a "pool-of-money" contract.

Long-term insurance is available either as part of a group or individual coverage, although most are currently purchased by individuals. Most policies cover skilled, custodial and intermediate long-term care services. A purchaser is wise not to consider a contract that does not cover each level of long-term care services.

A recent change in the U.S. federal tax law allows for a portion of a long-term insurance premium to be tax-deductible. This deduction increases with the insured's age.

Benefits under a long-term care contract are triggered in a tax-qualified policy when the insured becomes unable to perform a number of activities associated with normal daily living or suffers from a cognitive impairment that requires supervision.

Non tax-qualified policies usually offer more liberal eligibility criteria, which includes long-term benefits because of a medical necessity.

Long-term insurance can help pay for needed services, as well as protect against the risk of significant financial loss. It may also provide choices about services and where they are received. Normally, neither employer health insurance nor Medicare pays for significant long-term care expenses, although Medicare does pay for short-term skilled care. Medicaid, the federal/state health insurance for those with limited assets and income, does pay for long-term care, but patients must use most of their savings or assets before these benefits can be realized.

Viewpoints

Long-term insurance policies can be expensive and may be restrictive in what they provide. Before purchasing a policy, individuals should make certain that it is within their means and will meet their anticipated needs. Some policies allow policy holders to tap into survivor death benefits to use for health care needs. Several different policies should be compared in detail. Recommendations from elderly advocate organizations can be helpful. Young people with disabilities have fewer options for long-term insurance because many policies exempt individuals with a pre-existing condition.

Professional implications

Health care professionals should be aware of the pros and cons of long-term insurance and be able to answer patients' questions. Long-term insurance may involve special billing procedures.

Resources

Shelton, Phyllis. *Long-Term Care Planning Guide Version 2000.* Shelton Marketing Services, 2000.

PERIODICALS

Bern-Klug, Mercedes. "Health Insurance for People with Medicare." *Clinical Reference Systems* Annual 2000, p. 781.

Norrgard, Carolyn. "Long-term care insurance." *Clinical Reference Systems* Annual 2000, p. 988.

OTHER

American Association for Retired Persons (AARP) 601 E St., NW, Washington DC 20049. (800) 424-3410. <http://www.aarp.org>.

Jacqueline N. Martin, M.S.

Low-cholesterol diet *see* **Diet therapy**

Low-fat diet *see* **Diet therapy**

Low-phenylalanine diet *see* **Diet therapy**

Low-purine diet *see* **Diet therapy**

Low-salt diet *see* **Diet therapy**

Low back pain, physical therapy for *see* **Back and neck pain, physical therapy for**

Lower gastrointestinal exam *see* **Barium enema**

Lower limb orthoses

Definition

A lower limb orthosis is an external force system used to compensate or control for decreased or abnormal forces in the hip, knee, ankle, or foot.

Purpose

Orthoses may be used for any of the following reasons: to lend stability to a weak joint, correct or maintain alignment, control motion in the presence of abnormal tone, immobilize a body part, protect an inflamed joint, or provide proprioceptive feedback. Individuals who have upper or lower motor neuron dysfunction, inflammatory joint diseases, **sports injuries**, or skeletal deformities may use orthoses.

Description

Foot orthoses

Foot orthoses are fabricated for individuals who have abnormal joint alignment in the foot, causing inappropriate motion during stance and gait. Abnormal mechanics may lead to **pain** and increased stress in the joints of the foot, leg and even back. Custom foot orthoses are made based upon a cast of the individual's foot, following a thorough biomechanical assessment of stance and gait. Based on the findings, rigid, semi-rigid, or soft inserts are fabricated to fit into the client's shoe to provide support where needed, for example, under the arch, the metatarsals, and/or the heel. The University of California Biomechanics Laboratory (UCBL) orthosis is a specific custom-molded orthosis that snugly holds the heel and midfoot in optimal alignment with regards to mediolateral stability.

Ankle-foot orthoses (AFOs)

In adults and children with neuromotor dysfunction, AFOs can be used to maintain appropriate alignment, provide mediolateral stability, and help with toe clearance or heel rise during the gait cycle. The supramalleolar orthosis (SMO) evolved from the UCBL orthosis to address not only mediolateral stability, but also anterior-posterior issues, including foot clearance. It extends to the area above the malleoli, and may be solid or include a mechanical ankle joint.

Ankle-foot orthoses that extend to the area just below the knee provide more stability than the SMO, and may be either static or dynamic. Static AFOs prohibit ankle motion; the most common is the solid AFO. The solid AFO prevents foot drop during gait and also can help to control knee extension or hyperextension, depending on how the ankle is set. Dynamic AFOs may allow for plantarflexion and/or dorsiflexion of the ankle through the use of either a mechanical joint or the location of trimlines. Various methods, such as pin stops and check straps, can be used to limit the amount of plantarflexion or dorsiflexion allowed as well. These options provide versatility in setting the range of ankle motion for individuals who have some control and/or expected return of function.

A variety of ankle supports are also available for individuals with musculoskeletal function. Air casts provide stability to those rehabilitating from ankle sprains, while Achilles straps may be used for tendonitis. Night splints and arch straps may help with positioning in those with plantar fasciitis.

Knee-ankle-foot-orthoses (KAFOs)

A KAFO is used when the knee needs to be stabilized and an AFO is insufficient. For example, KAFOs may be used in patients who have had a stroke, **spinal cord injury** or traumatic injury to the limbs. A conventional KAFO consists of double metal uprights connected to the shoe via a stirrup. A thermoplastic KAFO is custom-formed for total contact to the patient's thigh and calf. A variety of knee joints are available to allow for or restrict flexion and extension movement.

Knee orthoses

There are three categories of orthoses that address musculoskeletal impairments at the knee joint. Athletes use prophylactic orthoses in hopes of preventing knee injury. Rehabilitative orthoses are used post-operatively to allow protected motion to occur at the knee joint.

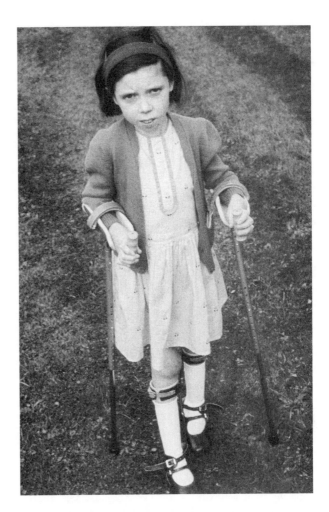

A girl with rheumatoid arthritis walks with the aid of braces. *(Photograph by John Moss. Photo Researchers, Inc. Reproduced by permission.)*

Functional orthoses are designed to provide stability and proprioceptive input to a patient returning to daily activities. Research is inconclusive on the effectiveness of prophylactic orthoses; however, studies do indicate that functional orthoses may be helpful in preventing further injuries in individuals who have already sustained an injury.

Hip-knee-ankle-foot orthoses (HKAFOs)

The hip guidance orthosis (HGO) and the reciprocating guidance orthosis (RGO) are two types of lumbosacral HKAFOs that can be used by adults or children to produce a reciprocal gait pattern. In both types, the user is braced from mid-trunk to the feet. These orthoses are most commonly used in children with myelomeningocele, but are also used by patients with traumatic **spinal cord** injury, **muscular dystrophy**, **cerebral palsy**, and **multiple sclerosis**.

Hip orthoses

Postoperative total hip orthoses sometimes are used after a total hip replacement in order to prevent the motions of hip flexion, adduction and internal rotation that can cause dislocation. In infants with developmental dysplasia of the hip, which causes hip instability, a Pavlik harness or hip abduction orthosis is used to position the hips in flexion and abduction to encourage desired bone development and prevent dislocation. Hip abduction orthoses are also used to treat children with Legg-Calve-Perthes disease.

Operation

Donning and doffing an orthosis can be a challenge at first, especially for children or for individuals with upper extremity impairments. The orthotist provides specific instructions for donning and doffing with the least difficulty. In addition, he or she provides instructions regarding the need to monitor skin for possible breakdown.

Maintenance

Orthotic maintenance may include resetting joint angles, which is usually done by an orthotist or a physical therapist under the direction of an orthotist. Screws in joint mechanisms also may loosen occasionally, and tightening can usually be done by the patient or caregiver at home with directions from the orthotist. As with operation, maintenance may vary depending on the type of orthosis, and users should follow the instructions of their orthotists.

Health care team roles

The patient, family, physician, orthotist and physical therapist all play important roles in orthotic intervention. The patient and family provide information about their lifestyles, home environment, and support network that allow for a realistic assessment of the ability to don, doff, care for and use an orthosis. The physician often plays an important role in identifying the need for an orthosis and preliminarily educating the patient about goals of orthotic intervention. The physical therapist and orthotist often cooperate in performing the preorthotic assessment. The physical therapist usually has important information regarding the patient's impairments and functional abilities, and may have an idea about what type of orthosis may be appropriate. The orthotist assesses limb function, takes necessary measurements for fabrication, and has extensive, up-to-date knowledge about what types of orthoses and components may best fit the patient's needs.

Training

The orthotist educates the patient about donning, doffing, caring for and using the orthosis. A wearing schedule is often provided for the patient to gradually grow accustomed to the orthosis. Because the physical therapist usually sees the patient regularly, he or she monitors the patient's progress with all aspects of orthotic intervention.

Resources

BOOKS

Lusaradi, Michelle M., and Caroline C. Nielsen. *Orthotics and Prosthetics in Rehabilitation.* Boston: Butterworth-Heinemann, 2000.

Nawoczenski, Deborah A. and Marcia E. Epler. *Orthotics in Functional Rehabilitation of the Lower Limb.* Philadelphia: W. B. Saunders Company, 1997.

PERIODICALS

Andrews, Karen L., and Kimberly A. Bouvette. "Anatomy for Management and Fitting of Prosthetics and Orthotics." *Physical Medicine and Rehabilitation: State of the Art Reviews* 10 (October 1996): 502-507.

ORGANIZATIONS

American Academy of Orthotists and Prosthetists. 526 King Street, Suite 201, Alexandria, VA 22314. (703) 836-0788. <http://www.oandp.org>.

Peggy Campbell Torpey, MPT

Lower limb prostheses

Definition

A lower limb prosthesis is an artificial replacement for any or all parts of the lower extremity (leg).

Purpose

A prosthesis is used to provide an individual who has an amputated limb with the opportunity to perform functional tasks, particularly ambulation (walking), which may not be possible without the limb. In 2000, there were more than 1.5 million people in the United States with amputations. Amputation surgery most often is performed due to complications of peripheral vascular disease or neuropathy; trauma is the second leading cause of amputation. Amputations performed because of tumor or congenital limb deficiency are less common.

Description

There are several levels of lower limb amputation, including partial foot, ankle disarticulation, transtibial (below the knee), knee disarticulation, transfemoral (above the knee), and hip disarticulation. The most common are transtibial (mid-calf) and transfemoral (mid-thigh). The basic components of these lower limb prostheses are the foot-ankle assembly, shank, socket, and suspension system.

Foot-ankle assembly

The foot-ankle assembly is designed to provide a base of support during standing and walking, in addition to providing shock absorption and push-off during walking on even and uneven terrain. Four general categories of foot-ankle assemblies are non-articulated, articulated, elastic keel, and dynamic-response. One of the most widely prescribed foot is the solid-ankle-cushion-heel (SACH) foot, due to its simplicity, low cost, and durability. It may be inappropriate, however, for active community ambulators and sports participants. Articulated assemblies allow motion at the level of the human ankle; this motion may occur in one or more planes, depending on whether it is a single-axis or multi-axis foot. These assemblies offer more mobility at the cost of less stability and increased weight. The elastic keel foot is designed to mimic the human foot without the use of mechanical joints; the dynamic-response foot is designed to meet the demands of running and jumping in athletic users.

Shank

The shank corresponds to the anatomical lower leg, and is used to connect the socket to the ankle-foot assembly. In an endoskeletal shank, a central pylon, which is a narrow vertical support, rests inside a foam cosmetic cover. Endoskeletal systems allow for adjustment and realignment of prosthetic components. In an exoskeletal shank, the strength of the shank is provided by a hard outer shell that is either hollow or filled with lightweight material. Exoskeletal systems are more durable than endoskeletal systems; however, they may be heavier and have a fixed alignment, making adjustments difficult.

Socket

The socket contacts the residual limb and disperses pressure around it. A hard socket offers direct contact between the limb and the socket, resulting in decreased friction, no liner bulk, easy cleaning, and increased durability. It is, however, difficult to fit and adjust in response to residual limb changes. A soft socket includes a liner as a cushion between the socket and residual limb. This provides additional protection for the limb but may increase friction and bulk. Transtibial socket types include: patellar tendon-bearing (PTB), silicone suction, energy-storing, or bent-knee designs. Transfemoral socket types include: quadrilateral, ischial containment, and contoured adducted trochanteric-controlled alignment method (CAT-CAM) designs. A prosthetic sock is usually worn to help cushion the limb from forces and accommodate for volume changes. Prosthetic socks are available in a variety of materials and thickness, and may be worn in layers to achieve the most comfortable fit.

Suspension

Suspension devices should keep the prosthesis firmly in place during use and allow comfortable sitting. Several types of suspension exist, both for the transtibial and transfemoral amputation. Common transtibial suspensions include sleeve, supracondylar, cuff, belt and strap, thigh-lacer, and suction styles. Sleeves are made of neoprene, urethane, or latex and are used over the shank, socket and thigh. Supracondylar and cuff suspensions are used to capture the femoral condyles and hold the prosthesis on the residual limb. The belt and strap method uses a waist belt with an anterior elastic strap to suspend the prosthesis, while the thigh-lacer method uses a snug-fitting corset around the thigh. The suction method consists of a silicone sleeve with a short pin at the end. The sleeve fits over the residual limb and the pin locks into the socket. With a transfemoral prosthesis, suction and several types of belt suspension also are available.

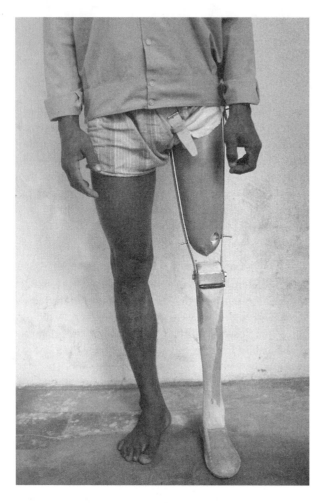

A man wears an artificial leg. *(Photograph by Andrew Holbrooke. Stock Market. Reproduced by permission.)*

Transfemoral amputations also provide the additional challenge of incorporating a prosthetic knee unit. The knee unit must be able to bend and straighten smoothly during ambulation, in addition to providing stability during weightbearing on that limb. Knees are available as single-axis, polycentric, weight-activated, manual-locking, hydraulic, and pneumatic units. Technology using microprocessors in knee units is becoming a reality, although costs can be prohibitive.

Operation

Use of an actual prosthesis usually follows a period of postoperative management that includes addressing issues of **pain**, swelling, and proper positioning. In addition, **physical therapy** for range of motion, strength, bed mobility, transfers, and single limb ambulation often takes place during the initial rehabilitation period. In some cases, an individual may be fitted with an immediate post-operative prosthesis to allow for early double-

limb ambulation. Many individuals will be fitted with a temporary prosthesis when the wound has healed. A temporary prosthesis allows for ambulation and continued shrinkage of the residual limb until a definitive prosthesis is fit.

When evaluating a prosthesis before use, the prosthetist and physical therapist should ensure that the inside of the socket is smooth and that all joints move freely. The socket should fit securely on the residual limb, and the overall prosthesis length should match the length of the intact leg. The patient must learn how to properly put on the residual limb sock and the prosthesis itself. A variety of techniques are used, depending on the type of socket and suspension system.

Maintenance

The user should be aware of how to properly care for and maintain the prosthesis, liner, and socks. Most plastic sockets and liners can be wiped with a damp cloth and dried. Socks should be washed and changed daily. Due to the wide variety of componentry and materials used in the fabrication of prostheses, the prosthetist should be the source for instructions regarding proper care and maintenance for each individual. In general, the patient should return to the prosthetist for any repairs, adjustments or realignments.

Health care team roles

The patient's primary care physician, surgeon, neurologist, prosthetist, physical and occupational therapists, nurses, and social worker are all important players in the multidisciplinary health care team. Surveys of patients with amputations have shown that the physical therapist, along with the physician and prosthetist, plays one of the most valued roles in providing information and help both at the time of amputation and following amputation. The entire team's input, along with the patient's input, is vital in determining whether a prosthesis should be fit and the specific prescription for the prosthesis. Input should be provided regarding the patient's medical history, premorbid level of function, present level of function, body build, range of motion, strength, motivation, and availability of familial and social support.

The physical therapist usually plays a major role in training an individual to walk with a prosthesis, and also is the health care professional who can evaluate prosthetic function immediately and over time. The physical therapist is trained in gait assessment and should watch for compensations and gait deviations that may indicate a problem with the prosthesis.

Training

The main goal of prosthetic training usually is smooth, energy-efficient gait. This includes the ability of the individual to accept weight on either leg, balance on one foot, advance each leg forward and adjust to different types of terrain or environmental conditions. Principles of motor learning often are used in training, progressing from simple to complex tasks. Individuals begin with learning to keep their bodies stable in a closed environment with no manipulation or variability. An example may be practicing standing balance on one or both legs. Mobility, environmental changes, and task variability are added slowly to further challenge the individual as tasks are mastered. In the end, an example of a more complex task practiced may be the ability walk in a crowded hallway while carrying an object in one hand. In addition to ambulation training, the patient also should be taught how to transfer to and from surfaces, assume a variety of positions such as kneeling or squatting, and manage **falls**. Depending upon the individual's previous and present level of function, use of a traditional cane, quad cane, or crutches may be indicated. Patient motivation, comorbidity, level of amputation and level of function are all factors in determining the outcome of rehabilitation.

Resources

BOOKS

Gailey, Robert S. *One Step Ahead: An Integrated Approach to Lower Extremity Prosthetics and Amputee Rehabilitation.* Miami: Advanced Rehabilitation Therapy, Inc., 1994.

Lusardi, Michelle M., and Caroline C. Nielsen. *Orthotics and Prosthetics in Rehabilitation.* Boston: Butterworth-Heinemann, 2000.

May, Bella J. *Amputations and Prosthetics: A Case Study Approach.* Philadelphia: F.A. Davis Company, 1996.

PERIODICALS

Hsu, Miao-Ju, et al. "Physiological Measurements of Walking and Running in People with Transtibial Amputations with 3 Different Prostheses." *Journal of Orthopedic and Sports Physical Therapy* 29 (Sept. 1999): 526-33.

Peggy Campbell Torpey, MPT

Lumbar puncture *see* Cerebrospinal fluid (CSF) analysis

Lumbosacral radiculopathy *see* Sciatica

Lung biopsy

Definition

Lung biopsy is a procedure by which a small sample of lung tissue is obtained for examination. Usually, it is examined under the **microscope** and also may be sent to the microbiological laboratory for culture. Microscopic examination is performed by pathologists.

Purpose

A lung biopsy is usually ordered to determine the cause of abnormalities that appear on chest x rays, such as nodules or infiltrates. Lung biopsies are performed to confirm a diagnosis of **cancer**, especially if malignant cells are detected in the patient's sputum or bronchial washing. In addition to evaluating lung tumors and their associated symptoms, lung biopsies may be used in the diagnosis of lung infections, especially **tuberculosis** and Pneumocystis **pneumonia**, drug reactions, and chronic diseases of the lung such as sarcoidosis.

A lung biopsy can be used for treatment as well as diagnosis. **Bronchoscopy**, a type of lung biopsy performed with a long slender instrument called a bronchoscope, can be used to clear a patient's air passages of secretions and to remove blockages from the airways. Today, flexible fiberoptic bronchoscopes, which are easier to use than rigid scopes, are used to perform most biopsies.

Precautions

As with any other biopsy, lung biopsies should not be performed on patients who have a tendency to bleed or abnormal **blood** clotting because of low platelet counts or prolonged prothrombin time (PT) or partial thromboplastin time (PTT). Platelets are small blood cells that play a role in the blood clotting process. PT and PTT measure how well blood clots. If they are prolonged, it might be unsafe to perform a biopsy because of the risk of bleeding. If the platelet count is lower than 50,000/cubic mm, the patient may be given a platelet transfusion as a temporary relief measure, and a biopsy can then be performed.

Description

Overview

The mediastinum separates the right and the left **lungs** from each other. The **heart**, the trachea, the lymph nodes, and the esophagus lie in the mediastinum. Lung biopsies may involve **mediastinoscopy**, as well as the lungs themselves.

Types of lung biopsies

Lung biopsies can be performed using a variety of techniques. A bronchoscopy is ordered if a lesion identified on the x ray seems to be located in the periphery of the chest. If the suspicious area lies close to the chest wall, a needle biopsy can be done. If both these methods fail to diagnose the problem, an open lung biopsy may be performed. When there is a question about whether the **lung cancer** has spread to the lymph nodes in the mediastinum, a mediastinoscopy is performed.

NEEDLE BIOPSY. About an hour before the needle biopsy procedure, a sedative is administered to the patient. The patient is mildly sedated but fully awake. An X ray technician takes a computerized axial tomography (CT) scan to identify the location of the suspicious areas. Markers are placed on the overlying skin to mark the biopsy site. The skin is thoroughly cleansed with an antiseptic solution, and a local anesthetic is injected to numb the area.

The physician then makes a small incision, about half an inch (1.25 cm) in length. The patient is asked to take a deep breath and hold it while the physician inserts the biopsy needle through the incision into the lung. When enough tissue has been obtained, the needle is withdrawn. Pressure is applied at the biopsy site and a sterile bandage is placed over the cut. The entire procedure takes between 30 and 45 minutes.

The patient may feel a brief sharp **pain** or some pressure as the biopsy needle is inserted. Most do not experience severe pain.

OPEN BIOPSY. Open biopsies are performed in a hospital operating room under **general anesthesia**. As with needle biopsies, patients are sedated before the procedure. An intravenous line is placed to give medications or fluids as necessary. A hollow tube, called an endotracheal tube, is passed through the mouth, into the airway leading to the lungs. It is used to convey the general anesthetic.

Once the patient is anesthetized, the surgeon makes an incision over the lung area, a procedure called a thoracotomy. Some lung tissue is removed and the incision is closed with sutures. The entire procedure usually takes about an hour. A chest tube is sometimes placed with one end inside the lung and the other end protruding through the closed incision. Chest tube placement is done to prevent the lungs from collapsing by removing the air from the lungs. The tube is removed a few days after the biopsy.

A **chest x ray** is done following an open biopsy, to check for a pneumothorax (lung collapse). The patient may experience some grogginess for a few hours after the procedure. Patients also may experience tiredness and muscle aches for a day or two, because of the general anesthesia. The throat may be sore because of the placement of the endotracheal tube. The patient may also have some pain or discomfort at the incision site, which can be relieved by pain medication.

VIDEO-ASSISTED THORASCOPIC SURGERY. A new technique, video-assisted thorascopic surgery (VATS), also can be used to biopsy lung and mediastinal lesions. VATS may be performed on selected patients in place of open lung biopsy. To perform a VATS procedure, the surgeon makes several small incisions in the patient's chest wall. A thorascope, a thin, hollow, lighted tube with a tiny video camera mounted on it, is inserted through one of the small incisions. The other incisions allow the surgeon to insert **surgical instruments** to retrieve tissue for biopsy.

MEDIASTINOSCOPY. The preparation for a mediastinoscopy is similar to that for an open biopsy. The patient is sedated and prepared for general anesthesia. The neck and the chest are cleansed with an antiseptic solution.

After the patient is anesthetized, an incision about two or three inches long is made at the base of the neck. A thin, hollow, lighted tube, called a mediastinoscope, is inserted through the incision into the space between the right and the left lungs. The surgeon removes any lymph nodes or tissues that look abnormal. The mediastinoscope is then removed, and the incision is sutured and bandaged. A mediastinoscopy takes about an hour.

Preparation

Before scheduling a lung biopsy, the physician performs a preoperative history and **physical examination**. An electrocardiogram (EKG) and laboratory tests may be performed before the procedure to check for clotting problems, anemia, and blood type, in case a transfusion becomes necessary.

Patient education

Patients who will undergo surgical diagnostic and treatment procedures should be encouraged to stop smoking. Patients able to stop smoking several weeks before surgical procedures have fewer postoperative complications.

Before any procedure is performed, the patient is asked to sign a consent form. The nurse may review the procedure and answer questions about the consent form or procedure. The nurse will advise the patient preparing for general anesthesia to refrain from eating or drinking anything for at least 12 hours before the biopsy.

Aftercare

Needle biopsy

Following a needle biopsy, the patient is allowed to rest comfortably. The nurse checks the patient's status at two-hour intervals. If there are no complications after four hours, then the patient can go home.

Patient education

Prior to discharge to home, the nurse instructs the patient about resuming normal activities. Patients are advised to rest at home for a day or two before resuming regular activities, and to avoid strenuous activities for a week after the biopsy.

Open biopsy, VATS, or mediastinoscopy

After an open biopsy, VATS, or mediastinoscopy, patients are taken to the recovery room for observation. If no complications develop, they are returned to the hospital room. Nursing care includes monitoring temperature, pulse **blood pressure** and respiration. **Fever** may indicate **infection**, and decreased breath sounds may be symptoms of pneumothorax. Sutures are usually removed after seven to 14 days.

If the patient has extreme pain, light-headedness, or difficulty breathing after an open biopsy, the physician should be notified immediately. The sputum may be slightly bloody for a day or two after the procedure. Heavy or persistent bleeding requires evaluation by the physician.

Complications

Needle biopsy

Needle biopsy is associated with fewer risks than open biopsy, because it does not involve general anesthesia. Rarely, the lung may collapse because of air that leaks in through the hole made by the biopsy needle. If a pneumothorax (lung collapse) occurs, a chest tube is inserted into the pleural cavity to re-expand the lung. Some hemoptysis (coughing up of blood) occurs in 5% of needle biopsies. Prolonged bleeding or infection may also occur, although these are very rare.

Open biopsy

Possible complications of an open biopsy include infection or pneumothorax. Death occurs in about 1 in 3000 cases. If the patient has very severe breathing problems before the biopsy, then breathing may be further

impaired following the operation. For patients with normal lung function before the biopsy, the risk of respiratory problems resulting from or following the procedure is very small.

Mediastinoscopy

Complications due to mediastinoscopy are rare; death occurs in fewer than one in 3000 cases. More common complications include pneumothorax or bleeding caused by damage to the **blood vessels** near the heart. Mediastinitis, infection of the mediastinum, may develop. Injury to the esophagus or larynx may occur. If the nerves leading to the larynx are injured, the patient may be left with a permanently hoarse voice. All of these complications are rare.

Results

Abnormal results of needle biopsy, VATS, and open biopsy may be associated with diseases other than cancer. Nodular lesions, while frequently cancerous, can also be the result of active infections such as tuberculosis, or may be healed scars from a previous infection. In a third of biopsies using a mediastinoscope, the lymph nodes that are biopsied prove to be cancerous. Abnormal results should always be considered in the context of the patient's medical history, physical examination, and other tests such as sputum examination, chest x rays, etc. before a definitive diagnosis is made.

Health care team roles

Fiberoptic bronchoscopy is performed by pulmonologists, physician specialists in pulmonary medicine. CT guided needle biopsy is done by interventional radiologists, physician specialists in radiological procedures. Thoracic surgeons perform open biopsy and VATS. Specially trained nurses, x ray, and laboratory technicians assist during the procedures and provide pre and postoperative education and supportive care.

Resources

BOOKS

"Bronchoscopy." In *The Merck Manual of Diagnosis and Therapy,* edited by Robert Berkow, et al. Rahway, NJ: Merck Research Laboratories, 1992.

Groenwald, S.L. et al. *Cancer Nursing Principles and Practice.* Sudbury, MA: Jones and Bartlett Publishers, 1997, pp.1273-1275.

Murphy, Gerald P., et al. *American Cancer Society Textbook of Clinical Oncology Second Edition* Atlanta, GA: The American Cancer Society, Inc., 1995, pp.223-234.

Otto, S.E. *Oncology Nursing.* St. Louis, MO: Mosby, 1997, pp. 317-318.

ORGANIZATIONS

American Cancer Society. 1599 Clifton Road, N.E., Atlanta, GA 30329. (800)227-2345.

American Lung Association. 1740 Broadway, New York, NY 10019-4374. (800)586-4872.

Cancer Research Institute. 681 Fifth Avenue, New York, NY 10022. (800)992-2623.

National Cancer Institute (National Institutes of Health). 9000 Rockville Pike, Bethesda, MD 20892. (800) 422-6237.

Barbara Wexler

Lung cancer

Definition

Lung **cancer** is a disease in which the cells of the lung tissues grow uncontrollably and form tumors. It is the leading cause of death from cancer among both men and women in the United States. The American Cancer Society estimates that in 2001 at least 169,500 new cases of lung cancer will be diagnosed, and that lung cancer will account for 28% of all cancer deaths—approximately 157,400 people.

Description

Types of lung cancer

There are two kinds of lung cancers, primary and secondary. Primary lung cancer starts in the lung itself. Primary lung cancer is divided into small cell lung cancer and non-small cell lung cancer, depending on how the cells look under the **microscope**. Secondary lung cancer is cancer that starts somewhere else in the body (for example, the breast or urinary bladder) and metastasizes (spreads) to the **lungs**. Identifying the type of lung cancer is important because treatment varies by type. For example, small cell cancers generally are treated with surgery. On the other hand, surgery is not generally considered beneficial for non-small cell cancers; they are treated with **chemotherapy**.

Small cell cancer was formerly called oat cell cancer, because the cells resemble oats in their shape. About a fourth of all lung cancers are small cell cancers. This is a very aggressive cancer and spreads to other organs within a short time. It is generally diagnosed in people who are heavy smokers. Non-small cell cancers account for the remaining 75% of primary lung cancers. They can be further subdivided into three categories.

Nearly 30% of non-small cell cancers are squamous cell carcinomas. Squamous cell carcinoma is most often found near the bronchi of patients with a history of smoking. Forty percent of non-small cell cancers are adenocarcinomas, most often found in the outer region of the lung. The remaining 10% are large-cell undifferentiated carcinomas. These rapidly spreading carcinomas may be found throughout the lung.

Incidence of lung cancer

Lung cancer is rare among young adults. It is usually found in people who are 50 years of age or older, the average age at diagnosis is 60. While the incidence of the disease is decreasing among white men, it is steadily rising among African-American men, and among both white and African-American women. This change is probably due to the increase in the number of smokers in these groups. In 1987, lung cancer replaced **breast cancer** as the number one cancer killer among women. Lung cancer is responsible for more deaths than the combined totals for cancers of the colon, breast, and prostate.

Causes and symptoms

Causes

SMOKING. Tobacco smoking is the leading cause of lung cancer. Ninety percent of lung cancers can be prevented by giving up tobacco. Smoking **marijuana** cigarettes is considered yet another risk factor for cancer of the lung. These cigarettes have a higher tar content than tobacco cigarettes. In addition, they are inhaled very deeply—as a result, the carcinogens in the smoke are held in the lungs for a longer time.

EXPOSURE TO ASBESTOS AND TOXIC CHEMICALS. Exposure to asbestos fibers, either at home or in the workplace, is also considered a risk factor for lung cancer. Studies show that compared to the general population, asbestos workers are seven times more likely to die from lung cancer. Asbestos workers who smoke increase their risk of getting lung cancer by 50-100 times. Besides asbestos, mining industry workers exposed to coal products or radioactive substances such as uranium, and workers exposed to chemicals such as arsenic, vinyl chloride, mustard gas, and other carcinogens also have a higher than average risk of contracting lung cancer.

ENVIRONMENTAL CONTAMINATION. High levels of radon, a radioactive gas that cannot be seen or smelled, pose a risk for lung cancer. This gas is produced by the breakdown of uranium, and does not present any problem outdoors. In the basements of some houses that are built over soil containing natural uranium deposits, however, radon may accumulate to dangerous levels. Other forms of environmental pollution (e.g., auto exhaust fumes) may also slightly increase the risk of lung cancer.

CHRONIC LUNG INFLAMMATION AND SCARRING. Inflammation and scar tissue are sometimes produced in the lung by diseases such as silicosis and berylliosis, which are caused by inhalation of certain **minerals**; **tuberculosis**; and certain types of **pneumonia**. This scarring may increase the risk of developing lung cancer.

FAMILY HISTORY. Although the exact cause of lung cancer is not known, people with a family history of lung cancer appear to have a slightly higher risk of contracting the disease.

Symptoms

Because lung cancers tend to spread very early, only 15% are detected in their early stages. The chances of early detection, however, can be improved by seeking medical care at once if any of the following symptoms appear:

- a cough that does not go away
- chest **pain**
- shortness of breath
- persistent hoarseness
- swelling of the neck and face
- significant weight loss that is not due to dieting or vigorous **exercise**; fatigue and loss of appetite
- bloody or brown-colored phlegm (sputum)
- unexplained **fever**
- recurrent lung infections, such as bronchitis or pneumonia

Diseases other than lung cancer may cause these symptoms. It is vital, however, for patients to consult a physician to rule out the possibility that they are the presenting symptoms of lung cancer.

If the lung cancer has spread to other organs, the patient may have other symptoms such as headaches, bone **fractures**, pain, bleeding, or **blood** clots. Early detection and treatment can increase the chances of a cure for some patients; for others, it can at least prolong life.

Diagnosis

Physical examination and initial tests

If lung cancer is suspected, the physician will take a detailed medical history to document the symptoms and assess the risk factors. The history is followed by a complete **physical examination**. The physician will examine the patient's throat to rule out other possible causes of hoarseness or coughing, and listen to the patient's breathing and the sounds made when the patient's chest and upper back are percussed (tapped). The physical examination, however, is not conclusive.

If there is reason to suspect lung cancer—such as a history of heavy smoking or occupational exposure to substances known to irritate the lungs—the physician may order a **chest x ray** to see if there are any masses in the lungs. Special imaging techniques, such as **PET** scans (**positron emission tomography**), CT (computerized axial tomography) scans or MRI (**magnetic resonance imaging**) may provide more precise information about the size, shape, and location of any tumors. X ray and other imaging techniques may be performed by a radiologic technician.

Sputum analysis

Sputum analysis involves microscopic examination of the cells that are either coughed up from the lungs, or are collected through a bronchoscope. Sputum analyses can diagnose at least 30% of lung cancers, some of which do not show up even on chest x rays. In addition, this laboratory test can help detect cancer in its very early stages, before it metastasizes (spreads) to other regions. The sputum test does not, however, provide any information about the location of the tumor and must be followed by other diagnostic tests.

Lung biopsy

Lung biopsy is the definitive diagnostic tool for cancer. It can be performed in several different ways. The physician can perform a **bronchoscopy**, which involves the insertion of a slender, lighted tube, called a bronchoscope, down the patient's throat and into the lungs. In addition to viewing the passageways of the lungs, the physician can use the bronchoscope to obtain samples of the lung tissue. In another procedure known as a needle biopsy, the location of the tumor is first identified using a CT scan or MRI. The physician then inserts a needle through the chest wall and collects a sample of tissue from the tumor. In the third procedure, known as surgical biopsy, the chest wall is opened up and a part of the tumor, or all of it, is removed. A pathologist, a physician who specializes in the study of diseased tissue, examines the tumor samples to identify the cancer type and stage.

Patient education

Patients who will undergo surgical diagnostic and treatment procedures should be encouraged to stop smoking. Patients able to stop smoking several weeks before surgical procedures have fewer postoperative complications.

Treatment

Treatment for lung cancer depends on the type of cancer, its location, and its stage. Staging is a process that describes if the cancer has metastasized and the extent of its spread. Lung cancer is staged at the time of diagnosis; this is called clinical staging. It usually is staged again following surgical intervention; this is called pathologic staging. When determining a course of treatment, the patient's age, medical history, and general state of health are taken into account. The most commonly used modes of treatment are surgery, radiation therapy, and chemotherapy.

Surgery

Surgery is not usually an option for small cell lung cancers, because they have usually spread beyond the lung by the time they are diagnosed. Because non-small cell lung cancers are less aggressive, however, surgery can be used to treat them. The surgeon determines the type of surgery, depending on how much of the lung is affected. Surgery may be the primary method of treatment, or radiation therapy and/or chemotherapy may be used to shrink the tumor before surgery is attempted.

Not all patients are candidates for surgery, especially the removal of an entire lung (pneumonectomy). For example, many smokers suffer from **emphysema** as well as lung cancer, and as a result have sharply reduced lung capacity. Spirometric testing may be performed to assess lung capacity. The forced expiratory volume in one second (FEV1) is a laboratory test that helps to determine whether patients will have adequate pulmonary function after resection.

There are three different types of surgical operations:

- Wedge resection. This procedure involves removing a small part of the lung. A wedge resection is done when the cancer is in a very small area and has not metastasized to any other chest tissues or other parts of the body.

- Lobectomy. A lobectomy is the removal of one lobe of the lung. The right lung has three lobes and the left lung has two lobes. If the cancer is limited to one part of the lung, the surgeon will perform a lobectomy.

- Pneumonectomy. A pneumonectomy is the removal of an entire lung. If the cancer cells have spread throughout the lung, and if the surgeon feels that removal of the entire lung is the best option for curing the cancer, a pneumonectomy will be performed.

Postoperative surgical nursing care includes monitoring temperature, pulse **blood pressure** and respiration. Fever may indicate **infection**; patients are vulnerable to bacterial and viral infections. Decreased breath sounds may be symptoms of pneumothorax. The pain that follows surgery can be relieved by medications. The tendency of surgical **stress** to weaken the patient's **immune system** is treatable with **antibiotics**, anti-viral medicines, and vaccines.

Patient education

Postoperative patient teaching encourages ambulation (walking), and reinforces patient and family understanding of surgical results and necessary follow-up.

Radiotherapy

Radiotherapy involves the use of high-energy rays to kill cancer cells. It is used either by itself or in combination with surgery or chemotherapy. Radiotherapy can be used to treat all types of cancer. The amount of radiation used depends on the size and the location of the tumor. There are two types of radiotherapy treatments, external beam radiation therapy and internal (or interstitial) radiotherapy. In external radiation therapy, the radi-

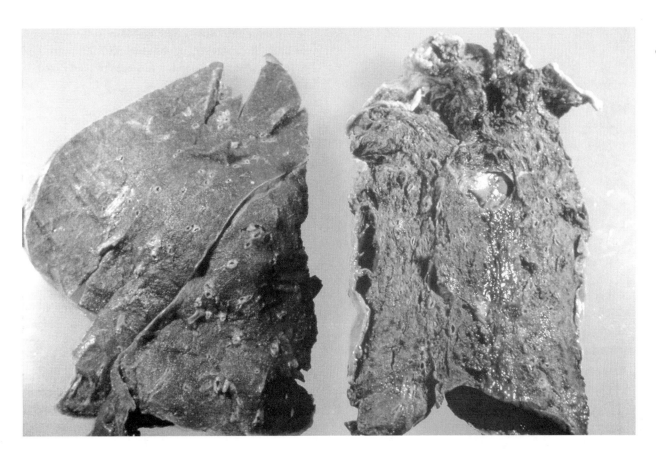

A normal lung (left) and the lung of a cigarette smoker (right). *(Photograph by A. Glauberman, Photo Researchers, Inc. Reproduced by permission.)*

ation is delivered from a machine positioned outside the body. Internal radiotherapy uses a small pellet of radioactive materials placed inside the body in the area of the cancer.

Radiation therapy may produce such side effects as tiredness, skin rashes, upset **stomach**, and **diarrhea**. Dry or sore throats, difficulty in swallowing, and loss of hair in the treated area are all minor side effects of radiation. Some side effects diminish or disappear either during the course of the treatment or after the treatment is over.

Patient education

Patient education by nurses and radiologic technicians includes measures to identify and manage side effects such as fatigue or radiodermatitis (skin condition resulting from radiotherapy).

Chemotherapy

Chemotherapy uses anti-cancer medications that are either given intravenously or taken by mouth. These drugs enter the bloodstream and travel throughout the body, killing cancer cells that have spread to different organs. Chemotherapy is used as the primary treatment

for cancers that have spread beyond the lung and cannot be removed by surgery. It may also be used in addition to surgery or radiation therapy.

Chemotherapy is tailored to each patient's needs. The prescribed regimen depends on the type of cancer, the extent of its spread, and the patient's general state of health. Most patients are given a combination of several different drugs. Besides killing the cancer cells, these drugs also harm normal cells. Hence, the dose has to be carefully adjusted to minimize damage to normal cells. Chemotherapy often has severe side effects, including nausea, vomiting, hair loss, anemia, weakening of the immune system, and sometimes **infertility**. Most of these side effects end when the treatment is over. Other medications can be given to lessen the unpleasant side effects of chemotherapy.

Patient education

Patient teaching helps patients and families to distinguish between anticipated side effects such as alopecia (hair loss), nausea, and constipation and the more serious side effects that require medical attention. Examples of

KEY TERMS

Alopecia—Hair loss.

Biopsy—The surgical removal and microscopic examination of living tissue for diagnostic purposes.

Bronchoscope—A thin, flexible, lighted tube that is used to view the air passages in the lungs.

Carcinogen—Any substance capable of causing cancer.

Chemotherapy—Treatment of cancer with synthetic drugs that destroy the tumor either by inhibiting the growth of cancerous cells or by killing them.

Lobectomy—Surgical removal of an entire lobe of the lung.

Metastasize—The spread of cancer cells from a primary site to distant parts of the body.

Pathologist—A physician who specializes in the diagnosis of disease by studying cells and tissues under a microscope.

Pneumonectomy—Surgical removal of an entire lung.

Pneumothorax—Collapse of the lung.

Radiation therapy—Treatment using high energy radiation from X-ray machines, cobalt, radium, or other sources.

Sputum—Mucus or phlegm that is coughed up from the passageways of the lungs.

Stage—A term used to describe the size and extent of spread of cancer.

Wedge resection—Removal of only a small portion of a cancerous lung.

side effects that can not be managed at home include bleeding, fever, and confusion or hallucinations.

Prognosis

If the lung cancer is detected before it has had a chance to spread to other organs, and if it is treated appropriately, at least 49% of patients can survive five years or longer after the initial diagnosis. Only 15% of lung cancers, however, are found at this early stage.

Improvements in surgical technique and the development of new approaches to treatment have markedly improved the one-year survival rate for lung cancer.

Slightly more than 40% of patients survive for at least a year after diagnosis, as opposed to 30% 25 years ago. The five-year survival rate for all stages of lung cancer is 14%.

Health care team roles

Lung cancer treatment involves an multidisciplinary team of health care professionals. In addition to primary care physicians, such as a family practitioner or an internist, the treatment team may include a pulmonologist, pathologist, radiologist, and thoracic surgeon as well as specialized nurses, radiologic and laboratory technicians, respiratory therapists, and dieticians.

Patient education

Before, during and after treatment, nurses and allied health professionals should inform and educate patients and families about the risks and complications of any planned diagnostic test, intervention, or treatment. Patients and families should be taught about some of the common side effects of treatment, including weight loss, malnutrition, increased risk of infection, pain, fatigue, and depression.

Prevention

The best way to prevent lung cancer is never to smoke or to quit smoking if one has already started. Secondhand smoke from tobacco should be avoided. Appropriate precautions should be taken when working with carcinogens (cancer-causing substances). Promoting healthy lifestyles, testing houses for the presence of radon gas, and asbestos abatement are also useful preventive strategies.

Patient education

The objectives of education are to prevent patients, especially children and adolescents, from smoking, and to encourage smokers to quit. Participation in smoking cessation programs should be encouraged and patients should be informed about the health risks of passive (secondhand) smoking. Patient education also should describe the role of environmental carcinogens such as asbestos and radon in the development of lung cancer.

Resources

BOOKS

Groenwald, S.L. et al. *Cancer Nursing Principles and Practice.* Sudbury, MA: Jones and Bartlett Publishers, 1997, pp.1260-1287.

Murphy, Gerald P., et al. *American Cancer Society Textbook of Clinical Oncology, Second Edition*. Atlanta, GA: The American Cancer Society, Inc., 1995, pp.220-234.

Otto, S.E. *Oncology Nursing*. St. Louis, MO: Mosby, 1997, pp. 312-343.

"Pulmonary Disorders: Tumors of the Lung." In *The Merck Manual of Diagnosis and Therapy,* edited by Robert Berkow, et al. Rahway, NJ: Merck Research Laboratories, 1992.

ORGANIZATIONS

American Cancer Society. 1599 Clifton Road, N.E., Atlanta, GA 30329. (800)227-2345.

American Lung Association. 1740 Broadway, New York, NY 10019-4374. (800)586-4872.

Cancer Research Institute. 681 Fifth Avenue, New York, NY 10022. (800)992-2623.

National Cancer Institute (National Institutes of Health). 9000 Rockville Pike, Bethesda, MD 20892. (800)422-6237.

Barbara Wexler

Lung function tests *see* **Pulmonary function test**

Lung perfusion and ventilation scan

Definition

A lung perfusion scan and ventilation study are two diagnostic imaging studies. A lung perfusion scan assesses **blood** flow to the **lungs**. A lung ventilation study reveals the distribution of air space within the lungs. These are two separate studies that are often performed sequentially. The tests are called by different names, including perfusion lung scan, aerosol lung scan, ventilation lung scan, xenon lung scan, ventilation/perfusion scanning (VPS), pulmonary scintiphotography, or most commonly, V/Q scan.

Purpose

Lung scans may be performed for patients with chest **pain**, for those coughing up blood (hemoptysis), or for those having difficulty breathing (dyspnea). A perfusion scan alone or both tests are frequently performed for patients with a suspected pulmonary embolism (blood clot in the lung) or for follow-up in patients with known pulmonary embolism. Lung scans are a sensitive method for demonstrating the presence of pulmonary disease but are not often specific for a certain disease. For example,

an abnormal scan may also be caused by chronic obstructive pulmonary disease (COPD), **asthma**, **pneumonia**, venous **hypertension**, pleural effusion, and cardiomegaly.

Precautions

The amount of radioactivity a person is exposed to during these tests is very low and is not harmful. However, if the patient has had other recent nuclear medicine tests, it may be necessary to wait until other radiopharmaceuticals have been cleared from the body so that they do not interfere with these tests.

Description

These tests are typically done in a hospital nuclear medicine department or out-patient radiology facility. Scans to diagnose pulmonary embolism are often done on an emergency basis. Most often, both studies are needed. Sometimes a perfusion scan is done without a ventilation scan. Rarely, a ventilation scan is done alone.

For a lung perfusion scan, the patient is injected intravenously with radioactive particles, known as Tc 99m MAA (macroaggregated albumin). The particles pass through the larger **blood vessels** and become temporarily trapped in small blood vessels. The images thus reflect blood perfusion in the lungs. Images are obtained anteriorly, posteriorly, laterally, and obliquely.

For a lung ventilation scan, the patient inhales a radioactive gas through a mask placed over the nose and mouth. Images of the ventilation lung scan show the distribution of the gas in the lungs. The test typically consists of three phases. The first stage is the initial, or ventilation stage, which reflects the rate of ventilation of the different lung segments. Second is the equilibrium stage, which represents gas volume of the lungs. The third stage is the wash-out phase, which demonstrates any gas trapping that may occur in obstructive diseases. Images are typically obtained posteriorly, although additional views may also be performed. Each test takes approximately 15 to 30 minutes. If possible, the patient usually sits up while the images are taken.

Preparation

To accompany the lung scan, the patient should have a **chest x ray** within 12 to 24 hours of the study. Otherwise, there is no special preparation needed for these tests. The patient may eat and drink normally before the procedure.

Aftercare

No special aftercare is needed. The patient may resume normal activities immediately.

Complications

There are no complications associated with these tests.

Results

Normally, there is a physiological relationship between the perfusion of the pulmonary blood vessels and their regional alveolar ventilation. An imbalance of this relationship as demonstrated by these studies reflect various respiratory diseases. Other diagnostic tests are often required to confirm a diagnosis.

Normal results for both tests show an even distribution of radioactive material in all parts of the lungs. For the lung perfusion scan, diminished or absent perfusion suggests decreased blood flow to that part of the lung, and possibly a pulmonary embolism. However, pneumonia, **emphysema**, or lung tumors can create readings on the lung perfusion scan that falsely suggest a pulmonary embolism is present. For the ventilation study, areas that show an increased accumulation of radioactive gas, particularly after the wash-out phase, suggests obstructive lung disease. Areas where there is decreased or absent radioactive gas flow suggests mechanical obstruction of air flow, such as an embolus. Certain combinations of abnormalities in lung perfusion and ventilation scans suggest pulmonary embolism.

Health care team roles

Both the lung perfusion and ventilation scans are performed by a nuclear medicine technologist. The technologist is trained to handle radioactive materials, operate the equipment, and process the data. The tests are interpreted by a radiologist who may specialize in nuclear medicine. Patients receive the results from their personal physician or the doctor who ordered the test.

Resources

BOOKS

Klingensmith III, M.D., Wm. C., Dennis Eshima, Ph.D., John Goddard, Ph.D. *Nuclear Medicine Procedure Manual 2000-2001.*

Pagana, Kathleen, and James Pagana. "Lung Scan." In *Mosby's Diagnostic and Laboratory Test Reference*, 2nd ed. St. Louis: Mosby, 1995, pp. 533-34.

"Scanning Tests." In *Illustrated Guide to Diagnostic Tests.* Springhouse: Springhouse Corp., 1996, pp. 679-82.

Zaret, Barry, ed. "Lung Scan." In *The Patient's Guide to Medical Tests.* New York: Houghton Mifflin, 1997, pp.138-40.

Christine Miner Minderovic, B.S., R.T., R.D.M.S.

Lungs

Definition

The two lungs are spongy and highly elastic organs of respiration in the pulmonary cavities of the thorax, where the aeration of **blood** occurs.

Description

Each lung has an irregular conical shape with a blunt top, called the apex, extending into the root of the neck. They have concave bottoms resting on the arc of the diaphragm, a mostly concave inner mediastinal surface that follows the lines of the pericardium, and a convex outer (costal) surface. The right lung is larger than the left, and consists of three lobes (upper, middle, and basal or lower). The left lung consists of two lobes, an upper and a basal, or lower, lobe.

Each lung consists of an exterior plasma coat comprised of an organ coat which folds back to make an interior lining for the chest cavity. The inner lung contains sub-serous areolar tissue with elastic fibers interspersed over the surface of the organ. The parenchyma, or functional part of the organ, is composed of secondary lobules (alveolar ducts) that differentiate into primary lobules (alveoli) consisting of **blood vessels**, lymphatics, nerves, and an alveolar duct that connects with air space.

The lung, as it relates to inspiration and expiration, has two distinct zones in which the lung passages convey air to the alveolar sacs. The zones relate to the two functions of these passages. One is for conducting air, and the other is for respiration. The parts of the conducting zone do not participate in gas transfer, rather they convey air to and from the respiratory zone. All of the parts of the respiratory zone can take part in gas transfer. However, the uppermost branches, such as the respiratory bronchioles, participate in respiration only in times of exertion.

The conducting zone starts at the trachea and branches out to the bronchi. The bronchi differentiate into bronchioles and then into terminal bronchioles. The respiratory zone starts after the terminal bronchioles at the respiratory bronchioles. These differentiate into the alveolar ducts, which terminate at the alveolar sacs. The lungs consist mainly of the tiny air containing alveolar sacs.

Function

The lung is the sole means of **gas exchange** in respiration. Air is brought into the body through the mouth or nose and trachea to the lung. There oxygen diffuses from the airspace of the alveoli into the blood stream and carbon dioxide diffuses from the blood into the alveoli's airspace.

The alveoli are small hollow sacs. Their ends connect to the lumens of the airways. The air adjacent to surfaces of the alveolar wall are lined by a single cell layer of flat epithelial cells called type I alveolar cells. In between type I cells are type II cells. They are thicker, and secrete a fluid called surfactant. In the alveolar walls this fluid and connective tissue fills the interstitial space and is interspersed with capillaries. In some places the interstitial space is nonexistent and the epithelial **cell membranes** are in direct contact with the capillaries. The blood in the capillaries is separated from the air by a single layer of flat epithelial cells. The surface area in a single alveoli is roughly the size of a small basketball court due to the undulating terrain of the type I and II epithelial cells. There are around 300 million alveoli in the adult male. Thus, there is a large surface area where the air and the blood stream are in close proximity. This large surface area is necessary for gas exchange to easily occur. The **respiratory system** also needs a continual supply of fresh air, which is supplied by the process of breathing.

The process of breathing is aided by the position of the lungs in the thorax (chest). The thorax is a closed chamber that extends from the neck muscles to the diaphragm. The diaphragm is a dome shaped sheet of skeletal muscle that separates the thorax from the abdomen. The sides of the thorax are bounded by connective tissue around the spine, ribs, intercostal muscles, and sternum.

A completely enclosed sac consisting of a thin sheet of cells, called the pleura, surround each lung. Between the pleura and the lung is interstitial fluid. As the diaphragm expands and contracts the intra-pleural pressure placed on the lungs causes the lung to inflate and deflate. Breathing allows a fresh supply of air and oxygen to enter the lung upon inflation and carbon dioxide to exit the lung upon deflation. It also causes a change in the pressure of the lung.

The epithelial surface from the conducting zone to the respiratory bronchioles is lined with cilia that continually beat in the direction of the pharynx. There are epithelial cells and glands on this surface that secrete mucus. This mucus catches particulate and bacterial matter, and the material (and mucus) is slowly moved by the cilia toward the pharynx. There it is either swallowed or coughed up as sputum. The epithelial layer also secretes another viscous fluid that allows the cilia to move mucus easily out of the lung.

Toxic substances can inhibit ciliary action. Agents like cigarette smoke can paralyze the cilia for extended periods of time. This inhibits the movement of mucus and particles out of the lungs. The suspension of this process can inhibit gas exchange and eventually cause prolonged oxygen deficiency.

Respiration

Respiration is the process by which the body takes in oxygen and emits carbon dioxide. The following is a summary of the steps of respiration:

- ventilation

- interchange of CO_2 and O_2 between alveolar air and blood in lung capillaries

- transport of CO_2 and O_2 through the bloodstream

- interchange of CO_2 and O_2 between blood in lung capillaries and alveolar air by diffusion

- use of O_2 and production of CO_2 by cells in **metabolism**

Ventilation is the interchange of air between the atmosphere and the alveoli by bulk flow. Bulk flow is the movement of air from a region of high pressure to one of low pressure. Bulk flow may be thought of as occurring between the outside air, the air in most of the lung, and the air in the alveolar sacs. Flow of some gases (especially oxygen and carbon dioxide) also occurs between the alveolar air and the blood. It is important to note that the pressure of individual gases is different in different types of air. For example, air going into the lungs is rich in oxygen and low in carbon dioxide. Air leaving the lungs is rich in carbon dioxide and low in oxygen. The different concentrations (or pressures) of individual gases are known as the partial pressures, and the partial

KEY TERMS

Interstitial space—The spaces found within organs and tissues.

Metabolism—A series of chemical and physiological changes in the body that either build larger molecules out of smaller molecules (anabolism) or break down larger molecules into smaller ones (catabolism).

Parenchyma—The active portion of an organ that fulfills its function (as opposed to purely structural portions of the organ).

Proteolysis—The breaking down of proteins by cleaving or hydrolyzing peptide bonds (the bonds connecting amino acids within the protein).

pressure of each individual gas adds up to the total pressure of the gas.

When air is inspired (taken in), it has a higher partial pressure of oxygen than the air already in the lung, and a lower partial pressure of carbon dioxide. Therefore, inspired air allows oxygen to flow from the area of highest pressure (inspired air) to the alveolar sacs (that have a lower partial pressure of oxygen), and into the bloodstream. The same inspired air has a low partial pressure of carbon dioxide, so carbon dioxide leaves the bloodstream (where it has a high partial pressure), enters the alveolar air (where the pressure is lower), and is passed onto the inspired air (where the partial pressure is even lower). Thus, carbon dioxide gas and oxygen gas both move from areas of highest pressure to lowest pressure in an attempt to reach a pressure (or concentration) equilibrium. This process is called gas exchange. After gas exchange has taken place, the air is expired, or expelled to rid the body of air that has a high concentration (partial pressure) of carbon dioxide gas. Then the process begins again.

Lung expansion and contraction

The concept of bulk flow (explained above) and Boyle's law explain the expansion and contraction of the lung. Boyle's law states that, at constant temperature, an increase in the volume of a container (lung) lowers the pressure of a gas, and a decrease in the container (lung) volume raises the pressure. Thus, when the volume of the lung expands, the pressure inside the lung is lowered, and when the volume of the lung contracts, the pressure inside the lung rises.

Inspiration occurs when the muscles of inspiration increase the volume of the thoracic cavity. The decrease in pressure in the cavity causes the lungs to expand to fill the cavity, which lowers the pressure inside the lung. Since air flows from areas of high pressure to low pressure, air fills the lungs to equalize the air pressure inside the lungs with the outside air, and inspiration occurs. The difference between the internal pressure in the lung and the pressure of the outside air is called the transpulmonary pressure.

During expiration, the muscles of inspiration relax, and the lung contracts. The decreased volume causes increased pressure inside the lungs, which results in air being expired, or expelled. In normal adults, expiration does not require any effort.

Role in human health

The lungs ability to extract oxygen from the atmosphere and supply it to the body's tissues is essential for metabolism and therefore for life. Disease and disorder can interfere with the body's normal function and slow a normally healthy person. Serious interference with the lung's function can cause hypoxia and even death.

Common diseases and disorders

Asthma is an intermittent disease characterized by a chronic inflammation of the airways, causing smooth **muscle contraction** in the airway. The causes vary from person to person and can include **allergies**, viral infections, environmental pollutants, mold, dust, dander, cigarette smoke, overexertion, and naturally released bronchiorestrictors. Ingested items such as food coloring, preservatives, and medications can trigger an attack.

Chronic obstructive pulmonary disease (COPD) refers to **emphysema**, chronic bronchitis, or a combination of the two. This category of disease is one of the major causes of death and disability in the world. These diseases restrict ventilation and the oxygenation of the blood.

Chronic bronchitis is characterized by excessive mucus production in the bronchi and chronic inflammatory changes in the small airways. The accumulation of mucus and thickening of inflamed airways obstruct the flow of air. It is primarily a result of cigarette smoking, although pollution may also play a role.

Emphysema is a major cause of hypoxia and is characterized by the destruction of the alveolar walls, and the atrophy and collapse of the lower airways. The lungs self-destruct through the secretion of proteolytic enzymes by white blood cells. Cigarette smoke stimulates the release of harmful enzymes and destroys the enzymes that normally protect against proteolysis. The proteolytic enzymes cause the breakdown of the alveolar walls. The damaged alveoli fuse and a gradual decrease in the surface area available for gas exchange results. Emphysema increases the work of breathing and, when severe enough, causes hypoventilation (inadequate ventilation). The obstruction caused by the collapse of the lower airways is accompanied with destruction of the lung's elastic tissues and the eventual collapse of the airways.

Pneumonia is normally caused by bacterial or viral **infection**. It can be triggered by the inhalation of toxic chemicals, chest trauma, yeast, rickettsiae, and **fungi**. It is the inflammation and compaction of the lung parenchyma. The alveolar spaces fill with mucus, inflammatory cells, and fibrin.

Tuberculosis is caused by the infection of *Mycobacterium tuberculosis*. It can affect most organs but is most commonly found in the lungs. The **bacteria** cause lesions to be formed on the lungs and spread to other tissues. Pulmonary tissue in motion will be chronically affected and may eventually be destroyed, if left untreated. The erosion of lung tissue into the blood vessels can result in life-threatening hemorrhages.

Other less common diseases of the lung include Legionnaire's disease, **cystic fibrosis**, histoplasmosis, coccidiomycosis, and *Mycobacterium avium* complex.

Resources

BOOKS

Bullock, John, et. al. *National Medical Series for Independent Study—Physiology.* Third ed. Williams & Wilkins, 1995.

Vander, Arthur et. al. *Human Physiology—the Mechanisms of Body Function.* Eighth ed. McGraw-Hill, 2001.

ORGANIZATIONS

The American Lung Association. 1740 Broadway, New York, NY, 10019. 212-315-8700. <http://www.lungusa.org/>.

OTHER

Thompson, B.H., W.J. Lee, J.R. Galvin, and J. S. Wilson. "Lung Anatomy." *Virtual Hospital.* University of Iowa Health Care. <http://www.vh.org/Providers/Textbooks/LungAnatomy/LungAnatomy.html>.

Sally C. McFarlane-Parrott

Luteinizing hormone test *see* **Pituitary hormone tests**

Lymphatic system

Definition

The lymphatic system is composed of a network of vessels that collects fluid and plasma **proteins** that leak out of capillaries and into the interstitial space. Lymphatic vessels return the lymph (fluid and plasma protein) back to the circulatory system through the veins.

Description

The lymphatic system is a secondary system of vessels that is distinct both in anatomy and function from the **blood** vessel capillaries of the circulatory system. Small lymphatic vessels (or "lymphatics") called lymphatic capillaries are found in almost all organs of the body except superficial layers of the skin, the **central nervous system**, endomysium of muscles, and the bone. These exceptions have a system of smaller vessels called prelymphatics. Fluid from prelymphatics returns to nearby lymphatic vessels, or the cerebral spinal fluid in the case of the central nervous system.

Lymphatic capillaries are made up of a single layer of endothelial cells. They are anchored to the surrounding connective tissue by special filaments called anchoring filaments. The system begins as a series of sacs. Each sac has a low hydrostatic pressure relative to the outside of the sac. At the end of the lymphatic capillaries there are endothelial valves. The valves form as a result of the slight overlap of the endothelial cells, and the overlapping edge has the ability to open inward. The valves open enough to allow fluid and plasma protein to pass into the lymphatic capillary.

Inside the lymph vessels are valves that prevent the backflow of lymph, a general name for the slightly opalescent fluid picked up by the lymphatics. Surrounding the lymphatics are smooth muscles that contract involuntarily to assist in the movement of lymph through the system. The lymphatic capillaries converge into larger lymph vessels. The larger lymph vessels pass through swellings called lymph nodes and then empty into one of two large lymph ducts. The lymph ducts empty into the venous circulatory system through either the right or left subclavian veins. Lymph from the right side of the head, arm and chest empties into the right subclavian vein. Lymph collected from the lower part of the body, and lymph from the left side of the head, arm and chest empties into the left subclavian vein. Both subclavian veins are located within the thorax underneath the clavicles, the thin bones located on the top part of the chest.

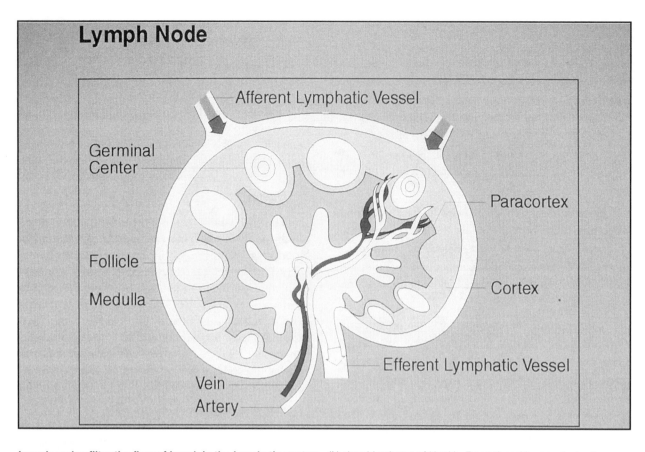

Lymph Node

Afferent Lymphatic Vessel

Germinal Center

Paracortex

Follicle

Medulla

Cortex

Efferent Lymphatic Vessel

Vein

Artery

Lymph nodes filter the flow of lymph in the lymphatic system. *(National Institutes of Health. Reproduced by permission.)*

At approximately 600 sites in the human body, lymphatic vessels converge into bundles of tissue called lymph nodes. The shape of a lymph node resembles a kidney bean and ranges in size from a few millimeters to a few centimeters. They are mostly found at the base of extremities such as the arms, legs and head. Many afferent lymphatics or vessels lead the lymph into the node at the larger curve of the bean shape and efferent lymphatics, fewer in number, take the lymph away from the node at the hilum, the depressed region of the bean shape. All nodes have a blood supply from the circulatory system running through them. The **blood vessels** enter and exit at the hilum. Inside the nodes are a honeycomb of lymph-filled sinuses that have macrophages and groupings of lymphocytes that produce antibodies.

As mentioned, lymph is the fluid flowing through the lymphatic system and originates from the interstitial spaces of the organs and tissues. Another element of the lymph is a type of cell of the **immune system** called a lymphocyte, which is a type of white blood cell. Lymphocytes mature in either the thymus (T-lymphocytes) or the bone marrow (B-lymphocytes), which are primary lymphoid organs The blood supply transports lymphocytes from their site of maturation (the thymus or bone marrow) to secondary lymphoid organs such as the lymph nodes, spleen, and tonsils. All lymphocytes in the adult originate in the bone marrow.

Function

Fluid enters organs and tissues from the arterial capillaries, and is eventually reabsorbed by the venous capillaries. However, not all of the fluid is reabsorbed by blood capillaries. About one tenth of the fluid is returned to the blood vessels via the lymphatic system. The lymphatic system reabsorbs about 2–4 qt (l) of fluid per day. Lymph composition is different depending on the site of origin. For example lymph collected from the gastrointestinal tract is high in fat that has been absorbed during digestion, and lymph collected from the bone marrow and thymus is high in lymphocyte concentration.

Lymph is collected when the pressure of the interstitial fluid and plasma proteins increases in the organs and tissues. Lymph pushes against the outside of the lymphatic valves and flows into the lymphatic capillary. This is called bulk flow. Valves are located throughout the lymphatic system approximately 0.15 in (38 mm) apart. Backflow is not possible in the lymphatics because the

Lymphatic System

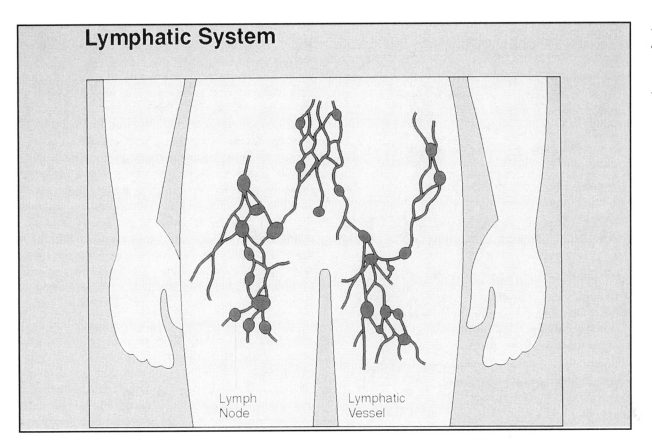

Lymph
Node

Lymphatic
Vessel

The lymph collected from the body's tissues is carried through the lymphatic vessels and lymph nodes. This illustration shows lymph nodes and vessels in the groin. (National Institutes of Health. Reproduced by permission.)

valves open in only one direction. Therefore, the lymphatic system runs in only one direction.

There are several factors the affect the rate at which lymph is collected. Interstitial fluid pressure affects the rate of flow of fluid into the lymphatic capillaries. Elevated capillary pressure, increased interstitial fluid pressure, and increased capillary permeability all contribute to an increase in the amount of interstitial pressure and the rate of lymph flow.

Smooth muscles around the lymphatic vessels act as lymphatic pumps, and their involuntary contractions affect the rate of lymph flow. As the lymphatic vessel swells with fluid, the smooth muscle around that portion senses the stretch and automatically contracts, pushing the lymph through the valve to the next chamber. The valve prevents backwards flow as the smooth muscle in the chamber contracts to send the lymph through the next valve into the next chamber. This process continues along the entire vessel until the lymph passes through the lymph nodes and into the subclavian vein.

Factors outside of the lymphatic system can also affect the rate of lymph flow by assisting in the pumping of lymph through the system. The following eternal factors can increase lymph flow: contraction of close **skeletal muscles**, movements made by other parts of the body, nearby arterial pulses, and compression of tissues by items outside of the body. Therefore, during periods of **exercise**, the lymphatic system is extremely active and the flow rate is high.

The terminal end of the lymphatic capillary also has a pump that can affect the rate of lymph flow. When the interstitial fluid pressure is high, the surrounding tissue expands. The anchoring filaments that are attached to the endothelial cells at the terminal end of the lymphatic capillary and to the connective tissue pull the capillary valves open, allowing inward flow of interstitial fluid. Then the internal lymphatic capillary pressure causes the valves to close and the smooth muscle in the first compartment to contract and push the lymph into the next chamber.

Contractile actomyosin filaments are also present in the end terminal of the lymphatic vessels. These filaments cause the rhythmic contraction of the terminal end of the lymphatic capillary. Therefore, they contribute to part of the initial pumping of lymph through the system.

KEY TERMS

B-lymphocytes (B-cells)—A type of white blood cell that originates in the bone marrow and recognizes foreign antigens (or proteins), secreting antibodies in an immune response.

Interstitial space—The spaces found within organs and tissues.

Lymph—The slightly opalescent fluid found within the lymphatic system.

Lymph nodes—Bean shaped swellings along the lymphatic vessels that contain macrophages and lymphocytes.

Lymphatics—The system of lymphatic vessels.

T-lymphocytes (T-cells)—A type of white blood cell that originates in the thymus and attaches themselves to foreign organisms, secreting lymphokines that kill the foreign organisms.

Tonsil—A collection of lymphocytes that form a mass in the back of the pharynx.

Role in human health

The lymphatic system has a variety of roles in human health ranging from returning fluid from organs back to the circulatory system, to an important part in the human **immune response**, to absorbing **lipids** from the intestines. The defining role of the lymphatic vessels is to return any fluid that has leaked from the capillaries and into the interstitial space back to the circulatory system through the veins. This is important because if fluid was retained in the tissues, the result in reduced blood volume and swelling of the tissues.

Another important role of the lymphatic system is the ability of plasma proteins to fit through the lymphatic valves and into the lymphatic capillary. Since most proteins have such a high molecular weight, they are unable to be reabsorbed by venous capillaries. With out the reabsorption of the plasma proteins, humans can die within 24 hours.

The lymphatic system also has an essential role in the process of digestion. Primarily, the lymphatic capillaries in the gastrointestinal tract are one of the main routes for **fats** to be absorbed. Fats enter the lymphatics before entering the blood stream.

High molecular weight proteins are not the only large substances that are absorbed. Microorganisms such as **bacteria** can also fit between the endothelial cells of the terminal end of the lymphatic capillary. As this occurs and the bacteria are transported to the next lymph node, the meshwork of the node and sinuses with in the node act as a filter, catching and trapping the foreign organisms. Once trapped, microorganisms can be attacked by the concentrated cells of the immune system. Macrophages may consume disease-causing bacteria, B-lymphocytes may come into contact with the antigens on the surface of the microorganism and stimulate antibodies, and T-lymphocytes called "killer" cells that attach themselves to the foreign organism and release a substance to destroy the organism. The destructive nature of the "killer" cells is enhanced by another T-lymphocyte called "helper" cells (T-helper cells also assist B-cells). If this system fails, then microorganisms are not destroyed, resulting in the spread of **infection** though the lymphatic system and extreme infection possibly leading to death.

Cancer cells that have lost adherence to, and break away from, the primary tumor are collected by the lymphatic system and filtered by latticework within the lymph nodes. Within the lymph node T-cells release substances called lymphokine (e.g. gamma interferor and interleukin 2) that may help destroy the cancer cells. Doctors use the lymph nodes as one factor of evaluation when determining the stage of the cancer. In other words, when determining how far the cancer has progressed at the time of diagnosis, the lymph nodes can be dissected to determine if cancer has spread (metastasized) from the original tumor or not. If cancer cells are present in the lymph nodes, then the cancer receives a higher stage and a less-optimistic diagnosis. In cancers that metastasize via the lymphatics, the lymph nodes where cancer cells are present are often removed. This is even more common when the lymph nodes in question are adjacent to the tumor, when the lymph nodes are located on the only lymphatic vessel present in the area of the tumor, or if no other lymphatics will be damaged during the removal.

Common diseases and disorders

Since the lymphatic system is responsible for draining excess fluid from tissues and organs, the most common symptom of diseases and disorders of the lymphatic system is swelling. For example, a disease known as elephantiasis, which is caused by a filarial worm infestation, involves the blockage of the lymphatics. When the lymphatics are blocked, fluid cannot be drained and swelling occurs in the affected areas. Administering ethyl-carbamazine drugs, elevating the area and wearing a compression stocking can treat elephantiasis.

Tonsillitis is another disease of the lymphatic system. Tonsillitis usually involves a bacterial or viral infection located within the tonsils. The tonsils are swollen, and the patient experiences a **fever**, **sore throat**, and difficulty swallowing. This can be treated by the use of **antibiotics** or through a surgical procedure called a tonsillectomy.

A condition common among individuals following surgery for **breast cancer** or **prostate cancer** is lymphedema. It is caused by blockage of lymph vessels or lymph nodes located near the surgical site and can result in swollen arms or legs. If microorganisms cause the swelling, then antibiotics are used as treatment. If microorganisms are not the cause, then compression garments and message therapy are used as treatment.

There are also cancers called lymphosarcomas and cancers of the lymph nodes that can affect the lymphatic system. The causes of these cancers are not known and there is not a consensus on what preventative measures can be taken to reduce the risk of developing these cancers. Symptoms of cancers affecting the lymphatic system include loss of appetite, energy, and weight, as well as swelling of the glands. As with many cancers, treatment includes surgical removal followed by adjuvant radiation and **chemotherapy**.

Resources

BOOKS

Braunwald, Eugene, et al. *Harrison's Principles of Internal Medicine,* 15th ed. New York: McGraw-Hill, 2001.

Lee, Richard G. M.D., et al. *Wintrob's Clinical Hematology,* 10th ed. Philadelphia: Lippincott Williams & Wilkins, 1999.

Vander, Arthur. *Human Physiology: The Mechanisms of Body Function,* Seventh ed. New York: WBC McGraw-Hill, 1998.

ORGANIZATIONS

Lymphatic Research Foundation. 941 N.E. 19th Avenue, Suite 305, Ft. Lauderdale, Florida, 33304-3071. (954)525-3510. <http://www.lymphaticresearch.org/>.

Sally C. McFarlane-Parrott

Lymphocyte typing *see* **Flow cytometry analysis**

Lymphomas *see* **Malignant lymphomas**

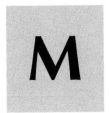

Macular degeneration

Definition

Macular degeneration is the progressive deterioration of a critical region of the retina called the macula. The macula is 3–5 mm and is responsible for central **vision**. This disorder leads to irreversible loss of central vision, although peripheral vision is retained. In the early stages, vision may be gray, hazy, or distorted.

Description

Macular degeneration is the most common cause of legal blindness in people over 60, and accounts for approximately 11.7% of blindness in the United States. About 28% of the population over age 74 is affected by this disease.

Age-related macular degeneration (ARMD) is the most common form of macular degeneration. It is also known as age-related maculopathy (ARM), aged macular degeneration, and senile macular degeneration. Approximately ten million Americans have some vision loss due to ARMD.

ARMD is subdivided into a dry (atrophic) and a wet (exudative) form. The dry form is more common and accounts for 70–90% of cases of ARMD. It progresses more slowly than the wet form and vision loss is less severe. In the dry form, the macula thins over time as part of the aging process and the pigmented retinal epithelium (a dark-colored cell layer at the back of the eye) is gradually lost. Words may appear blurred or hazy, and colors may appear dim or gray.

With wet ARMD, new **blood vessels** grow underneath the retina and distort the retina. These **blood** vessels can leak, causing scar tissue to form on the retina. The wet form may cause visual distortion and make straight lines appear wavy. A central blind spot develops.

The wet type progresses more rapidly and vision loss is more pronounced.

Less common forms of macular degeneration include:

• Cystoid macular degeneration: Vision loss in the macula due to fluid-filled areas (cysts) in the macular region. This may be a result of other disorders, such as aging, inflammation, or high myopia.

• Diabetic macular degeneration: Deterioration of the macula due to diabetes.

• Senile disciform degeneration (Kuhnt-Junius macular degeneration): A severe type of wet ARMD that involves hemorrhaging in the macular region. It usually occurs in people over 40 years old.

Causes and symptoms

Age-related macular degeneration is intrinsic to aging for some individuals, but not all. People with an ARMD-affected family member have an increased the risk for its development. A slightly higher incidence occurs in females, although males and females are considered to be equally at risk. Whites and Asians are more susceptible to developing ARMD than blacks, in whom the disorder is rare.

The cause of ARMD is thought to be arteriosclerosis in the blood vessels supplying the retina. Certain risks for the **heart** are considered similar risks to those that contribute to the development of macular degeneration. Smoking increases the risk of developing wet-type ARMD, and may increase the risk of developing dry-type as well. Dietary fat also increases the risk. In one study of older (age 45–84) Americans, signs of early ARMD were 80% more common in the group who ate the most saturated fat compared to those who ate the least. Low consumption of antioxidants, such as foods rich in **vitamin A**, is associated with a higher risk. It is generally believed that exposure to ultraviolet (UV) light may contribute to disease development, but this has not been proven conclusively.

A study reported in *Ophthalmology* in 2000 concluded that **hypertension**, thyroid hormones, and **antacids** are associated with certain types of ARMD. The issue of antacids is not widely recognized since no determination has yet been made regarding whether the antacids themselves lead to the disease, or whether it is the **stomach** problems that are a contributing factor. **Obesity** was also found to be a factor in this study.

The main symptom of macular degeneration is a central vision change. The patient may experience blurred central vision or a blank spot on the page when reading, visual distortion such as bending of straight lines, and images might appear smaller than is the actual object. Some patients notice a change in color perception, or abnormal light sensations. These symptoms can emerge suddenly and become progressively worse. Patients should be advised that a sudden onset of symptoms, particularly vision distortion, is an indication for immediate evaluation.

Diagnosis

Optometrists and ophthalmologists, with assistance from ophthalmic assistants, technicians and nurses, should carefully screen patients who are at risk for macular degeneration. These include patients older than 60; patients with hypertension or cardiovascular disease; cigarette smokers; patients with a first-degree family (sibling or maternal) history of vision loss from ARMD regardless of age; patients with aphakia or pseudophakia; or someone with a cataract, and patients with a history that indicates significant cumulative light exposure.

The ophthalmic assistant will take a careful history and log these risk factors. The patient then should have a complete ocular examination. Vision tests, performed by the physician or a skilled ophthalmic assistant, examine best corrected visual acuity, as well as near monocular visual acuity; refraction; biomicroscopy; tonometry; and stereoscopic fundus examination with pupillary dilation. Though rarely used even if ARMD is suspected, a central 10-degree computerized automated perimetry might be utilized along with fundus photography and laser ophthalmoscope scanning.

After preliminary testing, specific tests are performed to determine macular degeneration. To make the diagnosis, the doctor dilates the pupil with eye drops and examines the interior of the eye, examining the retina for the presence of drusen, small white-yellow spots in the macular area, and for gross changes in the macula such as thinning. The doctor also administers a visual field test to search for blank spots in the central vision. The doctor might order fluorescein **angiography** (intravenous injection of fluorescent dye followed by visual examination and photography of the back of the eye) to determine if blood vessels in the retina are leaking. Retinal pigmented epithelium (RPE) mottling that occurs, like the drusen, due to ateriorsclerotic changes of the macula decreasing the blood supply, can also be indicated through a thorough examination.

A central visual field test called an Amsler grid is usually given to patients who are suspected of having ARMD. It is a grid printed on a sheet of paper (also presented for home use every week). When viewing a central dot on the page, the patient should note if any of the lines appear to be wavy or missing. This could be an indication of fluid and the onset of wet ARMD. High-risk patients particularly will be urged to schedule more frequent checkups.

Although ophthalmologists and optometrists can accurately diagnose macular degeneration, attending physicians may want to consult with a retinal specialist for the best treatment protocols.

Treatment

While vision loss cannot be reversed, early detection is important because treatments are available that may halt or slow the progression of the wet form of ARMD. Some treatments for the dry form were still in early clinical trials in 2001.

In wet-type ARMD and in senile disciform macular degeneration, new capillaries grow in the macular region and leak. This leaking of blood and fluid causes a portion of the retina to detach. Blood vessel growth, called neovascularization, can be treated with laser photocoagulation in some cases, depending upon the location and extent of the growth. Argon or krypton lasers can destroy the new tissue and flatten the retina. This treatment is effective in about half the cases but results may be temporary. A concern exists that laser therapy causes the laser to destroy the photoreceptors in the treated area. If the blood vessels have grown into the fovea (a region of the macula responsible for fine vision), treatment may be impossible. Because capillaries can grow quickly, this form of macular degeneration should be handled as an emergency and treated immediately.

Photodynamic therapy (PDT) is a promising new treatment approved by the Food and Drug Administration in 2000. With PDT, the patient is given a light-activated drug intravenously with no damage to the retina. The drug, Visudyne, is absorbed by the damaged blood vessels. The affected area on the retina is exposed to a non-thermal laser light that activates the drug exactly 15 minutes after the infusion begins. It must be exactly 15 minutes for the treatment to be successful. The light chemically alters the drug, and any leakage from choroidal neovascularization (CNV) ceases. Patients require treatment every three months during the first year of therapy, and should be advised to avoid bright light or sun exposure for several days after therapy.

Another form of treatment for the wet form of ARMD is radiation therapy with either x rays, or a proton beam. Growing blood vessels are sensitive to treatment with low doses of ionizing radiation. The growth of nerve cells in the retina is stunted. They are insensitive and thus are not harmed by this treatment. External beam radiation treatment has shown promising results at slowing progression in limited, early trials.

Other therapies that are under study include treatment with alpha-interferon, thalidomide, and other drugs that slow the growth of blood vessels. Subretinal surgery also has shown promise in rapid-onset cases of wet ARMD. This surgery carries the risk of retinal detachment, hemorrhage, and acceleration of cataract formation. A controversial treatment called rheotherapy involves pumping the patient's blood through a device that removes some **proteins** and **fats**. As of 2001, this had not been proven to be safe or effective.

Consumption of a diet rich in antioxidants (beta carotene and the mixed carotenoids that are precursors of vitamin A, **vitamins** C and E, selenium, and **zinc**), or antioxidant nutritional supplements, may help prevent macular degeneration, particularly if started early in life. Research has shown that nutritional therapy can prevent ARMD or slow its progression once established.

Researchers also are working on therapies to treat the dry form of macular degeneration. Low-energy laser treatment for drusen is currently in clinical trials as of 2001. In this treatment the ophthalmologist uses a diode laser to reduce the drusen level. Some ophthalmologists were already performing this procedure "off-label," without FDA approval.

Another treatment, approved overseas but not in the United States, treats dry ARMD by implanting a miniaturized telescope to magnify objects in the central field of vision. This does not treat the disease, but aids the patient's vision in only the very severe cases of ARMD.

Prognosis

The dry form of ARMD is self-limiting and eventually stabilizes, with permanent vision loss. The vision of patients with the wet form of ARMD often stabilizes or improves even without treatment, at least temporarily.

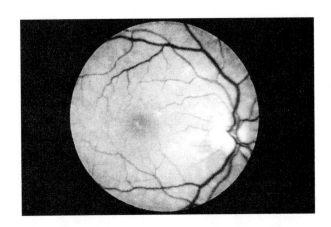

A slit-lamp view showing macular degeneration of the eye. (Custom Medical Stock Photo. Reproduced by permission.)

However, after a few years, patients with this type are usually left without acute central vision.

Many macular degeneration patients lose their central vision permanently and may become legally blind. However, macular degeneration rarely causes total vision loss. Peripheral vision is retained. Patients can compensate for central vision loss, even when macular degeneration renders them legally blind. Improved lighting and low-vision aids can help even if visual acuity is poor. Vision aids include special magnifiersallowing patients to read, and provide telescopic aids for long-distance vision. The use of these visual aids plus the retained peripheral vision assist in maintaining patient independence.

Health care team roles

Ophthalmic assistants, technicians, and nurses assist optometrists and ophthalmologists in testing for macular degeneration. Skilled ophthalmic staff take patient history and perform refraction; biomicroscopy; tonometry; stereoscopic fundus examination with pupillary dilation, only rarely; computerized automated perimetry; and fundus photography.

Registered ophthalmic nurses also play an important role in preparing patients for PDT. Only registered nurses and physicians are allowed to mix the drug used for PDT. RNs familiar with infusion are best-suited for this task. Nurses and ophthalmic staff also play an important role in PDT follow-up care. They are critical in issuing patient instructions to stay out of bright light and sunlight after treatment, and to wear sun-protective clothing for each treatment.

Patient education

Ophthalmic staff should reinforce the physician's instructions when assessing macular degeneration. They

KEY TERMS

Drusen—Tiny yellow dots on the retina that can be soft or hard and that usually do not interfere with vision.

Fovea—A tiny pit in the macula that is responsible for sharp vision.

Neovascularization—Growth of new capillaries.

Photoreceptors—Specialized nerve cells (rods and cones) in the retina that are responsible for vision.

Retina—The light-sensitive membrane at the back of the eye that images are focused on. The retina sends the images to the brain via the optic nerve.

should emphasize the importance of the Amsler grid and regular check-ups to monitor the progression of the disease.

Staff should also reaffirm doctor's orders with patients being treated with PDT. They should review that PDT is not a cure, but a slowing of the disease, and that retreatment is necessary for its success. Staff should also reinforce restrictions on patients' activities, such as staying out of direct sunlight or bright light for several days after PDT. They should also make follow-up calls to patients to ensure they are returning for PDT on time and to see if they have any questions about retreatment. Ophthalmic personnel should also be considerate of the age of most macular degeneration patients and provide large, easy-to-read instructions, and not rush them through the therapy or aftercare.

Prevention

Avoiding the risk factors for macular degeneration may help prevent it. This includes avoiding tobacco smoke and eating a diet low in saturated fat and rich in antioxidants. Some doctors suggest that wearing UV-blocking sunglasses reduces risk. Use of estrogen in post-menopausal women is associated with a lower risk of developing ARMD.

Resources

BOOKS

Norris, June, ed. *Professional Guide to Diseases,* 5th ed. Springhouse, PA: Springhouse Corporation, 1995.

Tierney, Lawrence M. Jr., Stephen J. McPhee, and Maxine A. Papadakis, eds. *Current Medical Diagnosis and*

Treatment, 37th ed. Stamford, CT: Appleton and Lange, 1998.

ORGANIZATIONS

American Academy of Ophthalmology (National Eyecare Project). P.O. Box 429098, San Francisco, CA. 94142-9098. (800)222-EYES. <http://www.eyenet.org>.

American Optometric Association. 243 North Lindbergh Blvd., St. Louis, MO 63141. (314) 991-4100. <http://www.aoanet.org>.

National Eye Institute. National Institutes of Health. Bethesda, Maryland. <http:://www.nei.nih.gov.publicaations/armd.htm>.

Prevent Blindness America. 500 East Remington Road, Schaumburg, IL 60173. (800) 331-2020. <http://www.prevent-blindness.org>.

OTHER

Angelucci, Diane. "Managing PDT." *Ophthalmology Management Online* <http://www.ophmanagement.com/archive_results.asp?loc=archive/03102000100458am.html>.

Kent, Christopher. "AMD Therapy New Hope for Treating Macular Degeneration" *Optometric Management Online* <http://www.optometric.com/archive_results.asp?loc=archive/0314200011121pm.html>.

"Macular Degeneration: A New Approach to Treating the Dry Form" *Ophthalmology Management Online* <http://www.ophmanagement.com/archive_results.asp?loc=archive/9899110732am.html>.

"National Study Finds Smoking, Hypertension, Antacid Use Associated with Macular Degeneration" *American Academy of Ophthalmology Online*. <http://www.eye-net.org/aaoweb1/Newsroom/1155_32019.cfm>.

Roach, Linda. "Retina/Vitreous: Laser to Drusen Offers Hope for Dry AMD" *EyeNet Magazine Online*. <http://www.eyenet.org/eyenet_mag/retina.html>.

Mary Bekker

Mad cow disease *see* **Creutzfeldt-Jakob disease**

Magnesium hydroxide *see* **Antacids**

Magnetic resonance angiography *see* **Magnetic resonance imaging**

Magnetic resonance imaging

Definition

Magnetic resonance imaging (MRI) is a unique and versatile medical imaging modality. Doctors can obtain highly refined images of the body's interior using MRI.

By using strong magnetic fields and pulses of radio waves to manipulate the natural magnetic properties in the body, this technique produces images not possible with other diagnostic imaging methods. MRI is particularly useful for imaging the **brain** and spine, as well as the soft tissues of joints and the interior structure of bones. The entire body can be imaged using MRI, and the technology poses few known health risks.

Purpose

MRI was developed in the 1980s. The latest additions to MRI technology are **angiography** (MRA) and spectroscopy (MRS). MRA was developed to study **blood** flow, while MRS can identify the chemical composition of diseased tissue and produce color images of brain function. The many advantages of MRI include:

• Detail. MRI creates precise images of the body based on the varying proportions of magnetically polarizable elements in different tissues. Very minor fluctuations in chemical composition can be determined. MRI images have greater subject contrast than those produced with standard x rays, computed tomography (CT), or ultrasound, all of which depend on the differing physical properties of tissues. This contrast sensitivity lets MRI distinguish fine variations in tissues deep within the body. It also is particularly useful for spotting and distinguishing diseased tissues (tumors and other lesions) early in their development. Often, doctors prescribe an MRI scan to more fully investigate earlier findings of the other imaging techniques.

• Scope. The entire body can be scanned, from head to toe and from the skin to the deepest recesses of the brain. Moreover, MRI scans are not adversely affected by bone, gas, or body waste, which can hinder other imaging techniques. (Although the scans can be degraded by motion such as breathing, heartbeat, and normal bowel activity.) MRI process produces cross-sectional images of the body that are as sharp in the middle as on the edges, even of the brain through the **skull**. A close series of these two-dimensional images can provide a three-dimensional view of a targeted area.

• Safety. MRI does not depend on potentially harmful ionizing radiation, as do standard x-ray and **CT scans**. There are no known risks specific to the procedure, other than for people who might have metal objects in their bodies.

Given all the advantages, doctors would undoubtedly prescribe MRI as frequently as ultrasound scanning, but the MRI process is complex and costly. The process requires large, expensive, and complicated equipment; a highly trained operator; and a doctor specializing in radiology. Generally, MRI is prescribed only when serious symptoms and/or negative results from other tests indicate a need. Many times an alternative imaging procedure is more appropriate for the type of diagnosis needed.

Doctors may prescribe an MRI scan of different areas of the body.

• Brain and head. MRI technology was developed because of the need for brain imaging. It is one of the few imaging tools that can see through bone (the skull) and deliver high quality pictures of the brain's delicate soft tissue structures. MRI may be needed for patients with symptoms of a **brain tumor**, stroke, or **infection** (like **meningitis**). MRI also may be needed when cognitive and/or psychological symptoms suggest brain disease (like Alzheimer's or Huntington's diseases, or **multiple sclerosis**), or when developmental retardation suggests a birth defect. MRI can also provide pictures of the sinuses and other areas of the head beneath the face.

• Spine. Spinal problems can create a host of seemingly unrelated symptoms. MRI is particularly useful for identifying and evaluating degenerated or herniated intervertebral discs. It can also be used to determine the condition of nerve tissue within the **spinal cord**.

• Joint. MRI scanning is often used to diagnose and assess joint problems. MRI can provide clear images of the bone, cartilage, ligaments, and tendons that comprise a joint. MRI can be used to diagnose joint injuries due to sports, advancing age, or arthritis. It can also be used to diagnose shoulder problems, like a torn rotator cuff. MRI can detect the presence of an otherwise hidden tumor or infection in a joint, and can be used to diagnose the nature of developmental joint abnormalities in children.

• Skeleton. The properties of MRI that allow it to see though the skull also allow it to view the interior of bones. It can be used to detect bone **cancer**, inspect the marrow for leukemia and other diseases, assess bone loss (**osteoporosis**), and examine complex **fractures**.

• The rest of the body. While CT and ultrasound satisfy most chest, abdominal, and general body imaging needs, MRI may be needed in certain circumstances to provide more detailed images or when repeated scanning is required. The progress of some therapies, like **liver cancer** therapy, need to be monitored, and the effect of repeated x-ray exposure is a concern.

Precautions

MRI scanning should not be used when there is the potential for an interaction between the strong MRI mag-

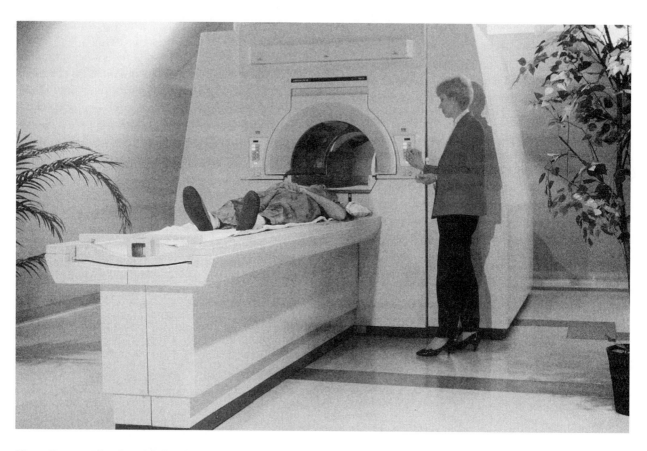

Magnetic resonance imaging (MRI) uses magnets and radio waves to make images of the body's organs, soft tissue, bone, and even blood flow. *(Jon Meyer/Custom Medical Stock Photo. Reproduced by permission.)*

netic field and metal objects that might be imbedded in a patient's body. The force of magnetic attraction on certain types of metal objects (including surgical steel and clips used to pinch off **blood vessels**) could move them within the body and cause serious injury. The movement would occur when the patient is moved into and out of the magnetic field. Metal may be imbedded in a person's body for several reasons.

- Medical. People with implanted cardiac **pacemakers**, metal aneurysm clips, or who have had broken bones repaired with metal pins, screws, rods, or plates must tell their radiologist prior to having an MRI scan. In some cases (like a metal rod in a reconstructed leg) the difficulty may be overcome.

- Injury. Patients must tell their doctors if they have bullet fragments or other metal pieces in their body from old **wounds**. The suspected presence of metal, whether from an old or recent wound, should be confirmed before scanning.

- Occupational. People with significant work exposure to metal particles (working with a metal grinder, for example) should discuss this with their doctor and radiologist. The patient may need prescan testing—usually

a single, standard x ray of the eyes to see if any metal is present.

Chemical agents designed to improve the image and/or allow for the imaging of blood or other fluid flow during MRA may be injected. In rare cases, patients may be allergic to or intolerant of these agents, and these patients should not receive them. If these chemical agents are to be used, patients should discuss any concerns they have with their doctor and radiologist.

The potential side effects of magnetic and electric fields on human health remain a source of debate. In particular, the possible effects on an unborn baby are not well known. Any woman who is, or may be, pregnant should carefully discuss this issue with her doctor and radiologist before undergoing a scan.

As with all medical imaging techniques, **obesity** greatly interferes with the quality of MRI.

Description

In essence, MRI produces a map of hydrogen atoms distributed in the body. Hydrogen is the simplest element known, the most abundant in biological tissue, and one that can be magnetically polarized. It will align itself within a strong magnetic field, like the needle of a compass. The earth's magnetic field is not strong enough to polarize a person's hydrogen atoms, but the superconducting magnet of an MRI machine can. The strength of the Earth's magnetic field is approximately 1 gauss. Typical field strength of an MRI unit, with a superconducting magnet is 1,500 gauss expressed as 1.5 kilogauss or 1.5 Tesla units. This comprises the "magnetic" part of MRI.

Once a patient's hydrogen atoms have been aligned in the magnet, pulses of very specific radio wave frequencies are used to jolt them out of alignment. The hydrogen atoms alternately absorb and emit radio wave energy, vibrating back and forth between their resting (polarized) state and their agitated (radio pulse) state. This comprises the "resonance" part of MRI.

The MRI equipment detects the duration, strength, and source location of the signals emitted by the atoms as they relax and translates the data into an image on a television monitor. The amount of hydrogen in diseased tissue differs from the amount in healthy tissue of the same type, making MRI particularly good at identifying tumors and other lesions. In some cases, chemical agents such as gadolinium can be injected to improve the contrast between healthy and diseased tissue.

A single MRI exposure produces a two-dimensional image of a slice through the entire target area. A series of these image slices closely spaced (usually less than half an inch) makes a virtual three-dimensional view of the area.

Magnetic resonance spectroscopy (MRS) is different from MRI because MRS uses a continuous band of radio wave frequencies to excite hydrogen atoms in a variety of chemical compounds other than water. These compounds absorb and emit radio energy at characteristic frequencies, or spectra, which can be used to identify them. Generally, a color image is created by assigning a color to each distinctive spectral emission. This comprises the "spectroscopy" part of MRS. MRS is still experimental and is available in only a few research centers.

Doctors primarily use MRS to study the brain and disorders, like epilepsy, **Alzheimer's disease**, brain tumors, and the effects of drugs on brain growth and **metabolism**. The technique is also useful in evaluating metabolic disorders of the muscles and nervous system.

Magnetic resonance angiography (MRA) is a variation on standard MRI. MRA, like other types of angiography, looks specifically at blood flow within vascular system, but does so without the injection of contrast agents or radioactive tracers. Standard MRI cannot detect blood flow, but MRA uses specific radio pulse sequences to capture usable signals. The technique is generally used in combination with MRI to obtain images that show both vascular structure and flow within the brain and head in cases of stroke, or when a blood clot or aneurysm is suspected.

Regardless of the exact type of MRI planned, or area of the body targeted, the procedure involved is basically the same and occurs in a special MRI suite. The patient lies back on a narrow table and is made as comfortable as possible. Transmitters are positioned on the body and the cushioned table that the patient is lying on moves into a long tube that houses the magnet. The tube is as long as an average adult lying down, and the tube is narrow and open at both ends. Once the area to be examined has been properly positioned, a radio pulse is applied. Then a two-dimensional image corresponding to one slice through the area is made. The table then moves a fraction of an inch and the next image is made. Each image exposure takes several seconds and the entire exam will last anywhere from 30-90 minutes. During this time, the patient is not allowed to move. If the patient moves during the scan, the picture will not be clear.

Depending on the area to be imaged, the radio-wave transmitters will be positioned in different locations.

• For the head and neck, a helmet-like hat is worn.

• For the spine, chest, and abdomen, the patient will be lying on the transmitters.

• For the knee, shoulder, or other joint, the transmitters will be applied directly to the joint.

Additional probes will monitor **vital signs** (like pulse, respiration, etc.).

The process is very noisy and confining. The patient hears a thumping sound for the duration of the procedure. Since the procedure is noisy, music supplied via earphones is often provided. Some patients get anxious or panic because they are in the small, enclosed tube. This is why vital signs are monitored and the patient and medical team can communicate between each other. If the chest or abdomen are to be imaged, the patient will be asked to hold his/her breath as each exposure is made. Other instructions may be given to the patient, as needed. In many cases, the entire examination will be performed by an MRI operator who is not a doctor. However, the supervising radiologist should be available to consult as necessary during the exam, and will view and interpret the results sometime later.

Open MRI units

Many adult patients and, especially children, become extremely claustrophobic when placed inside the confines of a full strength (1.5 Tesla) superconducting

KEY TERMS

Angiography—Any of the different methods for investigating the condition of blood vessels, usually via a combination of radiological imaging and injections of chemical tracing and contrasting agents.

Gadolinium—A very rare metallic element useful for its sensitivity to electromagnetic resonance, among other things. Traces of it can be injected into the body to enhance the MRI pictures.

Hydrogen—The simplest, most common element known in the universe. It is composed of a single electron (negatively charged particle) circling a nucleus consisting of a single proton (positively charged particle). It is the nuclear proton of hydrogen that makes MRI possible by reacting resonantly to radio waves while aligned in a magnetic field.

Ionizing radiation—Electromagnetic radiation that can damage living tissue by disrupting and destroying individual cells. All types of nuclear decay radiation (including x rays) are potentially ionizing. Radio waves do not damage organic tissues they pass through.

Magnetic field—The three-dimensional area surrounding a magnet, in which its force is active. During MRI, the patient's body is permeated by the force field of a superconducting magnet.

Radio waves—Electromagnetic energy of the frequency range corresponding to that used in radio communications, usually 10,000 cycles per second to 300 billion cycles per second. Radio waves are the same as visible light, x rays, and all other types of electromagnetic radiation, but are of a higher frequency.

magnet. This problem is often severe enough to prevent them from having an MRI scan performed. An alternative design, to the standard MRI unit is one where the magnet is comprised of two opposed halves with a large space in between. Units designed this way are known as open MRI machines. The advantage is, they can be used for patients who are claustrophobic. The disadvantage is, the field strength of the magnets is lower than with standard full strength machines, usually somewhere in the range of 0.2–0.5 Tesla. Lower strength magnetic fields require more time for image acquisition increasing the risks of

motion artifacts because patients need to remain still for longer periods of time.

Preparation

In some cases (such as for MRI brain scanning or an MRA), a chemical designed to increase image contrast may be given by the radiologist immediately before the exam. If a patient suffers from **anxiety** or claustrophobia, drugs may be given to help the patient relax.

The patient must remove all metal objects (watches, jewelry, **eye glasses**, hair clips, etc). Any magnetized objects (like credit and bank machine cards, audio tapes, etc.) should be kept far away from the MRI equipment because they can be erased. The patient cannnot bring their wallet or keys into the MRI machine. The patient may be asked to wear clothing without metal snaps, buckles, or zippers, unless a medical gown is worn during the procedure. The patient may be asked to remove any hair spray, hair gel, or cosmetics that may interfere with the scan.

Aftercare

No aftercare is necessary, unless the patient received medication or had a reaction to a contrast agent. Normally, patients can immediately return to their daily activities. If the exam reveals a serious condition that requires more testing and/or treatment, appropriate information and counseling will be needed.

Complications

MRI poses no known health risks to the patient and produces no physical side effects. Again, the potential effects of MRI on an unborn baby are not well known. Any woman who is, or may be, pregnant, should carefully discuss this issue with her doctor and radiologist before undergoing a scan.

Results

A normal MRI, MRA, or MRS result is one that shows the patient's physical condition to fall within normal ranges for the target area scanned.

Generally, MRI is prescribed only when serious symptoms and/or negative results from other tests indicate a need. There often exists strong evidence of a condition that the scan is designed to detect and assess. Thus, the results will often be abnormal, confirming the earlier diagnosis. At that point, further testing and appropriate medical treatment is needed. For example, if the MRI indicates the presence of a brain tumor, an MRS may be prescribed to determine the type of tumor so that aggressive treatment can begin immediately without the need for a surgical biopsy.

Health care team roles

The MRI examination is conducted by an MRI technologist and a radiologist. The MRI technologist is responsible for preparing the patient for the examination by making sure that all metallic objects have been removed and that the patient does not have any metallic implants that will be affected by the examination. It is recommended that a prescreening MRI questionnaire be developed and that all patients be required to complete the form prior to having an MRI. If necessary for the area being imaged, an intravenous contrast agent will be administered by either the technologist or a nurse. Nursing staff may also be present during the examination, depending on the medical condition of the patient. The radiologist oversees the selection of MRI imaging sequences and protocols and reviews the acquired images to be sure image quality is appropriate for diagnosis. The radiologist also provides the final interpretation of images and provides a report for any referring physicians.

Resources

BOOKS

Haaga, John R., et al., eds. *Computed Tomography and Magnetic Resonance Imaging of the Whole Body.* St. Louis, MO: Mosby, 1994.

Kevles, Bettyann Holtzmann. *Naked to the Bone: Medical Imaging in the Twentieth Century.* New Brunswick, NJ: Rutgers University Press, 1997.

Zaret, Barry L., et al., eds. *The Patient's Guide to Medical Tests.* Boston: Houghton Mifflin Company, 1997.

PERIODICALS

The Basics of MRI. Joseph P. Hornak, Ph.D., http//www.cis.rit.edu/htbooks/mri/.

Brief Introduction to FMRI. Copyright 1998, Steve Smith, FMRIB, <http://www.fmrib.ox.ac.uk/fmri_intro/>.

Kevles, Bettyann. "Body Imaging." *Newsweek* (Winter 97/98 Extra Millennium Issue): 74-76.

ORGANIZATIONS

American College of Radiology. 1891 Preston White Dr., Reston, VA 22091. (703) 648-8900. <http://www.acr.org.>.

American Society of Radiologic Technologists. 15000 Central Ave. SE, Albuquerque, NM 87123-3917. (505) 298-4500. <http://www.asrt.org>.

Center for Devices and Radiological Health. United States Food and Drug Administration. 1901 Chapman Ave., Rockville, MD 20857. (301) 443-4109. <http://www.fda.gov/cdrh>.

Stephen John Hage, AAAS, RT-R, FAHRA

▌Magnetic resonance imaging unit

Definition

A **magnetic resonance imaging** (MRI) unit uses a magnetic field, radiofrequency waves, and computerized image processing to produce cross-sectional images of the anatomy.

Purpose

An MRI unit has several diagnostic clinical applications, including:

- diagnosing diseases of the **central nervous system, brain,** and spine
- detecting musculoskeletal disorders and injuries
- identifying infectious diseases such as those associated with acquired **immunodeficiency** syndrome (AIDS)
- detecting metastatic **liver** disease
- imaging the cardiovascular system
- staging prostate, bladder, and uterine cancers
- studying bone marrow diseases
- imaging the breast adjunctive to conventional mammography

Some MRI units can perform magnetic resonance **angiography** (MRA), which is used to image vascular and arteriovenous malformations, thromboses, stenoses, and other vascular abnormalities. In particular, MRA is used for evaluating the carotid artery and cerebral vasculature in patients with suspected or known stroke. An MRI unit can also be used in conjunction with other imaging modalities such as computed tomography (CT) for localizing the treatment target for radiation treatment planning and prior to surgical treatment of tumors, including stereotactic radiosurgery and image-guided surgery. It is also possible to evaluate brain function associated with certain tasks such as language or **vision** using functional MRI.

MRI provides images with excellent contrast that allow clinicians to clearly see details of soft tissue, bone, joints, and ligaments. Because MRI does not use ionizing radiation to produce images, like radiography and CT, it is often the examination of choice for imaging the male and female reproductive systems, pelvis and hips, and urinary tract and bladder.

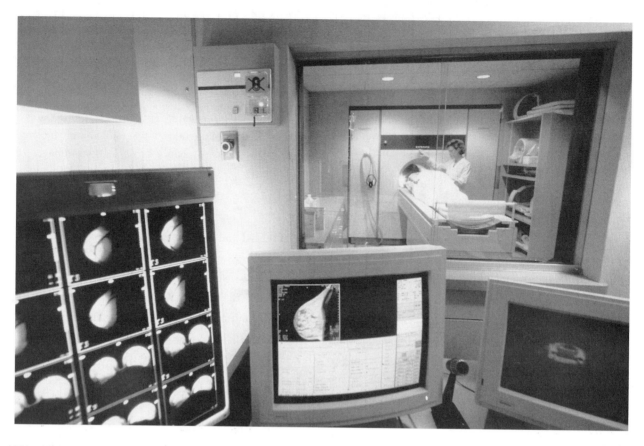

Magnetic resonance imaging system. *(Photograph by Mason Morfit. FPG International Corp. Reproduced by permission.)*

Description

MRI units are used in the radiology department and outpatient imaging centers for diagnostic imaging, in the emergency care and critical care settings to diagnose acute conditions such as stroke in the clinical research setting (especially for brain research), and in orthopedic practices. Large hospitals usually have one or more MRI units that are typically located in the radiology department or in a separate annex near the radiology and emergency departments.

An MRI unit consists of a magnet system, a radiofrequency (RF) transmitter/receiver system, a gradient system, a patient table, a computer workstation, and operator console. The magnetic strength of the magnet is measured in teslas (T), a unit of magnetic field strength, and ranges from 0.064–4 T, depending on the type of system. The magnetic field generated during an MRI examination is approximately 8,000 times stronger than the Earth's magnetic field. Principles of image production are based on the magnetic spin properties of hydrogen atoms in the body's tissues and fluids and how they behave in a magnetic field. Basically, hydrogen protons (particles located in the atom's nucleus) will align with an applied magnetic field and will spin perpendicular to the magnetic field when a radiofrequency pulse is added. When the pulse is terminated, protons relax back into alignment with the magnetic field, and this generates a radiofrequency signal that is received by the antenna coil. Different tissues such as those high in water and in fat will produce different signals that are then processed by the computer and converted into anatomical images. MRI protocols and imaging sequences are based on the different signals produced by different types and physiologic states of tissue.

The magnet system is contained in the gantry, which is a large square or round unit with a hole in the center (the bore) through which the patient table is moved. Magnets may be of three types: permanent magnet, resistive or superconducting electromagnet, and iron-core electromagnet. Permanent magnets are extremely heavy and thus require special construction; however, they do not require electrical power or cooling because they are constructed of magnetic alloys. They also have almost no fringe field (the magnetic field outside the magnet itself). Permanent magnets are limited to field strengths of 0.3 T or less. Resistive electromagnets use electrical coils to generate a magnetic field and thus require cooling water. Resistive magnets are limited to field strengths of 0.5 T.

Superconducting magnets use titanium alloy coils that require cooling with liquid helium or liquid nitrogen (cryogens). They can have field strengths of up to 2 T. Iron-core electromagnets use a combination of permanent and electromagnet technology, and require cooling water for operation. Field strengths are usually 0.3 or 0.4 T.

An MRI unit with a field strength less than 0.2 T is considered low field, an MRI unit with a field strength of 0.2 T to 1 T is considered mid field, and an MRI unit with a field strength greater than 1 T is considered high field. In general, high-field MRI units are capable of shorter imaging times and higher image quality and are preferred for many clinical applications.

The radiofrequency system transmits and receives signals using a coil that acts as an antenna. Separate coils are used for head and body imaging, and specially designed coils are used for imaging the spine, face, knee, breast, shoulder, and extremities. The gradient system produces magnetic fields in the direction of the primary field and perpendicular to the primary field in order to select the area for imaging and to register the location of signals received from the area imaged. The radiofrequency and gradient systems are turned on and off (pulsed) to control image contrast; these pulse patterns are called a pulse sequence. There are several different types of pulse sequences used, and they vary according to the duration, frequency, and timing of the pulses. Different pulse sequences are used to image different anatomic areas, and the pulse sequence is chosen based on the characteristics of the tissue being imaged such as fat content, water content, and anatomic area.

There are several different types of MRI units and MRI imaging methods:

- Conventional MRI units have long, closed bores that surround most of the patient's body during imaging.

- Short-bore MRI units were developed in response to patient claustrophobia and to retain the image-quality benefits of conventional systems, and have bore lengths that allow patients of average height to have much of their body outside the bore during imaging. The patient's head can then be outside the bore for exams not involving the brain and neck, thereby reducing claustrophobic reactions.

- Open MRI units were also developed in response to patient claustrophobia and to facilitate interventional procedures. They have bores that are open on most sides (sometimes columns are used to support the gantry). Open MRI units usually have low-field strengths.

- Dedicated extremity/head/breast MRI units have very small bores designed to accommodate imaging of limbs, joints, or the head, and are primarily used for orthopedic applications. A dedicated breast MRI system is also available.

- Mobile MRI units are installed in a specially designed trailer and driven to hospitals that do not have an MRI unit. Mobile MRI services are used frequently in rural areas.

- Functional MRI is an imaging technique that rapidly acquires images that display changes in cerebral **blood** flow in response to visual or auditory stimuli or motor tasks. This technique is used primarily for research to map the functional organization of the brain.

- Interventional and intraoperative MRI is a developing field that involves performing interventional procedures such as catheterization or guidewire insertion, and intraoperative guidance such as during neurosurgery, using a specially designed MRI unit. Open MRI units are being used for these applications due to their open-bore design, which facilitates patient access.

- MRI spectroscopy is an imaging technique used primarily in research that measures metabolites in the brain to evaluate brain tissue.

- Echoplanar MRI is an imaging technique that uses rapidly oscillating magnetic field gradients for image acquisition in less than 30 milliseconds. It is used to evaluate real-time cardiac and brain function, as well as muscle activity.

- MRI angiography is an imaging technique used to evaluate the **blood vessels**, for example, to detect aneurysms or atherosclerosis. Injection of a contrast agent is required.

- Diffusion tensor MRI is a relatively new imaging technique that tracks water molecules in the brain to detect abnormalities associated with stroke, **multiple sclerosis**, and other conditions.

Operation

An MRI unit is operated by the MRI technologist who prepares the patient for the examination, including administering any necessary intravenous contrast agents and positioning the patient on the table. Some examinations require the use of special surface coils (e.g., for head, knee, etc.) to focus the radiofrequency pulses on the area of interest. The MRI technologist places or attaches the appropriate coil and helps the patient onto the table. After the patient is properly positioned, the MRI technologist goes to the control room, which is adjacent to but separated from the MRI unit by a window, and initiates the imaging sequences selected by the radiologist. Usually, two to six imaging sequences are performed, each lasting approximately two to 15 minutes. The technologist instructs the patient via an intercom system when the scanning sequence is to begin and whether holding of breath or stillness is required. While the images are being acquired, the MRI technologist and radiologist review them on the computer workstation to make sure the image quality is sufficient for diagnosis.

Image artifacts may occur during image acquisition, and the technologist and radiologist should monitor acquired images for artifacts. Patient motion, respiratory motion, implants, signal loss, and improper unit settings can all cause artifacts to occur. Constantly occurring artifacts related to the unit's operation or magnetic field may require a service call from the manufacturer or testing by a medical physicist.

With regard to patient safety, there are no side effects associated with the magnetic field during an MRI examination, but, in general, MRI is not recommended for pregnant women. Patients with a pacemaker, cochlear implants, aneurysm clips, and other metallic implants must check with a physician before undergoing MRI due to the possible effects of the magnetic field on the implants. Patients who have been exposed to shrapnel or metal shavings (especially in the eye) may not be able to have an MRI; instances where the magnetic field caused movement of metal fragments in the body and subsequent patient injury have been reported. Because eyeshadow may contain metallic substances, patients undergoing MRI should not wear make-up during the examination.

Several incidents have occurred where patients undergoing MRI examinations received serious skin **burns** from contact with surface coils or monitoring cables. Therefore, the United States Food and Drug Administration (FDA) has issued precautions to prevent burns during MRI, including removal of unnecessary coils, cables, and leads before the scan is begun; frequent checking of coils, cables, and leads for frayed insulation or exposed wires; and a thorough check that cables and leads do not form loops, touch the sides of the magnet bore, or directly touch the patient.

The magnetic field requires that all medical equipment used in the MRI suite be MRI-compatible. For example, patient monitoring equipment, intravenous poles, **ventilators**, and contrast media injectors should have been tested and certified by the manufacturer as MRI-compatible. If interventional procedures are performed in the MRI suite, anesthesia units, surgical instrumentation, patient monitoring systems, and resuscitation equipment should all be MRI-compatible. The operation and performance of equipment that is not MRI-compatible may be affected by the magnetic field, or if the equip-

ment contains certain metals, it may be attracted to the magnet, causing equipment damage and presenting a safety problem. Because patients may be brought into the MRI suite on wheelchairs or with oxygen canisters, MRI staff should be sure that the magnetic field is not on during patient transfer. There have been several hazard reports of injury to patients and staff by oxygen canisters, wheelchairs, and other metal items when they were rapidly drawn to the magnet.

During the MRI examination, all patients, but particularly those under sedation or anesthesia or in critical condition, should be monitored using physiologic monitoring equipment, intercom systems, and video. Some patients may be claustrophobic during the examination or may experience **anxiety**. To alleviate these discomforts, an MRI-compatible music system and increased ventilation in the magnet bore can be installed.

Depending on the type of magnet, different types of shielding are required for the MRI suite. The performance of the MRI unit depends on the homogeneity, or uniformity, of the magnetic field, which may be disturbed by surrounding hospital equipment, metallic structures, and environmental factors. A process called shimming is used to improve the uniformity of the magnetic field, and is accomplished by using shim coils or ferromagnetic materials around the magnet. Shimming is usually done during installation or testing by physicists. The entire MRI suite may need to be shielded with different materials to insulate the magnet from outside interference or to prevent the magnet's fringe field from interfering with the operation of medical equipment in adjacent areas.

Maintenance

Because of the complexity of an MRI unit, a service contract covering parts replacement, preventive maintenance, and emergency repairs is usually purchased from the manufacturer or a third-party service organization. The **biomedical engineering** staff and/or the MRI technologist conduct periodic performance testing of image quality and other parameters. Surface coils should be cleaned and maintained according to manufacturer instructions. Many MRI units have special cooling system requirements, and storage and replenishment of cryogens (chemicals used for cooling the magnet system) is necessary. This is generally performed by the service provider or biomedical engineering staff.

Health care team roles

The MRI examination is conducted by an MRI technologist and a radiologist. The MRI technologist is responsible for preparing the patient for the examination by making sure that all metallic objects have been removed and that the patient does not have any metallic implants that will be affected by the examination. It is recommended that a prescreening MRI questionnaire be developed and that all patients be required to complete the form prior to having an MRI. If necessary for the area being imaged, an intravenous contrast agent will be administered by either the technologist or a nurse. Nursing staff may also be present during the examination, depending on the medical condition of the patient. The radiologist oversees the selection of MRI imaging sequences and protocols and reviews the acquired images to be sure image quality is appropriate for diagnosis. The radiologist also provides the final interpretation of images and provides a report for any referring physicians. For **cancer** cases, oncologists may also be involved in image review for treatment planning purposes. If interventional MRI procedures are performed, specialists such as a gastroenterologist, orthopedic surgeon, neurologist, or neurosurgeon may perform the procedures while the MRI unit is operated by the technologist.

Training

MRI technologists have completed special education programs in MRI physics, operation, and safety. All manufacturers of MRI units provide on-site, and sometimes off-site, training on the technical features and clinical applications of their systems. The American College of Radiology has developed an MRI site accreditation program, which requires that the MRI system, quality control procedures, MRI technologists, and radiologists be evaluated according to certain standards of performance. As of 2001, this accreditation was not mandatory, but many facilities undergo the process to demonstrate quality performance.

Resources

BOOKS

Dendy, P.P., and B. Heaton. *Physics for Diagnostic Radiology,* 2nd ed. Philadelphia, PA: Institute of Physics Publishing, 1999.

NessAiver, Moriel. *All You Really Need to Know about MRI Physics.* Baltimore, MD: Simply Physics, 1997.

PERIODICALS

Kanal, Emanual, ed. "MRI Safety." *Magnetic Resonance Imaging Clinics of North America* 6, no. 4 (November 1998).

Ladd, Mark E., Harald H. Quick, and Jorg R. Debatin. "Interventional MRA and Intravascular Imaging." *Journal of Magnetic Resonance Imaging* 12 (2000): 524-46.

Lewin, Jonathan S., Andrew Metzger, and Warren R. Selman. "Intraoperative Magnetic Resonance Image Guidance in

KEY TERMS

Aneurysm—Localized enlargement of an artery or vein.

Artifact—An artificial feature in an acquired MRI image.

Atherosclerosis—Hardening of the arteries, a form of heart disease.

Metabolites—Byproducts of metabolism that accumulate in brain tissue that is measured by MRI spectroscopy.

Teslas (T)—A unit of magnetic field strength.

Neurosurgery. *Journal of Magnetic Resonance Imaging* 12 (2000):512-24.

Sawyer-Glover, Anne M., and Frank G. Shellock. "Pre-MRI Procedure Screening: Recommendations and Safety Considerations for Biomedical Implants and Devices." *Journal of Magnetic Resonance Imaging* 12 (2000): 92-106.

Tempany, Clare M.C., and Barbara J. McNeil. "Advances in Biomedical Imaging." *Journal of the American Medical Association* 285, no. 5 (February 7, 2001): 562-67.

ORGANIZATIONS

American College of Radiology. 1891 Preston White Drive, Reston, VA 20191-4397. (800)227-5463. <http://www.acr.org>.

American Society of Radiologic Technologists (ASRT). 15000 Central Avenue SE, Albuquerque, NM 87123-2778. (800) 444-2778. <http://www.asrt.org>.

Clinical Magnetic Resonance Society. 2825 Burnet Avenue, Suite 2, Cincinnati, OH 45219. (800) 823-2677. <http://www.cmrs.com>.

International Society for Magnetic Resonance in Medicine. 2118 Milvia Street, Suite 201, Berkeley, CA 94704. (510) 841-1899. <http://www.ismrm.org>.

Radiological Society of North America. 820 Jorie Boulevard, Oak Brook, IL 60523-2251. (630) 571-2670. <http://www.rsna.org>.

OTHER

"Magnetic Resonance Imaging." *American Society of Radiologic Technologists.* <http://www.asrt.org/ patientpublic/MagneticResonance/ magneticresonanceimaging.htm>.

"MR Imaging (MRI)—Body." <http://www.radiologyinfo.org/content/ mr_of_the_body.htm>.

Jennifer E. Sisk, M.A.

Magnetic resonance spectroscopy *see* **Magnetic resonance imaging**

Malabsorption syndrome

Definition

Malabsorption syndrome is an alteration in the ability of the intestine to absorb nutrients adequately into the bloodstream.

Causes and symptoms

Protein, **fats**, and **carbohydrates** (macronutrients) normally are absorbed in the **small intestine**; the small bowel also absorbs about 80% of the 8.4–10.5 qt (8–10 l) of fluid ingested daily. There are many different conditions that affect fluid and nutrient absorption by the intestine. A fault in the digestive process may result from failure of the body to produce the enzymes needed to digest certain foods. Congenital structural defects or diseases of the **pancreas**, gall bladder, or **liver** may alter the digestive process. Inflammation, **infection**, injury, or surgical removal of portions of the intestine may also result in absorption problems; reduced length or surface area of intestine available for fluid and nutrient absorption can result in malabsorption. Radiation therapy may injure the mucosal lining of the intestine, resulting in **diarrhea** that may not become evident until several years later. The use of some **antibiotics** can also affect the **bacteria** that normally live in the intestine and affect intestinal function.

Risk factors for malabsorption syndrome include:

• family history of malabsorption or **cystic fibrosis**

• use of certain drugs such as mineral oil or other laxatives

• travel to foreign countries, which may introduce parasites into the body

• intestinal surgery

• excess alcohol consumption

Individuals may experience symptoms of malabsorption, the most common of which include:

• anemia, with weakness and fatigue due to inadequate absorption of **vitamin B₁₂**, **iron**, and **folic acid**

• diarrhea (sometimes explosive diarrhea with greasy, foul-smelling stools), steatorrhea (excessive amount of fat in the stool), and abdominal distention with cramps, bloating, and gas due to impaired water and carbohy-

drate absorption, and irritation from unabsorbed fatty acids

• **edema** (fluid retention in the body's tissues) due to decreased protein absorption

• malnutrition and weight loss due to decreased fat, carbohydrate, and protein absorption; weight may be 80–90% of usual weight despite increased oral intake of nutrients

• muscle cramping due to decreased **vitamin D**, **calcium**, and potassium levels

• muscle wasting and atrophy due to decreased protein absorption and metabolism

• perianal skin burning, itching, or soreness due to frequent loose stools

Irregular **heart** rhythms may also result from inadequate levels of potassium and other electrolytes. **Blood** clotting disorders may occur due to a **vitamin K** deficiency. Children with malabsorption syndrome often exhibit a failure to grow and thrive.

Several disorders can lead to malabsorption syndrome, including cystic fibrosis, chronic **pancreatitis**, lactose intolerance, and celiac disease (gluten enteropathy, non-tropical sprue).

Tropical sprue is a malabsorptive disorder that is uncommon in the United States, but seen more often in people from the Caribbean, India, or southeast Asia. Although its cause is unknown, the disorder is thought to be related to environmental factors, including infection, intestinal parasites, or possibly the consumption of certain food toxins. Symptoms often include a sore tongue, anemia, weight loss, along with diarrhea and passage of fatty stools.

Celiac disease, also known as non-tropical sprue, gluten enteropathy, or celiac sprue, is an inherited disorder resulting in malabsorption because of an allergic reaction after consumption of a protein called gluten. Gluten is found in wheat, rye, barley, and oats.

Whipple's disease is a relatively rare malabsorptive disorder that affects mostly middle-aged men. The cause of the disorder is possibly related to bacterial infection, resulting in nutritional deficiencies, chronic low-grade **fever**, diarrhea, joint **pain**, weight loss, and darkening of the skin's pigmentation. Other organs of the body may be affected, including the **brain**, heart, **lungs**, and eyes.

Short bowel syndromes—which may be present at birth (congenital) or the result of surgery—reduce the surface area of the bowel available to absorb nutrients and can also result in malabsorption syndrome.

Bacterial overgrowth that is triggered by intestinal diverticulosis, intestinal disorders, blind loops, fistulas, and strictures may cause malabsorption, resulting in fat malabsorption and flatulence.

Intestinal lymphangiectasia, also called idiopathic hypoproteinemia, is a disorder affecting children and young adults in which the lymph vessels supplying the lining of the small intestine become enlarged. Lymph vessel enlargement may be a birth defect or may have been due to inflammation of the pancreas, called pancreatitis or a condition called constrictive pericarditis, which is characterized by a stiffening of the sac around the heart (constrictive pericarditis). These conditions increase pressure on the **lymphatic system**. Symptoms of intestinal lymphangiectasia are severe edema, and perhaps nausea, vomiting, mild diarrhea, fatty stools, and abdominal pain. The number of lymphocytes in the blood may decrease. As well, cholesterol and protein levels in the blood are low.

Diagnosis

Doctors often suspect malabsorption syndromes when weight loss, diarrhea, and nutritional deficiencies occur despite eating a healthy and adequate diet. The diagnosis of malabsorption syndrome and identification of the underlying cause can require extensive diagnostic testing.

The first phase of diagnosis involves a thorough medical history and **physical examination** by a physician, who will then determine the appropriate laboratory studies and x rays. A 72-hour stool collection may be ordered for fecal fat measurement; increased fecal fat in the stool indicates malabsorption. A biopsy of the small intestine may be done to assist in differentiating between malabsorption syndrome and small bowel disease. Pancreatic function tests are often conducted since pancreatic disorders are a common cause of malabsorption syndromes. Ultrasound, computed tomography scan (CT scan), **magnetic resonance imaging** (MRI), **barium enema**, or other x rays to identify abnormalities of the gastrointestinal tract and pancreas may also be ordered.

To diagnose intestinal lymphangiectasia, an intravenous injection of radioactive-labeled albumin may be ordered. Excessive protein is lost if abnormal amounts of the radioactive substance appear in the stool. Enlarged lymph vessels are indicated by a biopsy of the small intestine.

Laboratory studies of the blood may include:

- Serum cholesterol: May be low due to decreased fat absorption and digestion.
- Serum sodium, potassium, and chloride: May be low due to electrolyte losses with diarrhea.

- Serum calcium: May be low due to vitamin D and amino acid malabsorption.
- Serum protein and albumin: May be low due to protein losses.
- Serum **vitamin A** and carotene: May be low due to bile salt deficiency and impaired fat absorption.
- D-xylose test: Decreased excretion may indicate malabsorption.
- Schilling test: May indicate malabsorption of vitamin B_{12}.

Treatment

Fluid and nutrient monitoring and replacement is essential for any individual with malabsorption syndrome. Hospitalization may be required when severe fluid and electrolyte imbalances occur. Consultation with a dietitian to assist with nutritional support and meal planning is helpful. If the patient is able to eat, the diet and supplements should provide bulk and be rich in carbohydrates, **proteins**, fats, **minerals**, and **vitamins**. The patient should be encouraged to eat several small meals throughout the day, avoiding fluids and foods that promote diarrhea. Intake and output should be monitored, along with the number, color, and consistency of stools.

The individual with malabsorption syndrome must be monitored for **dehydration**, including dry tongue, mouth, and skin; increased thirst; low, concentrated urine output; or feeling weak or dizzy when standing. Pulse and **blood pressure** should be monitored for increased or irregular pulse rate, or hypotension (low blood pressure). The individual should also be alert for signs of nutrient, vitamin, and mineral depletion, including nausea or vomiting; fissures at corner of mouth; fatigue or weakness; dry, thinning hair; easy bruising; tingling in fingers or toes; and numbness or burning sensation in legs or feet. Fluid volume excess, as a result of diminished protein stores, may require fluid intake restrictions. The physician should also be notified of any shortness of breath.

Other specific medical management for malabsorption syndrome is dependent upon the cause. Treatment for tropical sprue consists of folic acid supplements and long-term antibiotics. Depending on the severity of the disorder, this treatment may be continued for six months or longer. Whipple's disease also may require long-term use of antibiotics such as tetracycline. Management of some individuals with malabsorption syndrome may require injections of vitamin B_{12} and oral iron supplements. The doctor may also prescribe enzymes to replace missing intestinal enzymes, or antispasmodics to reduce abdominal cramping and associated diarrhea. People with cystic fibrosis and chronic pancreatitis require pan-

KEY TERMS

Anemia—A decrease in the number of red blood cells in the bloodstream, characterized by pallor, loss of energy, and generalized weakness.

Atrophy—A wasting away of a tissue or organ, often caused by insufficient nutrition.

Biopsy—A tissue sample removed from the body for examination under the microscope.

Constrictive pericarditis—A condition that is characterized by a stiffening of the sac around the heart, which leads to increased pressure on the lymphatic system.

Cystic fibrosis—A hereditary genetic disorder that occurs most often in Caucasians. Thick, sticky secretions from mucus-producing glands cause blockages in the pancreatic ducts and the airways.

Edema—An excessive accumulation of fluid in the tissue spaces.

Gluten enteropathy—A hereditary malabsorption disorder caused by sensitivity to gluten, a protein found in wheat, rye, barley, and oats; also called non-tropical sprue or celiac disease.

Intestines—Also known as the bowels; intestines are divided into the large and small intestines, extending from the stomach to the anus.

Short bowel syndrome—A condition in which the bowel is not as long as normal, either because of surgery or because of a congenital defect.

Steatorrhea—An excessive amount of fat in the stool.

creatic supplements. Those with lactose intolerance or gluten enteropathy will have to modify their diets to avoid foods that they cannot properly digest.

Intestinal lymphangiectasia is treated by correcting the cause of the lymph vessel enlargement. For instance, treating constrictive pericarditis may relieve pressure on the lymph vessels. Some people improve by eating a low-fat diet and taking supplements of certain triglycerides, which are absorbed directly into the blood and not through the lymph vessels. If only a small part of the intestine is affected, it can be removed surgically.

Prognosis

The expected course for the individual with malabsorption syndrome varies, depending on the cause. The onset of symptoms may be slow and difficult to diagnose. Treatment may be long, complicated, and changed often for optimal effectiveness. Patience and a positive attitude are important in controlling or curing the disorder.

Health care team roles

The health care team should familiarize patients with their condition and the methods of dealing most effectively with their malabsorption syndrome. Physicians will typically take charge of the patient's care, ordering tests and medications. Nurses are involved in the daily care of the patient, including administering medicines. Clinical laboratory scientists and medical technologists peform laboratory tests on blood or fecal samples. Radiologic technologists perform many of the imaging studies used in diagnosis.

Prevention

Many malabsorption syndromes are hereditary. Genetic screening may prevent passing on the genes to unborn children. For infants or children, the best means of prevention of some of these hereditary conditions are by early detection at routine well-baby examinations and periodic follow-ups with school-aged and adolescent children. In some cases, however, prevention of malabsorption syndromes can consist of simply avoiding foods or substances that cause the patient an allergic reaction and/or gastrointestinal distress. Careful monitoring is necessary to prevent additional illnesses caused by nutritional deficiencies. Impure water sources should be avoided when traveling to prevent parasitic infection.

Resources

BOOKS

Institute of Medicine. *Dietary Reference Intakes: Applications in Dietary Assessment.* Washington, D.C.: National Academy Press, 2001.

Institute of Medicine. *Dietary Reference Intakes: Risk Assessment (Compass Series).* Washington, D.C.: National Academy Press, 1999.

Larson-Duyff, Roberta. *The American Dietetic Association's Complete Food & Nutrition Guide.* New York: John Wiley & Sons, 1998.

Kelsen, David, Bernard Levin, and Joel Tepper. *Principles and Practice of Gastrointestinal Oncology.* Philadelphia: Lippincott Williams & Wilkins Publishers, 2001.

Mahan, L. Kathleen, and Sylvia Escott-Stump. *Krause's Food, Nutrition, & Diet Therapy.* London: W. B. Saunders Co., 2000.

Monahan, Frances, and Marianne Neighbors. *Medical-Surgical Nursing: Foundations for Clinical Practice.* Philadelphia: W. B. Saunders Co., 1998.

Rodwell-Williams, Sue. *Essentials of Nutrition and Diet Therapy.*) London: Mosby-Year Book, 1999.

Speakman, Elizabeth, and Norma Jean Weldy. *Body Fluids and Electrolytes,* 8th ed. London: Mosby Incorporated, 2001.

PERIODICALS

Jeppesen, Palle B., et al. "Differences in Essential Fatty Acid Requirements by Enteral and Parenteral Routes of Administration in Patients with Fat Malabsorption." *American Journal of Clinical Nutrition* (1999): 70: 78-84.

Misbah, S.A., and N. P. Mapstone. "Whipple's Disease Revisited." *Journal of Clinical Pathology* (2000): 53: 750-55.

Murphy, Jane, et al. "Fat Malabsorption in Cystic Fibrosis Patients." *American Journal of Clinical Nutrition* (1999): 70: a943-a944.

ORGANIZATIONS

American Dietetic Association. 216 W. Jackson Blvd., Chicago, IL 60606-6995. (312) 899-0040. <http://www.eatright.org/>.

Food and Nutrition Information Center Agricultural Research Service, USDA. National Agricultural Library, Room 304, 10301 Baltimore Avenue, Beltsville, MD 20705-2351. (301) 504-5719. (301) 504-6409. <http://www.nal.usda.gov/fnic/>. fnic@nal.usda.gov.

OTHER

"Malabsorption." 2001. <http://www.thriveonline.com>.

Crystal Heather Kaczkowski, M.Sc.

Malabsorption tests

Definition

Malabsorption tests are done to determine if a patient has dietary malabsorption or maldigestion and to help differentiate between these two conditions. Malabsorption occurs when the gastrointestinal (GI) tract cannot take up a dietary compound. This is caused by the loss of function of the cells responsible for absorption. Maldigestion occurs when an important digestive enzyme or tissue is lacking or not functioning correctly. This may be caused by genetic disorders, injury to the tissue that provides the enzyme (i.e. the **pancreas**), alterations in pH that make the enzymes inactive, or to surgery. In general, clinicians speak of both disorders as malabsorption disorders since they both result in a lack of absorption of nutrients.

Purpose

Malabsorption tests are generally used to determine why someone is malnourished or is experiencing gastrointestinal upset. Some malabsorption tests are used as a last resort because the testing procedures are complicated. The physician first needs to rule out other disorders such as ulcers in the **stomach** and intestine. In the population, the elderly are at the greatest risk for developing malabsorption disorders. Before ordering malabsorption tests, physicians may do a general screen for malnutrition. This can include tests for **proteins** that reflect nutritional status such as serum albumin and prealbumin (transthyretin); tests for serum **calcium, vitamin B$_{12}$,** folate, **iron,** and **vitamin D** to detect a deficiency of **vitamins** or **minerals**; and a peripheral **blood** smear to detect anemia, which may have a related cause.

The absorptive capacity of the gastrointestinal tract is staggering. In general, we absorb hundreds of grams of **carbohydrates,** over 100 grams of fat and 50-100 grams of amino acids per 24-hour period. This is accomplished by the mucosal cells lining the intestine. These surfaces contain many villi, small projections that increase the surface area of the intestinal wall. It is estimated the average adult human intestine has the absorptive surface area of a tennis court. Different parts of the GI tract have different functions and nutrients are broken down and absorbed in different parts.

Carbohydrate digestion begins in the mouth with salivary amylase and continues in the stomach via the action of the stomach and low pH. In the **small intestine,** pancreatic amylase and intestinal enzymes such as lactase complete carbohydrate hydrolysis, forming simple sugars that are absorbed. Any undigestible carbohydrate (fiber) is excreted in the feces. Fat digestion and absorption is very efficient, with very little fat found in the feces. Pancreatic and gastric lipases are the enzymes most responsible for the breakdown of triacylglycerides (triglycerides) into small glycerides and free fatty acids. The action of lipase requires bile salts and bile acids that are also needed to emulsify the **fats.** The free fatty acids and small glycerides produced by the hydrolysis of triglycerides are absorbed in the intestine and converted by the mucosal cells into chlyomicrons. Protein digestion begins in the stomach with the action of hydrochloric acid and pepsin, and continues in the intestine via the activity of pancreatic and intestinal proteases such as trypsin, chymotrypsin, and carboxypeptidase. The dipeptides and amino acids produced from protein hydrolysis are absorbed via complex mechanisms by the intestinal epithelial cells.

Malabsorption of nutrients can cause painful GI symptoms and over time cause malnutrition. Patients lose vitamins and minerals along with basic nutrients. Some malabsorption syndromes can cause **dehydration** since they produce **diarrhea**. Diagnosing the cause of malabsorption is difficult, and doctors will try many different testing approaches. Malabsorption can be caused by many things including:

- Pancreatic insufficiency, caused by inflammation of the pancreas (**pancreatitis**), obstruction of the pancreatic duct, pancreatic **cancer**, inherited deficiency of pancreatic enzymes.

- Defective stimulation of the stomach due to illness or surgery. Muscles in the stomach need to contract to mix up the food with digestive enzymes and acid.

- Elevated pH of stomach acid (hypoacidity or achlorhydria).

- Lack of bile acids due to obstruction (gallstones or tumors) or due to **liver** disease.

- Bacterial overgrowth in the lower intestine.

- Food **allergies** such as celiac disease.

- Inflammation of the intestines or colon, such as colitis, **Crohn's disease**, inflammatory bowel syndrome.

- Parasitic infections, such as Whipple's disease or tropical sprue.

- Lack of enzymes in the intestine. For example, lactase deficiency causes lactose intolerance, a very common cause of malabsorption in adults.

- Surgical removal of parts of the intestine due to disease, or surgery to decrease the size of the stomach to promote weight loss.

- Diseases such as diabetes, **AIDS**, **cystic fibrosis**, thyroid disease, and alcoholism.

Symptoms of malabsorption are varied because the disorder effects so many systems. General symptoms may include loss of appetite (anorexia), weight loss, fatigue, shortness of breath, dehydration, low **blood pressure**, and swelling (**edema**). Nutritional disorders may cause anemia (lack of iron, folate and vitamin B_{12}), bleeding tendency (lack of **vitamin K**), or bone disease (lack of vitamin D). Gastrointestinal symptoms include flatulence, stomach distention, borborygmi (rumbling in the bowels), discomfort, diarrhea, steatorrhea (excessive fat in stool) and frequent bowel movements.

Precautions

Most malabsorption tests require a blood sample collected by venipuncture. The nurse or phlebotomist must follow **universal precautions** for the prevention of transmission of bloodborne pathogens. Most of the tests done to measure malabsorption are relatively safe but do require some effort on the patient's part. Many require an overnight fast. Some patients who need malabsorption tests may be malnurished or dehydrated. Clinicians should watch for low blood pressure, weakness, thirst, concentrated urine (dehydration), and dizziness. Some tests require ingestion of highly concentrated nutrients that may be difficult for the patient to digest. Asking patients to collect urine or feces over a long time period can cause problems with compliance. It is important to make sure the patient understands the test and why he or she must comply. Clinical laboratories will reject any samples that appear to have been collected or stored incorrectly.

Description

Breath hydrogen test

The breath hydrogen test is used to measure two things, carbohydrate malabsorption such as lactose intolerance and bacterial overgrowth. Hydrogen is produced by bacterial fermentation of unabsorbed carbohydrates in the intestines. Bacterial overgrowth can occur in this situation because there is a large food supply. The hydrogen produced goes into the blood stream and is excreted through the **lungs**. The test is done using a gas chromatograph, an apparatus that can separate compounds from one another based on their chemical composition. The patient is asked to fast overnight, and his or her breath is collected in a plastic syringe at the start of the test. The patient is then given something to eat depending on what is being evaluated. If the doctor suspects that the patient has trouble absorbing carbohydrates, then he or she may be given rice, glucose or fructose. If lactose intolerance is suspected, the patient is given a food containing lactose such as milk. For general bacterial overgrowth tests, the patient will be given glucose. The patient's breath will be collected in a plastic syringe every thirty minutes for the next two to five hours, depending on the test. The syringe will be capped and sent to the laboratory for analysis. The test is simple and non-invasive and while not diagnostic, it gives the doctor an idea of what may be wrong.

D-xylose absorption test

D-xylose is a sugar that is not normally found in the blood. It can be easily absorbed by healthy intestinal cells without the aid of pancreatic enzymes, and is poorly metabolized so that at least 50% of the dose is excreted in the urine within 24 hours. This test is a good general screen for malfunction of absorption, and helps to differentiate intestinal malabsorption syndromes (reduced D-xylose absorption) from pancreatitis (normal D-xylose absorption). Adults are given an oral dose (usually 25 grams) of D-xylose. A five-hour timed urine sample is collected, and a blood sample is collected two hours after the dose is given. Children are given a 5 gram dose of D-xylose, and a blood sample is collected one hour after the dose is given. Adults should excrete at least 25% of the dose in the five-hour urine sample, and have a two-hour blood level of at least 25 mg/dL. Children should have a one-hour blood level of at least 20 mg/dL. The D-xylose test will be normal if the patient has normal absorptive capacity in the intestine, or if the patient has malabsorption that is caused by a pancreatic problem. It will be low if the patient has celiac disease, tropical sprue, Crohn's disease, advanced AIDs, or pellegra (**niacin** deficiency).

Tests for celiac disease

Celiac disease is a disorder characterized by antibodies to gluten, a protein found in wheat. The disease produces lesions in the intestine and decreases the tissue's ability to absorb many different nutrients. Patients have diarrhea and lose weight over time. The lesions will improve when foods containing gluten are removed from the diet. Tests for this disease involve drawing the patient's blood and testing for the presence of three antibodies, antigliadin, antiendomysium, and antireticulin antibodies. Patients with celiac disease are followed closely by their doctors, even after dietary changes, because they are more prone to developing intestinal cancers and intestinal ulcerations.

Stool fat testing

Stool fat testing, measuring fats in the feces, is a sensitive way to determine if the patient has fat malabsorption but the test does not differentiate between pancreatic and intestinal causes. Fat is normally absorbed very efficiently by the intestinal cells. High levels of fat in the feces causes steatorrhea, a type of feces that appears pale in color and greasy. Before the test, the patient is put on a high fat diet, consuming between 50-150 g/day of fat for three days. The patient must collect their feces over the next 72 hours using a 1-gallon paint can that can be well sealed. The fecal sample must be refrigerated to prevent any bacterial action. Fecal fat analysis is performed by first weighing the sample and then extracting the **lipids** with an organic solvent. The extraction solvent is evaporated and the dry weight of the fat that remains is measured. Normal absorption of fat is indicated by a fecal fat level of less than or equal to 7 grams per day.

A more simple but less accurate way to measure fat absorption is to count the fat droplets in a well mixed sample of the stool specimen using a **microscope** and a neutral fat stain. Another simplified screening test is the fat tolerance test called the butterfat or the fatty meal test.

The patient is asked to fast overnight and is given 1 gram of fat per kg of body weight. This is a substantial amount of fat and usually is given as 1 gram of butter per Kg spread on a piece of toast or as 6 ounces of corn oil. Blood is drawn before the dose and again three and six hours afterwards. The fasting, three-hour and six-hour plasma samples are analyzed for triglyceride concentration. Normal absorption is indicated by at least a 50% increase in triglycerides over the fasting level.

Preparation

The patient should be advised about the test he or she is taking and what the testing procedure involves. It is important with all tests, except the celiac antibody tests, that the patient fasts overnight. This allows the clinician to determine a "baseline" or starting value. Patients who are required to collect a 72-hour fecal sample must seal the sample well and keep it refrigerated to prevent any degradation.

Aftercare

Some patients may feel sick after the procedures since they are being exposed to compounds that they may have trouble absorbing. Nurses should be careful to discuss any side effects with the patient beforehand, and the patient should be given the smallest amount of substance possible to avoid problems. In addition, patients may be malnourished and need something to eat and drink once the procedure is over.

Complications

The hydrogen breath test may not be accurate if the patient is a smoker, has pulmonary disease, is not fasting or is hyperventilating. Patients being measured for bacterial overgrowth must not only fast overnight, but avoid fiber-rich foods for three days before the test. Patients taking the fecal fat test must remain on a high fat diet before and during the test.

Falsely low results with the D-xylose test will be seen if the pateint has been vomiting, has gastric stasis, fluid build up (ascites), fluid retention (edema) or bacterial overgrowth. There is a decrease in urinary excretion of D-xylose with aspirin, colchicine, digitalis, MAO inhibitors, food consumption, neomycin and opiates. In addition, excretion is lower in those with impaired renal function and in elderly patients.

Results

D-xylose absorption should be greater than 1.2 g/5 hours with a 5 g dose of D-xylose and 4.0 g/5 hours in an

KEY TERMS

Absorption—Process of taking up digested food substances into the cells and blood stream of the body.

Carbohydrate—A macromolecule (large molecule) that is made of sugars or starch.

Diarrhea—Excessive production of feces. This is usually due to a large amount of water in the stool.

Fats—A macromolecule that is not soluble in water. Fats are also called lipids.

Gastrointestinal—Having to do with the stomach and intestines.

Gluten—One of the proteins found in wheat products.

Lactase—An enzyme that breaks down lactose.

Lipase—An enzyme that breaks down fats.

Mucosa—The cells lining the digestive tract. These cells secrete mucus to protect themselves from digestion.

Protease—An enzyme that breaks down proteins.

Protein—A macromolecule that is made of amino acids.

Steatorhhea—Feces that contain a high level of fat due to poor fat absorption in the GI tract.

Villi—Projections of tissue into the intestine that increase the surface area.

adult given a 25 g dose of D-xylose. Fecal fat should be less than 7 g/day in adults and less than 2 g/day in a child. Hydrogen breath test results are based on the baseline value, which in most people should be extremely low. The results are measured in parts per million and the actual numbers depend on the sugar or carbohydrate given. Abnormal results with the celiac tests are any antibodies measured since healthy people do not generate antibodies to gluten protein.

Health care team roles

Malabsorption tests are ordered by a physician. The malabsorption tests call for a skilled team of nurses and dieticians who administer the tests. Clinical laboratory scientists/medical technologists perform malabsorption tests, and the physician interprets the result.

Resources

BOOKS

Burtis, Carl A. and Edward R. Ashwood. *Tietz Textbook of Clinical Chemistry.* Philadelphia: W.B. Saunders Company, 1999.

Kaplan, Lawrence A. and Amadeo J. Pesce. *Clinical Chemistry Theory, Analysis and Correlation.* St. Louis: Mosby Publishing, 1996.

Jane E. Phillips, Ph.D.

Malaria

Definition

Malaria is a serious, infectious disease spread by certain mosquitoes. It is most common in tropical climates. It is characterized by recurrent symptoms of chills, **fever**, and an enlarged spleen. The disease can be treated with medication, but it often recurs. Malaria is endemic (occurs frequently in a particular locality) in many third world countries. Isolated, small outbreaks sometimes occur within the boundaries of the United States.

Description

Malaria is not a serious problem in the United States. Within the last decade, only about 1,200 cases have been reported each year in this country, mostly by people who were infected elsewhere. Locally transmitted malaria has occurred in California, Florida, Texas, Michigan, New Jersey, and New York City. While malaria can be transmitted in **blood**, the American blood supply is not screened for malaria. Widespread malarial epidemics are far less likely to occur in the United States, but small, localized epidemics could return to the western world.

The picture is far more bleak outside the territorial boundaries of the United States. A recent government panel warned that disaster looms over Africa from the disease. Malaria infects between 300 and 500 million people every year in Africa, India, southeast Asia, the Middle East, Oceania, and Central and South America. About 2 million of the infected die each year. Most of the cases and almost all of the deaths occur in sub-Saharan Africa. At the present time, malaria kills about twice as many people each year as does **AIDS**. As many as half a billion people worldwide are left with chronic anemia due to malaria **infection**. In some parts of Africa, people battle up to 40 or more separate episodes of malaria in their lifetimes. The spread of malaria is becoming even more serious as the parasites that cause malaria develop resistance to the drugs used to treat the condition.

Causes and symptoms

Human malaria is caused by four different species of a parasite called plasmodium: *Plasmodium falciparum* (the most deadly), *P. vivax, P. malariae,* and *P. ovale.* The last two are fairly uncommon. Many animals can get malaria but human malaria does not spread to animals. In turn, animal malaria does not spread to humans.

A person gets malaria when bitten by a female mosquito who is looking for a blood meal and is infected with the malaria parasite. The parasites enter the blood stream and travel to the **liver**, where they multiply. When they re-emerge into the blood, symptoms appear. By the time a person shows symptoms, the parasites have reproduced very rapidly, clogging **blood vessels** and rupturing blood cells.

Malaria cannot be casually transmitted directly from one person to another. Instead, a mosquito bites an infected person and then passes the infection on to the next human it bites. It is also possible to spread malaria via contaminated needles or in blood transfusions. This is why all blood donors are carefully screened with questionnaires for possible exposure to malaria.

The amount of time between the mosquito bite and the appearance of symptoms varies, depending on the strain of parasite involved. The incubation period is usually between eight and 12 days for falciparum malaria, but it can be as long as a month for the other types. Symptoms from some strains of *P. vivax* may not appear until eight to 10 months after the mosquito bite occurred.

The primary symptom of all types of malaria is the "malaria ague" (chills and fever). In most cases, the fever has three stages, beginning with uncontrollable shivering for an hour or two, followed by a rapid spike in temperature (as high as 106°F, or 41.1°C), which lasts for three to six hours. Then, just as suddenly, the affected person begins to sweat profusely, which will quickly bring down the fever. Other symptoms may include fatigue, severe headache, or nausea, and vomiting. As the sweating subsides, an individual typically feels exhausted and falls asleep. In many cases, this cycle of chills, fever, and sweating occurs every other day, or every third day, and may last for between a week and a month. Those with the chronic form of malaria may have a relapse as long as 50 years after the initial infection.

Falciparum malaria is far more severe than other types of malaria because the parasite attacks all red blood cells, not just the young or old cells, as do other types. It causes the red blood cells to become very "sticky." A person with this type of malaria can die within hours of the first symptoms. The fever is prolonged. So many red blood cells are destroyed that they block the blood vessels in vital organs (especially the **kidneys**), and the spleen becomes enlarged. There may be **brain** damage, leading to **coma** and convulsions. The kidneys and liver may fail.

Malaria in **pregnancy** can lead to premature delivery, **miscarriage**, or stillbirth.

Certain kinds of mosquitoes (called anopheles) can pick up the parasite by biting an infected human. (The more common kinds of mosquitoes in the United States do not transmit the infection.) This is true for as long as that human has parasites in the blood. Since strains of malaria do not protect against each other, it is possible to be re-infected with the parasites again and again. It is also possible to develop a chronic infection without developing an effective **immune response**.

Diagnosis

Malaria is diagnosed by examining blood under a **microscope**. The parasite can be seen in the blood smears on a slide. These blood smears may need to be repeated over a 72-hour period to make an accurate diagnosis. Antibody tests are not usually helpful because many people developed antibodies from past infections, and the tests may not be readily available.

Anyone who becomes ill with chills and fever after being in an area where malaria exists must see a doctor and mention the recent travel to endemic areas. A person with the above symptoms who has been in a high-risk area should insist on a blood test for malaria. The doctor may believe the symptoms are just the common flu virus. Malaria is often misdiagnosed by North American doctors who are not used to seeing the disease. Delaying treatment of falciparum malaria can be fatal.

Treatment

Falciparum malaria is a medical emergency that must be treated in a hospital. The type of drugs, the method of giving them, and the length of the treatment depend on where the malaria was contracted and how sick is the affected person.

For all strains except falciparum, the treatment for malaria is usually chloroquine (Aralen) by mouth for three days. Those falciparum strains suspected to be resistant to chloroquine are usually treated with a combination of quinine and tetracycline. In countries where quinine resistance is developing, other treatments may include clindamycin (Cleocin), mefloquin (Lariam), or sulfadoxone/pyrimethamine (Fansidar). Most persons

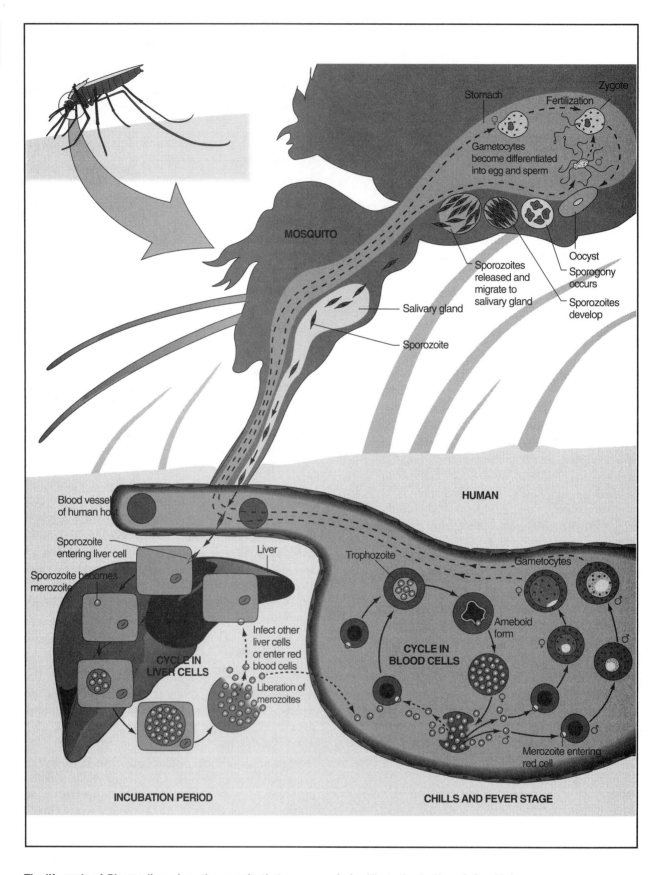

The life cycle of *Plasmodium vivax*, the parasite that causes malaria. *(Illustration by Hans & Cassidy.)*

GALE ENCYCLOPEDIA OF NURSING AND ALLIED HEALTH

receive an antibiotic for seven days. Those who are very ill may need intensive care and intravenous (IV) malaria treatment for the first three days.

Anyone who acquired falciparum malaria in the Dominican Republic, Haiti, Central America west of the Panama Canal, the Middle East, or Egypt can still be cured with chloroquine. Almost all strains of falciparum malaria in Africa, South Africa, India, and southeast Asia are now resistant to chloroquine. In Thailand and Cambodia, there are strains of falciparum malaria that have some resistance to almost all known drugs.

A person with falciparum malaria needs to be hospitalized and given antimalarial drugs in different combinations and doses depending on the resistance of the strain. The individual may need IV fluids, red blood cell transfusions, **kidney dialysis**, and assistance breathing.

A drug called primaquine may prevent relapses after recovery from *P. vivax* or *P. ovale*. These relapses are caused by a form of the parasite that remains in the liver and can reactivate months or years later.

Another new drug, halofantrine, is available abroad. While it is licensed in the United States, it is not marketed in this country and it is not recommended by the Centers for Disease Control and Prevention in Atlanta, Georgia.

Preventing mosquito bites while in the tropics is an important way to avoid malaria.

Alternative treatment

The Chinese herb qiinghaosu (the western name is artemisinin) has been used in China and southeast Asia to fight severe malaria, and became available in Europe in 1994. Because this treatment often fails, it is usually combined with another antimalarial drug (mefloquine) to boost its effectiveness. It is not available in the United States and other parts of the developed world due to fears of its toxicity, in addition to licensing and other issues.

A western herb called wormwood (*Artemesia annua*) that is taken as a daily dose can be effective against malaria. Protecting the liver with herbs like goldenseal (*Hydrastis canadensis*), Chinese goldenthread (*Coptis chinensis*), and milk thistle (*Silybum marianum*) can be used as preventive treatment.

Prognosis

If treated in the early stages, malaria can be cured. Those who live in areas where malaria is epidemic, however, can contract the disease repeatedly, never fully recovering between bouts of acute infection.

Health care team roles

Physicians, assisted by laboratory technicians, usually make a diagnosis of malaria. Nurses may provide prevention education and support during recovery from malaria ague.

Prevention

Several researchers are currently working on a malarial vaccine, but the complex life cycle of the malaria parasite makes it difficult. A parasite has much more genetic material than a virus or bacterium. For this reason, a successful vaccine has not yet been developed.

Malaria is an especially difficult disease to vaccinate against because the parasite goes through several separate stages. One recent, promising vaccine appears to have protected up to 60% of people exposed to malaria. This was evident during field trials for the drug that were conducted in South America and Africa. It is not yet commercially available.

The World Health Association (WHO) has been trying to eliminate malaria for the past 30 years by controlling mosquitoes. Their efforts were successful as long as the pesticide DDT killed mosquitoes and antimalarial drugs cured those who were infected. Today, however, the problem has returned a hundredfold, especially in Africa. Because both the mosquito and parasite are now extremely resistant to the insecticides designed to kill them, governments are now trying to teach people to take antimalarial drugs as a preventive medicine and avoid being bitten by mosquitoes.

Travelers to high-risk areas should use insect repellent containing DEET for exposed skin. Because DEET is toxic in large amounts, children should not use a concentration higher than 35%. DEET should not be inhaled. It should not be rubbed onto the eye area, on any broken or irritated skin, or on children's hands. It should be thoroughly washed off after coming indoors.

Individuals who use the following preventive measures get fewer infections than those who do not:

- Between dusk and dawn, remain indoors in well-screened areas.

- Sleep inside pyrethrin or permethrin repellent-soaked mosquito nets.

- Wear clothes over the entire body.

Anyone visiting endemic areas should take antimalarial drugs starting a day or two before leaving the United States. The drugs used are usually chloroquine or mefloquine. This treatment is continued through at least four weeks after leaving the endemic area. However,

Malaria

KEY TERMS

Arteminisinins—An antimalarial family of products derived from an ancient Chinese herbal remedy. Two of the most popular varieties are artemether and artesunate, used mainly in southeast Asia in combination with mefloquine.

Chloroquine—This antimalarial drug was first used in the 1940s, until the first evidence of quinine resistance appeared in the 1960s. It is now ineffective against falciparum malaria almost everywhere. However, because it is inexpensive, it is still the antimalarial drug most widely used in Africa. Native individuals with partial immunity may have better results with chloroquine than a traveler with no previous exposure.

Mefloquine—An antimalarial drug that was developed by the United States Army in the early 1980s. Today, malaria resistance to this drug has become a problem in some parts of Asia (especially Thailand and Cambodia).

Quinine—One of the first treatments for malaria, quinine is a natural product made from the bark of the Cinchona tree. It was popular until being superseded by the development of chloroquine in the 1940s. In the wake of widespread chloroquine resistance, however, it has become popular again. It or its close relative quinidine can be given intravenously to treat severe falciparum malaria.

Sulfadoxone/pyrimethamine (Fansidar)—This antimalarial drug developed in the 1960s is the first drug tried in some parts of the world where chloroquine resistance is widespread. It has been associated with severe allergic reactions due to its sulfa component.

even those who take antimalarial drugs and are careful to avoid mosquito bites can still contract malaria.

International travelers are at risk for becoming infected. Most Americans who have acquired falciparum malaria were visiting sub-Saharan Africa. Travelers in Asia and South America are less at risk. Travelers who stay in air conditioned hotels on tourist itineraries in urban or resort areas are at lower risk than backpackers, missionaries, and Peace Corps volunteers. Some people in western cities where malaria does not usually exist may acquire the infection from a mosquito carried onto a jet. This is called airport or runway malaria.

Resources

BOOKS

Humphreys, Margaret. *Malaria in the United States: Poverty, Race, and Public Health.* Baltimore: Johns Hopkins University Press, 2001.

Krause, Peter J. "Malaria." In *Nelson Textbook of Pediatrics, 16th ed.,* edited by Richard E. Behrman et al. Philadelphia: Saunders, 2000, 1049-1052.

Krogstad, Donald J. "Malaria." In *Cecil Textbook of Medicine, 21st ed.,* edited by Goldman, Lee and Bennett, J. Claude. Philadelphia: W.B. Saunders, 2000, 1947-1951.

Poser, Charles M. and Bruyn, G.W. *An Illustrated History of Malaria.* New York: Parthenon Publishing Group, 1999.

White, Nicholas J. and Bremen, Joel G. "Malaria and Other Diseases Caused by Red Blood Cell Parasites." In *Harrison's Principles of Internal Medicine, 14th ed.,* edited by Anthony S. Fauci, et al. New York: McGraw-Hill, 1998, 1180-1189.

PERIODICALS

Albrecht, H., Lennox, J., del Rio, C. "Quinidine and malaria." *Archives of Internal Medicine* 161, no. 8 (2001): 1118-1119.

Arya, S.C. "Limitations of Rapid Tests for Malaria Diagnosis by Travelers." *Journal of Travel Medicine* 7, no. 6 (2000): 340-342.

Etchegorry, M.G., Matthys F., Galinski M., White N.J., Nosten F. "Malaria Epidemic in Burundi." *Lancet* 357, no. 9261 (2001): 1046-1047.

Kerr, C. "Malaria Vaccine News." *Trends in Microbiology* 9, no. 5 (2001): 202-207.

Lawler, S. "Boost for Development of Malaria Vaccine." *Trends in Cellular Biology* 11, no. 4 (2001): 151-157.

Marshall, H. "Vaccine Prevents Malaria Parasite from Infecting Mosquitoes." *Trends in Immunology* 22, no. 3 (2001): 125-132.

Smith, T.A., Leuenberger, R., Lengeler, C. "Child Mortality and Malaria Transmission Intensity in Africa." *Trends in Parasitology* 17, no. 3 (2001): 145-149.

Taverne, J. "Malaria, HIV and Mosquito Control on the Web." *Trends in Parasitology* 17, no. 3 (2001): 155-156.

Taylor-Robinson, A. "Immunity to Malaria Increases During puberty." *Trends in Parasitology* 17, no. 5 (2001): 213-215.

Taylor-Robinson, A. "Rationale for Malaria Anti-toxin Therapy." *Trends in Parasitology* 17, no. 3 (2001): 119-124.

ORGANIZATIONS

Centers for Disease Control and Prevention, 1600 Clifton Road, Atlanta, GA 30333. (404) 639-3534 or (800) 311-3435. <http://www.cdc.gov/nchstp/tb/faqs/qa.htm>; <http://www.cdc.gov/netinfo.htm>.

Pan American Health Organization, 525 Twenty-third Street, NW, Washington, D.C. 20037. (202)974-3000. Fax: (202)974-3663. <http://www.paho.org/>; webmaster@paho.org.

World Health Organization, Communicable Diseases, 20 Avenue Appia, 1211 Geneva 27, Switzerland. +41 (22) 791 4140. Fax: +41 (22) 791 4268. <http://www.who.int/gtb/>, tuberculosis@who.org.

OTHER

Centers for Disease Control and Prevention. <http://www.cdc.gov/travel/malinfo.htm> and <http://www.cdc.gov/ncidod/dpd/parasites/malaria/default.htm>.

Malaria Foundation International. <http://www.malaria.org/>.

Malaria Vaccine Initiative. <http://www.malariavaccine.org/>.

Medical Research Programme of South Africa. <http://www.malaria.org.za/>.

National Institutes of Health. <http://mim.nih.gov/>.

World Health Organization Malaria Fact Sheets. <http://www.who.int/health-topics/malaria.htm> and <http://www.who.int/inf-fs/en/fact094.html. >.

World Health Organization Tropical Disease Research. <http://www.wehi.edu.au/MalDB-www/who.html>.

L. Fleming Fallon, Jr., M.D., Dr.P.H.

Male infertility *see* **Infertility**

Male reproductive system *see* **Reproductive system, male**

Malignant lymphomas

Definition

Malignant lymphomas are a group of cancers in which cells of the **lymphatic system** become abnormal and start to grow uncontrollably and spread (metastasize) throughout the body. Because lymph tissue is in many parts of the body, lymphomas can start in almost any organ of the body. Lymphomas are classified as being either non-Hodgkin's lymphoma or Hodgkin's disease.

Description

The lymph system is made up of ducts or tubules that carry lymph to all parts of the body. Lymph is a milky fluid that contains the lymphocytes or white **blood** cells, as well as protein and waste products. These are the infection-fighting cells of the blood. Small pea-shaped organs are found along the network of lymph vessels. These are called the lymph nodes, and their main function is to make and store lymphocytes. Clusters of lymph nodes are found in the pelvis region, underarm, neck, chest, and abdomen. The spleen, the tonsils, and the thymus are part of the lymphatic system.

The lymphocyte is the main cell of the lymphoid tissue. There are two main types of lymphocytes: the T lymphocyte and the B lymphocyte. Lymphomas develop from these two cell types. B cell lymphomas are more common among adults; while among children, the incidence of T and B cell lymphomas is almost equal.

The T and the B cell perform different jobs within the **immune system**. When an infectious bacterium enters the body, the B cell makes **proteins** called "antibodies." These antibodies attach themselves to the **bacteria** and flag them for destruction by other immune cells. The T cells help protect the body against **viruses**. When a virus enters the cell, it generally produces certain proteins that are projected on the surface of the infected cell. T cells recognize these proteins and produce certain substances (cytokines) that destroy the infected cells. Some of the cytokines made by the T cells attract other cell types, which are capable of digesting the virus-infected cell. The T cells can also destroy some types of cancerous cells.

Lymphomas can be divided into two main types: Hodgkin's lymphoma or Hodgkin's disease, and non-Hodgkin's lymphomas. The two are distinguished by cell type and have similar symptoms. Non-Hodgkin's lymphomas are more common, with at least 30 different types. Hodgkin's primarily affects individuals 15–40 years of age, while Non-Hodgkin's occurs mainly in persons between the ages of 30–70.

Lymphomas are grouped (staged) by how aggressively they grow—slow growing (low grade, mostly found in B-cell types), intermediate growing (seen in both B-cell and T-cell types), and rapidly growing (high grade, seen in both B-cell and T-cell types)—and how far they spread. Lymphomas are also staged by the Roman numerals I, II, III, and IV. These stages indicate the following:

- Stage I. There is only one **cancer** site. No bone marrow involvement found.

- Stage II. Two sites are found, either above or below the diaphragm. There is no bone marrow involvement.

- Stage III. Sites are found above and below the diaphragm, but there is still no bone marrow involvement.

- Stage IV. The bone marrow is involved and the cancer cells have metastasized beyond the lymphatic system.

A majority of non-Hodgkin's lymphomas begin in the lymph nodes. About 20% start in other organs, such as the **lungs**, **liver**, or the gastrointestinal tract. Malignant lymphocytes multiply uncontrollably and do not perform their normal functions. Hence, the body's ability to fight infections is affected. In addition, these malignant cells may crowd the bone marrow and, depending on the stage,

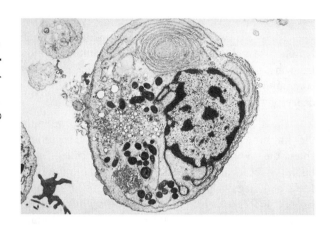

A close-up view of a malignant lymph cell. *(Custom Medical Stock Photo. Reproduced by permission.)*

prevent the production of normal red blood cells, white blood cells, and platelets. A low red blood cell count causes anemia, while a reduction in the number of platelets makes the person susceptible to excessive bleeding. Cancerous cells can also invade other organs through the circulatory system of the lymph, causing those organs to malfunction.

In 2001, an estimated 56,200 Americans received a diagnosis of non-Hodgkin's lymphoma, and approximately 16,300 people died from malignant lymphomas. It is the fifth most common cancer in the country (not including nonmelanoma skin cancers). The incidence of non-Hodgkin's lymphoma has nearly doubled since the 1970s; however, during the 1990s the rate began to decline. The increase was related both to an actual increase in the number of cases as well as improved methods of detecting the disease. Over 95% of non-Hodgkin's lymphomas occur in adults, with the average age at diagnosis being in the early 40s. The disease more commonly occurs in men than women, and whites are affected to a greater extent than Asian Americans or African Americans.

Causes and symptoms

The exact cause of non-Hodgkin's lymphomas is not known. However, the incidence has increased significantly in recent years. Part of the increase is due to the **AIDS** epidemic. Individuals infected with the AIDS virus have a higher likelihood of developing non-Hodgkin's lymphomas.

People exposed to certain pesticides and ionizing radiation have a higher than average chance of developing this disease. For example, an increased incidence of lymphomas has been seen in survivors of the atomic bomb explosion in Hiroshima, and in people who have undergone aggressive radiation therapy. People who suf-

fer from immune-deficient (**immunodeficiency**) disorders and those who have been treated with immune suppressive drugs for transplants or for conditions such as rheumatoid arthritis and autoimmune diseases are at an increased risk for this disease.

Some studies have shown a loose association between retroviruses, such as HTLV-I, and some rare forms of lymphoma. The Epstein-Barr virus has been linked to Burkitt's lymphoma in African countries. However, a direct cause-and-effect relationship has not been established.

The symptoms of lymphomas are often vague and non-specific. The signs and symptoms may differ, depending on the location of the involvement. Patients may experience loss of appetite, weight loss, nausea, vomiting, abdominal discomfort, and indigestion. The patient may complain of a feeling of fullness, which is a result of enlarged lymph nodes in the abdomen. Sometimes the abdomen can become so swollen it may resemble **pregnancy** in a woman. Pressure or **pain** in the lower back is another symptom. In the advanced stages, the patient may have bone pain, headaches, constant coughing, and abnormal pressure and congestion in the face, neck, and upper chest. Some may have fevers and night sweats. In most cases, patients go to the doctor because of the presence of swollen glands in the neck, armpits, or groin area. Since all the symptoms are common to many other illnesses, it is essential to seek medical attention if any of the conditions persist for two weeks or more. Only a qualified physician can correctly diagnose whether the symptoms are due to lymphoma or some other ailment.

Diagnosis

Like all cancers, lymphomas are best treated when found early. However, it is often difficult to diagnose lymphomas. There are no screening tests available; and, since the symptoms are non-specific, lymphomas are rarely recognized in their early stages. Detection often occurs by chance during a routine **physical examination**.

When the doctor suspects lymphoma, a complete medical history is taken and a thorough physical examination is performed. Enlargement of the lymph nodes, liver, or spleen may suggest lymphomas. Blood tests will determine the cell counts and obtain information on how well the organs, such as the kidney and liver, are functioning.

A biopsy of the enlarged lymph node is the most definitive diagnostic tool for staging purposes. The doctor may perform a bone marrow biopsy. During the biopsy, a cylindrical piece of bone and marrow fluid is removed. They are generally taken out of the hipbone. These samples are sent to the laboratory for examination. In addition to diagnosis, the biopsy may also be repeated during the treatment phase of the disease to see if the lymphoma is responding to therapy.

Once the exact form of lymphoma is known, it is then staged to determine how aggressive it is, and how far it has spread. Staging is necessary to plan appropriate treatment.

Conventional imaging tests, such as x rays, computed tomography scans (**CT scans**), **magnetic resonance imaging** (MRI), and abdominal sonograms, are used to determine how far the disease has spread.

Rarely, a lumbar puncture or a spinal tap is performed to check if malignant cells are present in the fluid surrounding the **brain**. In this test, the physician inserts a needle into the epidural space at the base of the spine and collects a small amount of spinal fluid for microscopic examination.

Treatment

Much progress has been made in the treatment of non-Hodgkin's lymphoma. Treatment options for lymphomas depend on the type of lymphoma and its present stage. In most cases, treatment consists of **chemotherapy**, **radiotherapy**, or a combination of the two methods.

Chemotherapy is the use of anti-cancer drugs to kill cancer cells. In non-Hodgkin's lymphomas, combination therapy, which involves the use of multiple drugs, has been found more effective than single drug use. The treatment may last about six months, but in some cases may last as long as a year. The drugs may either be administered intravenously or given orally in the form of pills. If cancer cells have invaded the **central nervous system**, then chemotherapeutic drugs may be injected, through a needle in the brain or back, into the fluid that surrounds the brain. This procedure is known as intrathecal chemotherapy.

Radiation therapy, where high-energy ionizing rays are directed at specific portions of the body, such as the upper chest, abdomen, pelvis, or neck, is often used for treatment of lymphomas. External radiation therapy, where the rays are directed from a source outside the body, is the most common mode of radiation treatment.

Stem cell transplantation is used in cases where the lymphomas do not respond to conventional therapy, or in cases where the patient has had a relapse or suffers from recurrent lymphomas. However, one study done in the Netherlands suggested that patients may do just as well with a standard chemotherapy regimen rather than the transplant.

There are two ways of performing stem cell transplantation. In a procedure called "allogeneic stem cell transplant," a donor is found whose cells match that of the patient. The donor can be a twin (best match), a sibling, or a person who is not related at all. High-dose chemotherapy or radiation therapy is given to eradicate the lymphoma. The donor stem cells are then given to replace those destroyed by the therapy.

In "autologous stem cell transplantation," some of the patient's own stem cells are collected, "purged" of lymphoma cells, and frozen. High-dose chemotherapy and radiation therapy are given. The stem cells that were taken and frozen are then thawed and put back into the patient's body to replace the destroyed marrow. One of the serious risks of autologous stem cell transplants is that it is possible for some of the lymphoma cells to remain even after purging the stem cells.

There are no proven alternative treatments for non-Hodgkin's lymphoma. However, many complementary therapies, including **vitamins** and herbal remedies, massage, and acupuncture, may help persons going through treatment to better cope with the side effects they might experience. Because many of these therapies have not been studied thoroughly, it is not known which ones may be potentially harmful or helpful. Therefore, the patient with lymphoma should be advised to speak with their health care professional prior to trying any alternative or complementary treatment.

Prognosis

Like all cancers, the prognosis for lymphoma depends on the stage of the cancer, and the patient's age and general health. When all the different types and stages of lymphoma are considered together, only 50% of patients survive five years or more after initial diagnosis. This is because some types of lymphoma are more aggressive than others. Patients with T-cell lymphomas generally have a worse prognosis than those with B-cell types.

The five-year survival rate for those with non-Hodgkin's lymphoma rose from 31% in 1960 to 51% in 1994. The overall survival rate among children, 78%, is definitely better than among older people. About 90% of the children diagnosed with early stage disease survive five years or more, while only 60%–70% of adults diagnosed with low grade lymphomas survive for five years or more.

KEY TERMS

Antibodies—Proteins made by the B lymphocytes in response to the presence of infectious agents such as bacteria or viruses in the body.

Autoimmune disease—A disease caused by a person's own antibodies or T cells that attack molecules, cells, or tissues.

Biopsy—The surgical removal and microscopic examination of living tissue for diagnostic purposes.

Growth factors (cytokines)—Chemicals made by the cells that act on other cells to stimulate or inhibit their function. Cytokines that stimulate growth are called "growth factors."

Metastasize—The spread of a disease, such as a cancer, from its original site to another part of the body.

Health care team roles

Many members of the health care team will work with the lymphoma patient. The primary physician may initially suspect lymphoma and order the appropriate diagnostic workup. The surgeon performs the biopsy, and the pathologist confirms the cellular diagnosis. Various x-ray and lab technicians will perform other imaging studies. Specially trained nurses administer chemotherapy and will instruct the patient on all aspects of his diagnosis and treatment. The patient may see both a medical and radiation oncologist, depending upon the specifics of the treatment ordered. Registered nurses also provide part-time family education.

Prevention

Although many cancers may be prevented by making diet and life style changes which reduce risk factors, there is currently no known way to prevent lymphomas. Protecting oneself from developing AIDS, which may be a risk factor for lymphomas, is the only preventive measure that can be practiced.

No special tests are available for early detection of non-Hodgkin's lymphomas. Paying prompt attention to the signs and symptoms of this disease and seeing a doctor if the symptoms persist are the best strategies for an early diagnosis of lymphoma. Early detection affords the best chance for a cure.

Resources

BOOKS

Beers, Mark H. and Robert Berkow, eds. *The Merck Manual of Diagnosis and Therapy.* 17th ed. Whitehouse Station, NJ: Merck and Company, Inc., 1999.

PERIODICALS

"Bexxar Highly Effective First-Line Treatment" *Vaccine Weekly* (June 7, 2000).

Gottlieb, Scott. "Bone Marrow Transplants Show No Benefit For Non-Hodgkin's Lymphoma" *British Medical Journal* (January 20, 2001): 127.

ORGANIZATIONS

American Cancer Society. (800) ACS-2345. <http://www.cancer.org>.

The Leukemia and Lymphoma Society of America, Inc. 1311 Mamaroneck Ave, White Plains, NY 10605. (914)949-5213. <http://www.leukemia-lymphoma.org>.

Lymphoma Research Foundation. 8800 Venice Boulevard, Suite 207, Los Angeles, CA 90034. (310)204-7040. <http://www.lymphoma.org>.

National Cancer Institute. Building 31, Room 10A31, 31 Center Drive, MSC 2580, Bethesda, MD 20892-2580. (800)4CANCER. <http://www.nci.nih.gov>.

Deanna Swartout-Corbeil, R.N.

Malignant melanoma

Definition

Malignant melanoma is a type of skin tumor that is characterized by the cancerous growth of melanocytes, which are cells that produce a dark pigment called melanin.

Description

Overview

Cancer of the skin is the most common type of cancer and continues to grow in incidence. Skin cancer starts in the top layer of skin (the epidermis) but can grow down into the lower layers, the dermis and the subcutaneous layer. There are three main types of cells located in the epidermis, each of which can become cancerous. Melanocytes are the pigmented cells that are scattered throughout the skin, providing protection from ultraviolet (UV) light. Basal cells rest near the bottom of the epidermis and the layer of cells that continually grow to replace skin. The third type of epidermal cell is the squamous cells which make up most of the cells in human skin.

Melanoma

Malignant melanoma is the most serious type of skin cancer. It develops from melanocytes. Although melanoma is the least common skin cancer, it is the most aggressive. It spreads (metastasizes) to other parts of the body—especially the **lungs** and liver—as well as invading surrounding tissues. Melanomas in their early stages resemble moles. In Caucasians, melanomas appear most often on the trunk, head, and neck in men and on the arms and legs in women. Melanomas in African Americans, however, occur primarily on the palms of the hand, soles of the feet, and under the nails. Melanomas appear only rarely in the eyes, mouth, vagina, or digestive tract. Although melanomas are associated with exposure to the sun, the greatest risk factor for developing melanoma may be genetic. People who have a first-degree relative (parent, sibling or child) with melanoma have an increased risk up to eight times greater of developing the disease.

Basal cell cancer

Basal cell cancer is the most common type of skin cancer, accounting for about 75% of all skin cancers. It occurs primarily on the parts of the skin exposed to the sun and is most common in people living in equatorial regions or areas of high ozone depletion. Light-skinned people are more at risk of developing basal cell cancer than dark-skinned people. This form of skin cancer is primarily a disease of adults; it appears most often after age 30, peaking around age 70. Basal cell cancer grows very slowly. If it is not treated, however, it can invade deeper skin layers and cause disfigurement. This type of cancer can appear as a shiny, translucent nodule on the skin or as a red, wrinkled and scaly area.

Squamous cell cancer

Squamous cell cancer is the second most frequent type of skin cancer. It arises from the outer keratinizing layer of skin, so named because it contains a tough protein called keratin. Squamous cell cancer grows faster than basal cell cancer; it is more likely to metastasize to the lymph nodes as well as to distant sites. Squamous cell cancer most often appears on the arms, head, and neck. Fair-skinned people of Celtic descent are at high risk for developing squamous cell cancer. This type of cancer is rarely life-threatening but can cause serious problems if it spreads and can also cause disfigurement. Squamous cell cancer usually appears as a scaly, slightly elevated area of damaged skin.

Other skin cancers

Besides the three major types of skin cancer, there are a few other relatively rare forms. The most serious of these is Kaposi's sarcoma (KS), which occurs primarily in persons who have **AIDS** or older males of Mediterranean descent. When KS occurs with AIDS it is usually more aggressive. Other types of skin tumors are usually nonmalignant and grow slowly. These include:

• Bowen's disease. This is a type of skin inflammation (dermatitis) that sometimes looks like squamous cell cancer.

• Actinic or solar keratosis. This is a sunlight-damaged area of skin that sometimes develops into cancer.

• Keratoacanthoma. A keratoacanthoma is a dome-shaped tumor that can grow quickly and appear like squamous cell cancer. Although it is usually benign, it should be removed.

Risk factors

SUN EXPOSURE. Most skin cancers are associated with the amount of time that a person spends in the sun and the number of sunburns received, especially if they occurred at an early age. Skin cancer typically does not appear for 10-20 years after the sun damage has occurred. Because of this time lag, skin cancer rarely occurs before **puberty** and occurs more frequently with age.

MOLES. The number of moles (nevi) on a person's skin is related to the likelihood of developing melanoma. There are three types of nevi: not cancerous (benign); atypical (dysplastic); or birthmark (congenital). All three types of nevi have been associated with a higher risk of developing melanoma. Sometimes the moles themselves can become cancerous. Usually, however, the cancer is a new growth that occurs on normal skin.

HEREDITY. The tendency to develop skin cancer also tends to run in families. As has already been mentioned, there appears to be a significant genetic factor in the development of melanoma.

Causes and symptoms

Skin cancer begins to develop when a change or mutation occurs in one of the cells of the skin, causing it to grow without control. This mutation can be caused by ultraviolet (UV) light; most skin cancers are thought to be caused by overexposure to UV light from the sun. The incidence of severe, blistering sunburns is particularly closely related to skin cancer, more so when these **burns** occur during childhood. Exposure to ionizing radiation, arsenic, or polycyclic hydrocarbons in the workplace also

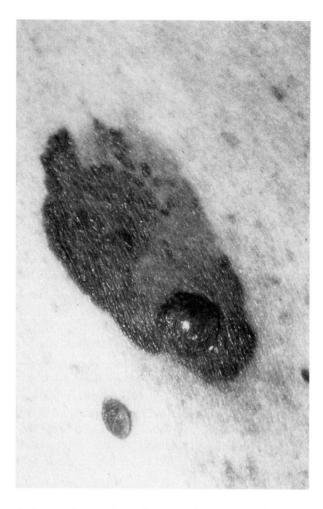

A close-up image of a malignant melanoma on patient's back. *(Custom Medical Stock Photo. Reproduced by permission.)*

- Asymmetry. A normal mole is round, whereas a suspicious mole is unevenly shaped.

- Border. A normal mole has a clear-cut border with the surrounding skin, whereas the edges of a suspect mole are often irregular.

- Color. Normal moles are uniformly tan or brown, but cancerous moles may appear as mixtures of red, white, blue, brown, purple, or black.

- Diameter. Normal moles are usually less than 0.20 in (5 mm) in diameter. A skin lesion greater than 0.25 in (0.6 cm) across may be suspected as cancerous.

There are two systems used in staging melanomas. The first is Clark's, which bases staging on the level of invasion, or which tissues the tumor has penetrated (i.e. which skin layer). The other is the American Joint Committee on Cancer. The second system is sometimes called the TNM system, which stands for tumor-nodes-metastasis, after the three major phases in cancer progression. Most experts generally agree that the thickness of the tumor is more accurate than the level of invasion for predicting prognosis (the outcome of the disease and estimated chance of recovery) and choosing an appropriate treatment.

Diagnosis

A person who has a suspicious-looking mole or area of skin should consult a doctor. In many cases, the person's primary care physician will make a referral to a doctor who specializes in skin diseases (a dermatologist). The dermatologist will carefully examine the lesion for the characteristic features of skin cancer. If further testing seems necessary, the dermatologist will perform a skin biopsy by removing the lesion under **local anesthesia**. Because melanomas tend to grow in diameter, as well as downwards into the epidermis and fatty layers of skin, a biopsy sample that is larger than the mole will be taken. This tissue is then analyzed under a **microscope** by a specialist in diseased organs and tissues (a pathologist). The pathologist makes the diagnosis of cancer and determines how far the tumor has grown into the skin. The evaluation of the progression of the cancer is called staging. Staging refers to how advanced the cancer is and is determined by the thickness and size of the tumor. Additional tests will also be done to determine if the cancer has moved into the lymph nodes or other areas of the body. These tests might include **chest x ray**, computed tomography scan (CT scan), **magnetic resonance imaging** (MRI), and **blood** tests.

appears to stimulate the development of skin cancers. The use of psoralen for treatment of psoriasis may be associated with the development of squamous cell cancer. Skin cancers are also more common in immunocompromised persons, such individuals with AIDS or those who have undergone organ transplants.

The first sign of skin cancer is usually a change in an existing mole, the presence of a new mole, or a change in a specific area of skin. Any change in a mole or skin lesion, including changes in color, size, or shape, tenderness, scaliness, or itching should be suspected of being skin cancer. Areas that bleed or are ulcerated may be signs of more advanced skin cancer. By doing a monthly self-examination, a person can identify abnormal moles or areas of skin and seek evaluation from a qualified health professional. The ABCD rule provides an easy way to remember the important characteristics of moles when one is examining the skin:

Treatment

Surgery

The primary treatment for skin cancer is to cut out (excise) the tumor or diseased area of skin. Surgery usually involves a simple excision using a scalpel to remove the lesion and a small amount of normal surrounding tissue. A procedure known as microscopically controlled excision can be used to examine each layer of skin as it is removed to ensure that the proper amount is taken. Depending on the amount of skin removed, the cut is either closed with stitches or covered with a skin graft. When surgical excision is performed on visible areas, such as the face, cosmetic surgery may also be performed to minimize the scar. Other techniques for removing skin tumors include burning, freezing with dry ice (cryosurgery), or **laser surgery**. For skin cancer that is localized and has not spread to other areas of the body, excision may be the only treatment needed.

Nonsurgical approaches

Although **chemotherapy** is the normal course of therapy for most other types of advanced cancer, it is not usually effective and not usually used for advanced skin cancer. For advanced melanoma that has moved beyond the original tumor site, the local lymph nodes may be surgically removed. Immunotherapy in the form of interferon or interleukin is being used more often with success for advanced melanoma. There is growing evidence that radiation therapy may be useful for advanced melanoma. Other treatments under investigation for melanoma include **gene therapy** and **vaccination**. Recent studies have shown that the use of a vaccine prepared from a person's own cancer cells may be useful in treating advanced melanoma. For people previously diagnosed with skin cancers, the chances of getting additional skin cancers are high. Therefore, regular monthly self-examination, as well as frequent examinations by a dermatologist, are essential.

Alternative treatment

There are no established alternative treatments for skin cancer. Immunotherapy, which strengthens the **immune system**, is an approach that may prove valuable in the future. Preventive measures that can be helpful include minimizing exposure to the sun and sunburn, eating a diet high in antioxidants and supplementation with antioxidant nutrients.

Prognosis

The prognosis for skin cancer depends on several factors, the most important of which are the invasiveness of the tumor and its location. The prognosis is good for localized skin cancers that are diagnosed and treated early. For basal cell cancer and squamous cell cancer, the cure rate is close to 100%, although most people with these forms will have recurrent skin cancer. For localized melanoma, the cure rate is approximately 95%. The prognosis worsens with larger tumors. Melanoma that has spread to the lymph nodes has a 5-year survival rate of 54%; advanced melanoma has a survival rate of only 13%. When melanoma has spread to other parts of the body, it is generally considered incurable. The median length of survival is six months.

Health care team roles

A physician makes an initial diagnosis. A dermatologist and pathologist may confirm the diagnosis. A surgeon removes most lesions. A plastic and reconstructive surgeon may repair or minimize surgical scars. Nurses and nurse practitioners will participate in prevention education with patients.

Prevention

Prevention is the best way to approach skin cancer. Avoiding unnecessary sun exposure, from such sources as sun lamps and tanning salons, is relatively simple. Parents of small children should protect them against the risk of sunburn. Precautions include avoiding high sun, when the rays of the sun are most intense (between 11 A.M. and 1 P.M.). In addition, persons living at high elevations need to take extra precautions because the intensity of UV radiation increases by 4% with every 1,000-ft (305-m) rise above sea level. When outdoors protective clothing should be worn, covering exposed skin. Sunglasses with UV protective coating should also be worn.

There is presently some debate about the ability of sunscreen to protect against skin cancer. Some scientists believe that gradual exposure to the sun, in order to develop a mild tan, may offer the best protection from skin cancer. Skin cancer has also been related to diets that are high in fat. Decreasing the amount of fat consumed may also help to decrease the risk of skin cancer.

Resources

BOOKS

Balch, Charles M. *Cutaneous Melanoma, 3rd ed.* St. Louis, Quality Medical Publishing, 1998.

Buchan, John and Roberts, Daffyd Lloyd. *Pocket Guide to Malignant Melanoma.* New York, Blackwell Science, 2000.

KEY TERMS

Biopsy—Removal of a small piece of tissue for examination. This is done under local anesthesia and removed by either using a scalpel or a punch, which removes a small cylindrical portion of tissue.

Cryosurgery—The use of extreme cold to destroy tissue in treating skin cancer.

Dermatologist—A doctor who specializes in skin diseases.

Epidermis—The outermost layer of skin.

Interferon—A group of proteins that have an effect on immune function and appear to have an anti- tumor effect in some persons.

Melanin—A dark pigment that is found in certain skin cells and helps to protect the skin from ultraviolet light.

Melanocyte—A specialized skin cell that produces melanin.

Metastasis—The movement of cancer cells from one area of the body to another through the blood or the lymph vessels.

Pathologist—A specialist in diseased organs and tissues.

Staging—The process of classifying and evaluating the progression of a cancer.

TNM staging—A staging system for classifying cancers developed by the American Joint Committee on Cancer. The initials stand for tumor, nodes, and metastasis.

Darmstadt, Gary L. "Tumors of the skin." In *Nelson Textbook of Pediatrics, 16th ed.,* edited by Richard E. Behrman et al. Philadelphia: W.B. Saunders, 2000, 2051-2053.

Parker, Frank. "Skin diseases of general importance." In *Cecil Textbook of Medicine, 21st ed.,* edited by Goldman, Lee and Bennett, J. Claude. Philadelphia: W.B. Saunders, 2000, 2276-2298.

Poole, Catherine M. and Guerry, DuPont. *New Haven, CT, Yale University Press, 1998.*

Schofield, Jill R. and Robinson, William A. *What You Really Need to Know About Moles and Melanoma.* Baltimore: Johns Hopkins University Press, 2000.

Smithson, William A. "Cancer of the skin." In *Nelson Textbook of Pediatrics, 16th ed.,* edited by Richard E. Behrman et al. Philadelphia: Saunders, 2000, 1566-1567.

Sober, Arthur J., Koh, Howard K., Tran, N-LT and Washington, Carl V. "Melanoma and other skin cancers." In *Harrison's Principles of Internal Medicine, 14th ed.,* edited by Anthony S. Fauci, et al. New York: McGraw-Hill, 1998, 543-549.

PERIODICALS

Bedikian A.Y., Plager C., Stewart J.R., O'Brian C.A., Herdman S.K., Ross M., Papadopoulos N., Eton O., Ellerhorst J., Smith T. "Phase II evaluation of bryostatin-1 in metastatic melanoma." *Melanoma Research* 11, no. 2 (2001): 183-188.

Hillner B.E., Kirkwood J.M., Agarwala S.S. "Burden of illness associated with metastatic melanoma." *Cancer* 91, no. 9 (2001): 1814-1821.

Lucci A., Citro H.W., Wilson L. "Assessment of knowledge of melanoma risk factors, prevention, and detection principles in Texas teenagers." *Journal of Surgical Research* 97, no. 2 (2001): 179-183.

Naylor M.F. "Melanoma vaccines." *Dermatology Online Journal* 6, no. 1 (2000): 5-9.

Shore R.E. "Radiation-induced skin cancer in humans." *Medical and Pediatric Oncology* 36, no. 5 (2001): 549-554.

Taran J.M., Heenan P.J. "Clinical and histologic features of level 2 cutaneous malignant melanoma associated with metastasis." *Cancer* 91, no. 9 (2001): 1822-1825.

ORGANIZATIONS

American Academy of Dermatology, 930 N. Meacham Road, PO Box 4014, Schaumburg, IL 60168-4014. (847) 330-0230. Fax: (847) 330-0050. <http://www.aad.org>.

American Melanoma Foundation, 3914 Murphy Canyon Road, Suite A132, San Diego, CA 92123. (858) 277-4426. <http://www.melanomafoundation.org/homepage.html>. sunsmartz@melanomafoundation.org.

Melanoma Education Foundation, 7 Jones Road, Peabody, MA 01960. <http://www.skincheck.com/#Site%20Content>. MEF@skincheck.org.

Melanoma Research Foundation, 23704-5 El Toro Rd., #206, Lake Forest, CA 92630. Phone/Fax: (800) 673-1290. mrf@melanoma.org.

National Cancer Institute, Building 31, Room 10A31, 31 Center Drive, MSC 2580, Bethesda, MD 20892-2580. (800) 422-6237 or (301) 435-3848. ttp://www.nci.nih.gov/.

Skin Cancer Foundation, 245 5th Avenue Suite 1403, New York, NY 10016. (800) 754-6490. Fax: (212) 725-5751. <http://www.skincancer.org/melanoma/>, info@skincancer.org.

OTHER

American Academy of Dermatology. <http://www.aad.org/SkinCancerNews/WhatIsSkinCancer/ABCDMel.html>.

Melanoma Foundation of Australia. <http://www.med.usyd.edu.au/medicine/melanoma/>.

National Library of Medicine. <http://www.nlm.nih.gov/medlineplus/melanoma.html>.

National Melanoma Foundation. <http://www.nationalmelanoma.org/>.

University of California-Davis. <http://matrix.ucdavis.edu/tumors/new/tutorial-intro.html>.

University of Maryland. <http://umm.drkoop.com/conditions/ency/article/001442.htm>.

University of Pennsylvania. <http://cancer.med.upenn.edu/disease/melanoma/>.

L. Fleming Fallon, Jr., M.D., Dr.P.H.

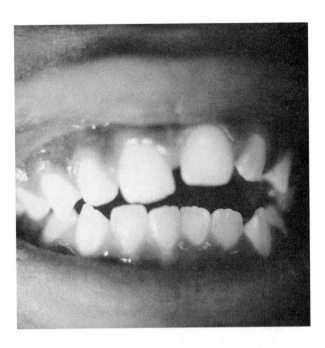

A close-up of person's mouth and teeth. The teeth are misarranged due to excessive thumb sucking. *(Custom Medical Stock Photo. Reproduced by permission.)*

Malocclusion

Definition

Malocclusion is an abnormality in the way the upper and lower teeth fit together in biting or chewing. The word malocclusion literally means "bad bite." The condition may also be referred to as an irregular bite, crossbite, or overbite.

Description

Malocclusion may be seen as crooked, crowded, or protruding teeth, or disproportionately smaller or larger jaws. Malocclusion can affect a person's appearance, speech, and ability to eat. Usually by age seven, enough of the permanent teeth have come in for dentists to identify current malocclusion and anticipate future problems if teeth and bone are left untreated. Adults and children can be successfully treated for most problems related to malocclusion.

Causes and symptoms

Malocclusions are most often inherited, but may be acquired. Inherited conditions include too many or too few teeth; too much or too little space between teeth; irregular mouth, jaw size, and shape; and atypical formations of the jaws and face, such as a cleft palate. Malocclusions may be acquired from habits like finger or thumb sucking, tongue thrusting, premature loss of teeth from an accident or dental disease, and medical conditions such as enlarged tonsils and adenoids that lead to mouth breathing.

Malocclusions may not have symptoms, or they may produce **pain** from increased stress on the oral structures.

Teeth may show abnormal signs of wear on the chewing surfaces or decay in areas of tight overlap. Chewing may be difficult. Left untreated, crooked or crowded teeth can become worse, sometimes requiring costly treatment to correct serious problems that develop over time. Orthodontic problems can contribute to conditions that cause tooth decay and gum disease. They can also help cause abnormal wear of tooth surfaces, inefficient chewing function, excessive stress on gum tissue and supporting bone, as well as jaw misalignment, resulting in headaches and face or neck pain.

Diagnosis

Malocclusion is most often found during a **dental examination** or screening. A dentist or dental hygienist checks a patient's occlusion by watching how the teeth make contact when the patient bites down normally. The dentist asks the patient to bite down on a piece of coated paper placed between the upper and lower teeth; this paper will leave colored marks at the points of contact. When malocclusion is suspected, photographs and x rays of the face and mouth may be taken for further study. To confirm the presence and extent of malocclusion, the dentist makes a plaster study model of the patient's teeth from impressions. These models duplicate the fit of the teeth and are very useful in treatment planning.

KEY TERMS

Braces—An orthodontic appliance consisting of brackets cemented to the surface of each tooth and wires of stainless steel or nickel titanium alloy. Braces treat malocclusion by gradually changing the position of the teeth.

Impression—An imprint of the upper or lower teeth made in a pliable material that sets. When this material has hardened, it may be filled with plaster, plastic, or artificial stone to make an exact model of the teeth.

Occlusion—The way the upper and lower teeth fit together in biting or chewing.

Retainer—An orthodontic appliance worn to stabilize teeth in a new position.

Space maintainer—An orthodontic appliance worn to prevent adjacent teeth from moving into the space left by an unerupted or prematurely lost tooth.

Treatment

Malocclusion may be remedied by orthodontic treatment. Orthodontics is a specialty of dentistry that manages the growth, prevention, and correction of abnormal dental and facial relationships. Braces are the most commonly used **orthodontic appliances** in the treatment of malocclusion.

Braces apply constant gentle force to slowly change the position of the teeth, straightening them and properly aligning them with the opposing teeth. Braces consist of removable or fixed (cemented or bonded to the teeth) brackets, made of metal, ceramic, or plastic.

In most cases, braces are not removable for daily tooth brushing, so the patient must be especially diligent about keeping the mouth clean and removing bacterial plaque that is easily trapped, in order to prevent tooth decay. Foods that are crunchy should be avoided to minimize the risk of breaking the appliance. Hard fruits, vegetables, and breads must be cut into bite-sized pieces before eating. Foods that are sticky, including chewing gum, should be avoided because they may pull off the brackets or weaken the cement. Carbonated beverages may also weaken the cement, as well as contribute to tooth decay. Teeth should be brushed immediately after eating sweet foods. Special floss threaders are available to make flossing easier.

If overcrowding is creating malocclusion, one or more teeth may be extracted (surgically removed), giving other teeth room to move. If a tooth has not yet erupted or is prematurely lost, the orthodontist may insert an appliance called a space maintainer to keep the other teeth from moving out of their natural position. In severe cases of malocclusion, surgery may be necessary and the patient would be referred to yet another specialist, an oral or maxillofacial surgeon.

Once the teeth have been moved into their new position, the braces are removed and a retainer is worn until the teeth stabilize in that position. Retainers do not move teeth, they only hold them in place.

Orthodontic treatment is the only effective treatment for malocclusion not requiring surgery. However, depending on the cause and severity of the condition, an orthodontist may be able to suggest other appliances as alternatives to braces. Experts recommend early treatment, which can help to guide the growth of the jaw, regulate the widths of the dental arches, correct thumb, finger, and other sucking habits, enhance swallowing and speech, and improve personal appearance and self-esteem. Adults are candidates for orthodontics to correct malocclusion, as well. Healthy teeth can be moved to more desirable positions at any age.

Alternative treatment

There are some techniques of craniosacral therapy that can alter structure. This therapy may allow correction of some cases of malocclusion. If surgery is required, pre- and post-surgical care with natural remedies, as well as vitamin and mineral supplements, may enhance recovery. Night guards and stress management are sometimes recommended to ease the strain on the jaw and to limit teeth grinding.

Prognosis

Depending on the cause and severity of the malocclusion and the appliance used in treatment, a patient should expect correction of the condition to take one to three years. Interceptive, or early treatment procedures, might take months or more. The time required to correct malocclusion depends on the growth of the patient's mouth and face, patient cooperation, and the extent of the problem.

Health care team roles

The general dentist or dental hygienist, during preventive oral care, is often the first health professional to see evidence of a malocclusion. The general dentist usually determines a patient's need to have the problem looked at by a specialist, such as an orthodontist. Dental assistants are ancillary personnel used in dentists' or orthodontists' offices to assist in the procedures.

Prevention

Malocclusion is preventable at times. It can be prevented by space maintenance and may be minimized by controlling habits such as finger or thumb sucking. Initial consultation with an orthodontist before a child is seven years old may lead to appropriate management of the growth and development of the child's dental and facial structures, circumventing many of the factors contributing to malocclusion.

Resources

ORGANIZATIONS

Academy of General Dentistry. 211 East Chicago Ave., Chicago, IL 600611. (312) 440-4800. <http://www.agd.org>.

American Association of Oral and Maxillofacial Surgeons. 9700 West Bryn Mawr Avenue, Rosemont, IL 60018-5701. (847) 678-6200. <http://www.aaoms.org>.

American Association of Orthodontists. 401 N. Lindbergh Blvd. St. Louis, MO 63141-7816. (314) 993-1700. <http://www.aaortho.org>.

OTHER

OrthoFind. (310) 328-2020. <http://www.orthofind.com>.

Interview with Dr. Leslie Seldin, practicing general dentist and spokesperson for the American Dental Association. Office address: 40 Central Park. New York, NY 10019-1413. (212) 246-2398.

Lisette Hilton

Malpractice

Definition

Malpractice is defined as improper or negligent practice by a lawyer, physician, or other professional who injures a client or patient. The fields in which a judgment of malpractice can be made are those that require training and skills beyond the level of most people's abilities. Medical malpractice is defined as a wrongful act by a physician, nurse, or other medical professional in the administration of treatment— or at times, the omission of medical treatment, to a patient under his or her care. Although dentists, architects, accountants, and engineers are also liable to malpractice suits, most lawsuits of this type in the United States involve medical malpractice.

Negligence can result from a lack of knowledge or skill, or from failure to exercise reasonable judgment in the application of professional knowledge or skill. Lack or failure is determined by comparing the action in question with what a similar practitioner would reasonably be expected to do in the same circumstances.

In law, malpractice is classified as a tort, which is a wrongful act resulting in injury to another's person, property, or reputation. In a tort, the injured party is entitled to seek compensation for the injury. All torts, including malpractice, have three features:

• a person who has a duty of care toward others

• a failure to exercise due care

• an injury or financial damages caused by the failure

Description

The American Nurses Association estimates that there are 1–3 million health care errors in United States hospitals per year. In the past, only physicians were sued for malpractice, but as of 2001, nurses and other allied health professionals are being named with increasing frequency as defendants in lawsuits. This focus on shared responsibility can be attributed to a number of factors.

The responsibilities of nurses and allied health professionals are continually expanding to include more risk and more patient contact without a physician present. In some clinic settings, **advanced practice nurses** have prescriptive authority and can perform many of the same functions as a physician. This expansion increases the liklihood of lawsuits against nonphysician health care providers.

In 2001, limits on staffing and a shortage of qualified nurses have increased demands on the time and attention of health care professionals. Even conscientious workers may find themselves making mistakes when under increased pressure to do more with fewer resources. This pressure leads to errors resulting from breakdowns in communication as well.

In addition, the advent of the Internet has produced a patient population that is more knowledgeable about health care and more aware of the risks and benefits of treatment. Health care providers are no longer regarded as "always knowing what's best." Easy access to health care information enables patients to judge for themselves if they are receiving reasonable care or not.

The legal process of malpractice suits

When a patient wishes to sue a medical professional for malpractice, he or she must first consult an attorney. Most malpractice attorneys work on a contingent fee

KEY TERMS

Contingent fee—A method of compensation in which an attorney is paid only if damages are awarded to the client. Contingent fees are usually a percentage of the gross amount of the award.

Defendant—The party sued or accused in a court of law.

Plaintiff—The party initiating a lawsuit in a court of law.

Prescriptive authority—Legal authority granted to advanced practice nurses to prescribe medication.

Tort—A wrongful act that causes injury to another person's body, property, or reputation, for which the injured party is entitled to seek compensation. Malpractice is classified as a tort in the legal system of the United States.

basis. This term means that the attorney is paid only if the patient recovers damages from the professional. The attorney usually receives a percentage of the gross award—sometimes as high as 30–40%.

The attorney will obtain a detailed medical history from the patient, including the names of all physicians and hospitals who have treated him or her. The most important step is securing a medical expert. The attorney will consult someone certified in the relevant medical specialty in order to determine whether there is sufficient evidence that the defendant medical professional did indeed injure the patient.

If the medical expert concludes that there is evidence of malpractice, a lawsuit is filed. If the plaintiff and the defendant cannot resolve their differences outside of court, the case will go to trial before a judge and jury.

Proving medical malpractice

Four elements must be proven in court in order for a verdict of malpractice, or negligence, to be issued. These include legal duty; breach of duty; causation; and damages.

Legal duty to the patient is initiated upon establishment of a provider-patient relationship. For example, if treatment is begun, a contract is implied to exist between the health care provider and the patient. If health care professionals assist at the scene of an accident, they are covered under Good Samaritan law if the assistance is given freely and in a situation where other medical personnel and equipment are not immediately available. In most states, there is no legal duty to assist in such a situation, although there may be an ethical or moral duty. Good Samaritan law offers protection against litigation for simple negligence in order to encourage health care professionals to stop at accident scenes, but any action considered gross negligence is not protected.

Breach of duty is determined by comparing the action in question with the established standard of care. These standards are developed by the Joint Commission on Accreditation of Healthcare Organizations (JCAHO) and State Nurse Practice Acts, and are communicated by professional associations, professional journals and textbooks, job descriptions, and organization policies and procedures.

Proving causation requires evidence that the health care provider's negligence directly caused injury or harm to the patient. Even if breach of duty can be established, malpractice is not proven unless causation is confirmed.

The last step in proving malpractice is verifying that the patient suffered disability, disfigurement, **pain**, suffering, or financial loss as a result of negligence. In some states, any of the defendants may be required to pay 100% of the award, even if they were only slightly negligent in comparison to the other defendants. This rule is gradually being abolished, however, and usually liability is distributed based on degree of fault.

Viewpoints

Since there has been a trend to include nurses and allied health professionals in medical malpractice suits, the question of liability insurance must be addressed. Nurses and allied health professionals are usually covered by liability insurance provided by their employer, and many professionals consider this coverage sufficient. Others, however, encourage purchasing a personal policy as well for the following reasons:

• The employer's policy may not cover the total award.

• Employer coverage may not apply after job termination.

• Agency workers are not usually covered by hospital policies.

• Personal policies may also cover attorney fees, transportation, and paid time off from work.

Some professionals may think that having personal liability insurance makes them more likely to be sued; however, this is not true. If a health care worker is involved in a negligent situation in any way, they can be named in the lawsuit. The plaintiff's lawyer may not investigate the defendants for personal insurance; and even if the lawyer does make an investigation, the jury is not allowed to have that information.

Some nurses and allied health professionals may decide not to have personal liability insurance "because it costs too much." The average yearly cost of a nursing policy with a liability limit of $1,000,000 is approximately $90. That's relatively inexpensive protection from having to pay out of one's own pocket for damages awarded in a lawsuit.

Professional implications

The obvious professional implications of malpractice include the reasons for lawsuits against nurses and allied health professionals; and ways to avoid being named in a suit.

Reasons for lawsuits against nurses and allied health professionals

Nurses and allied health care professionals have a duty to question physician orders that are inappropriate or unclear. If they do not ask such questions, and a patient is harmed as a result of an inappropriate order, the nurse or allied health professional is just as liable for damages as the physician. The same is true for verbal orders. Verbal orders should be accepted only in emergency situations, and the physician should write and sign the order immediately afterwards. Telephone orders can be accepted by a **registered nurse** or pharmacist, but should be signed by the physician as soon as possible.

If a patient's status changes and the physician is not notified, the nurse is liable for damages that may occur. These changes include change in physical status, critical laboratory values, and critical information that the physician should ask for but doesn't. If a medical resident is managing the patient, the attending physician must still be notified.

Documentation is crucial. Specifics should be documented about the patient's condition, who was notified and what was said, the interventions implemented, and the outcomes of care. A favorite phrase in health care is "If it wasn't documented, it wasn't done," and that's exactly how the court will view the patient's chart in a lawsuit.

Other common reasons for lawsuits against nurses include:

• failure to secure the patient's safety

• failure to properly assess the patient

• failure to perform a procedure according to established standards of care

• failure to administer medication properly

Ways to avoid being named in a lawsuit

Nurses and allied health care professionals who are conscientious and who exercise good judgment are usually successful at avoiding negligent practice. Not every situation can be completely controlled, however, especially when other physicians or health care professionals are involved. The American Nurses Association is a strong advocate for patient safety and has proposed whistle-blower protection for nurses and allied health care professionals who report unsafe patient care practices. Whistle-blower protection legislation has been addressed at the state and federal levels.

There is another simple way to lessen the chance of being included in a lawsuit: give compassionate care. It's been established that patients who file lawsuits tend to sue people who have made them angry. Often, the real issue for patients is that they feel they have not been heard or treated with respect. One study (Beckman, et al., 1994) reviewed 45 malpractice cases against a large medical center and found that in 71% of the cases, plaintiffs stated that they had a negative relationship with the caregivers. The issues included feelings of abandonment; feeling that discomfort had been ignored; not receiving explanations about the care given or expected outcomes; and feeling that the patient's or family's opinions were discounted.

In another situation, a defense attorney for health care providers found that a plaintiff refused to name a certain nurse in the lawsuit, even though the nurse was clearly negligent. The plaintiff felt that this nurse was the only one who gave compassionate care.

Effective communication, compassionate care, and treating patients with dignity increases both patient and professional satisfaction. The end result is patients who are less likely to initiate lawsuits, and health care workers who are less likely to end up in court.

Resources

PERIODICALS

Beckman, H.B., et al. "The Doctor-Patient Relationship and Malpractice: Lessons from Plaintiff's Depositions." *Archives of Internal Medicine* 154, no.12 (1994): 1365.

Calloway, S. "Preventing Communication Breakdowns." *RN* 64, no. 1(2001): 71-72, 74.

Crane, Mark. "NPs and PAs: What's the malpractice risk?" *Medical Economics* 77, no. 6 (March 20, 2000).

Helm, A., and N. Kihm. "Is Professional Liability Insurance for You?" *Nursing* 31, no. 1 (2001): 48.

Martin, G.A. "ARNA Workplace Advocacy Newsletter. Torts-R-Us." *Arkansas Nursing News* 17, no. 4 (2001): 16-18.

Mock, K. "Keep Lawsuits at Bay with Compassionate Care." *RN* 64, no. 5 (2001): 83-84, 86.

ORGANIZATIONS

American Bar Association (ABA). 750 North Lake Shore Drive, Chicago, IL 60611. (312) 988-5000 or (800) 964-4253.

American Nurses Association. 600 Maryland Ave. SW, 100 W., Washington, DC 20024. (800) 274-4ANA. <http://www.nursingworld.org>.

OTHER

Allied Health Professionals Policy.HCPro. 2001. <http://www.credentialinfo.com/cred/pandp/ahppolicy.cfm> (July 28, 2001).

Abby Wojahn, R.N.,B.S.N.,C.C.R.N.

Mammography

Definition

Mammography is the study of the breast using x-rays. The actual test is called a mammogram. It is an x-ray of the breast which shows the fatty, fibrous and glandular tissues. There are two types of mammograms. A screening mammogram is ordered for women who have no problems with their breasts. It consists of two x-ray views of each breast: a craniocaudal (from above) and a mediolateral oblique (from the sides). A diagnostic mammogram is for evaluation of abnormalities in either men or women. Additional x rays from other angles, or special coned views of certain areas are taken.

Purpose

The purpose of screening mammography is **breast cancer** detection. A screening test, by definition, is used for patients without any signs or symptoms, in order to detect disease as early as possible. Many studies have shown that having regular mammograms increases a woman's chances of finding breast **cancer** in an early stage, when it is more likely to be curable. It has been estimated that a mammogram may find a cancer as much as two or three years before it can be felt. The American Cancer Society (ACS) guidelines recommend an annual screening mammogram for every woman of average risk beginning at age 40. Radiologists look specifically for the presence of microcalcifications and other abnormalities that can be associated with malignancy. New digital mammography and computer aided reporting can automatically enhance and magnify the mammograms for easier finding of these tiny calcifications.

The highest risk factor for developing cancer is age. Some women are at an increased risk for developing breast cancer, such as those with a positive family history of the disease. Beginning screening mammography at a younger age may be recommended for these women.

Diagnostic mammography is used to evaluate an existing problem, such as a lump, discharge from the nipple, or unusual tenderness in one area. It is also done to evaluate further abnormalities that have been seen on screening mammograms. The radiologist normally views the films immediately and may ask for additional views such as a magnification view of one specific area. Additional studies such as an ultrasound of the breast may be performed as well to determine if the lesion is cystic or solid. Breast-specific **positron emission tomography** (**PET**) scans as well as in MRI (**magnetic resonance imaging**) may be ordered to further evaluate a tumor, but mammography is still the first choice in detecting small tumors on a screening basis.

Precautions

Screening mammograms are not usually recommended for women under age 40 who have no special risk factors and a normal physical breast examination. A mammogram may be useful if a lump or other problem is discovered in a woman aged 30-40. Below age 30, breasts tend to be "radiographically dense," which means the breasts contain a large amount of glandular tissue which is difficult to image in fine detail. Mammograms for this age group are controversial. An ultrasound of the breasts is usually done instead since it gives no radiation to the patient.

Description

A mammogram may be offered in a variety of settings. Hospitals, outpatient clinics, physician's offices, or other facilities may have mammography equipment. In the United States only places certified by the Food and Drug Administration (FDA) are legally permitted to perform, interpret, or develop mammograms. Mammograms are taken with dedicated machines using high frequency generators, low kvp, molybdenum targets and specialized x-ray beam filtration. Sensitive high contrast film and screen combinations along with prolonged developing enable the visualization of minute breast detail.

In addition to the usual paperwork, a woman will be asked to fill out a questionaire asking for information on her current medical history. Beyond her personal and family history of cancer, details about menstruation, previous breast surgeries, child bearing, birth control, and hormone replacement therapy are recorded. Information about breast self-examination (BSE) and other breast health issues are usually available at no charge.

At some centers, a technologist may perform a **physical examination** of the breasts before the mammogram. Whether or not this is done, it is essential for the technologist to record any lumps, nipple discharge, breast **pain** or other concerns of the patient. All visible scars, tattoos and nipple alterations must be carefully noted as well.

Clothing from the waist up is removed, along with necklaces and dangling earrings. A hospital gown or similar covering is put on. A small self-adhesive metal marker may be placed on each nipple by the x-ray technologist. This allows the nipple to be viewed as a reference point on the film for concise tumor location and easier centering for additional views.

Patients are positioned for mammograms differently, depending on the type of mammogram being performed:

- Craniocaudal position (CC): The woman stands or sits facing the mammogram machine. One breast is exposed and raised to a level position while the height of the cassette-holder is adjusted to the same level. The breast is placed mid-film with the nipple in profile and the head turned away from the side being x-rayed. The shoulder is relaxed and pulled slightly backward while the breast is pulled as far forward as possible. The technologist holds the breast in place and slowly lowers the compression with a foot pedal. The breast is compressed between the film holder and a rectangle of plastic (called a paddle). The breast is compressed until the skin is taut and the breast tissue firm when touched on the lateral side. The exposure is taken immediately and the compression released. Good compression can be uncomfortable, but it is very necessary. Compression reduces the thickness of the breast, creates a uniform density and separates over-lying tissues. This allows for a detailed image with a lower exposure time and decreased radiation dose to the patient. The same view is repeated on the opposite breast.

- Mediolateral oblique position (MLO): The woman is positioned with her side towards the mammography unit. The film holder is angled parallel to the pectoral muscle, anywhere from 30-60 degrees depending on the size and height of the patient. The taller and thinner the patient the higher the angle. The height of the machine is level with the axilla (armpit). The arm is placed at the top of the cassette-holder with a corner touching the armpit. The breast is lifted forward and upward and compression is applied until the breast is held firmly in place by the paddle. The nipple should be in profile and the opposite breast held away if necessary by the patient. This procedure is repeated for the

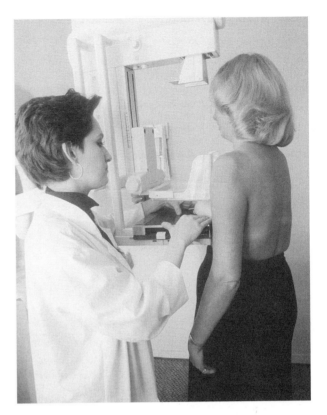

Mammography can detect breast cancer before it can be felt, increasing the chances that it can be treated successfully. *(D. Weinstein/Custom Medical Stock Photo. Reproduced by permission.)*

other breast. A total of four x-rays, two of each breast, are taken for a screening mammogram. Additional x-rays, using special paddles, different breast positions, or other techniques may be taken for a diagnostic mammogram.

The mammogram may be seen and interpreted by a radiologist right away, or it may not be reviewed until later. If there is any questionable area or abnormality, extra x-rays may be recommended. These may be taken during the same appointment. More commonly, especially for screening mammograms, the woman is called back on another day for these additional films.

A screening mammogram usually takes approximately 15-30 minutes. A woman having a diagnostic mammogram can expect to spend up to an hour for the procedure.

The cost of mammography varies widely. Many mammography facilities accept "self referral." This means women can schedule themselves without a physician's referral. However, some insurance policies do require a doctor's prescription to ensure payment. **Medicare** will pay for annual screening mammograms for all women over age 39.

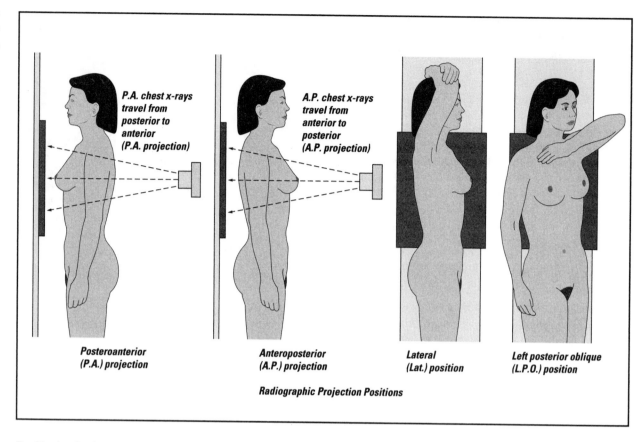

P.A. chest x-rays
travel from
posterior to
anterior
(P.A. projection)

A.P. chest x-rays
travel from
anterior to
posterior
(A.P. projection)

**Posteroanterior
(P.A.) projection**

**Anteroposterior
(A.P.) projection**

**Lateral
(Lat.) position**

**Left posterior oblique
(L.P.O.) position**

Radiographic Projection Positions

Positioning for breast x rays. *(Delmar Publishers, Inc. Reproduced by permission.)*

Preparation

The compression or squeezing of the breast necessary for a mammogram is a concern of many women. Mammograms should be scheduled when a woman's breasts are least likely to be tender. One to two weeks after the first day of the menstrual period is usually best. Some women with sensitive breasts also find that stopping or decreasing **caffeine** intake from coffee, tea, colas, and chocolate for a week or two before the examination decreases any discomfort. Women receiving hormone therapy may also have sensitive breasts. Over-the-counter pain relievers are recommended an hour before the mammogram appointment when pain is a significant problem.

Women should not put deodorant, powder, or lotion on their upper body on the day the mammogram is performed. Particles from these products can get on the breast or film holder and may show up as abnormalities on the mammogram. Most facilities will have special wipes available for those patients who need to wash before the mammogram.

Aftercare

No special aftercare is required.

Complications

The risk of radiation exposure from a mammogram is considered minimal and not significant. Experts are unanimous that any negligible risk is by far outweighed by the potential benefits of mammography. Patients who have breast implants must be x-rayed with caution and compression is minimally applied so that the sac is not ruptured. Special techniques and positioning skills must be learned before a technologist can x-ray a patient with breast implants.

Some breast cancers do not show up on mammograms, or "hide" in dense breast tissue. A normal (or negative) study is not a guarantee that a woman is cancer-free. The false-negative rate is estimated to be 15-20%, higher in younger women and women with dense breasts.

False positive readings are also possible. Breast biopsies may be recommended on the basis of a mammogram, and find no cancer. It is estimated that 75-80% of all breast biopsies resulted in benign (no cancer present) findings. This is considered an acceptable rate, because recommending fewer biopsies would result in too many missed cancers.

Results

A mammography report describes details about the x ray appearance of the breasts. It also rates the mammogram according to standardized categories, as part of the Breast Imaging Reporting and Data System (BIRADS) created by the American College of Radiology (ACR). A normal mammogram may be rated as BIRADS 1 or negative, which means no abnormalities were seen. A normal mammogram may also be rated as BIRADS 2 or benign findings. This means there are one or more abnormalities but they are clearly benign (not cancerous), or variations of normal. Some kinds of calcifications, enlarged lymph nodes or obvious cysts might generate a BIRADS 2 rating.

Many mammograms are considered borderline or indeterminate in their findings. BIRADS 3 means either additional images are needed, or an abnormality is seen and is probably (but not definitely) benign. A follow-up mammogram within a short interval of six to twelve months is suggested. This helps to ensure that the abnormality is not changing, or is "stable." Only the affected side will be x-rayed at this time. Some women are uncomfortable or anxious about waiting, and may want to consult with their doctor about having a biopsy. BIRADS 4 means suspicious for cancer. A biopsy is usually recommended in this case. BIRADS 5 means an abnormality is highly suggestive of cancer. A biopsy or other appropriate action should be taken.

Health care team roles

The mammographic x-ray technologist works closely with the radiologist. Films of high quality must be taken so the radiologist can make an accurate diagnosis. The technologist also assists the radiologist when performing biopsies or fine needle aspirations. Analysis of the specimen will be carried out in the laboratory by the medical laboratory technician. It is important for the technologist to fill out the proper laboratory forms. Biopsies performed in the operating room will sometimes require a magnified x-ray of the specimen itself. The technologist must work in conjunction with the surgeon and operating room nurses to make sure the specimen is x-rayed immediately and than returned for further analysis.

All radiology technologists must be certified according to a recognized standard such as that of the American Society of Registered Radiology Technologists. The MQSA, or Mammography Quality Standards Act,

KEY TERMS

Breast biopsy—A procedure where suspicious tissue is removed and examined by a pathologist for cancer or other disease. The breast tissue may be obtained by open surgery, or through a needle.

Craniocaudal—Head to tail, x-ray beam directly overhead the part being examined.

Radiographically dense—An abundance of glandular tissue, which results in diminished film detail.

enforced by the FDA, ensures that all mammographic x-ray technologists receive adequate training and continued education to perform special techniques such as mammography of patients with breast implants. It is also part of the technologist's or nurse's job to perform quality assurance and to keep statistics to ensure FDA compliance.

Patient education

The mammography technologist must be empathetic to the patient's modesty and **anxiety**. He or she must explain that compression is necessary to improve the quality of the image but does not harm the breasts. Patients will be very anxious when additional films are requested. Explaining that an extra view will give the radiologist more information will help to eases the patient's tension. One in eight women in North America will develop breast cancer. Educating the public on monthly breast self-examinations and yearly mammograms will help in achieving an early diagnosis and therefore a better cure.

Resources

PERIODICALS

Carmen, Ricard, R. T. R. *Mammography: Techniques and Difficulties.* O.T.R.Q., 1999.

Gagnon, Gilbert. *Radioprotection in Mammography.* O.T.R.Q., 1999.

Ouimet, Guylaine, R. T. R. *Mammography: Quality Control.* O.T.R.Q., 1999.

ORGANIZATIONS

American Cancer Society (ACS), 1599 Clifton Rd., Atlanta, GA 30329. (800) ACS-2345. <http://www.cancer.org>.

Federal Drug Administration (FDA), 5600 Fishers Ln., Rockville, MD 20857. (800) 532-4440. <http://www.fda.gov>.

National Cancer Institute (NCI) and Cancer Information Service (CIS), Office of Cancer Communications, Bldg.

31, Room 10A16, Bethesda, MD 20892. (800) 4-CAN-CER (800) 422-6237. Fax: (800) 624-2511 or (301) 402-5874. <http://cancernet.nci.nih.gov>, cancermail@cips.nci.nih.gov.

Lorraine K. Ehresman

Managed care plans

Definition

Managed care plans are health care delivery systems that integrate the financing and delivery of health care. Managed care organizations generally negotiate agreements with providers to offer packaged health care benefits to covered individuals.

Description

A majority of insured Americans belong to a managed care plan, a health care delivery system that applies corporate business practices to medical care in order to reduce costs and streamline care. The managed care era began in the late 1980s in response to skyrocketing heath care costs, which stemmed from a number of sources. Under the fee-for-service, or indemnity, model that preceded managed care, doctors and hospitals were financially rewarded for using a multitude of expensive tests and procedures to treat patients. Other contributors to the high cost of health care included the **public health** advances after World War II that lengthened the average life span of Americans—putting increased pressure on the health care system, and efforts by providers to adopt state-of-the-art diagnostic and treatment technologies as they became available.

Managed care companies attempted to reduce costs by negotiating lower fees with clinicians and hospitals in exchange for a steady flow of patients, developing standards of treatment for specific diseases, requiring clinicians to get plan approval before hospitalizing a patient (except in the case of an emergency), and encouraging clinicians to prescribe less expensive medicines. Many plans offer financial incentives to clinicians who minimize referrals and diagnostic tests, and some even apply financial penalties, or disincentives, on those deemed to have ordered unnecessary care. The primary "watchdog" and accreditation agency for managed care organizations is the National Committee for Quality Assurance (NCQA), a non-profit organization that also collects and disseminates health plan performance data.

Three basic types of managed care plans exist: health maintenance organizations (HMOs), preferred provider organizations (PPOs), and point-of-service (POS) plans.

- HMOs, in existence for over 50 years, are the best known and oldest form of managed care. Participants in HMO plans must see a primary care provider, who may be a physician or an advanced practice **registered nurse** (APRN) in order to receive care from a specialist. Four types of HMOs exist: the Staff Model, Group Model, Network Model, and the Independent Practice Association (IPA). The Staff Model hires clinicians to work on site. The Group Model contracts with group practice physicians on an exclusive basis. The Network Model resembles the group model except participating physicians can treat patients who are not plan members. The Independent Practice Association (IPA) contracts with physicians in private practice to see HMO patients at a prepaid rate per visit as a part of their practice.

- PPOs are more flexible than HMOs. Like HMOs, they negotiate with networks of physicians and hospitals to get discounted rates for plan members. But, unlike HMOs, PPOs allow plan members to seek care from specialists without being referred by a primary care practitioner. These plans use financial incentives to encourage members to seek medical care from providers inside the network.

- POSs are a blend of the other types of managed care plans. They encourage plan members to seek care from providers inside the network by charging low fees for their services, but they add the option of choosing an out-of-plan provider at any time and for any reason. POS plans carry a high premium, a high deductible, or a higher co-payment for choosing an out-of-plan provider.

Viewpoints

Several managed care theories, such as those stressing continuity of care, prevention, and early intervention are applauded by health care practitioners and patients alike. But managed care has come under fire by critics who feel patient care may be compromised by managed care cost-cutting strategies, such as early hospital discharge and use of financial incentives to control referrals, which may make clinicians too cautious about sending patients to specialists. In general, the rise of managed care has shifted decision-making power away from plan members, who are limited in their choices of providers, and away from clinicians, who must concede to managed-care administrators regarding what is a medically necessary procedure. Many people would like to see managed care restructured to remedy this inequitable distribution of power. Such actions would maximize consumer choice and allow health care practitioners the freedom to provide the best care possible. According to the American Medical Association, rejection of care resulting from managed care stipulations should be subjected to an independent appeals process.

Professional implications

The health care industry today is dominated by corporate values of managed care and is subject to corporate principles such as cost cutting, mergers and acquisitions, and layoffs. To thrive in such an environment, and to provide health care in accordance with professional values, health care practitioners must educate themselves on the business of health care, including hospital operations and administrative decision-making, in order to influence institutional and regional health care policies. A sampling of the roles available for registered nurses in a managed care environment include:

- *Primary care provider.* The individual responsible for determining a plan of care, including referrals to specialists.

- *Case manager.* This person tracks patients through the health care system to maintain continuity of care.

- *Triage nurse.* In a managed care organization, triage nurses help direct patients through the system by determining the urgency and level of care necessary and advising incoming patients on self care when appropriate.

- *Utilization/Resource reviewer.* This individual helps manage costs by assessing the appropriateness of specialized treatments.

According to an American Nursing Association statement, it is difficult to predict the effect of the managed care revolution on the nursing profession, but the profession will benefit from building broad nursing coalitions at the state and federal levels to publicize nursing's views on patient care issues, and to monitor developing trends in the industry, including the impact of proposed mergers and acquisitions of health care institutions on the provision of care.

Resources

PERIODICALS

Simon, S., et al. "Views of Managed Care: A Survey of Students, Residents, Faculty, and Deans at Medical Schools in the United States." *The New England Journal of Medicine* 12 (1999): 340.

ORGANIZATIONS

Agency for Health Care Research and Quality. 2101 E. Jefferson St., Suite 501. Rockville, MD 20852. (301) 594-1364.

American Association of Managed Care Nurses. PO Box 4975, Glen Allen, VA 23058-4975. (804)-747-9698. <http://www.aamcn.org/joinaamcn.htm>.

American Medical Association. The Council on Ethical and Judicial Affairs. 515 N. State Street, Chicago, IL 60610. (312) 464-4823. <http://www.ama-assn.org/ama/pub/category/2498.html>.

American Nurses Association (ANA). 600 Maryland Avenue, SW, Suite 100 West, Washington, DC 20024. (800) 274-4ANA. <http://www.nursingworld.org>.

Center for Bioethics at the University of Pennsylvania. Suite 320, 3401 Market Street, Philadelphia, PA 19104-3308. (215) 898-7136. <http://bioethics.org>.

National Committee for Quality Assurance. 2000 L St. NW, Washington, DC 20036. (202) 955-3500. <http://www.ncqa.org>.

National Student Nurses Association (NSNA). 555 West 57th Street, New York, NY 10019. (212) 581-2211. <http://www.nsna.org>.

OTHER

American Medical Association. *Principles of Managed Care.* <http://www.ama-assn.org/advocacy/principl.htm>.

American Nurses Association. "Nursing's Agenda for Health care Reform." *NursingWorld.* <http://www.nursingworld.org/readroom/rnagenda.htm>.

Health Care in Chaos: Will We Ever See Real Managed Care? *American Nurses Association Continuing Education Module.* <http://www.nursingworld.org/mods/mod3/cemc1.htm>.

Ann Quigley

Manic depression *see* **Bipolar disorder**

Manual therapy *see* **Joint mobilization and manipulation**

Marijuana

Definition

Marijuana is prepared from the leaves and flowering tops of *Cannabis sativa*, the hemp plant, which contains a number of pharmacologically active principles, called cannabinoids.

Description

Marijuana is most popularly used for its euphoric properties. Its many nicknames include grass, pot, Mary Jane, reefer, and cannabis, which is derived from *Cannabis sativa*, the scientific name for hemp.

The beneficial effects of marijuana's most active ingredient, tetrahydrocannabinol (THC), include the lowering of intraocular pressure, which may help control glaucoma, and the relief of **pain**, nausea, and appetite loss among **chemotherapy** and **AIDS** patients.

Marijuana's short-term effects are psychological and physical, usually lasting for three to five hours after a person has smoked marijuana. The psychological reaction, more commonly known as a high, involves changes in the user's feelings and thoughts. These changes are primarily caused by THC, which affects **brain** function.

The effects of marijuana's high vary for each individual. In most cases the high consists of a dreamy, relaxed state in which users seem more aware of their senses and feel that time is moving slowly. Sometimes, however, marijuana produces feelings of panic and dread. Reactions vary according to the concentration of THC, the setting in which marijuana is used, and the user's expectations, personality, and mood.

Marijuana's short-term physical effects include reddening of the eyes and rapid heartbeat. The drug interferes with the individual's judgment, coordination, and short-term **memory**.

Long-term effects are not completely known. Marijuana use affects memory and motivation. Some chronic users experience bronchitis, coughing, and chest pains. Among males marijuana use can reduce sperm production and testosterone level. Among females it can cause menstrual irregularity and reduced fertility. Extended marijuana use often has a psychological impact and may result in the loss of interest in, for example, school, work, and social activities. Some regular marijuana users become dependent on it.

Marijuana affects psychomotor performance. The effects depend on the nature of the task and the individual's experience with marijuana. Cannabinoids, especially THC, can impact **immune response**, either enhancing or diminishing it.

Human volunteers performing auditory attention tasks while smoking marijuana show impaired performance, which is associated with substantial reduction in **blood** flow to the brain's temporal lobe. However, marijuana smoking increases blood flow in other brain regions, such as the frontal lobes and lateral cerebellum. Although some studies purported to show structural changes in the brains of heavy marijuana users, these results have not been replicated with more sophisticated techniques. Nevertheless, some studies have found subtle defects in the performance of cognitive tasks among heavy marijuana users.

THC narrows bronchi and bronchioles and produces inflammation of the mucous membranes. Marijuana smoke contains many of the same chemicals and tars of tobacco smoke and therefore increases the risk of **lung cancer**.

Although a distinctive marijuana withdrawal syndrome has been identified, it is mild and short-lived. Symptoms include restlessness, irritability, mild agitation, insomnia, sleep disturbance, nausea, and cramping.

Viewpoints

Marijuana has been used as a medicine and intoxicant for thousands of years. In the United States, marijuana use has been prohibited by state and local laws since the early 1900s, and by federal law since 1937. In spite of these laws, use of the drug became widespread during the 1960s and 1970s. Between 1969 and 1978, the federal and many state governments reduced the criminal charge for possession of small amounts of marijuana from a felony to a misdemeanor. Some states even substituted fines for jail sentences. Use of marijuana in the United States declined from the mid-1970s through the early 1990s. In the mid-1990s, however, marijuana use again began to rise.

The Institute of Medicine recently released its findings on the medical merits of marijuana. Initially commissioned by the Office of National Drug Control Policy in 1997, the study concluded that cannabinoids, marijuana's active components, can be useful in treating pain, nausea and appetite loss caused by advanced **cancer** and AIDS. For very ill patients with no other treatment options, investigators recommended short-term use of smoked marijuana under strict medical oversight. However, the Institute of Medicine found that the drug's benefits were hampered by the toxicity of smoking, and that marijuana's future lay in the development of synthetic cannabinoids and in smokeless delivery systems—ideally an asthma-type inhaler. Finally, researchers found no conclusive evidence that recommending marijuana medicinally would increase general use.

Proponents of medical marijuana cite scientific research indicating the potential therapeutic value of cannabinoid drugs, primarily THC, for pain relief, control of nausea and vomiting, and appetite loss that often accompany cancer and AIDS. However, proponents lament the fact that the emphasis on pharmaceutical research will delay treatment because research and development for new drugs can cost $300 million and only about one in five are approved.

In 1985, the U.S. Food and Drug Administration approved Marinol, a capsule containing THC, as a prescription drug. However, Marinol takes from one to several hours to take effect and many patients experience severe side effects. Since 1996, voters in Arizona,

California, Oregon, several other states, and the District of Columbia have passed laws allowing medical use of marijuana.

Opponents focus their arguments on marijuana's addictive potential and other health problems.

Professional implications

Because marijuana is a crude THC delivery system that also delivers harmful substances, smoked marijuana should generally not be recommended for medical use. Nevertheless, marijuana is widely used by certain patient groups, which raises both safety and efficacy issues. Marijuana's future as a medicine lies in its isolated components, the cannabinoids and their synthetic derivatives. Isolated cannabinoids provide more reliable effects than crude plant mixtures.

The accumulated data suggest a variety of indications, particularly for pain relief, antiemesis, and appetite stimulation. For patients such as those with AIDS or who are undergoing chemotherapy, and who suffer simultaneously from severe pain, nausea, and appetite loss, cannabinoid drugs might offer broad-spectrum relief not found in any other single medication. The therapeutic effects of cannabinoids are most well established for THC, marijuana's primary psychoactive ingredient. Although marijuana smoke delivers THC and other cannabinoids it also delivers harmful substances, including most of those found in tobacco smoke. In addition, plants contain a variable mixture of biologically active compounds and cannot be expected to provide a precisely defined drug effect. For those reasons there seems to be little future in smoked marijuana as a medically approved medication.

While clinical trials are the route to developing approved medications, they are also valuable for other reasons. For example, the personal medical use of smoked marijuana to treat certain symptoms is sufficient reason to advocate clinical trials to assess the degree to which the symptoms or course of diseases are affected. Trials testing the safety and efficacy of marijuana use are an important component to understanding the course of a disease, particularly diseases such as AIDS. The argument against the future of smoked marijuana for treating any condition is not that there is no reason to predict efficacy but that there is risk. That risk could be overcome by the development of a non-smoked rapid-onset delivery system for cannabinoid drugs.

In addition to smoking, there are other means of cannabinoid delivery. Inhalers eliminate smoke toxicity while maintaining quick bloodstream entry. Pills are legal and smokeless, however, they can take over an hour to enter bloodstream and some patients cannot tolerate the concentrated dose.

The psychological effects of cannabinoids, such as **anxiety** reduction, sedation, and euphoria can influence their potential therapeutic value. Those effects are potentially undesirable for certain patients, although they may be beneficial for others. In addition, marijuana's psychological effects can complicate the interpretation of other aspects of the drug's effect.

Since marijuana smoke contains many of tobacco smoke's harmful components, it is important to consider the relationship between habitual marijuana smoking and lung disease. Given a cigarette of comparable weight, as much as four times the amount of tar can be deposited in the **lungs** of marijuana smokers as in the lungs of tobacco smokers. Marijuana smoke's carcinogenicity is an important concern.

Alveolar macrophages protect lungs against infectious microorganisms, inhaled foreign substances, and tumor cells. Marijuana smoking reduces the ability of alveolar macrophages to kill **fungi**, pathogenic **bacteria**, and tumor target cells. The reduction in ability to destroy fungal organisms is similar to that observed in tobacco smokers.

Marijuana smoke and oral THC can cause tachycardia (fast **heart** beat). In some cases **blood pressure** increases while a person is in a reclining position but decreases inordinately on standing, resulting in postural hypotension or decreased blood pressure, which may cause dizziness and faintness.

Advances in cannabinoid science have revealed a wealth of new opportunities for the development of medically useful cannabinoid-based drugs. The accumulated data suggest a variety of indications, particularly for pain relief, antiemesis, and appetite stimulation. For patients such as those with AIDS or who are undergoing chemotherapy, and who suffer simultaneously from severe pain, nausea, and appetite loss, cannabinoid drugs might offer broad-spectrum relief not found in any other single medication.

The risks of smoking marijuana should be considered before recommending its use to any patient with pre-existing immune deficits, including AIDS patients, cancer patients, and those receiving immunosuppressive therapies.

The argument against the future of smoked marijuana for treating any condition is not the absence of efficacy but the risk. That risk could be overcome by the development of a non-smoked, rapid-onset delivery system for cannabinoid drugs.

Resources

BOOKS

Gabriel N., Sutin, K., and Harvey, D., eds. *Marijuana and Medicine.* Humana Press, 1999.

Joy J., Watson, S., and Benson, J., eds. *Marijuana and Medicine: Assessing the Science Base.* Institute of Medicine, 1999.

Mack, A. and Joy, J. *Marijuana As Medicine?: The Science Beyond the Controversy.* National Academy Press, 2000.

PERIODICALS

Kalb, C., Wingert, P., Rosenberg, D., Underwood, A., and Hammer, J. "No Green Light Yet: A long-awaited report supports medical marijuana. So now what?" *Newsweek* Section: Nation; Subsection: Medicine (March 29, 1999): 35.

Sohn, E. "Is grass a proven tonic?" *U.S. News & World Report* (May 28, 2001).

ORGANIZATIONS

Campaign to Legalise Cannabis International Association. Cannabis Campaigner's Guide, Up-to-Date Chronology of Cannabis Hemp. <http://www.paston.com.uk/uses/webbooks/chronol.html>.

Center for Cardiovascular Education, Inc. Smoking Marijuana Increases Heart Attack Risk. Heart Information Network. <http://www.heartinfo.org/news2000/marijuana061400.htm>.

Bill Asenjo, Ph.D., C.R.C.

Maslow's hierarchy of needs

Definition

Maslow's hierarchy of needs is a theory of motivation and personality developed by the psychologist Abraham H. Maslow (1908-1970). Maslow's hierarchy explains human behavior in terms of basic requirements for survival and growth. These requirements, or needs, are arranged according to their importance for survival and their power to motivate the individual. The most basic physical requirements, such as food, water, or oxygen, constitute the lowest level of the need hierarchy. These needs must be satisfied before other, higher needs become important to individuals. Needs at the higher levels of the hierarchy are less oriented towards physical survival and more toward psychological well-being and growth. These needs have less power to motivate persons, and they are more influenced by formal education and life experiences. The resulting hierarchy of needs is often depicted as a pyramid, with physical survival needs located at the base of the pyramid and needs for self-actualization located at the top.

Description

Maslow's hierarchy specifies the following levels:

- *Physiological needs:* These are the basic requirements for human physical survival. They include such essentials as food, water, shelter, oxygen, and sleep. When these needs are unmet, human beings will focus on satisfying them and will ignore higher needs.

- *Safety needs:* Once the individual's basic physical needs are met, his or her needs for safety emerge. These include needs for a sense of security and predictability in the world. The person tries to maintain the conditions that allow him or her to feel safe and avoid danger. Maslow thought that inadequate fulfillment of these needs might explain neurotic behavior and other emotional problems in some people.

- *Love and belonging needs:* When the individual's physiological and safety needs are met, needs for love and belongingness emerge. These needs include longings for an intimate relationship with another person as well as the need to belong to a group and to feel accepted. Maslow emphasized that these needs involve both giving and receiving love.

- *Esteem needs:* Esteem needs include both self-esteem and the esteem of others. Self-esteem is the feeling that one is worthwhile, competent, and independent. The esteem of others involves the feeling that other people respect and appreciate the person. Once the person has satisfied his or her basic needs, concerns about worthiness emerge. The focus becomes not just surviving, but doing well according to meaningful communal standards.

- *Self-actualization needs:* These are the needs associated with realizing one's full potential. As these needs emerge, the person focuses on doing what he or she is meant to do in life—developing his or her talents and abilities to their fullest extent.

Other human needs

Maslow described other needs that did not fit into his hierarchy. These included cognitive needs, such as curiosity and scientific interest, as well as aesthetic needs, which include the need for beauty and order. As Maslow studied self-actualizing individuals, he also discovered a range of needs that extend beyond self-actualization. He called these needs transcendence needs or B-values. They refer to needs to contribute to human welfare and to find higher meanings in life. Although transcendence needs are usually described as lying somewhere beyond the need for self-actualization, these needs are not included in most formulations of Maslow's needs hierarchy.

While Maslow described human needs as a hierarchy, he allowed for some departures from the strict order of his needs hierarchy. He stated that lower needs must be reasonably well satisfied in order for the person to focus on higher needs, but he noted that complete satisfaction of a given need may not be possible or necessary. He indicated that most people would show a range of need satisfaction levels at any given time. For example, a person might be 85% satisfied in the area of physiological needs, 60% satisfied in the area of safety needs, 45% satisfied in the area of love and belongingness needs, and so on. Maslow also noted situations in which lower needs might be ignored in favor of higher needs, as when an artist sacrifices comfort and security in order to pursue aesthetic goals, or when a student postpones looking for a romantic partner in order to earn high grades and get into a prestigious graduate program. Maslow thought, however, that these departures from a strict hierarchy did not invalidate his general theory.

The historical context of Maslow's theories

At the time Maslow developed his theory in the early 1960s, psychology was dominated by two views of human behavior, the psychoanalytic and the behaviorist. The psychoanalytic view emphasized unconscious conflicts and drives, drawing many of its concepts from case studies of neurotic people. The behaviorist view emphasized the role of learning and derived many of its principles from observations of animal behavior. Maslow pointed out that the psychoanalysts had failed to consider the behavior of healthy human beings, while the behaviorists were too mechanistic and largely ignored subjective experience. He thought that no theory of human personality could be complete without a thorough study of healthy functioning, so he set out to examine the conscious motivations and experiences of healthy individuals. One important finding was that psychologically healthy people were more likely to report what Maslow called "peak experiences." A peak experience, according to Maslow, is one in which the individual loses a sense of time and place and experiences a momentary feeling of unity with the universe. It is a particularly intense form of growth experience.

Maslow's perspective, together with similar approaches proposed by Carl Rogers, Gordon Allport, and others, came to be known as the "third force" in psychology. Because of their focus on the positive, growth-oriented aspects of human behavior, these views are also described as humanistic theories of behavior. They stim-

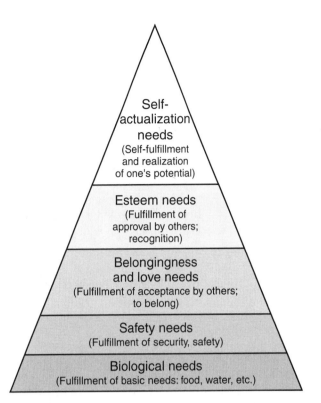

Maslow's hierarchy of needs. *(EPD Photos. Courtesy Gale Group.)*

ulated the emergence and rapid growth of the human potential movement of the late 1960s and early 1970s.

Viewpoints

Maslow's theory and the other humanistic theories have had an important impact on psychology as well as in other fields. By emphasizing positive aspects of human behavior, these theories provide a framework for understanding human behavior outside the context of mental illness and dysfunction. Humanistic approaches to behavior allow for the possibility of growth and achievement, in addition to providing useful explanations for some forms of maladjustment that do not fit the traditional understanding of neurosis and mental illness. The humanistic viewpoint has been very influential on **psychotherapy** and counseling, and many therapists identify themselves as humanistic in orientation.

Maslow's need hierarchy provides a helpful way to understand human motivation in many settings. Maslow proposed many changes in business management in order to make workplaces more responsive to the needs of workers. He called his ideas "eupsychian management," emphasizing the potential for human growth in the workplace. A small body of research has shown modest support for some of Maslow's concepts. Maslow's hierarchy

KEY TERMS

Behaviorism—The theory that human or animal psychology can be accurately studied only through analysis of objectively observable and quantifiable behaviors, in contrast to subjective mental states.

Humanistic psychology—An approach to psychology that emphasizes the special qualities and potential of human beings. It emphasizes the positive qualities in people, rather than the characteristics of maladaptive or unhealthy individuals.

Peak experience—An awe-inspiring emotional experience, characterized by a sense of timelessness, unity, and wonder. Maslow found that self-actualizing people were more likely to have peak experiences, but that ordinary individuals could have these experiences as well.

Self-actualization—The development of one's full potential as a person through creativity, independence, spontaneity, and a grasp of the real world.

Self-esteem—A sense of competence, achievement, and self-respect. Maslow felt that the most stable source of self-esteem is genuine accomplishment rather than public acclaim or praise.

Transcendence needs—Needs or values that go beyond the need for self-actualization. These values involve a higher purpose and concern for the good of the community rather than personal welfare.

of needs is also used in medical and social welfare settings, providing a set of theoretical guidelines for understanding the concerns of people suffering from physical illness, disabilities, or other life problems. In addition to these settings, the theory is frequently applied in educational and career counseling, in which it is used to help clients select appropriate goals for their lives.

Maslow's theory has been criticized because it is difficult to evaluate objectively. Many of the phenomena that Maslow describes are subjective and difficult to quantify. Most studies rely on self-reported data, which are notoriously subject to distortion and inaccuracies. Because studies based on Maslow's concepts often focus on value-laden topics, it is also difficult for researchers to remain objective. Maslow acknowledged these difficulties himself, but thought that human potential was so important that it should be explored without regard to current limitations of scientific accuracy.

The field of personality theory has changed considerably over the 30 years since Maslow's death in 1970. The cognitive behaviorist approach has become increasingly influential, answering some of Maslow's criticisms of earlier psychoanalytic and behaviorist theories. Humanistic theories have become less popular in academic and research settings, with newer approaches generating more research topics. Nonetheless, Maslow's theory, with its positive emphasis, remains influential, particularly in such applied settings as counseling, industrial management, and health care.

Professional implications

Maslow's understanding of human motivation has had an important influence in the fields of nursing and allied health. The needs hierarchy provides a useful framework for understanding patients, and this framework has been incorporated into several important theories of medical and nursing care. One major approach to nursing theory has been described as a "needs" approach, and it relies on Maslow's need hierarchy as well as the developmental theories of Erik Erikson. Needs-oriented theories emphasize the nurse's role in helping the patient to meet his or her physiological and psychosocial needs. Although more recent theories have moved away from this position, the needs hierarchy has been useful in helping care providers look for the "big picture" of a given patient's situation. A description of Maslow's needs hierarchy is still included in many textbooks for students of nursing and allied health.

As the realities of health care in a managed care environment have affected medical professionals, Maslow's theory has also found a role in human resource management for health care. The needs hierarchy offers one approach to such human resource issues as quality assurance, employee burnout, and job satisfaction. By understanding the larger set of needs that health care providers bring to their professions, human resource managers can do a better job of coping with and planning for problems that arise in the medical workplace. Maslow's ideas remain influential because they make sense of a certain range of human behavior.

On the other hand, Maslow's emphasis on a strict hierarchical ordering of human needs has not held up well in other respects because it has never been empirically substantiated. The connections between motivation and external behavior in human beings are more complex than Maslow's theory allows. People strive to satisfy simultaneous needs for love, safety, self-esteem, etc. Moreover, people who have their "lower" needs met in a satisfactory fashion do not invariably seek the fulfilment of "higher" needs, as the behavior of many wealthy or famous individuals indicates. In addition, the drive to satisfy "higher" needs takes precedence over "lower" needs more frequently than Maslow thought. In sum, human beings are influenced by a wide range of needs and motives. For some people, love, safety, and security are paramount values, while others are motivated by desires for power and dominance. Lastly, human beings are shaped to a considerable extent by their cultures, and cultures differ widely in the sets of values that they emphasize and transmit to their members. For example, the very notion of a "self" is more consistently individualistic in Western societies, whereas it incorporates family relationships in Eastern cultures. Maslow's hierarchy of needs reflects the values of twentieth-century Western middle-class males; it is not culture-neutral and is therefore not universally applicable to all periods of human history or to all contemporary societies.

Resources

BOOKS

Burger, Jerry M. *Personality*. 5th ed. Belmont, CA: Wadsworth/Thomson Learning, 2000.

Goble, Frank G. *The Third Force: The Psychology of Abraham Maslow.* New York: Grossman Publishers, 1970.

Maslow, Abraham H. *Motivation and Personality*. 2nd ed. New York: Harper and Row, 1970.

Maslow, Abraham H. *Toward a Psychology of Being*. 2nd ed. New York: Van Nostrand Reinhold, 1968.

Meleis, Afaf I. *Theoretical Nursing: Development and Progress.* 2nd ed. Philadelphia: J. B. Lippincott Co., 1991.

Sargent, S. Stansfeld. "Abraham H. Maslow (1908-1970)." *International Encyclopedia of Psychiatry, Psychology, Psychoanalysis, & Neurology*. Vol. 7. Ed. Benjamin B. Wolman. New York: Aesculapius Publishers, Inc., 1977.

Smither, Robert D. *The Psychology of Work and Human Performance.* 2nd ed. New York: HarperCollins, 1994.

PERIODICALS

Crapanzano, S. "Motivation, morale, education, and leadership." *Pelican News* 56 (March 2000): 6.

Zimberg, Stephen E., and Dolores G. Clement. "Physician motivation, satisfaction and survival."*Medical Group Management Journal* 44 (July/August 1997): 19-26; 63.

ORGANIZATIONS

American Psychological Association. 750 First Street, NE, Washington, DC 20002. (800) 374-2721.

Denise L. Schmutte, Ph.D.

Massage therapy

Definition

Massage therapy is the scientific manipulation of the soft tissues of the body for the purpose of normalizing those tissues and consists of manual techniques that include applying fixed or movable pressure, holding, and/or causing movement of or to the body.

Origins

Massage therapy is one of the oldest health care practices known to history. References to massage are found in Chinese medical texts more than 4,000 years old. Massage has been advocated in Western health care practices at least since the time of Hippocrates, the "Father of Medicine." In the fourth century B.C. Hippocrates wrote, "The physician must be acquainted with many things and assuredly with rubbing" (the ancient Greek term for massage was rubbing).

The roots of modern, scientific massage therapy go back to Per Henrik Ling (1776–1839), a Swede, who developed an integrated system consisting of massage and active and passive exercises. Ling established the Royal Central Gymnastic Institute in Sweden in 1813 to teach his methods.

Modern, scientific massage therapy was introduced in the United States in the 1850s by two New York physicians, brothers George and Charles Taylor, who had studied in Sweden. The first clinics for massage therapy in the United States were opened by two Swedish physicians after the Civil War period. Doctor Baron Nils Posse operated the Posse Institute in Boston and Doctor Hartwig Nissen opened the Swedish Health Institute near the Capitol in Washington, D.C.

Although there were periods when massage fell out of favor, in the 1960s it made a comeback in a different way as a tool for **relaxation**, communication, and alternative healing. Today, massage is one of the most popular healing modalities. It is used by conventional, as well as alternative, medical communities and is now covered by some health insurance plans.

Benefits

Generally, massage is known to affect the circulation of **blood** and the flow of blood and lymph, reduce muscular tension or flaccidity, affect the nervous system through stimulation or sedation, and enhance tissue healing. These effects provide a number of benefits:

• reduction of muscle tension and stiffness

- relief of muscle spasms

- greater flexibility and range of motion

- increase of the ease and efficiency of movement

- relief of **stress** and aide of relaxation

- promotion of deeper and easier breathing

- improvement of the circulation of blood and movement of lymph

- relief of tension-related conditions, such as headaches and eyestrain

- promotion of faster healing of soft tissue injuries, such as pulled muscles and sprained ligaments, and reduction in **pain** and swelling related to such injuries

- reduction in the formation of excessive scar tissue following soft tissue injuries

- enhancement in the health and nourishment of skin

- improvement in posture through changing tension patterns that affect posture

- reduction in stress and an excellent stress management tool

- creation of a feeling of well-being

- reduction in levels of **anxiety**

- increase in awareness of the mind-body connection

- promotion of a relaxed state of mental awareness

Massage therapy also has a number of documented clinical benefits. For example, massage can reduce anxiety, improve pulmonary function in young **asthma** patients, reduce psycho-emotional distress in persons suffering from chronic inflammatory bowel disease, increase weight and improve motor development in **premature infants**, and may enhance **immune system** functioning. Some medical conditions that massage therapy can help are: **allergies**, anxiety and stress, arthritis, asthma and bronchitis, **carpal tunnel syndrome** and other repetitive motion injuries, chronic and temporary pain, circulatory problems, depression, digestive disorders, **tension headache**, insomnia, myofascial pain, **sports injuries**, and temporomandibular joint dysfunction.

Description

Massage therapy is the scientific manipulation of the soft tissues of the body for the purpose of normalizing those tissues and consists of a group of manual techniques that include applying fixed or movable pressure, holding, and/or causing movement of or to the body. While massage therapy is applied primarily with the hands, sometimes the forearms or elbows are used. These techniques affect the muscular, skeletal, circulatory, lym-phatic, nervous, and other systems of the body. The basic philosophy of massage therapy embraces the concept of *vis Medicatrix naturae*, which is aiding the ability of the body to heal itself, and is aimed at achieving or increasing health and well-being.

Touch is the fundamental medium of massage therapy. While massage can be described in terms of the type of techniques performed, touch is not used solely in a mechanistic way in massage therapy. One could look at a diagram or photo of a massage technique that depicts where to place one's hands and what direction the stroke should go, but this would not convey everything that is important for giving a good massage. Massage also has an artistic component.

Because massage usually involves applying touch with some degree of pressure and movement, the massage therapist must use touch with sensitivity in order to determine the optimal amount of pressure to use for each person. For example, using too much pressure may cause the body to tense up, while using too little may not have enough effect. Touch used with sensitivity also allows the massage therapist to receive useful information via his or her hands about the client's body, such as locating areas of muscle tension and other soft tissue problems. Because touch is also a form of communication, sensitive touch can convey a sense of caring—an essential element in the therapeutic relationship—to the person receiving massage.

In practice, many massage therapists use more than one technique or method in their work and sometimes combine several. Effective massage therapists ascertain each person's needs and then use the techniques that will meet those needs best.

Swedish massage uses a system of long gliding strokes, kneading, and friction techniques on the more superficial layers of muscles, generally in the direction of blood flow toward the **heart**, and sometimes combined with active and passive movements of the joints. It is used to promote general relaxation, improve circulation and range of motion, and relieve muscle tension. Swedish massage is the most commonly used form of massage.

Deep tissue massage is used to release chronic patterns of muscular tension using slow strokes, direct pressure, or friction directed across the grain of the muscles. It is applied with greater pressure and to deeper layers of muscle than Swedish, which is why it is called deep tissue and is effective for chronic muscular tension.

Sports massage uses techniques that are similar to Swedish and deep tissue, but are specially adapted to deal with the effects of athletic performance on the body and

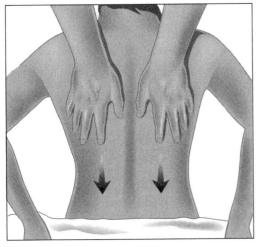

Basic Effleurage

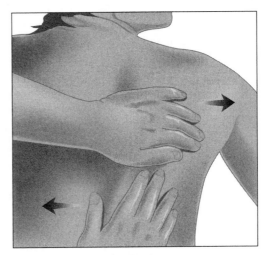

Rolling Petrissage

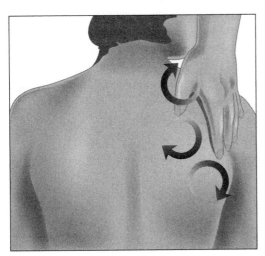

Circular Friction

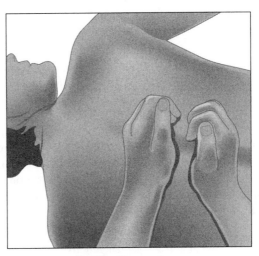

Beating Percussion

Four basic massage techniques. In basic effleurage, keep firm contact with the skin as you stroke down your partner's back. In rolling petrissage, push the heel of one hand across your partner's back, while you pull and lift the skin with the fingers of the other. In circular friction, rotate your thumb in small circles on the ropelike tissues of your partner's back. In beating percussion, use a loose fist to gently beat the fleshy areas of the body. *(Illustration by Electronic Illustrators Group.)*

the needs of athletes regarding training, performing, and recovery from injury.

Neuromuscular massage is a form of deep massage that is applied to individual muscles. It is used primarily to release trigger points (intense knots of muscle tension that refer pain to other parts of the body), and also to increase blood flow. It is often used to reduce pain. Trigger point massage and myotherapy are similar forms.

Acupressure applies finger or thumb pressure to specific points located on the acupuncture meridians (channels of energy flow identified in Asian concepts of anatomy) in order to release blocked energy along these meridians that causes physical discomforts, and re-balance the energy flow. **Shiatsu** is a Japanese form of acupressure.

The cost of massage therapy varies according to geographic location, experience of the massage therapist, and length of the massage. In the United States, the average range is from $35–60 for a one hour session. Massage therapy sessions at a client's home or office may cost more due to travel time for the massage therapist. Most sessions are one hour. Frequency of massage sessions can vary widely. If a person is receiving massage for a specific problem, frequency can vary widely based on the condition, though it usually will be once a week. Some people incorporate massage into their regular personal health and fitness program. They will go for massage on a regular basis, varying from once a week to once a month.

The first appointment generally begins with information gathering, such as the reason for getting massage therapy, physical condition and medical history, and other areas. The client is asked to remove clothing to one's level of comfort. Undressing takes place in private, and a sheet or towel is provided for draping. The massage therapist will undrape only the part of the body being massaged. The client's modesty is respected at all times. The massage therapist may use an oil or cream, which will be absorbed into the skin in a short time.

To receive the most benefit from a massage, generally the person being massaged should give the therapist accurate health information, report discomfort of any kind (whether it's from the massage itself or due to the room temperature or any other distractions), and be as receptive and open to the process as possible.

Insurance coverage for massage therapy varies widely. There tends to be greater coverage in states that license massage therapy. In most cases, a physician's prescription for massage therapy is needed. Once massage therapy is prescribed, authorization from the insurer may be needed if coverage is not clearly spelled out in one's policy or plan.

Preparations

Going for a massage requires little in the way of preparation. Generally, one should be clean and should not eat just before a massage. One should not be under the influence of alcohol or non-medicinal drugs. Massage therapists generally work by appointment and usually will provide information about how to prepare for an appointment at the time of making the appointment.

Precautions

Massage is comparatively safe. However, it is generally contraindicated, i.e., it should not be used if a person has one of the following conditions: advanced heart diseases, **hypertension** (high **blood pressure**), phlebitis, thrombosis, embolism, kidney failure, **cancer** if massage would accelerate metastasis (i.e., spread a tumor) or damage tissue that is fragile due to **chemotherapy** or other treatment, infectious diseases, contagious skin conditions, acute inflammation, infected injuries, unhealed **fractures**, dislocations, frostbite, large hernias, torn ligaments, conditions prone to hemorrhage, and psychosis.

Massage should not be used locally on affected areas for the following conditions: rheumatoid arthritis flare up, eczema, goiter, and open skin lesions. Massage may be used on the areas of the body that are not affected by these conditions.

In some cases, precautions should be taken before using massage for the following conditions: **pregnancy**, high fevers, **osteoporosis**, diabetes, recent postoperative cases in which pain and muscular splinting (i.e., tightening as a protective reaction) would be increased, apprehension, and mental conditions that may impair communication or perception. In such cases, massage may or may not be appropriate. The decision on whether to use massage must be based on whether it may cause harm. For example, if someone has osteoporosis, the concern is whether bones are strong enough to withstand the pressure applied. If one has a health condition and has any hesitation about whether massage therapy would be appropriate, a physician should be consulted.

Side effects

Massage therapy does not have side effects. Sometimes people are concerned that massage may leave them too relaxed or too mentally unfocused. To the contrary, massage tends to leave people feeling more relaxed and alert.

Research and general acceptance

Before 1939, more than 600 research studies on massage appeared in the main journals of medicine in English. However, the pace of research was slowed by medicine's disinterest in massage therapy.

Massage therapy research picked up again in the 1980s, as the growing popularity of massage paralleled the growing interest in complementary and alternative medicine. Well designed studies have documented the benefits of massage therapy for the treatment of acute and chronic pain, acute and chronic inflammation, chronic lymphedema, nausea, muscle spasm, various soft tissue dysfunctions, anxiety, depression, insomnia, and psycho-emotional stress, which may aggravate mental illness.

Premature infants treated with daily massage therapy gain more weight and have shorter hospital stays than infants who are not massaged. A study of 40 low-birth-weight babies found that the 20 massaged babies had a 47% greater weight gain per day and stayed in the hospital an average of six days less than 20 infants who did not receive massage, resulting a cost savings of approximately $3,000 per infant. Cocaine-exposed, preterm infants given massage three times daily for a 10 day period showed significant improvement. Results indicated that massaged infants had fewer postnatal complications and exhibited fewer stress behaviors during the 10 day period, had a 28% greater daily weight gain, and demonstrated more mature motor behaviors.

A study comparing 52 hospitalized depressed and adjustment disorder children and adolescents with a control group that viewed relaxation videotapes, found massage therapy subjects were less depressed and anxious, and had lower saliva cortisol levels (an indicator of less depression).

Another study showed massage therapy produced relaxation in 18 elderly subjects, demonstrated in measures such as decreased blood pressure and heart rate and increased skin temperature.

A combination of massage techniques for 52 subjects with traumatically induced spinal pain led to significant improvements in acute and chronic pain and increased muscle flexibility and tone. This study also found massage therapy to be extremely cost effective, with cost savings ranging from 15–50%. Massage has also been shown to stimulate the body's ability to naturally control pain by stimulating the **brain** to produce endorphins. **Fibromyalgia** is an example of a condition that may be favorably affected by this effect.

A pilot study of five subjects with symptoms of tension and anxiety found a significant response to massage therapy in one or more psycho-physiological parameters of heart rate, frontalis and forearm extensor electromyograms (EMGs) and skin resistance, which demonstrate relaxation of muscle tension and reduced anxiety.

Lymph drainage massage has been shown to be more effective than mechanized methods or diuretic drugs to control lymphedema secondary to radical mastectomy, consequently using massage to control lymphedema would significantly lower treatment costs. A study found that massage therapy can have a powerful effect upon psycho-emotional distress in persons suffering from chronic inflammatory bowel disease. Massage therapy was effective in reducing the frequency of episodes of pain and disability in these patients.

Massage may enhance the immune system. A study suggests an increase in cytotoxic capacity associated with massage. A study of chronic fatigue syndrome subjects found that a group receiving massage therapy had lower depression, emotional distress, and somatic symptom scores, more hours of sleep, and lower epinephrine and cortisol levels than a control group.

Training and certification

The generally accepted standard for training is a minimum of 500 classroom hours. Training should include anatomy, physiology, pathology, massage theory and technique, and supervised practice. Most massage therapists also take additional courses and workshops during their careers.

In the United States, massage therapists are currently licensed by 29 states, the District of Columbia, and a number of localities. Most states require 500 or more classroom hours of training from a recognized training program and passing an examination.

A national certification program was inaugurated in June 1992 by the National Certification Board for Therapeutic Massage and Bodywork (NCBTMB). The NCBTMB program is accredited by the National Commission for Certifying Agencies, the chief outside agency for evaluating certification programs. Those certified can use the title Nationally Certified in Therapeutic Massage and Bodywork (NCTMB). Most states use the NCBTMB exam for their licensing exams.

A national accreditation agency, the Commission on Massage Therapy Accreditation, designed according to the guidelines of the U.S. Department of Education, currently recognizes about 70 training programs. The Accrediting Commission of Career Schools and Colleges of Technology and the Accrediting Council for Continuing Education and Training also accredit massage training programs.

Resources

BOOKS

Beck, Mark F. *Milady's Theory and Practice of Therapeutic Massage*. Milady Publishing, 1994.

Capellini, Steve. *Massage Therapy Career Guide for Hands-On Success*. Milady Publishing, 1998.

Downing, George. *The Massage Book*. New York: Random House, 1998.

Loving, Jean E. *Massage Therapy: Theory and Practice*. Appleton & Lange, 1998.

PERIODICALS

Field, T., W. Sunshine, M. Hernandez-Reif, and O. Quintino. "Chronic fatigue syndrome: massage therapy effects on depression and somatic symptoms in chronic fatigue syndrome." *Journal of Chronic Fatigue Syndrome* (1997): 43-51.

Ironson, G., T. Field, F. Scafidi, and M. Hashimoto. "Massage therapy is associated with enhancement of the immune system's cytotoxic capacity." *International Journal of Neuroscience* (February 1996): 205-217.

Joachim, G. "The effects of two stress management techniques on feelings of well-being in patients with inflammatory bowel disease." *Nursing Papers* (1983): 4, 5-18.

Kaarda, B., and O. Tosteinbo. "Increase of plasma beta-endorphins in connective tissue massage." *General Pharmacology* (1989): 487-489.

Scafidi, F., T. Field, A. Wheeden, S. Schanberg, C. Kuhn, R. Symanski, E. Zimmerman, and E. S. Bandstra. "Cocaine exposed preterm neonates show behavioral and hormonal differences." *Pediatrics* (June 1996): 851-855.

Weintraub, M. "Shiatsu, Swedish muscle massage, and trigger point suppression in spinal pain syndrome." *American Massage Therapy Journal* 31, Summer 1992:3; 99-109.

ORGANIZATIONS

American Massage Therapy Association. <http://www.amta-massage.org>.

Elliot Greene

Mastitis

Definition

Mastitis is an **infection** of the ducts of the breast. It usually only occurs in women who are breastfeeding their babies.

Description

In the process of breastfeeding, the unaccustomed pull and tug by the infant suckling at the breast may

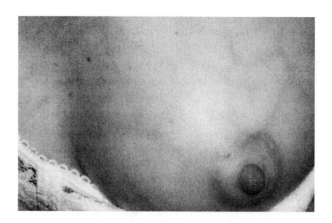

Mastitis is usually caused by bacterial infection through damaged nipples during breastfeeding. Mastitis can also be caused by a hormone imbalance and usually occurs at puberty or in the newborn. *(Photograph by Dr. P. Marazzi, Photo Researchers, Inc. Reproduced by permission.)*

result in the mother's nipples may becoming sore, cracked, or slightly abraded. This creates a tiny opening in the breast, through which **bacteria** can enter. The presence of milk, with high sugar content, gives the bacteria an excellent source of **nutrition**. Under these conditions, the bacteria are able to multiply, until they are plentiful enough to cause an infection within the breast.

Mastitis is most likely to occur in the fifth and sixth week of the postpartum period. Studies indicate an incidence of mastitis from 6–33% of all women who have a history of breastfeeding.

Causes and symptoms

The most common bacteria causing mastitis is *Staphylococcus aureus*, but sometimes *Escherichia coli* is responsible. In rare instances, *Streptococcus* can also induce an episode of mastitis. In 25–30% of people, *Staphylococcus aureus* is present on the skin, lining normal, uninfected nostrils. It is probably this bacteria, clinging to the baby's nostrils, that is available to create infection when an opportunity (i.e., a crack in the nipple) presents itself. A sluggish flow of milk and trauma to the nipples are the main contributing factors to the development of mastitis. Fatigue, **stress**, and returning to work may also predispose a nursing mother to developing the condition.

Diagnosis

The clinic, midwife, or office of the physician will most likely receive a call from the mother at home. The condition rarely occurs in the hospital. She will likely report general malaise, fatigue, headache, chills, an increased **heart** rate, and flu-like symptoms. Usually, only one breast is involved. An area of the affected breast becomes swollen, red, hard, and painful. A red streak may be evident. Often, the location of the infection is in the upper, outer quadrant, which is the location of most of the glandular tissue.

Lumps in the breasts may result from plugged milk ducts. Plugged ducts can contribute to mastitis. If the mother describes **pain** in both breasts, then the condition might be engorgement of the breasts, as opposed to mastitis, which almost always occurs unilaterally.

A definitive diagnosis of the offending pathogen involves obtaining a sample of breast milk from the infected breast. A culture is done to identify the pathogen. In practice, however, laboratory studies are done infrequently because antibiotic therapy is initiated before results are returned, and insurance companies may not cover the cost of the tests.

Treatment

A penicillinase-resistant penicillin or a cephalosporin, for six to 10 days, can both be used to treat mastitis. Low doses of erythromycin or trimethoprin-sulfamethoxazole over an extended period of time have been used to treat chronic mastitis. Breastfeeding should be continued, because the rate of **abscess** formation in the infected breast increases sharply among women who stop breastfeeding during a bout of mastitis. Some symptoms of mastitis respond solely to frequent breastfeeding and pumping, without requiring antibiotic therapy. Most practitioners allow women to take acetaminophen while nursing, to relieve both **fever** and pain. Since almost all drugs the mother takes appear in her breast milk, any medication taken by breastfeeding women must also be safe for the baby. Warm, moist compresses applied to the affected breast can be soothing. Increasing fluid intake and bed rest are also recommended.

Prognosis

Prognosis for uncomplicated mastitis is excellent. A small percentage of women with mastitis will end up with an abscess within the affected breast. This complication will require a surgical procedure to drain the pus. In the case of a small abscess, aspiration with a needle under the direction of ultrasound may be the preferred method of treatment. A larger abscess requires an incision be made into the affected area, so that drainage can occur. A drain in the wound may be placed to facilitate further drainage. Manual expression of the site allows for elimination of pus and milk. The wound normally heals in one to two weeks.

KEY TERMS

Abscess—A persistent pocket of pus.

Lactation consultant—A health care provider who is certified in managing the breastfeeding concerns of mothers.

Health care team roles

The **registered nurse** (R.N.) and **lactation** consultant are frequently the first to speak with the mother who has mastitis. Rapid diagnosis, followed by treatment, can prevent the formation of an abscess. It is imperative to help the mother understand that continuation of breastfeeding is part of successful management of mastitis. It should be emphasized to her that abrupt cessation will actually worsen the problem.

Patient education

When counseling a mother who has mastitis, the health care provider should encourage her to breastfeed frequently and to use a breast pump if the baby does not adequately empty the breast. The mother should be instructed to start each nursing session by breastfeeding her baby on the breast that is not affected, because the baby's initial sucks will be the most vigorous ones. Once the baby switches to the affected breast, the milk will have already started to flow in "letdown reflex," and the baby's sucking will be less painful. The health care provider should instruct the mother to rest, increase her fluid intake, and take medications as prescribed.

Prevention

To prevent mastitis, mothers should breastfeed frequently, ensuring adequate emptying of each breast at least every other nursing session. Handwashing is important in decreasing the chance of spreading bacteria to the breasts. Mothers should also be instructed to avoid wearing tight bras, skipping feedings, and becoming overly tired.

Resources

BOOKS

Biancuzzo, Marie. *Breastfeeding the Newborn.* Herndon, VA: Mosby, 1999.

Cunningham, F. Gary, et al., eds. *Williams Obstetrics.* Stamford, CT: Appleton & Lange, 1997.

Riordan, Jan, and Kathleen Auerbach. *Breastfeeding and Human Lactation.* Boston, MA: Jones and Bartlett, 1999.

ORGANIZATIONS

LaLeche League International. 1400 N. Meacham Rd., Schaumburg, IL 60173-4048. (847) 519-7730 or (800) LALECHE. <http://www.lalecheleague.org>.

Nadine M. Jacobson

MD *see* **Muscular dystrophy**

Mean corpuscular hemoglobin *see* **Red blood cell indices**

Mean corpuscular volume *see* **Red blood cell indices**

Mechanical circulation support

Definition

Mechanical circulatory support is used to treat patients with advanced **heart failure**. A mechanical pump is surgically implanted to provide pulsatile or non-pulsatile flow of **blood** to supplement or replace the blood flow generated by the native **heart**. Types of circulatory support pumps include pneumatic and electromagnetic pumps. Rotary pumps, which are also available, propel blood by axial or centrifugal force, or by the use of positive displacement roller pumps.

Purpose

Heart failure causes low cardiac output, which results in inadequate **blood pressure** and reduced blood flow to the **brain**, **kidneys**, heart, and/or **lungs**. Pharmaceutical and palliative surgical treatments are typically exhausted before mechanical circulatory support is initiated. The extent of failure exhibited by one or both ventricles of the heart determines if univentricular or biventricular support is required. In either case, blood flow is supplemented or replaced by a mechanical circulatory support device. The device works by removing blood from the inlet of the ventricle(s) and reinjecting it at the outlet of the ventricle(s) in order to increase blood pressure and blood flow to the brain, kidneys, heart, and lungs.

The Abiomed and Thoratec devices along with the intra-aortic balloon pump (IABP), centrifugal pump, and extracorporeal membrane oxygenation (ECMO) are systems that are meant to sustain the patient until the heart recovers. If recovery does not occur, or is not expected,

then heart transplantation becomes the desired course of treatment. In this case intermediate- to long-term mechanical circulatory support devices are available. These longer-term devices include ECMO, Thoratec, Novacor, HeartMate, and Cardiowest products.

Description

Tertiary care facilities have the staff and equipment to provide treatment for heart failure patients, with the use of mechanical circulatory support devices. Short-, intermediate-, and long-term support requires bedside monitoring of the equipment and patient throughout treatment. The specialized nature of the equipment and intensive patient care requires dedicated staff who are able to provide continuous bedside treatment.

In most instances, patients receive pharmaceuticals that anticoagulate the blood by blocking the clotting factors from interacting with the foreign surfaces of the device and each other. Frequent laboratory testing determines the proper amount of medication required to prevent blood clots. To mimic the lining of **blood vessels**, some surfaces of the device attract native cells, which stick to the device surface, thereby eliminating the need for anticoagulation.

Blood flow generated by these devices is able to sustain blood pressure and flow to the heart, kidneys, **liver**, and brain. Temporary assist devices sustain vital organ tissues in situations where recovery of the heart function is anticipated. Long-term support devices sustain patients until a donor heart is available for transplantation.

Venoarterial ECMO circulatory support provides cardiopulmonary bypass. Both cardiac and pulmonary function can be supplemented with this device. The complexity of care and highly trained staff with specialized equipment limit the availability of ECMO to tertiary care facilities. Surgical cannulation is venoarterial, using the femoral or intrathoracic vessels. **Postoperative care** in the critical care unit requires dedicated bedside staffing.

Short- to intermediate-term devices

VENOARTERIAL ECMO. The positive displacement roller head pump provides pulsatile or non-pulsatile blood flow to the systemic circulation. Tubing connected to the venous cannula carries blood to the roller pump. The roller assembly rotates and engages the tubing, which is then compressed against the pump's housing, propelling blood ahead of the roller head. Rotational frequency and tubing inner diameter determine blood flow. Blood flow to the lungs is reduced as blood is drained from the venous circulation. Blood pumped by the left ventricle is also reduced as blood is returned directly to the systemic circulation. The heart is allowed to rest, pumping less blood than needed to maintain pressure and flow to the vital organs. An oxygenator is placed after the roller pump in the circuit. **Gas exchange** occurs prior to return of the blood to the arterial circulation.

As cardiac function improves, flow from ECMO support is reduced, allowing the heart to gradually resume normal function. The cannulae are surgically removed from the patient once the heart can maintain adequate cardiac output. Systemic anticoagulation is required throughout the length of support, and often leads to complications of stroke and coagulapathies. Long-term use of ECMO is limited since the patient is immobilized and sedated during treatment.

IABP. Ease of insertion for placement in the aorta makes the IABP the most often used univentricular assist device. Tertiary care centers provide this service in the **cardiac catheterization** laboratory, operating room, critical care unit, and emergency room. Secondary care level hospitals can also employ this technology. Well-trained staff are required to monitor equipment at regular intervals and troubleshoot problems.

Left ventricular support with the IABP reduces the workload of the heart and increases blood flow to the vital organs. Once in position, the IABP times the inflation and deflation of the balloon catheter to the electrocardiogram or arterial blood pressures waveform. Helium or carbon dioxide gases are used to fill the balloon, although low molecular weight helium is preferred because it can be transported rapidly. Carbon dioxide has the advantage that it is highly soluble in the blood in case of balloon rupture. The balloon inflates during diastole to deliver increased oxygen saturated blood to the heart. Blood flow is also increased to the arteries distal to the balloon, since flow is not occluded in either direction. Deflation of the balloon occurs prior to systole. Less contractile force is required for the heart to eject blood against a decreased afterload.

With recovery of the heart, the device is timed to inflate with every second or third heart beat. The catheter is removed, non-surgically, when the heart can sustain blood pressure and systemic blood flow. Therapeutic anticoagulation is achieved with minimal pharmaceutical anticoagulant throughout the treatment. The device can be in place up to several weeks, but duration is limited because the patient must be immobilized during the treatment.

CENTRIFUGAL PUMPS. Centrifugal pumps are able to provide uni-ventricular or bi-ventricular support to the ventricles. Blood is removed from the left or right atrium and returned to the aorta or pulmonary artery, respectively, therefore surgery is required to place the device.

Tertiary care facilities have the staff and equipment to provide treatment to heart failure patients with the use of mechanical circulatory support devices. Post-operative care in critical care units requires continuous monitoring by dedicated staff.

The cannulae are passed through the chest wall to attach to a pump that is magnetically coupled to the control unit, which is kept at the patient's bedside during treatment. The centrifugal force draws blood into the device and propels it to the arterial cannula. Rotational speed determines the amount of blood flow, which is measured by a flowmeter. If rotational frequency is too low, blood may flow in the wrong direction since the system is non-occlusive in nature.

As the heart recovers, flow is decreased from the centrifugal pump until the device can be removed. The native heart is then able to maintain blood pressure and flow. Anticoagulant is delivered continuously during treatment with a centrifugal pump, and patient immobilization limits the length of support to several weeks.

Intermediate- to long-term devices

When short-term support devices, such as ECMO, IABP, and the centrifugal pump are ineffective to sustain the patient to recovery or organ transplantation, a medium or long-term device is required. An advantage of treatment with a medium to long-term device is that it allows the patient to be mobile. In some instances patients have been able to leave the hospital for continued treatment at home with the implanted device. Complete recovery of the heart has been demonstrated in 5–15% of patients being supported as a bridge to organ transplantation.

PNEUMATIC PULSATILE. Pneumatically driven pulsatile paracorporeal mechanical circulatory support devices provide pulsatile support for the left or right ventricle, or both. Devices implanted in at least 100 patients by January 2001 include Abiomed, Thoratec, HeartMate, and Cardiowest brands. Staff are trained to monitor and troubleshoot equipment, thus limiting use to tertiary care facilities.

Cannulation of the left or right atrium, along with the aorta or pulmonary artery, respectively, requires a surgical approach. The cables that connect to the control center are tunneled out of the chest wall and the housing is typically implanted in the chest cavity, except Abiomed, which remains extracorporeal. The rigid outer housing encloses two compartments separated by a flexible boundary. Valves located at the inlet and outlet of the device direct the path of blood flow from high to low pressure, preventing back flow after ejection. Inflation of the gas chamber creates pressure in the blood chamber,

KEY TERMS

Anticoagulant—Pharmaceuticals to prevent clotting proteins and platelets in the blood to be activated to form a blood clot.

Cannulae—Tubes that provide access to the blood once inserted into the heart or blood vessels.

Cardiac—Of or relating to the heart.

Cardiac output—The liter per minute blood flow generated by contraction of the heart.

Cardiopulmonary bypass—Diversion of blood flow away from the right atrium and return of blood beyond the left ventricle, to bypass the heart and lungs.

Console—A freestanding device that monitors, measures, and controls parameters associated with the mechanical circulatory support device it operates.

Extracorporeal—Circulation of blood outside of the body.

Intracorporeal—Circulation of blood inside the body.

Paracorporeal—Circulation of blood near or close to the body.

which opens the outlet valve. Blood is then ejected until the chamber empties and pressure in the chamber decreases, closing the outlet valve. The inlet valve opens when the pressure is low enough in the blood chamber. Blood fills from the atrium and the inlet valve closes once the blood volume has increased the pressure. The cycle repeats itself when the controller fills the gas chamber again. The ejection is not typically timed to that of the native heart. The heart is emptied of blood by the assist device so there is little ejection from the native heart.

Removal of the device occurs at the time of cardiac transplant, unless the native heart has healed during support. Anticoagulation is achieved by low doses of pharmaceuticals. Some patients regain mobility while assisted by these devices.

ELECTRICAL PULSATILE. Novacor and HeartMate make devices that run electrically. Pusher plates activate the compression of the blood chamber for pulsatile blood flow. Cannulation and cable positioning are the same as for pneumatic devices. Valves are required for direction of blood flow and operation is the same as for pneumatic mechanical circulatory support. Electronic connections that use magnetic induction to cross the skin barri-

er, rather than cables tunneled through the chest wall decrease the risk of **infection**.

DESTINATION THERAPIES. Destination therapies intended to supplement or permanently replace the native heart are provided by chronic implantation of the mechanical circulatory support system. The Nimbus/TCI IVAS, the Jarvik 2000 IVAS, and DeBakey Micromed IVAS axial flow pumps are expected to achieve "first generation" chronic device trials in the United States. Low volume centrifugal pump technology includes the AB-180 Circulatory Support System, the HeartMate III LVAD, and the CorAide centrifugal blood pump. Pulsatile assist devices include the Thoratec Intracorporeal Ventricular Assist Device (IVAD), the Novacor II, the Worldheart HeartSaver VAD, and the Arrow Lionheart VAD. Total artificial hearts (TAH), made by Abiomed (AbioCor) and Penn State/3M, will replace the native heart. Upon removal of the native heart the TAH will be attached to the major blood vessels, thereby supplying blood pressure and flow to both the pulmonary and systemic circulation. No blood contact will be required with the Abiomed Heart Booster. The next five years, beyond 2001, expect to find these products in clinical trials, offering patients not eligible for organ transplantation a promising future.

Operation

The operator powers up the control console as equipment in the surgical field is inserted into the patient. Any tubing that will be connected to the patient is filled with crystalloid solution, which displaces any air that would be harmful to the patient if it entered the bloodstream. Once all sterile connections are complete, the physician will request that mechanical circulatory support be initiated. Rotational frequency is then increased or pneumatic pumping commences. Initial adjustments may be frequent, but decrease as the patient stabilizes.

Maintenance

Electrical maintenance is performed biannually to check consoles for leakage currents exceeding 100 mAmps. The Joint Commission on Accreditation of Healthcare Organizations (JCAHO) requires documentation of all electrical and mechanical maintenance activities. Specific manufacturer maintenance protocols must be followed to prevent mechanical failure. Physician orders provide the nursing and allied health staff with specific treatment instructions for maintenance of the patient on the support device.

Health care team roles

The physician, nursing, and allied health staff work as a team when patients are treated with mechanical circulatory support. Support initiation requires clear communication by the device operator of changes in device status that will alert the team to the changing condition of the patient. Once stable, the patient is transported to the intensive care unit (ICU). Any change in patient status is reported to the physician. Around-the-clock bedside care is provided by nursing staff trained to operate the mechanical circulatory support, or by nursing staff and an allied health professional trained in the operation of the particular mechanical circulatory support device in use.

Training

A circulation technologist earns a certificate of completion from a program accredited by the Commission on Accreditation of Allied Health Education Programs (CAAHEP). A bachelor's degree is required before entering the certification program, or is achieved by the time of completion of the certificate-granting program. Registered nurses usually receive in-service training from a circulation technologist, an experienced nurse, or a manufacturer representative. A respiratory therapist can pursue additional training as an ECMO specialist. Those who receive on-the-job training may also provide support services. Electrical and mechanical maintenance of the control unit is provided by biomedical engineers, who hold an associates or undergraduate degree in engineering.

Resources

BOOKS

DeBakey, Michael, and Antonio M. Gotto. *The New Living Heart.* Holbrook: Adams Media Corporation, 1997.

Gravelee, Glenn P., Richard F. Davis, Mark Kurusz, Joe R. Utley. *Cardiopulmonary Bypass: Principles and Practice, Second Edition.* Philadelphia: Lippincott Williams & Wilkins, 2000.

PERIODICALS

Stevenson, Lynne W. and Robert L. Kormos, et al. "Mechanical Cardiac Support 2000: Current Applications and Future Trial Design." *The Journal of Heart and Lung Transplantation* (January 2001): 1-38.

ORGANIZATIONS

Commission on Accreditation of Allied Health Education Programs. 1740 Gilpin Street, Denver, CO 80218. (303) 320-7701. <http://www.caahep.org>.

Extracorporeal Life Support Organization (ELSO). 1327 Jones Drive Suite 101, Ann Arbor, MI 48105. (734) 998-6600. <http://www.elso.med.umich.edu/>.

Joint Commission on Accreditation of Health Organizations. One Renaissance Boulevard, Oakbrook Terrace, IL 60181. (630) 792-5000. <http://www.jcaho.org/>

OTHER

"Spare Hearts: A Houston Chronicle Four-Part Series." *The Houston Chronicle,* October 1997. <http://www.chron.com/content/chronicle/metropolitan/heart/index.html>.

Allison Spiwak

Mechanical traction *see* **Spinal traction**

Mechanical ventilation *see* **Ventilation assistance**

Median nerve entrapment *see* **Carpal tunnel syndrome**

Mediastinoscopy
Definition

Mediastinoscopy is a surgical procedure that allows physicians to view areas of the mediastinum, the cavity behind the breastbone that lies between the **lungs**. The organs in the mediastinum include the **heart** and its vessels, the lymph nodes, trachea, esophagus, and thymus.

Mediastinoscopy is most commonly used to detect or stage **cancer**. It is also ordered to detect **infection**, and to confirm diagnosis of certain conditions and diseases of the respiratory organs. The procedure involves insertion of an endotracheal tube, followed by a small incision in the chest. A mediastinoscope is inserted through the incision. The purpose of this equipment is to allow the physician to directly see the organs inside the mediastinum, and to collect tissue samples for laboratory study.

Purpose

This procedure allows direct visualization of the tissues and organs in the chest cavity behind the sternum (breastbone) and is used to detect or evaluate infections and various types of cancers. Originally the aim of mediastinoscopy was to retrieve tissue samples for microscopic analysis. Other indications for the procedure are diagnosing pulmonary lesions and predicting the benefit of surgery. Mediastinoscopy is often the diagnostic method of choice for detecting lymphoma, including Hodgkin's disease. Diagnosis of sarcoidosis (a chronic lung disease) and the staging of **lung cancer** can also be accomplished through mediastinoscopy. The lymph nodes in the mediastinum are likely to show if lung cancer has spread beyond the lungs (metastatis). Mediastinoscopy allows a physician to observe and extract a sample from the nodes for further study. Involvement of these lymph nodes can indicate the diagnosis and staging of lung cancer.

Alternatives to mediastinoscopy, such as computed tomography (CT), **magnetic resonance imaging** (MRI), and new developments in ultrasonography, have resulted in a decrease in the number of mediastinoscopies performed. In addition, fine-needle aspiration and core-needle biopsy procedures coupled with new techniques in thoracoscopy have brought alternative possibilities in examining mediastinal masses. As of 2000, the choice of procedures is one of the most controversial issues in the staging of lung cancer.

Precautions

Since mediastinoscopy is a surgical procedure, it should only be performed when the benefits of the exam's findings outweigh the risks of surgery and anesthesia. Patients who previously had mediastinoscopy should not receive it again if there is scarring present from the first exam.

Mediastinoscopy is contraindicated in those patients who have a superior vena cava obstruction, due to the risk of hemorrhage. The procedure is also contraindicated for patients with a **tracheotomy**.

Description

Mediastinoscopy is usually performed in a hospital under **general anesthesia**. An endotracheal tube is inserted first, after **local anesthesia** is applied to the throat. Once the patient is under general anesthesia, a small incision is made usually just below the neck. The surgeon may clear a path and feel the patient's lymph nodes first to evaluate any abnormalities within the nodes. Next, the physician will insert the mediastinoscope through the incision. The scope is a narrow, hollow tube with an attached light, which allows the surgeon to see inside the area. The surgeon can insert tools through the hollow tube to help perform the exam. A sample of tissue from the lymph nodes or one of the organs can be extracted and sent for study under a **microscope** or on to a laboratory for further testing.

In some cases, analysis of the tissue sample that shows malignancy will suggest the need for immediate surgery while the patient is already prepared and under anesthesia. In other cases, the surgeon will complete the visual study and tissue extraction and stitch the small incision closed. The patient will remain in the surgery recovery area until it is determined that the effects of anesthesia have lessened and it is safe for the patient to leave the area. The entire procedure should take about an hour, not counting preparation and recovery time. Studies have shown that mediastinoscopy is a thorough and cost-effective diagnostic tool with less risk than some other procedures. Mediastinoscopy has been shown to be an effective and safe technique for biopsy of mediastinal masses in the pediatric population.

Preparation

Patients should sign a consent form after having reviewed the risks of mediastinoscopy and known risks or reactions to anesthesia. The patient should have nothing to eat or drink after midnight the day of the procedure, or at least 8 hours before the exam. A local anesthetic may be applied to the throat to ease discomfort during placement of the endotracheal tube.

Aftercare

Following mediastinoscopy, patients will be carefully monitored for changes in **vital signs** or indications of complications of the procedure or the anesthesia. A patient may have a **sore throat** from the endotracheal tube and temporary chest **pain**, soreness, or tenderness at the site of incision.

Complications

Complications from the actual mediastinoscopy procedure are relatively rare. Risks to internal organs consist of puncture of the esophagus, trachea, or the **blood vessels** in the area. Air leaks from the lung can also occur and occasionally require additional treatment. Infection and hemorrhage are other rare complications. The usual risks associated with general anesthesia apply to this procedure. General anesthesia is safe for most patients, but it is estimated to cause major or minor complications in 3–10% of those having surgery of all types.

Results

In the majority of procedures performed to diagnose cancer, a normal result would involve evidence of normal lymph nodes and no tumors. In the case of lung cancer staging, results are related to the severity and progression of the cancer.

If the lymph nodes are malignant, this indicates that a cancer such as lymphoma (including Hodgkin's disease), lung cancer, or esophageal cancer are present.

Health care team roles

Either a surgeon or a trained pulmonary specialist performs this procedure. An anesthesiologist will obtain a medical history and supervise the anesthesia for the procedure. A Certified **Registered Nurse** Anesthetist (CRNA) may work under the direction of the anesthesiologist. Operating room personnel include the scrub person and a circulator. Depending on the facility, there may be unlicensed assistive personnel (UAPs) in attendance, as well.

Patient education

After the procedure, the patient will experience some pain and soreness at the incision site, and possibly a sore throat from the endotracheal tube. Pain at the incision site may last for up to two weeks after the procedure. Patients should be instructed that there will be a small scar wherever the instruments were inserted. There will be a small dressing over the incision. The incision site must be kept clean and dry for 48 hours, and then patients may shower.

Patients should notify their health care provider if they develop any of these symptoms:

- redness at the incision site
- drainage of **blood** or pus from the incision site
- fever more than 101°F (38.3 °C)
- progressive swelling at the incision site

Resources

BOOKS

Fraser, R. S., and P. D. Pare. "Endoscopy and Diagnostic Biopsy Procedures." In *Diagnosis of Diseases of the Chest.* 4th ed., vol. I. Philadelphia: W.B. Saunders Company, 1999.

George, Ronald, Richard Light, Michael Matthay, and Richard Matthay. "Lung Neoplasms." In *Chest Medicine: Essentials of Pulmonary and Critical Care Medicine.* 4th ed. Philadelphia: Lippincott, 2000.

Pagana, Kathleen D., and Timothy J. Pagana. *Diagnostic Testing and Nursing Implications.* 5th ed. St. Louis: Mosby, 1999.

PERIODICALS

Glick, R. D., and I. A. Pearse. "Diagnosis of Mediastinal Masses in Pediatric Patients Using Mediastinoscopy and the Chamberlain Procedure." *Journal of Pediatric Surgery* 34, no. 4 (April 1999): 559–64.

Hammoud, Z. T., and R. C. Anderson. "The Current Role of Mediastinoscopy in the Evaluation of Thoracic Disease."*Journal of Thoracic and Cardiovascular Surgery* 118, no. 5 (November 1999): 894–9.

KEY TERMS

Endotracheal—Within the trachea, which is commonly known as the windpipe.

Hodgkin's disease—A malignant disorder of lymph tissue (lymphoma) that appears to originate in a particular lymph node and later spreads to the spleen, liver, and bone marrow.

Mediastinum—The mass of organs and tissues separating the lungs. It contains the heart and large vessels, trachea, esophagus, thymus, lymph nodes, and connective tissue.

Sarcoidosis—A chronic disease known for development of nodules in the lungs, skin, lymph nodes, and bones.

Superior vena cava—The principal vein that drains the upper portion of the body.

Tracheotomy—Incision of the trachea through the skin and muscles of the neck.

ORGANIZATIONS

American Cancer Society. 1599 Clifton Rd. NE, Atlanta, GA 30329. (800) ACS-2345. <http://www.cancer.org >.

American College of Chest Physicians. 3300 Dundee Rd, Northbrook, IL 60062-2348. (800) 343-2227. <http://www.chestnet.org>.

American Lung Association. 1740 Broadway, New York, NY 10019-4374. (800) LUNG-USA. <http://www.lungusa.org>.

OTHER

Harvard Medical School Family Health Guide. 8 August 2001. <http://www.health.harvard.edu/fhg/ diagnostics/mediastinoscopy/mediastinoscopy.shtml>.

Maggie Boleyn, RN, BSN

▌Medicaid

Definition

Medicaid is a federal-state entitlement program for low-income citizens of the United States. The Medicaid program is part of Title XIX of the Social Security Act that became law in 1965. Medicaid offers federal matching funds to states for costs incurred in paying healthcare providers for serving covered individuals. State partici-

KEY TERMS

Categorically needy—A term that describes certain groups of Medicaid recipients who qualify for the basic mandatory package of Medicaid benefits. There are categorically needy groups that states participating in Medicaid are required to cover, and others that the states have the option to cover.

DHHS—The Department of Health and Human Service. It is a federal agency that distributes funds for Medicaid.

Entitlement—A program that creates a legal obligation on the federal government to any person, business, or government entity that meets the legally defined criteria. Medicaid is an entitlement both for eligible individuals and for the states that decide to participate in it.

Federal poverty level (FPL)—The federal government's definition of poverty used as the reference point for Medicaid eligibility for certain groups of beneficiaries. The FPL is adjusted every year to allow for inflation.

HCFA—Health Care Financing Administration. A federal agency that provides guidelines for the Medicaid program.

Medically needy—A term that describes a group whose coverage is optional with the states because of high medical expenses. These persons meet Medicaid's category requirements (they are children or parents or elderly or disabled) but their income is too high to qualify them for "categorically needy" coverage.

Supplemental Security Income (SSI)—A federal entitlement program that provides cash assistance to low-income blind, disabled, and elderly people. In most states, people receiving SSI benefits are eligible for Medicaid.

pation is voluntary, but since 1982 all 50 states have chosen to participate in Medicaid.

Description

Medicaid benefits

Medicaid benefits cover basic health care and long-term care services for eligible persons. About 59% of Medicaid spending covers hospital and other acute care services. The remaining 41% pays for nursing home and long-term care.

States that choose to participate in Medicaid must offer the following basic services:

- hospital care, both inpatient and outpatient
- nursing **home care**
- physicians' services
- laboratory and diagnostic x-ray services
- immunizations and other screening, diagnostic, and treatment services for children
- family planning
- health center and rural health clinic services
- nurse midwife and nurse practitioner services

Participating states may offer the following optional services and receive federal matching funds for them:

- prescription medications
- institutional care for the mentally retarded
- home- or community-based care for the elderly, including case management
- personal care for the disabled
- dental and **vision** care for eligible adults

Because the participating states are allowed to design their own benefits packages as long as they meet federal minimum requirements, Medicaid benefits vary considerably from state to state. About half of all Medicaid spending covers groups of people and services above the federal minimum.

Eligibility for Medicaid

Medicaid covers three major groups of low-income Americans:

- Parents and children. In 1997 Medicaid covered 21 million low-income children—one-fifth of all children in the United States—and 8.6 million low-income adults in families with children. Most of these low-income adults are women.

- The elderly. In 1997 Medicaid covered 4 million adults over the age of 65. Medicaid is the largest single purchaser of long-term and nursing home care in the United States. In 1997, Medicaid paid for 38% of the $115 billion spent on long-term care and 47% of the $83 billion spent on nursing home care.

- The disabled. About 17% of Medicaid recipients are blind or disabled. Most of these are eligible for Medicaid because they receive assistance through the Supplemental Security Income (SSI) program.

All Medicaid recipients must have incomes and resources below specified eligibility levels. These levels vary from state to state depending on the local cost of living and other factors. For example, in 1999 the federal poverty level (FPL) was determined to be $13,880 for a family of three on the mainland of the United States, but $15,970 in Hawaii and $17,360 in Alaska.

In most cases, persons must be citizens of the United States to be eligible for Medicaid, although legal immigrants may qualify in some circumstances depending on their date of entry. Illegal aliens are not eligible for Medicaid except for emergency care.

A person must fit into an eligibility category to receive Medicaid even if their income is low. Childless couples and single childless adults who are not disabled or elderly are not eligible for Medicaid.

Medicaid costs

Medicaid is by far the government's most expensive general welfare program. In 1966, Medicaid accounted for 1.4% of the federal budget, but by 2001 its share had risen to nearly 9%. Combined federal and state spending for Medicaid takes nearly 20 cents of every tax dollar. The federal government covers about 57% of Medicaid's costs, with the states paying for the remaining 43%.

As of 2001, Medicaid's costs rise at an average annual rate of 7.9%. The federal government spent $107 billion on Medicaid in fiscal year (FY) 1999, a sum that is expected to rise to $159 billion in 2004. The states spent $81 billion to cover Medicaid costs in FY 1999. These costs are projected to increase to $120 billion by FY 2004.

Although 50% of all Medicaid beneficiaries are children, most of the money (72%) goes for services for the elderly and disabled. The single largest portion of Medicaid money pays for long-term care for the elderly. Only 17% of Medicaid funds are spent on services for children.

There are several factors involved in the steep rise of Medicaid costs:

• The rise in the number of eligible individuals. As the life span of most Americans continues to increase, the number of elderly individuals eligible for Medicaid also rises. The fastest-growing age group in the United States is people over 85.

• The price of medical and long-term care. Advances in medical technology, including expensive diagnostic imaging, keep these costs high.

• The increased use of services covered by Medicaid.

• The expansion of state coverage from the minimum benefits package to include optional groups and optional services.

Viewpoints

The need to contain Medicaid costs is considered one of the most problematic policy issues that legislators will face in the coming years. In addition, the complexity of the Medicaid system, its vulnerability to billing fraud and other abuses, the confusing variety in the benefits packages available in different states, and the time-consuming paperwork are other problems that disturb taxpayers and legislators alike.

Professional implications

Medicaid has increased the demand for health care services in the United States without greatly improving the **quality of health care** for low-income Americans. On the one hand, Medicaid's position as the largest health insurer in the United States means that it affects the employment of several hundred thousand health care workers. In 1997, Medicaid payments went to over 5,000 hospitals, 3,000 **nursing homes**, 7,000 homes for the mentally retarded, 670 community health clinics, and 550 managed care plans— all of which provide employment for thousands of health care providers, administrators, and support staff. On the other hand, participation in Medicaid is optional for physicians and nursing homes. Many do not participate in the program because the reimbursement rates are low. As a result, many low-income people who are dependent on Medicaid must go to overcrowded facilities where they often receive substandard health care.

Resources

BOOKS

Morris, Virginia. "Paying the Way." *How to Care for Aging Parents.* New York: Workman Publishing, 1996.

ORGANIZATIONS

Health Care Financing Administration. United States Department of Health and Human Services. 200 Independence Avenue SW, Washington, D.C. 20201. <http://www.hcfa.gov>.

Kaiser Commission on Medicaid and the Uninsured. 1450 G Street NW, Suite 250, Washington, DC 20005. (202) 347-5270. Fax: (202) 347-5274. <http://www.kff.org>.

National Center for Policy Analysis. 655 15th Street NW, Suite 375, Washington, DC 20005. (202) 628-6671. Fax: (202) 628-6474. <http://www.ncpa.org>.

United States Department of Health and Human Services. 200 Independence Avenue SW, Washington, D.C. 20201. <http://www.hhs.gov>.

Kaiser Commission on Medicaid and the Uninsured. *Medicaid: A Primer.* Washington, DC: Kaiser Commission on Medicaid and the Uninsured, 1999.

Peggy Elaine Browning

Medical assisting

Definition

Medical assisting involves supporting physicians and other health care staff in a variety of administrative and clinical duties.

Description

Medical assistants are not to be confused with physician assistants who examine, diagnose, and treat patients under the supervision of a physician. Medical assistants support physicians and other health care staff through administrative and clinical duties. The scope of their duties varies according to the size of the facilities in which they work. For example, in a large office, the medical assisting duties may be divided among a number of staff, one arranging for hospital or outside laboratory testing for patients, another scheduling appointments, with still others handle only insurance forms, keep patient records, do the bookkeeping, or are involved with direct care of the patient. Small offices may require the medical assistant to do most of these duties or to share them with one other administrative person.

Clinical duties are subject to the state laws in which the medical assistant works. Some of these duties include taking patient medical histories, preparing patients for medical exams and other procedures, taking patients' **vital signs**, taking x rays, taking and preparing laboratory specimens such as drawing **blood**, and performing basic lab tests in the office. Medical assistants may also be responsible for disposing of contaminated supplies and sterilizing equipment. They may prepare and administer medications, authorize drug refills, remove sutures, and change dressings.

Specialists may employ medical assistants who have training in their specific fields. Among these are podiatrists, ophthalmologists, and chiropractors. Podiatric medical assistants take x rays, make casts of feet, and assist podiatrists in surgery. Ophthalmic medical assistants administer **vision** tests, test eye function, administer eye-drops, maintain **surgical instruments**, and assist ophthalmologists in surgery.

All medical assistants deal with the public, and many directly with patients. They must be neat and well groomed and have a pleasant manner. They must be able to put patients at ease and explain to them medical procedures and medication requirements.

Medical assistants may advance to office manager or other administrative support positions. They may also qualify to teach medical assisting.

Work settings

Medical assistants work in clean, well-lighted offices and hospitals, interacting with patients, co-workers, and supervisors daily. Most medical assistants (about 65% in 1998) are employed in physicians' offices, while about 20% work in hospitals, **nursing homes**, and other related health care facilities. All others work in the offices of chiropractors, ophthalmologists, and podiatrists.

Education and training

There is no formal licensing for medical assistants, and on-the-job training was considered the norm in the past. In 2001, employers are beginning to require that medical assistants have formal training. Medical assisting programs can be found in vocational/technical high schools, technical colleges, community and junior colleges, and in universities and colleges. Most technical programs offer a certificate or diploma after one year of study. Two-year programs offer an associate degree.

The course of study incorporates two main areas: administrative and clinical. The administrative emphasis is on computer technology, accounting, record keeping, medical transcription, and insurance processing. The clinical area involves course work on laboratory techniques, clinical procedures, pharmaceuticals, medication administration, **first aid**, and universal sterilization precautions.

Accredited programs are certified by the Commission on Accreditation of Allied Health Education Programs and the Accrediting Bureau of Health Education Schools. In 1999, there were 590 schools accredited by these organizations. The Committee on Accreditation for Ophthalmic Medical Personnel accredited 14 others.

Among the certificates that verify a standard of competency for medical assistants are the Certified Medical Assistant (the American Association of Medical Assistants), Registered Medical Assistant (the American Medical Technologists), and the Podiatric Medical Assistant Certified (the American Society of Podiatric Medical Assistants). The Joint Commission on Allied Health Personnel in Ophthalmology offers three certificates: Ophthalmic Medical Assistant, Certified Ophthalmic Technician, and Certified Ophthalmic Medical Technologist.

Advanced education and training

With additional training, medical assistants may enter other related health fields such as medical technology.

Future outlook

The employment outlook for medical assistants will be increasing over the next decade. Demand for medical assistants is expected to increase faster than the average for all occupations through 2008. It is expected to be one of the 10 fastest growing occupations in the United States. This is due to the increased number of group medical practices, clinics, and related health care facilities that will require assistants. Due to the flexibility of the medical assistant's job focus, medical assistants will be highly sought after. Private outpatient settings will experience the most growth. Formally trained medical assistants will be in high demand.

Currently, earnings range from $14,000 to $24,000, with the average being around $21,000 annually. Private medical practices and hospitals have the highest salary range. This is expected to increase with demand.

Resources

BOOKS

Fremgen, Bonnie F. *Essentials of Medical Assisting: Administrative and Clinical Competencies.* Upper Saddle River, NJ: Brady Prentice Hall, 1998.

Occupational Outlook Handbook, First Edition. US Department of Labor, 2000.

Primm, Russell E. *Medical Assistant.* Mankato, MN: Capstone High/Low Books, 1998.

ORGANIZATIONS

The American Association of Medical Assistants. 20 North Wacker Dr., Suite 1575, Chicago, IL 60606-2903. <http://www.aama-ntl.org>.

Registered Medical Assistants of American Medical Technologists. 710 Higgins Rd., Park Ridge, IL. 60068-5765. <http://www.amtl.com>.

Janie F. Franz

Medical billing

Definition

Medical billing is the process of collecting fees for medical services. A medical bill is called a claim.

Purpose

The purpose of medical billing is to ensure that the provider receives fair payment for services rendered. Payment should reflect the services performed and should be received in a timely manner.

Precautions

There are laws regarding medical billing procedures. Staff members involved in collecting fees must be aware of these regulations.

Some of these laws are:

• The Fair Debt Collection Act. This federal law dictates how and when to collect a debt. It protects patients and consumers from unlawful threats.

• The Health Insurance Portability and Accountability Act of 1996 (HIPAA) contains an administrative portion that increases the efficiency of data exchange for healthcare financial transactions and protects the privacy of electronic data transmission. This protection is especially important for confidential patient records. Violators are subject to financial penalties.

Description

Medical billing may be handled directly by the physician and his or her staff, or it may be administered by a third party. The third party is an independent contractor or company that specializes in handling medical billing.

Physician fees

A physician sets fees for his or her services. There are some important concepts in fee-setting. One is usual, reasonable, and customary (UCR). Usual fees represent the fair value of a service; customary rates are similar to those of other physicians; and reasonable rates meet the criteria for the other two factors.

Another method used in setting fees is the Resource-Based Relative Value Scale (RBRVS), which examines the relative value of a service and relates it to geographic peculiarities. This method considers the time and skills needed to perform a service, intensity of the service, office (overhead) expenses, and the **malpractice** insurance premiums that the physician pays. The geographic differences allow for consideration of health care cost variations around the nation.

It is recommended that fees be discussed with the patient in advance of treatment. Often, the medical office personnel are called upon to do this. If any co-payments are due, they are collected at the time of service.

Fees may be adjusted for certain payors, such as managed care companies (HMOs, PPOs, etc.). In these cases, physicians and managed care companies negotiate fees for various services. Sometimes certain patients receive discounts. This practice may be enforced when the patient works in the health care field.

Basic bookkeeping

There are a few systems that help physician office staffs keep records. A day sheet is a record of all transactions that occurred in one day. This information is placed into a board called a pegboard. Each patient's card, called a ledger card, is also inserted into the peg board. It contains a record of his or her charges, credits, and payments. This legal document should be held as long as the patient's medical record. The information, including patient's name, diagnosis, treatments, charges, payments, and credits, are entered into a pre-printed bill called a superbill.

The medical claim

When a service such as an office visit is complete, the staff begins preparing the claim or sends the patient information to a third party for billing. A physician's office will send out a claim if that physician accepts assignment of benefits. To accept assignment of benefits, the physician must receive the patient's signature allowing his or her office to receive payment directly from the insurance company.

Claim preparation begins with proper coding. Medical procedures and diagnoses have codes. The Current Procedural Terminology (CPT), developed in 1966 by the American Medical Association, lists medical procedures and corresponding codes. Each medical procedure has a code that is listed in a CPT manual. The book is divided into sections so that similar procedures appear in the same area.

The major sections of the CPT book are:

- evaluation/management
- anesthesia
- surgery
- radiology
- pathology and laboratory
- medicine

In addition to procedure codes, there are codes for diagnoses, called ICD-9 codes. This practice was established in 1983 when **Medicare** began using diagnosis-related groups (DRGs). An ICD-9 book lists each diagnosis within the DRGs. Each DRG corresponds to a fee.

Coding must be accurate because it determines reimbursement.

Health plans issue identification numbers to providers. This number is placed on claim forms so that payors can quickly and accurately identify providers.

The medical claim also contains important information, such as:

- provider name, address, telephone number, and ID number
- name of insurance plan and group number
- ID number of insurance holder
- patient's name, date of birth
- insured person's name, date of birth
- patient's address and telephone number
- insured person's address and telephone number
- relationship between patient and insured person
- other health insurance the patient may have
- patient's medical condition, and whether it was related to a job automobile accident, or other type of accident
- other information, such as the patient's history of related illness, may need to appear on the claim

The use of computer software allows medical offices to submit claims electronically. This method shortens the time between filing the claim and reimbursement.

Payment

Medical bills may be paid by the patient or by third party payors, such as private insurance company, a managed care company, or a government insurance program such as Medicare. Often, the patient pays for a portion of the care (co-payment or deductible), and an insurance or managed care company is billed for the remaining fees. In some cases, patients may ask to pay their portion over time, and credit may be extended to them. The medical office may charge interest as long as the patient has been informed. This practice is called truth-in-lending. Credit laws vary by state.

Payment received from an insurance or managed care company contains a document called the explanation of benefits (EOB). This statement explains what was paid and what services were not covered and is sent to the provider and the patient. A service may not be covered if a patient has not met his or her yearly deductible. In this case, the provider bills the patient for his or her fee. It is common to bill patients once a month.

When a payment arrives, it is important to endorse it right away. This can be done with a rubber stamp that contains the name of the provider and the bank account number. Endorsing is a form of protection because only the provider who endorsed it can cash the check in the event it is lost or stolen. The provider should have a deposit procedure.

Complications

Complications impact bill collection. Accurate coding, standard office procedures, and good communication within a provider group minimize complications.

Overdue payments

In some cases, a patient may not pay his or her bill within a month or by the claim's due date. A document called an aging schedule lists overdue accounts. The information includes the patient's name, amount due, payments received, and comments. An account is aged beginning with the billing date rather than the date the procedure was performed. Eighty percent of fees should be collected within a month of billing. If this number falls to 50% or less, collection procedures should be examined.

A patient must be reminded of an overdue bill. This can be done with a written notice, phone call, or during the next office visit.

KEY TERMS

Adjustment—Changes to a standard fee. Changes may be made because of managed care agreements or other discounts.

Aging schedule—A list of overdue medical accounts calculated from date of original bill to current date.

Claim—Medical bill.

Diagnostic related groups (DRGs)—Diagnosis categories that are used when doing physician or hospital billing. Each diagnosis is placed into the appropriate category.

Managed care—A type of health plan with a network of providers and pre-arranged fee schedule. Examples include a health maintenance organization (HMO) or preferred provider organization (PPO).

Payor—One who pays a medical claim. A third party payor is an entity other than the patient, such as the insurance company.

Provider—Health team professional or entity (hospital) that offers care.

Denied claims

If the insurance or managed care company's EOB indicates that the claim is denied, it is important to determine why this happened. The claim should be double-checked to determine if an error has occurred. If the patient is not entitled to coverage, he or she is billed when the monthly billings are sent out.

Fraud

Medicare has the right to audit a physician's office and examine its billing practices. Errors in claims are checked to determine the presence of fraudulent practices. A medical office must not bill for services that were not performed and must not inaccurately code a service to receive a higher level of payment. These practices are examples of fraud.

Health care professionals who report fraud are called whistle-blowers. The Federal Claims Act protects and reward these individuals when they report Medicare fraud. States also have anti-fraud regulations.

Collecting fees after a patient's death

If a patient has died, the physician may collect fees from his or her estate. Since death is followed by a period of grief, it is recommended that the physician's office wait before sending a final statement to the patient's next of kin as indicated on the chart.

Health care team roles

Clear communication within a provider group helps ensure that claims are properly coded, patients are informed of fees, and fair reimbursement is billed and received. The physician must be questioned if there is any doubt that a service was performed or if the diagnosis is not clear.

The team involved in billing includes the physician, office manager, nurse, receptionist, medical assistant, and insurance clerk, with these billing-related duties:

- Performs billable service: physician, nurse, medical assistant.

- Explains fees/billing: physician, receptionist, nurse, medical assistant, insurance clerk.

- Prepares day sheet, ledger, superbill: nurse, medical assistant, insurance clerk.

- Files (sends out) claim: insurance clerk.

- Reminds patient of overdue payment: receptionist, nurse, medical assistant, insurance clerk.

- Communicates with insurance companies: receptionist, medical assistant, nurse, insurance clerk.

Resources

BOOKS

Hosley, Julie B., Shirley A. Jones, Elizabeth A. Molle-Matthews. *Lippincott's Textbook for Medical Assistants.* Philadelphia: Lippincott-Raven Publishers, 1997.

Jones, Marleeta K. *St. Anthony's ICD-9 CM Code Book, Volumes 1,2,3.* Reston, VA: St. Anthony's Publishing, 1997.

ORGANIZATIONS

American Medical Association. 515 N. State Street, Chicago, IL 60610. (312) 464-5000. <http://www.ama-assn.org>.

Health Care Financing Association. 7500 Security Boulevard, Baltimore, MD 21244. (410) 786-3000. <http://www.hcfa.gov>.

OTHER

Goldsmith, Connie. "Blowing the Whistle: Laws protect nurses who report healthcare fraud." *NurseWeek* (May 18, 2000): <http://www.nurseweek.com/features/00-05/whistle.html>.

Rhonda Cloos, R.N.

Medical chart

Definition

The medical chart is a confidential document that contains detailed and comprehensive information on the individual patient and their care experience.

Purpose

The purpose of the medical chart is to serve as both a medical and legal record of patient clinical status, care, history, and caregiver involvement. The detailed information contained in the chart is intended to provide a of the patient's clinical condition by detailing diagnoses, treatments, tests and response to treatment, as well as any other factors that may affect the clinical state of the patient.

Description

The term medical chart or medical record is a general description of a collection of information on a patient. However, different clinical settings and systems utilize different forms of documentation to achieve this purpose. As technology progresses, more institutions are adopting computerized systems that aid in clear documentation, enhanced access, and efficient storage of patient records.

New uses of technology have also raised concerns about confidentiality. Confidentiality, or patient privacy, is an important principle related to the chart. Whatever system may be in place, it is essential that the health care provider protect the patient's privacy by limiting access to authorized individuals only. Generally, physicians and nurses write most frequently in the chart. The documentation by the clinician who is leading treatment decisions (usually the physician) often focuses on diagnosis and prognosis, while the documentation by the nursing team generally focuses on patient responses to treatment and details of day-to-day progress. In many institutions the medical and nursing staff may complete separate forms or areas of the chart specific to their disciplines.

Other on-staff health care professionals that have access to the chart include physician assistants; social workers; psychologists; nutritionists; physical, occupational, speech, or respiratory therapists; and consultants. It is important that the various disciplines view the notes written by other specialties in order to form a complete picture of the patient and provide continuity of care. Quality assurance and regulatory organizations, legal bodies, and insurance companies may also have access to the chart for specific purposes such as documentation, institutional audits, legal proceedings, or verification of information for care reimbursement. It is important to know the institution's policies regarding chart access in order to ensure the privacy of the patient.

The medical record should be stored in a predesignated, secure area and discussed only in appropriate and private clinical areas. The patient has a right to view and obtain copies of his or her own record. Special state statutes may cover especially sensitive information such as psychiatric, communicable disease (i.e., HIV), or substance abuse records. Institutional and government policies govern what is contained in the chart, how it is documented, who has access, and policies for regulating access to the chart and protecting its integrity and confidentiality. In cases where chart contents need to be accessed by individuals outside of the immediate care system, the patient or patient representative is asked for written permission to release records. Patients are often asked to sign these releases so that caregivers in new clinical settings may review their charts.

Operation

Documentation in the medical record begins when the patient enters the care system, which may be a specific place such as a hospital or a program such as a home health care service. Frequently the facility will request permission to obtain copies of previous records so that they have complete information on the patient. Although chart systems vary from institution to institution, there are many aspects of the chart that are universal. Frequently used chart sections include:

- Admission paperwork: includes legal paperwork such as living will or health care proxy, consents for admission to the facility or program, demographics, and contact information.

- History and physical: contains comprehensive review of patient's medical history and physical exam.

- Orders: contains medication and treatment orders by the doctor, nurse practitioner, physician assistant, or other qualified health care team members.

- Medication record: records all medication administered.

- Treatment record: documents all treatments received, such as dressing changes or respiratory therapy.

- Procedures: summarizes diagnostic or therapeutic procedures, i.e., **colonoscopy** or open-heart surgery.

- Tests: provides reports and results of diagnostic evaluations, such as laboratory tests and **electrocardiography** or radiography images or summaries.

- Progress notes: includes regular notes on the patient's status by the interdisciplinary care team.

- Consultations: contains notes from specialized diagnosticians or care providers.

- Consents: includes permissions signed by patient for procedures, tests, or access to chart. May also contain releases, such as the release signed by the patient when leaving the facility against medical advice (AMA).

- Flow records: tracks specific aspects of patient care that occur on a routine basis, using tables or chart format.

- Care plans: documents treatment goals and plans for future care within the facility or following discharge.

- Discharge: contains final instructions for the patient and reports by the care team before the chart is closed and stored following patient discharge.

- Insurance information: lists health care benefit coverage and insurance provider contact information.

These general categories may be further divided for the individual facility's purposes. For example, a psychiatric facility may use a special section for psychometric testing, or a hospital may provide sections specifically for operations, x-ray reports, or electrocardiograms. In addition, certain details such as **allergies** or do not resuscitate orders may be displayed prominently (i.e., on large colored stickers or special chart sections) on the chart in order to communicate uniquely important information. It is important for the health care provider to become familiar with the charting systems in place at his or her specific facility or program.

It is important that the information in the chart be clear and concise, so that those utilizing the record can easily access accurate information. The medical chart can also aid in clinical problem solving by tracking the patient's baseline, or status on admission; orders and treatments provided in response to specific problems; and patient responses. Another reason for the standard of clear documentation is the possibility of the legal use of the record, when documentation serves as evidence in exploring and evaluating the patient's care experience. When medical care is being referred to or questioned by the legal system, the chart contents are frequently cited in court. For all of these purposes, certain practices that protect the integrity of the chart and provide essential information are recommended for adding information and maintaining the chart. These practices include:

- Include date and time on all records.

- Include full patient name and other identifiers (i.e., medical record number, date of birth) on all records.

- Mark continued records clearly (i.e., if note continued on reverse of page).

- Sign each page of documentation.

KEY TERMS

Consultation—Evaluation by an expert or specialist.

Continuity—Consistency or coordination of details.

Discipline—In health care, a specific area of preparation or training, i.e., social work, nursing, or nutrition.

Documentation—The process of recording information in the medical chart, or the materials in a medical chart.

Interdisciplinary—Consisting of several interacting disciplines that work together to care for the patient.

Objective—Not biased by personal opinion

Prognosis—Expected outcome of an illness or injury.

Regulatory organization—Organization designed to maintain or control quality in health care, such as the Joint Commission on Accreditation of Healthcare Organizations (JCAHO), Department of Health (DOH), or the Food and Drug Administration (FDA).

Subjective—Influenced by personal opinion or experience.

- Use blue or black non-erasable ink on handwritten records.

- Keep records in chronological order.

- Prevent disposal or obliteration of any records.

- Note documentation errors and correct clearly, i.e., by drawing one line through the error and noting presence of error, initialing the area.

- Avoid excess empty space on the page.

- Avoid abbreviations or use only universally accepted abbreviations.

- Avoid other unclear documentation, such as illegible penmanship.

- Avoid including contradictory information. For example, if a nurse documents that a patient has complained of abdominal **pain** throughout the shift, while the physician documents that the patient is free of pain, these discrepancies should be discussed and clarified.

- Provide objective rather than subjective information. For example, do not allow personality conflicts between staff to enter into the notes. All events involving the patient should be described as objectively as possible, i.e., describe a hostile patient by simply stating the facts, such as what the patient said or did and surrounding circumstances or response of staff, without using derogatory or judgmental language.

- Document any occurrence that might affect the patient. Only documented information is considered credible in court. Undocumented information is considered questionable since there is no written record of its occurrence.

- Always use current date and time with documentation. For example, if adding a note after the fact, it can be labeled "addendum" and inserted in correct chronological order, rather than trying to insert the information on the date of the actual occurrence.

- Record actual statements of patients or other individuals in quotes.

- Never leave the chart in an unprotected environment where unauthorized individuals may read or alter the contents.

Several methods of documentation have arisen in response to the need to accurately summarize the patient experience. In the critical care setting, flow records are often used to track the frequent patient evaluations, checks of equipment, and changes of equipment settings that are required. Flow records also offer the advantages of displaying a large amount of information in a relatively small space and allowing for quick comparison. Flow records can also save time for the busy clinician by allowing completion of checklists versus narrative notes.

Narrative progress notes, while more time consuming, are often the best way to capture specific information about the patient. Some institutions require only charting by exception (CBE), which requires notes for significant or unusual findings only. While this method may decrease repetition and lower required documentation time, most institutions that use CBE notes also require a separate flow record that documents regular contact with the patient. Many facilities or programs require notes at regular intervals even when there no significant occurrence, i.e., every nursing shift. Frequently used formats in patient notes include SOAP (Subjective, Objective, Assessment, Plan) notes. SOAP notes use a subjective patient statement to capture an important aspect of care, then follow with a key objective statement regarding the patient's status, a description of the patient assessment, and a plan for how to address patient problems or concerns. Focus charting and PIE (problem-intervention-evaluation) charting use similar systems of notes that begin with a particular focus such as a patient concern or a **nursing diagnosis**. Nursing diagnoses are often used as guides to nursing care by focusing on individual patient needs and responses to treatment. An example of a nursing diagnosis would be "Fluid volume deficit" for a patient that is dehydrated. The notes would then focus on assessment for **dehydration**, interventions to address the problem, and a plan for continued care, such as measurement of input and output and intravenous therapy.

Maintenance

Current medical charts are maintained by the health care team and usually require clerical assistance, such as the unit clerk in the hospital setting. No alterations should be made to the record unless they are required to clarify or correct information and are clearly marked as such. After patient discharge, the **medical records** department of a facility checks for completeness and retains the record. Sometimes the record will be made available in another format, i.e., recording paper charts on microfilm or computer imaging. Institutional and state laws govern storage of charts on- and off-site and length of storage time required.

Health care team roles

All members of the health care team require thorough understanding of the medical chart and documentation guidelines in order to provide thorough care and maintain a clear, concise, and pertinent record. Health care systems often employ methods to guarantee thorough and continuous use and review of charts across disciplines. For example, nursing staff may be required to sign below every new physician order to indicate that this information has been communicated, or internal quality assurance teams may study groups of charts to determine trends in missing or unclear documentation. In legal settings, health care team members may be called upon to interpret or explain chart notations as they relate to the individual legal case.

Training

Thorough training is essential prior to independent use of the medical chart. Whenever possible, the new clinician should spend time reviewing the chart to get a sense of organization and documentation format and style. Training programs for health care professionals often include practice in writing notes or flow charts in mock medical records. Notes by trainees are often initially cosigned by supervisors to ensure accurate and relevant documentation and document appropriate supervision.

Resources

BOOKS

Marrelli, T. M., and Deborah S. Harper. *Nursing Documentation Handbook, 3rd ed.* St. Louis: Mosby Inc., 2000.

Mastering Documentation, 2nd ed. Springhouse, Pennsylvania: Springhouse Corporation, 1999.

Katherine L. Hauswirth, APRN

Medical codes and oaths *see* **Ethical codes and oaths**

Medical electrodes

Definition

The medical electrode transfers the energy of ionic currents in the body into electrical currents that can be amplified, studied, and used to help make diagnoses.

Purpose

Medical electrodes permit surface quantification of internal ionic currents, yielding an ordinarily non-invasive test for a variety of nervous, muscular, ocular, cardiac, and other disorders that might otherwise have required surgical means to verify their presence. For instance, muscular exams using electrodes may produce evidence of diminished muscle strength and can discriminate between primary muscle disorders and neurologically-based disorders, in addition to detecting if a muscle is truly weak or seems so due to other reasons. The electrodes are typically easy to use, fairly cheap, disposable (or easily sterilizable), and often unique in the tasks they help to perform. The essential role of the electrode is to provide ideal electrical contact between the patient and the apparatus used to measure or record activity.

Description

Medical electrodes are generally comprised of a lead (for conduction of electrical current), a metal electrode, and electrode-conducting paste or gel for surface electrodes. There is also often a metal (for good electrical contact) snap for the lead to snap into place so that the electrode can be disposable while the lead can be reused.

Electrodes can be classified into many groupings; those useful for EEG, for example, follow:

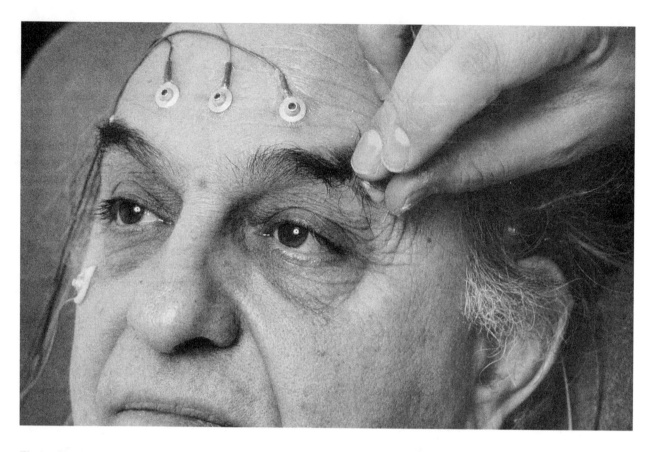

Electrodes are placed to monitor this man's brain activity for Alzheimer's research. *(SIU BioMed/Custom Medical Stock Photo. Reproduced by permission.)*

- disposable electrodes (both types, without gel and pre-gelled)
- reusable disc electrodes (gold, silver, stainless steel, or tin)
- headbands
- saline-based electrodes, which include various kinds

Electromyography requires more specialized needle electrodes that must be capable of piercing the skin.

Electrodes are used for diverse procedures and check-ups in the health setting. Combined with monitoring systems, they can be powerful predictors of disease and disorders. Some of the main types of exams utilizing medical electrodes include:

- Electrocardiography (ECG/EKG): Evaluates the electrical activity of the **heart**. It may be used to assess heart rate and regularity, in addition to damage, effects of drugs, and devices. ECG is also popularly used to determine the size and position of the chambers of the heart as they relate to the onset of various forms of heart disease. Diagnostic ECG may require 12 to 15 surface electrodes, while monitoring ECG usually employs three to five.

- Electroencephalography (EEG): Helps to identify specific irregularities in the **brain**. Brain wave patterns can be recorded and observed by positioning typically 10 to 20 electrodes upon the scalp of the patient in different areas and measuring ionic, electrical waves of neuronal activity.

- Electromyography (EMG): Assesses muscular response to electrical activity in innervated muscle. Utilizes needle electrodes that are inserted through the skin into relevant muscle fibers.

- Electonystagmography (ENG): Records eye movements graphically by placing metal electrodes above, below, and to the side of the appropriate eye, in addition to a ground electrode on the forehead. Eye motion is then recorded relative to the ground electrode location. Testing is usually performed to verify the presence of nystagmus.

- Electroretinography (ERG): Operates with an electrode positioned onto the cornea of the eye to record the electrical response of retinal rods and cones. Electrodes measure retinal electrical response to the impingement of light in order to assess a probable retinal disorder (both hereditary and acquired) and whether it may require surgery.

Offshoot technologies of electrodes, as of July 2001, are veering toward multi-functional processes. One original electrode application boasts hands-free defibrillator capabilities in addition to its normal electrode functions in ECG. It should also be noted that, using a voltage or current generator, electrical stimulation can be applied to precise areas of the body using medical electrodes (in addition to their more conventional utility in measuring ionic currents).

Operation

Prior to performing EMG, ENG, and ERG tests, adults need not take any special precautions, except to inform their medical provider of any medications they take. EEG patients should thoroughly wash their hair the night before and use nothing in their hair (such as hair spray, lotions, or oils) on the day of the test. Discontinuance of medications may be necessary and patients should avoid **caffeine** for at least eight hours prior to the test. ECG patients should inform the provider of any medications taken, in addition to refraining from ingesting cold water and from exercising immediately before the test. Removal of all jewelry is also required.

Since the role of medical electrodes is generally for monitoring of electrical impulses, there is no risk of shock. Electrical stimulation using electrodes carries more risk because electricity is delivered to the body and should thus only be performed by personnel with an understanding of the risks involved (especially electrical) and how to avoid them. Knowledge of the ground electrodes and how to use them is strictly required and differs for different systems.

Maintenance

Maintenance of electrodes, if they are not disposable, involves sterilization and checking to ensure that the electrode is electrically viable by following the manufacturer's instructions.

Health care team roles

Doctors, nurses, or other technicians may need to perform tests involving medical electrodes. Often the technician or nurse applies the electrodes in patterns conforming to testing standards (i.e., Einthoven's triangle).

Training

Electrode placement is essential and thus must be known well enough to position electrodes correctly to

---

KEY TERMS

Einthoven's triangle—An ECG reference system with the subject's heart presumed to be the center of an equilateral triangle (both physically, in that electrodes are placed in form of a triangle on the body, and figuratively, in the mathematical measurement techniques used to assess a patient's cardiac health) formed by three bipolar limb leads. Can be used to diagnose various disorders of the heart. Named after Wilhelm Einthoven, the Dutch electrocardiographer who advanced these recording techniques.

Nystagmus—Rapid, repetitive involuntary movements of the eyes.

Retinal rods and cones—The two types of light-sensitive photoreceptor cells in the retina.

Saline—Containing a salt, or of the nature of a salt.

---

obtain viable data on many different types of patients. Since each procedure is unique, training must be appropriate to the specific procedure being performed. Electrode impedances may be checked to ensure superior electrical contact; the optimal values should be listed in the manufacturer's manual.

In using electrodes, the technician should follow the guidelines set in the manufacturer's manual, because electrode handling is not conserved over all electrode types and applications. The following general guidelines have been adapted from Biomedical Life Systems (as of July 2001), a major manufacturer of medical electrodes, but do not apply to all types of electrodes:

- Electrodes, gel, and tape (for securing the electrode) should not be applied over broken skin.

- Body hair should be trimmed or shaved where electrodes are going to be applied.

- Carbon electrodes should be cleaned with mild soap and water to remove skin oils, gel, and dirt.

- Skin should be cleaned before and after applying electrodes.

- Cleaning lead wires with mild soap and water will prevent them from becoming brittle.

Resources

PERIODICALS

Mroz, A., M. Borchardt, C. Diekmann, K. Cammann, M. Knoll, and C. Dumchat. "Disposable Reference Electrode." *The Analyst* 123, no. 6. (June 1998): 1373–6.

Medical Electrodes (ECG, EEG, EMG, ENG, ERG).
<http://www.nlm.nih.gov/medlineplus>.

Bryan Ronain Smith

Medical emergency kit *see* **First aid kit**

Medical ethics

Definition

Medical ethics refers to the discussion and application of moral values and responsibilities in the areas of medical practice and research. While questions of medical ethics have been debated since the beginnings of Western medicine in the fifth century B.C., medical ethics as a distinctive field came into prominence only since World War II. This change has come about largely as a result of advances in medical technology, scientific research, and telecommunications. These developments have affected nearly every aspect of clinical practice, from the confidentiality of patient records to end-of-life issues. Moreover, the increased involvement of government in medical research as well as the allocation of health care resources brings with it an additional set of ethical questions.

Description

The Hippocratic tradition

Medical ethics generally traces its origins to the ancient Greek physician Hippocrates (460–377 BC), who is credited with defining the first ethical standard in medicine: "Do no harm." The oath attributed to Hippocrates was traditionally recited by medical students as part of their medical school's graduation ceremonies. A modernized version of the Hippocratic Oath that has been approved by the American Medical Association (AMA) reads as follows:

You do solemnly swear, each by whatever he or she holds most sacred

That you will be loyal to the Profession of Medicine and just and generous to its members

That you will lead your lives and practice your art in uprightness and honor

That into whatsoever house you shall enter, it shall be for the good of the sick to the utmost of your power,

your holding yourselves far aloof from wrong, from corruption, from the tempting of others to vice

That you will exercise your art solely for the cure of your patients, and will give no drug, perform no operation, for a criminal purpose, even if solicited, far less suggest it

That whatsoever you shall see or hear of the lives of men or women which is not fitting to be spoken, you will keep inviolably secret

These things do you swear. Let each bow the head in sign of acquiescence

And now, if you will be true to this your oath, may prosperity and good repute be ever yours; the opposite, if you shall prove yourselves forsworn.

Religious traditions and medical ethics

Ancient Greece was not the only premodern culture that set ethical standards for physicians. Both Indian and Chinese medical texts from the third century B.C. list certain moral virtues that practitioners were to exemplify, among them humility, compassion, and concern for the patient's well-being. In the West, both Judaism and Christianity gave extensive consideration to the importance of the physician's moral character as well as his duties to patients. In Judaism, medical ethics is rooted in the study of specific case histories interpreted in the light of Jewish law. This case-based approach is known as casuistry. In Christianity, ethical reflection on medical questions has taken the form of an emphasis on duty, moral obligation, and right action. In both faiths, the relationship between the medical professional and the patient is still regarded as a covenant or sacred bond of trust rather than a business contract. In contemporary Buddhism, discussions of medical ethics reflect specifically Buddhist understandings of suffering, the meaning of human personhood, and the significance of death.

The Enlightenment and the nineteenth century

The eighteenth century in Europe witnessed a number of medical as well as general scientific advances, and the application of scientific principles to medical education led to a new interest in medical ethics. The first book on medical ethics in English was published by a British physician, Thomas Percival, in 1803. In the newly independent United States, Benjamin Rush—a signer of the Declaration of Independence as well as a physician—lectured to the medical students at the University of Pennsylvania on the importance of high ethical standards in their profession. Rush recommended service to the poor as well as the older Hippocratic virtues of honesty and justice.

In the middle of the nineteenth century, physicians in the United States and Canada began to form medical societies with stated codes of ethics. These codes were drawn up partly because there was no government licensing of physicians or regulation of medical practice at that time. The medical profession felt a need to regulate itself as well as set itself apart from quacks, faith healers, homeopaths, and other practitioners of what would now be called alternative medicine. The AMA, which was formed in 1847, has revised its Code of Ethics from time to time as new ethical issues have arisen. The present version consists of seven principles. The Canadian Medical Association (CMA) was formed in 1867 and has a Code of Ethics with 40 guidelines for the ethical practice of medicine.

Viewpoints

Theoretical approaches to medical ethics

PHILOSOPHICAL FRAMEWORKS. Since the early Middle Ages, questions of medical ethics have sometimes been discussed within the framework of specific philosophical positions or concepts. A follower of Immanuel Kant (1724–1804), for example, would test an ethical decision by the so-called categorical imperative, which states that one should act as if one's actions would serve as the basis of universal law. Another philosophical position that sometimes appears in discussions of medical ethics is utilitarianism, or the belief that moral virtue is based on usefulness. From a utilitarian perspective, the best decision is that which serves the greatest good of the greatest number of people. An American contribution to philosophical approaches to medical ethics is pragmatism, which is the notion that practical results, rather than theories or principles, provide the most secure basis for evaluating ethical decisions.

CASUISTRY. Casuistry can be defined as a case-based approach to medical ethics. An ethicist in this tradition, if confronted with a complicated ethical decision, would study a similar but simpler case in order to work out an answer to the specific case under discussion. As has already been mentioned, casuistry has been used as a method of analysis for centuries in Jewish medical ethics.

THE "FOUR PRINCIPLES" APPROACH. Another approach to medical ethics was developed in the 1970s by a philosopher, Tom Beauchamp, and a theologian, James Childress, who were working in the United States. Beauchamp and Childress drew up a list of four principles that they thought could be weighed against one another in ethical decision-making in medicine. The four principles are:

- the principle of autonomy, or respecting each person's right to make their own decisions
- the principle of beneficence, or doing good as the primary goal of medicine
- the principle of nonmaleficence, or refraining from harming people
- the principle of justice, or distributing the benefits and burdens of a specific decision fairly

One limitation of the "Four Principles" approach is that different persons involved in an ethical decision might well disagree about the relative weight to be given to each principle. For example, a patient who wants to be taken off a life-support system could argue that the principle of autonomy should be paramount, while the clinical staff could maintain that the principles of beneficence and nonmaleficence are more important. The principles themselves do not define or imply a hierarchical ranking or ordering.

Current issues in medical ethics

One well-known writer in the field of medical ethics has recently written an article listing what he considers "cutting-edge" topics in medical ethics. While space does not permit discussion of these subjects here, they serve as a useful summary of the impact of technology and globalization on medical ethics in the new millennium:

- End-of-life care. Medical advances that have led to a dramatic lengthening of the life span for adults in the developed countries and a corresponding increase in the elderly population have made end-of-life care a pressing issue.
- Medical error. The proliferation of new medications, new surgical techniques, and other innovations means that the consequences of medical errors are often very serious. All persons involved in health care have an ethical responsibility to help improve the quality of care.
- Setting priorities. The fair allocation of health care resources is one example of setting priorities.
- Biotechnology. Medical ethicists are still divided over the legitimacy of stem cell research, cloning, and other procedures that advances in biotechnology have made possible.
- "eHealth." The expansion of the Internet and other rapid changes in information technology have raised many questions about the confidentiality of electronic **medical records** as well as the impact of online education on medical training.
- Global **bioethics**. Global bioethics represents an attempt to consider the ethical problems confronting the poorer countries of the world, rather than concen-

KEY TERMS

Casuistry—A case-based approach to medical ethics.

Categorical imperative—The principle that one should act in such a way that one's deeds could become universal rules of conduct.

Ethics—A system or set of moral principles; also, the study of values relating to human conduct.

Hippocratic Oath—The ethical oath attributed to Hippocrates that is used as a standard for care by physicians worldwide.

Pragmatism—A philosophical position that regards practical results, rather than abstract principles or theories, as the essential criterion of moral value.

Utilitarianism—An ethical position based on the premise that usefulness is the best measure of moral worth, and that ethical decisions should promote the good of the largest number of persons.

trating on medical issues from the perspective of the wealthy countries. Of the 54 million deaths that occur each year around the world, 46 million occur in low- and middle-income countries.

Professional implications

One implication for physicians is the importance of studying ethical issues during one's professional education. Many medical, dental, and nursing schools now include courses in their curricula that deal with such topics as moral decision-making, definitions of life and death, the ethical complexities of professional-patient relationships, and the moral safeguards of medical research. As of 2000, more than 25 universities in the United States and Canada offer graduate degrees in medical ethics.

A second implication is recognizing the necessity of interdisciplinary conversation and cooperation. Physicians can benefit from the insights of scholars in the social sciences, philosophy, theology, law, and history. At the same time, they have much to offer professionals in other fields on the basis of their clinical experience.

Resources

BOOKS

Brody, Baruch A., et al. *Medical Ethics: Codes, Opinions, and Statements*. New York: BNA Books, 2000.

Burkhardt, Margaret A., and Alvita K. Nathaniel. *Ethics and Issues in Contemporary Nursing*. Albany, NY: Delmar Publishers, 1998.

Davis, Anne J., et al. *Ethical Dilemmas and Nursing Practice*. Paramus, NJ: Prentice Hall, 1996.

Dubler, Nancy N. "Legal and Ethical Issues." *The Merck Manual of Geriatrics*. 2nd ed. Whitehouse Station, NJ: Merck Research Laboratories, 2000.

PERIODICALS

Hughes, James J., and Damien Keown. "Buddhism and Medical Ethics: A Bibliographic Introduction." *Journal of Buddhist Ethics* 7 (2000): 1-12.

Sabatini, Margaret M. "Health Care Ethics: Models of the Provider-Patient Relationship." *Dermatology Nursing* (June 1998): 201-206.

Singer, Peter A. "Medical Ethics (Clinical review)." *British Medical Journal* 321 (July 29, 2000): 282-285.

Wolinsky, Howard. "Steps Still Being Taken to Undo Damage of 'America's Nuremberg.'" *Annals of Internal Medicine* (August 15, 1997).

ORGANIZATIONS

American Medical Association, Council on Ethical and Judicial Affairs. 535 North Dearborn St., Chicago, IL 60610. (312) 645-5000.

American Nurses Association. 600 Maryland Ave. SW, Ste. 100 West, Washington, DC 20024. (800) 274-4262. <http://www.nursingworld.org>.

American Society of Bioethics and Humanities. 4700 W. Lake, Glenview, IL 60025. (847) 375-4745. <http://www.asbh.org>.

Canadian Medical Association. 1867 Alta Vista Drive, Ottawa ON K1G 3Y6. (613) 731-8610 x2307 or (888) 855-2555. Fax (613) 236-8864. <cmamsc@cma.ca>.

Institute for Jewish Medical Ethics. Hebrew Academy of San Francisco, San Francisco, CA. (415) 752-7333 or (800) 258-4427. <http://www.ijme.org>.

National Bioethics Advisory Commission. 6705 Rockledge Drive, Suite 700, Rockville, MD 20892. (310) 402-4242. <http://www.bioethics.gov>.

OTHER

Canadian Medical Association. *Code of Ethics of the Canadian Medical Association*. Policy statement approved by the CMA Board of Directors, October 15, 1996.

Ken R. Wells

Medical gases

Definition

A medical gas is defined as one that is manufactured, packaged, and intended for administration to a patient in anesthesia, therapy, or diagnosis. Title 21 of the Code of Federal Regulations (CFR) designates medical gases as drugs, and mandates the Secretary of the Treasury and the Secretary of Health and Human Services to promulgate regulations for the efficient enforcement of the Federal Food, Drug, and Cosmetic Act (FDA)(drug portion of 21 CFR). Such other regulatory bodies as the Department of Transportation (DOT) and national organizations [e.g., the Compressed Gas Association (CGA) and the National Fire Protection Association (NFPA)] write regulations and standards for compressed gases. Medical gases are considered prescription drugs because their use as drugs is unsafe without the supervision of a licensed practitioner or by properly instructed emergency personnel. Regulations regarding the purity of these substances are established by the United States Pharmacopeia/National Formulary (USP/NF).

Purpose

Medical gases are used within hospital settings for many purposes. They include the following elements and compounds:

- Oxygen, used to provide supplemental oxygen to the **respiratory system**; in dentistry in combination with **nitrous oxide**; and as an emergency standby.

- Nitrous oxide, used as an anesthetic agent in surgery; mixed with oxygen to help patients relax during dental procedures; and in cryosurgery (the use of extreme cold to destroy tissue).

- Nitrogen, used to provide pneumatic pressure in medical equipment; to prevent combustion and other chemical reactions; and as a component of many gas mixtures.

- Carbon dioxide, used to inflate areas of the body for "keyhole" surgery (small incisions made to accommodate **surgical instruments**); mixed with air or oxygen to stimulate breathing; and in cryosurgery or testing tooth sensitivity in dentistry.

- Medical air, used in administering breathing treatments and as a mixing component for other respiratory gases.

- Helium, used in breathing mixtures for patients with impaired lung functions.

Since medical gases are the most frequently administered drugs in the United States, the FDA is attempting to heighten both consumer and industry awareness about this specialized category of regulated products. Such related delivery hardware as regulators and tubing is also regulated as medical devices.

Description

Cylinder markings

For the transport and delivery of a cylinder of compressed gas to a provider, the cylinder must have designated markings permanently affixed to its neck to identify the regulatory body governing the use of the cylinder; the service pressure; the serial number; the date of manufacture; the last test date; a stick-on label identifying its contents; its hazard class and color code (green for oxygen, blue for nitrous oxide, yellow for air). The cylinder is equipped with a valve threaded into it that is specifically designed only for the specific type of medical gas the cylinder is designated to contain.

Pin index safety system

The pin index safety system is used to prevent a cylinder of compressed gas from being filled with the wrong gas, or to prevent the connection of the wrong cylinder to a yoke on an anesthesia machine or to a pipeline within an institution. This system consists of three holes drilled in the valve of the gas cylinder that mate with matching pins on the yoke of the pipeline or anesthesia machine. The large central opening is the gas outlet of the cylinder. The other two holes are drilled to comply with the specifications of the safety system for the gas the cylinder is designed to contain. Despite the design of the safety system, it is not completely proof against mixups. Incidents have been reported of hospital personnel removing an oxygen fitting from an empty vessel, installing it on a nitrogen vessel and attaching it to the oxygen supply system in an institution. Patient deaths have been reported as resulting from such incidents.

Safety of hospital employees

In addition to concerns about patient safety, medical gases pose safety hazards to hospital personnel as well. The National Safety Council (NSC) has stated that hospital employees are 41% more likely to lose time from work because of injury or illness than employees in other fields. Hospital employees who work in or around laboratories or operating rooms are more likely to be injured by exposure to medical gases than workers in other areas. The highest risks are related to waste anesthetic gases, which result from inadequate maintenance of anesthesia machines or from poor work practices during the administration of anesthesia. The symptoms of acute exposure to waste anesthetic gases include drowsiness, depression, headaches, nausea, irritability, and loss of coordination. Chronic exposure can result in **liver** or kidney disease, **cancer**, or **miscarriage**.

KEY TERMS

Compressed medical gas—Any liquefied or vaporized gas alone or in combination with other gases.

Cryogenic vessel—A metal container designed to hold liquefied compressed medical gases at extremely low temperatures.

Cylinder—A metal container designed to hold compressed medical gases at a high pressure.

Manifold—A pipe or chamber with several openings for funneling the flow of liquids or gases.

Regulator—A mechanism that controls the flow of a medical gas.

Operation

Storage and transport of liquid oxygen

Pipelines serve as a convenient and economical method for the distribution of medical gases throughout a health care institution by reducing the number of gas cylinders required. This reduction contributes to the cleanliness of the facility, simplifies gas delivery, decreases the cost of the gas, and serves to decrease the number of personnel injuries related to the movement of heavy gas tanks. Liquid oxygen, stored at a temperature between -230– -283°F (-150°– -175°C) in double-walled stainless steel containers built to withstand a pressure of 250 lb per square inch gauge (psig), is the system used by most health care facilities for the main supply of this gas. Since liquid oxygen can vaporize rapidly with an abrupt rise in temperature to create dangerously high pressure, the bulk oxygen container must be located away from the institution for safety reasons. An underground pipeline, fitted with protective casings in areas of high surface loads, is used to transport the oxygen to the main facility's distribution system. Alarm systems are used to monitor the condition and operation of the liquid oxygen container. To avoid misfillings of oxygen containers, hose connections must be noninterchangeable. A high-pressure cylinder manifold system with an automatic switch-over valve serves as a reserve supply of liquid oxygen.

Storage and transport of liquid nitrous oxide

Cylinders of liquefied nitrous oxide connected to a gas manifold usually serve as the supply of this medical gas for facilities. The manifold controls the release of nitrous oxide from each tank. The gas is reduced to a working pressure of 45–55 psig before entering the main pipeline. Like liquid oxygen, liquid nitrous oxide has an automatic switch-over valve for a reserve bank of cylinders. These banks of gas cylinders are located in a designated storage room, which is usually adjacent to the facility's loading dock. To prevent cross-filling of tanks or rupture of the pipeline, a system of check valves, shutoff valves and pressure relief valves is employed.

Installation and inspection specifications

Pipelines in health care facilities must be constructed from hard-drawn seamless medical gas type tubing. All pipelines delivered to these facilities must also be cleaned for oxygen service, permanently labeled, and capped. Supports for the pipelines must have a copper finish if the support is to make contact with the copper tubing. Only qualified technicians should undertake all welding of medical pipelines. Shutoff valves are required throughout a facility's pipeline system; in particular, those that service a patient area should also have a pressure gauge. A newly installed pipeline system must be cleaned in accordance with set regulations before it is tested. The NFPA requires that both the installer and the user corroborate the findings of the pipeline testing before it is used with patients; and a record of these test results must be kept on file by the facility. Although this testing is designed to ensure the medical gas pipeline system is safe for patients, regulations addressing the requirements for the companies that perform the testing and the certification of pipeline systems have not been established. The American Hospital Association, however, does provide recommendations and verifications for the choice of a company to perform the inspection.

Operating rooms

Noninterchangeable outlets for medical gases located in operating rooms may be placed on the ceilings or walls. Each one must be color-coded and labeled with the name or chemical symbol of the medical gas it delivers. Automatic closing mechanisms in the outlet of each pipeline will prevent the leakage of gas when the mating end of the transfer hose is absent. The end of each hose used to connect the pipelines to an anesthesia machine must be color-coded and provided with a gas-specific noninterchangeable connection. Three gas sources supply an anesthesia machine:

- a storage container of liquid oxygen backed up by a reserve supply of oxygen in a cylinder

- liquid nitrous oxide in a cylinder

- medical air, supplied by gas cylinders or generated on site by compressors

Building codes

States regulate and enforce building codes regarding these pipelines but the variability of these codes are extreme. Some states have separate codes for each county or even for different regions within a large city. The NFPA has updated standards for the pipelines of health care facilities. In addition, the American Welding Society, the Manufacturers' Standardization Society of the Valve and Fittings Industry, the American Society of Mechanical Engineers, and the American National Standard Institute (ANSI) all have set standards for their installation, design and testing. With such varied coding, an enforcement mechanism is quite difficult. National standardization may come about only through the issue of medical liability.

Maintenance

Written procedures must be established for the testing intervals and maintenance of the pipelines as well as policies indicating procedures to be instituted for a shutdown. The American Hospital Association and the NFPA should be contacted regarding maintenance recommendations. The tests and procedures performed by the pipeline installer include:

- Pressurizing the pipeline to 1.5 times the working pressure for 24 hours, with each joint being checked for leaks.

- Blowing out the pipelines with oil-free nitrogen, pressurizing the pipelines to 1.2 times the working pressure for 24 hours and rechecking for leaks.

- Placing a white cloth over the outlets of the pipeline and intermittently purging it until the cloth is no longer discolored.

- Checking each pipeline with nitrogen and every outlet for the delivery of the labeled gas.

System users must repeat most of these tests and continue to ensure that each outlet is delivering the labeled medical gas. Further inspections of the manifolds, medical air compressors and alarms should be routinely performed. FDA inspectors are mandated to inspect gas liquefaction and container plants every other year.

Health care team roles

Biomedical technicians are the primary caretakers of medical gas pipelines within a health care facility. They are usually responsible for accepting medical gas deliveries and validating the contents of the delivery as well as its date and source. They should conduct scheduled shutdowns; establish protocol; maintain written policies and procedures; and remain informed of new standardized recommendations within the medical gas supply industry. They must also ensure that persons working under them have the proper training to identify medical gas cylinders, connection valves, regulators, and the distribution system within a facility.

Respiratory therapists primarily utilize oxygen from outlets within patient areas or from individual cylinders. They are responsible for checking the labels on any cylinders they use. They should also be aware of their duties in the event of a shutdown.

Certified **registered nurse** anesthetists and anesthesiologists should be aware of the location of the banks of gas cylinders and know the personnel responsible for changing them. They should also be knowledgeable about the workings of the cylinder bank and be able to troubleshoot the system with the biomedical technicians. Lastly, they should know the symptoms of exposure to waste anesthetic gases and the proper methods of treatment.

Training

All employees handling medical gases should be alerted to the possible hazards associated with their use. These personnel should be trained to recognize the various medical gas labels and to examine all labels carefully. Personnel who receive medical gas deliveries should be trained to store medical grade products separately from industrial grade products. The storage area for these medical grade products should be well defined, with one area for receiving full cryogenic vessels and another area for storing empty vessels. All personnel responsible for changing or installing cryogenic vessels must be trained to connect medical gas vessels properly. They must understand how vessels are connected to the oxygen supply system and be alerted to the serious consequences of altering the connections. Emphasis must be placed on the fact that the fittings on these vessels should not be changed under any circumstances. If a cryogenic vessel fitting does not form a good connection with the oxygen supply system fitting, the supplier should be contacted immediately. The vessel should be returned to them for correction of the problem. Finally, before the medical gas is introduced into the system, a knowledgeable person should ensure that the correct vessel has been connected properly. Every opportunity should be taken to promote the importance of properly handling medical gases to all personnel and especially those who are directly involved with handling them.

Resources

ORGANIZATIONS

Food and Drug Administration. 5630 Fishers Lane, Room 1061, Rockville, MD 20852. <http://www.fda.gov>.

National Fire Protection Association (NFPA). 1 Batterymarch Park, Quincy, MA 02269-9101. (617) 770-3000 or (800) 344-3555. Fax: (617) 770-0700. <http://www.nfpa.org>.

OTHER

FDA Public Health Advisory. *Guidance for Hospitals, Nursing Homes, and Other Health Care Facilities.* March 2001.

Occupational Safety and Health Administration (OSHA). *OSHA Technical Manual,* Section VI, Chapter 1, "Hospital Investigations: Health Hazards." Washington, DC: United States Department of Labor, 2001.

United States Food and Drug Administration. <http://www.fda.gov/cder/dmpq/freshair.htm>.

Linda K. Bennington, CNS

Medical history *see* **Health history**

Medical laboratories

Definition

The medical laboratory, also called the clinical laboratory or the pathology laboratory, provides diagnostic testing services for physicians to help identify the cause of disease and changes produced in the body by disease conditions. Medical laboratories are classified as either clinical pathology laboratories, which analyze **blood**, urine, culture products, and other body fluids; or anatomical (or surgical) pathology laboratories, which analyze tissue or organ samples obtained during surgery or **autopsy** and cervical and body fluid samples obtained by biopsy or lavage. A typical hospital medical laboratory will be called the Department of Pathology (investigation of disease-related processes) and will offer both types of testing. Medical laboratories of various sizes, offering a variety of testing services, can be found in acute-care hospitals, medical centers, doctor's offices and group practices, skilled nursing facilities, and long-term care facilities. Commercial medical laboratories operate as independent businesses and serve as testing facilities for physicians and for companies engaged in medical or pharmaceutical research. Additional commercial laboratories that specialize in a specific type of testing such as genetic, drug, and fertility testing also serve the medical community. Reference laboratories are often established by universities, state governments, organizations, and companies to provide more comprehensive testing or to perform more difficult tests not needed routinely.

Purpose

Medical laboratory science, or medical technology, is an important part of diagnostic medicine. It uses sophisticated instruments and methods to evaluate hundreds of body processes that occur constantly as body organs do their work. Combinations of laboratory tests are needed to help diagnose a patient's condition. Clinical pathology evaluates disease by identifying (qualitative testing) and measuring (quantitative testing) chemical substances found in blood, urine, spinal fluid, sputum, feces, and other body fluids. **Bacteria** and sometimes **viruses** are grown and identified in culture products (samples of blood, urine, sputum, **wounds**, etc. that are transferred onto culture media and incubated until they grow enough to be identified). Biochemical substances such as hormones, enzymes, **minerals**, and other chemicals produced in the body can be measured, as well as chemicals ingested (eaten with food or consumed as medications or poisons) or produced as waste products.

Normal levels or reference levels of these substances are determined by performing the tests on large numbers of people and establishing a typical range of results expected in the absence of disease. These reference ranges are often gender and age specific and will vary from laboratory to laboratory depending upon the methods used. A level that is higher or lower than normal gives physicians information about a patient's condition at the time of testing and may help physicians diagnose a disorder or disease in that patient. Measuring changes in the levels of chemicals may also help to monitor changes in the patient's condition during and after treatment. For example, a substance produced by the prostate gland called prostate specific antigen is used to screen for **prostate cancer**. Following treatment, the physician will request that this test be performed because complete removal of the tumor will cause the blood level to return to normal. Following demonstration of successful treatment, the test will be performed at regular intervals to detect any recurrence of the tumor.

Anatomical pathology identifies either the cause of disease or, through autopsy, the consequences of disease (cause of death). Samples of cells, tissues, or organs obtained during surgery or autopsy are examined macroscopically (by the naked eye) and microscopically (by powerful microscopes). Advances in the relatively new sciences of genomics (study of DNA and RNA) and proteomics (study of molecular **proteins**), cell genetics, and molecular analysis may also be performed to better understand the origins of disease in individuals.

Anatomical pathology gives doctors the most definitive information on the disease process causing a patient's symptoms, illness, or death. Results of anatomical pathology depend upon the qualified opinion of a pathologist, a physician trained and experienced in identifying the causes of disease and changes in body chemistry or tissues in the presence of disease. The anatomical pathology report is written in appropriate detail for the testing physician, and will be used along with clinical data to determine the stage (extent) and prognosis (outlook) of the disease.

Doctors order laboratory tests to make, confirm, or rule out a diagnosis, to select or monitor therapy (drugs, **physical therapy**, surgery, etc.), to monitor a patient's progress during therapy and help determine a prognosis for the patient. A single test is usually not enough to confirm a diagnosis. Combinations of laboratory tests are used along with the patient's history, **physical examination**, and diagnostic imaging exams (such as x ray, MRI, CAT scans, and ultrasound) to make a definitive diagnosis. Laboratory screening tests are often performed on apparently healthy patients to make sure they have no underlying disease. Test profiles are also designed that combine a series of related tests (such as a hematology profile or chemistry profile) or organ-related tests (such as a cardiac profile, **liver** profile, or thyroid profile) to get a broad view of a patient's condition. More specific testing is usually required to make a definitive diagnosis.

Description

Testing laboratories rely on well defined technical procedures, complex precise instruments, and a variety of automated and electronic equipment to do diagnostic testing. Tests are performed by medical technologists, technicians, and laboratory assistants. The technical staff works under the direction of a pathologist, who interprets the results of the laboratory tests. Laboratories, laboratory equipment, and testing personnel are evaluated and accredited by national scientific organizations and government agencies, including the American Society of Clinical Pathologists (ASCP) and the Joint Commission on Accreditation of Healthcare Organizations (JCAHO). This accreditation process helps to standardize lab procedures, establish quality control standards, and ensure that labs provide physicians with accurate and timely test results.

The medical laboratory is typically divided into sections that perform related groups of tests. The standard laboratory sections include, but are not limited to:

- Clinical chemistry: the study of body chemistry and the detection and measurement of chemicals such as hormones, enzymes, proteins, **fats**, **vitamins**, minerals, metals, and drugs. The chemistry department has sub-specialties that include enzymology, **toxicology**, and immunochemistry.

- Hematology: the study of red and white blood cells, including their concentration and morphology(appearance and stages of growth), and the measurement of hemoglobin (iron-bearing protein in the blood) and other substances in the blood that may help diagnose bleeding and coagulation problems, anemia, **infection**, and various other illnesses including **cancer**. In large laboratories it is common practice to combine the automated components of both clinical chemistry and hematology into one section that is staffed by personnel who are skilled in both disciplines.

- Microbiology: the study of microorganisms, and the isolation and identification of disease-causing bacteria, yeasts, **fungi**, parasites, and viruses. Microbiologists also determine the antibiotic susceptibility of pathogenic bacteria that are grown from clinical specimens.

- Immunology: the study of the body's **immune system** and immune processes that mediate and regulate the body's defense against bacteria, viruses, and foreign cells or antigens (proteins). Immunology is also the section of the laboratory that tests for organ transplant compatiblity, a specialized area called histocompatibility testing, and autoimmune disease (i.e., an immunological response to one's own tissues). In addition, a branch of immunology called serology measures the concentration of specific antibodies that indicate infectious disease, previous exposure to a pathogen, or immunity resulting from **vaccination**.

- **Urinalysis**: the examination of urine and the study of waste products that are eliminated by the **kidneys** may indicate or help explain metabolic or kidney disease processes and monitor treatment with therapeutic drugs. Urinalysis also includes the analysis of cells, crystals, and other objects that enter the urine or are formed by the kidney or urinary tract.

- Every clinical laboratory will offer testing capabilities within these categories. All hospitals that perform surgery will also have an immunohematology department, which comprises the blood bank and those tests that are used to determine whether blood from a donor will be compatible with the intended recipient. In addition, the blood bank technologists perform tests to detect antibodies on red blood cells, store blood and blood products, and prepare blood products for transfusion. The blood bank also performs therapeutic bleeding or removal of specific blood components for some patients.

Smaller laboratories, such as those in doctors' offices, will perform routine testing and screening tests

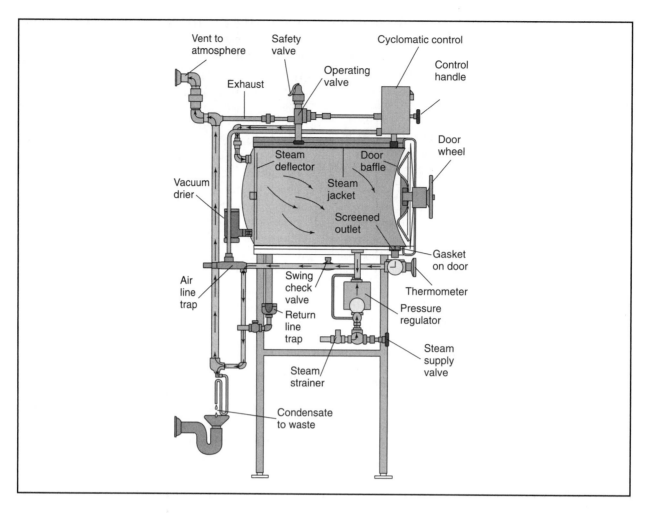

A steam autoclave is used to disinfect lab equipment. *(Delmar Publishers, Inc. Reproduced by permission.)*

related to the physician's specialty, usually testing blood and urine samples only, and will still need the hospital or independent testing laboratories for special diagnostic tests. Smaller laboratories generally use state-of-the-art equipment and automated instruments that are designed for less testing volume and that are less complex than those used in larger laboratories.

While some tests are performed manually, medical laboratories depend upon computer-controlled automated equipment for as many tests as possible to keep up with the volume and variety of tests ordered. Multichannel analyzers are commonly used to perform clinical chemistry tests. These large, complicated instruments are computer-controlled to perform many separate chemistry tests simultaneously (often called a chemistry panel or profile) on each patient's sample. The goal of such automation is to reduce the amounts of sample required; reduce the amount of chemicals (reagents) needed per test; reduce the time of analysis; eliminate contamination and error that results from excessive sam-

ple handling; and reduce the number of technologists needed to perform the testing. The precise operation of automated systems provides a higher degree of precision avoiding the differences in operator technique that increases the variance of manual testing methods. Computer-calculated results have been shown to be far more reliable than results subject to human manipulation, which is more likely to introduce transcription and random computational errors. Cost savings achieved through automation are important to both the testing facility and the patient. Time savings are important to the testing physicians and unit nurses who are waiting for test results to make critical patient-care decisions.

Laboratory computerization also includes laboratory information systems (LIS) that can access patient information and allow reporting of test results directly to the patient's record. Patient orders and test results can be viewed on a terminal or printed out in a comprehensive record, showing daily or hourly results side by side for comparison. This is especially valuable to physicians and nurses who are monitoring the patient's treatment. Results may be reported more quickly when the LIS interfaces with the healthcare facility's medical information system (MIS), which displays results on computer terminals in point-of-care nursing units, or transfers the information to the testing physician's office.

Hundreds of different types of tests are performed daily in the medical laboratory using different methods on a variety of special instruments. The demand for both rapid and reliable results has led to increased reliance on automation and to new portable testing methods that can be performed at the bedside or other point-of-care. Some of the most common automated testing methods are:

- Automated general chemistry analyzer (automated spectrophotometry. Most automated tests performed on multichannel analyzers use this technique. The instrument consists of components that perform all of the steps of a manual procedure. Robotic arms may be used to convey the samples from the centrifuge to the analyzer and bar code readers are used to input test order and patient information directly to the analyzer's computer. Sample and reagents are added to reaction cells in precise amounts, mixed mechanically, and incubated at constant temperature for a specific period of time. The chemical reaction typically results in production of a colored product. The color intensity (absorbance) is determined by the instrument's optical system or spectrophotometer. The instructions for how to perform each different test (i.e., sample volume, reagent volume, incubation time, wavelengths for analysis) are stored in the computer's **memory**. The computer also stores calibration information needed to calculate results, and quality control data that is needed to validate instrument performance. Reaction cells may be disposable or cleaned and reused by an automated wash system on the analyzer. In addition to optical analysis, these instruments usually have electrochemical sensors for analysis of electrolytes such as sodium and potassium. The test menu is usually large, for example 40 to 60 different analytes that can be measured in any order or combination. Smaller, single-channel spectophotometers are also used in doctor's offices, clinics, and nursing units to perform a more restrictive number of procedures. Another type of light measuring instrument called a reflectance photometer is often used to read dry reagent strip urine or dry slide chemistry tests.

- Immunoassays. This comprises a wide range of laboratory methods that utilize specific antibodies to facilitate a measurement. Immunoassay platforms are incorporated into several large autoanalyzers (automated chemistry analyzers), and are used to identify minute amounts of analytes (substances analyzed in blood, urine or body fluids), which include hormones, drugs, tumor markers, specific proteins, and cardiac markers. Some systems also support immunological tests to identify bacterial and viral antigens and allergens (responsible for **allergies**). The technology is based upon the measurement of antigen-antibody complexes and usually involves the use of a label such as an enzyme, radioactive isotope, or fluorescent molecule to measure the amount of immune complexes formed. New technology allows the selection of individual tests in any order or combination without the need to change reagents or instrument settings manually.

- Electrophoresis. Electrically charged particles of varying size and electrical charge, will move at different rates under the influence of an electric field. These differences can be measured by a technique called electrophoresis. The process permits separation of similar molecules such as proteins with different net charges or of different sizes. Serum protein electrophoresis separates proteins found in blood serum, the clear portion of a blood sample after it clots. It is used as an aid to the diagnosis of diseases such as multiple myeloma, acute and chronic inflammation, kidney disease, liver disease, and nutritional disorders. Immunofixation electrophoresis uses the separation of proteins in conjunction with specific antibodies to help diagnose multiple myeloma (a malignant disease) and **immunodeficiency** states that occur in disorders such as **AIDS**. Hemoglobin electrophoresis separates the red pigment in blood cells to diagnose certain **anemias** and blood disorders.

- Chromatography. Substances can be separated and identified on the basis of their molecular size or chemical properties (how they interact). High performance liquid chromatography (HPLC), thin-layer chromatography, and gas-liquid chromatography each use a different type of medium to separate drugs, certain proteins, amino acids, **lipids**, organic acids, and hormones in blood or urine. Various detectors can be used to measure the quantity of the analytes following their separation.

- Mass spectrometry. This technology is coupled to gas chromatography in order to conclusively identify a compound based upon its unique chemical structure. The mass spectrometer is most often used to confirm positive **drug tests** performed by immunoassay. Mass spectrometry equipment is highly specialized and the testing is more likely offered by an independent laboratory specializing in this technique than by a hospital laboratory. Pharmaceutical companies often requires this type of testing on thousands of samples in the research and development of therapeutic drugs.

Analyte—A chemical substance in body fluids, cells, or tissues that is the subject of laboratory investigation.

Biochemistry—The study of biochemical origins of humans in health, growth, nutrition, and disease.

Clinical chemistry—A broad field of analytical techniques that detect and measure chemicals in body fluids, cells, or tissues, such as enzymes, hormones, proteins, drugs, or other naturally occurring chemicals or those either ingested or used to treat disease.

Diagnostic medicine—Diagnostic medicine is the scientific study of body fluids, tissues, and organs to diagnose disease, monitor the course of disease, and monitor the response to treatment, particularly drug therapy.

Enzymes—Important naturally occurring biological catalysts present in the body. They enhance all body processes, including growth, maturation, and reproduction, and can be detected and measured in body fluids to diagnose and monitor disease. Synthetic enzyme reagents (not manufactured in the body) can be used as markers or labels in tests for other analytes.

Fluorescence—A phenomenon exhibited by molecules that absorb light energy and then give off the energy as light of a longer wave length. Fluorescent technology is a measurement technique used in clinical laboratory procedures and equipment.

Immunoassay—This type of assay is a measurement technique that uses binding reactions between different types of proteins, one protein being an antigen, the other an antibody that attaches to it. Known amounts of either antigen or antibody are combined with a blood sample or other body fluid to attract the analyte of interest and allow it to be detected and measured. Antigen-antibody reactions can be measured using enzyme technology, fluorescence, or radioisotopes.

Immunology—The scientific study of the immune system, which the body's defense system against bacteria, viruses, foreign cells (as in transfusion or transplantation). Immune reactions in the body involve antigen-antibody reactions that can be detected and evaluated using similar antigen-antibody technology.

Markers—Also called labels or tags. They attach to analytes in patient samples and allow them to be detected and measured by various measurement techniques using light, heat, or radioactivity. The term also refers to analytes that signal the presence of a specific diseaase. For example, troponin I is a maker for a heart attach because it is liberated from myocardial cells following infarction.

Pathology—The scientific study of the causes and consequences of disease.

Reagents—Reagents are chemical preparations (compounds) used to perform laboratory tests or used in the operation of laboratory equipment.

• Atomic absorption and ion-selective electrodes. These techniques are used to measure trace metals and electrolytes, respectively. Atomic absorption spectrophotometry is an optical method that converts ions to atoms and then measures the absorbance of a wavelength of light by the atoms. Metals most commonly measured are lead, **zinc**, mercury, selenium, and **copper**. Ion selective electrodes are sensors that produce a small potential difference (voltage) in response to specific ions. This technique is accurate but not as sensitive as atomic absorption spectrophotometry. Therefore, it is used for measuring ions that are relatively abundant in blood such as sodium, potassium, chloride, hydrogen ions, magnesium, **calcium**, and lithium.

• Automated blood cell counters. Hematology laboratories count red and white blood cells, measure hemoglobin (the iron-bearing protein in blood), and determine the hematocrit (the volume percentage of blood occupied by the red cells), as well as other tests reported in a **complete blood count** (CBC). These tests can all be performed on an automated hematology system. Some automated systems can also identify each type of white cell in what is called a differential blood test. This automated system and its results are useful in diagnosing anemias, infections, leukemia and other blood disorders related to various types of cancer, and for general health screening.

• Flow cytometry. A flow cytometer is a more specialized type of cell counter that can differentiate, count, and in some cases sort specific subpopulations of cells. Flow cytometers make use of some of the rapidly expanding tools and molecular diagnostics. Fluorescent labeled antibodies are used to tag the cells of interest and these cells are counted as they flow in single file past through an aperature into which a laser is focused. The laser stimulates the fluorochrome to emit light of a specific color. Light filters and detectors respond to the specific colors and the instrument's computer processes the resulting electrical signals to determine the cell count. Two rapidly advancing biosciences, genomics and proteomics, are being applied to flow cytometry to permit measurement of the DNA content of cells to determine if they are benign or cancerous.

Operation

Clinical instruments use a variety of measuring technologies to evaluate patient samples, but the principles of operation between analyzers share some fundamental characteristics. All methods on all instruments must undergo a preliminary evaluation of precision and accuracy to demonstrate that they meet the manufacturer's claims for analytical performance. All methods must be calibrated on a regular basis by analyzing samples of known concentration to which the measured signals from patient samples are compared. All methods must be validated using quality control specimens on a daily basis. The quality control sample is made of the same composition as patient samples and has an expected concentration that is specific for the method of assay. When results for quality control samples do not fall within the expected range, the operator must institute correction actions before patient specimens can be analyzed and reported. Automated instruments have intricate computerized monitoring systems and software codes that signal the operator when results are likely to be invalid. The operator must troubleshoot these problems and perform whatever steps are required to facilitate successful measurement of affected patient samples. Every test result is reviewed and evaluated with respect to quality control performance and its reasonableness before it is electronically transferred to the LIS for reporting.

Maintenance and safety

Laboratory personnel often are trained in the operation and maintenance of new equipment by the manufacturers of each type of instrument. Technologists are responsible for calibrating measuring devices such as pipets, equipment such as centrifuges, as well as all instruments. In addition, all incubators, refrigerators, and freezers are monitored for temperature accuracy and electrical lines are checked for current leakage and unstable voltage. All reagents are dated, examined for contamination, and stored in a manner than complies with safety regulations and manufacturer specifications. Instruments, equipment, glassware, and work surfaces are regularly cleaned and disinfected. Gloves, leak-proof gowns, and other forms of barrier protection are utilized to reduce the risk of transmission of bloodborne pathogens and exposure to chemical and physical agents that may be harmful. While large hospitals may rely on staff biomedical engineers to perform some maintenance and instrument repairs, the laboratory personnel are responsible for day-to-day operation, cleaning and maintenance procedures. Each laboratory must maintain records of equipment calibration, cleaning and maintenance, and a manual of all laboratory procedures and policies. Laboratory operations, facilities, and services are inspected by external accrediting agencies that evaluate compliance by the laboratory with the Clinical Laboratory Improvement Act of 1988 (CLIA 88) as well as their own standards.

Health care team roles

Physicians order diagnostic tests from the medical laboratory to help diagnose and treat their patients. When an order is received by the laboratory, either on a manual lab request form or through the hospital MIS, the lab will first obtain the proper type of sample. This may involve drawing blood (venipuncture), which is typically performed by a phlebotomist (person who specializes in venipuncture). Samples such as urine, feces, sputum, or tissue usually are obtained by nurses or physicians in the nursing unit. Surgical samples will be delivered to the lab by surgical technicians. Some samples, such as single or 24-hour urine samples, are brought to the lab by patients themselves (if they are outpatients). Laboratory personnel are responsible for checking all specimens received in order to determine that they are properly labeled and collected in the proper container. Personnel responsible for specimen processing will separate the blood components if required and store the sample at the proper temperature prior to testing. Technologists or technicians perform the analysis, evaluate the test system using quality control procedures, and review each result before reporting it. Inappropriate specimens are rejected, and suspicious results may require repeat testing using a new sample. Critical values and stat requests must be called immediately to the ordering physician. Some physicians have issued a written request for follow-up testing when results are abnormal. Timely communication between the laboratory staff and the primary care provider is essential for effective utilization of laboratory tests and results.

Training

Laboratory medicine is a well developed field based upon natural and physical sciences that requires education in medical science, techniques and research methods. Pathologists are physicians (MDs) who have completed four years of medical school, followed by a residency in a pathology laboratory. Medical laboratory technologists, technicians, and assistants who work in all fields of medical laboratory science are educated and trained at various levels. Those with more education will have greater technical and administrative decision-making responsibilities in the laboratory. Some may have advanced degrees (Ph.D. or M.S.) in sciences such as biochemistry or immunology. Certified technologists are required to have a Bachelor of Science degree and to have successfully completed an accredited laboratory training program. Their course of study typically includes anatomy, physiology, molecular biology, organic and biochemistry, immunology, microbiology, mathematics and statistics. Professional laboratory training includes courses in hematology, diagnostic and pathogenic microbiology, clinical immunology, immunohematology, and clinical biochemistry and urinalysis. A clinical practicum (internship) is typically required either as part of the baccalaureate degree or afterwards. After this training, graduates will be eligible for certification by examination by the American Society of Clinical Pathologists (ASCP) or National Certification Agency for Clinical Laboratory Personnel (NCA). Certified clinical laboratory technicians earn an associate degree from an accredited medical laboratory technician program. The program will include a clinical practicum as part of the training. Following this graduates are eligible for certification by examination by the American Society of Clinical Pathologists (ASCP) or National Certification Agency for Clinical Laboratory Personnel (NCA). Some vocational schools offer basic education and training for medical laboratory assistants, allowing graduates to perform some laboratory procedures and assist more skilled laboratory personnel.

Resources

BOOKS

Henry, J. B. *Clinical Diagnosis and Management by Laboratory Methods.* 20th edition. St. Louis: W. B. Saunders, 2001.

ORGANIZATIONS

American Society for Clinical Laboratory Science (ASCLS). 7910 Woodmont Avenue, Ste. 530, Bethesda, MD 20814. (301) 657-2768. <http://www.ascls.org>.

American Society of Clinical Pathologists (ASCP). 40 West Harrison Street, Chicago, IL 60612 (312). 738-1336. <http://www.ascp.org>.

OTHER

Medical Laboratory Observer (MLO) <http://www.mlo-online.com/article-ind/articles.html>.

L. Lee Culvert

▮ Medical laboratory technology

Definition

Medical laboratory technology is the branch of medical science responsible for performing laboratory investigations relating to the diagnosis, treatment, and prevention of disease.

Description

Laboratory scientists (medical and clinical technologists as well as medical and clinical laboratory technicians) facilitate the diagnosis of diseases, as well as the implementation and monitoring of therapies to treat disease. Laboratory scientists are responsible for examining and analyzing **blood**, body fluids, tissues, and cells in an effort to help clinicians determine the underlying cause of an illness, the stage of a disease, or the effectiveness of therapy. To accomplish their objectives, laboratory scientists perform a wide variety of laboratory tests, often with the aid of complex, computerized, and automated instrumentation.

Tests performed by laboratory scientists include:

- Microbiology tests that isolate and identify pathogenic **bacteria**, yeast, **fungi**, parasites, and **viruses** and determine antibiotic sensitivity.

- Chemistry tests that measure the chemical content of plasma, body fluids and cells including electrolytes, glucose, **lipids**, **proteins**, hormones, enzymes, trace metals, drugs, and toxins.

- Blood banking tests, such as typing, antibody screening, and cross matching, that are used to identify and prepare blood components that are compatible for transfusion.

- Immunology tests that are used to determine a person's ability to resist infections, diagnose autoimmune diseases, **allergies**, and infectious diseases, and determine tissue compatibility for organ transplantation.

- Hematology tests that count and classify blood cells, diagnose blood diseases, diagnose **bleeding disorders**, and monitor anticoagulant therapy.

- Histology procedures that prepare specimens for microscopic examination by pathologists.

- Cytology procedures such as the Pap smear test, which identify cancerous changes within cells.

- Cytogenetic procedures which identify abnormal chromosome counts, morphology, and disease genes.

Over the past few decades the proliferation of laboratory automation has significantly decreased the hands-on nature of the work. Today, many experienced laboratory scientists spend more time analyzing results, developing and modifying procedures, and establishing and monitoring quality control programs than they do performing tests.

Work settings

An article published in the July 1999 issue of *Medical Laboratory Observer* reported that "in general, medical technologists and medical laboratory technicians are stable professionally." Laboratory scientists in their study, which was conducted in 1998 and 1999, had been employed at their current lab for 12 years and had been in the lab profession for 21 years. This job stability may be due in part to job flexibility. Because many large hospitals and reference laboratories operate 24 hours a day, seven days a week, they offer opportunities for laboratory scientists to work full or part-time, days, evenings, or nights. However, smaller hospitals with a more limited staff often require their laboratory scientists to rotate shifts, while others place laboratory workers on call several nights a week or on weekends to ensure coverage during an emergency situation. Working an occasional weekend and holiday is also quite common.

Clinical laboratories are well lit and clean, and the work is not physically demanding or particularly dangerous. That said, in a typical day most laboratory scientists will spend a significant portion of their day on their feet and be exposed to odiferous reagents and specimens, some of which will be infectious.

Wages for laboratory personnel are rising and correlate with the level of education and training. According a survey conducted by the American College of Clinical Pathologists, the median annual salary for a staff medical technician in 2000 was $29,120, an increase of 8.5% since 1998. In contrast, the median annual salary for a staff medical technologist in 2000 was $37,232, an increase of 11.9% since 1998. For both technicians and technologists, salaries on the coasts were higher than elsewhere in the United States.

As the MLO article and others have reported, the majority of laboratory scientists work full-time in hospitals, reference and physician office laboratories. However, there are also numerous employment opportunities for laboratory scientists in forensic, environmental and food industry laboratories. In addition, manufacturers of home diagnostic testing kits and laboratory equipment and supplies seek experienced technologists to work in product development, marketing, and sales.

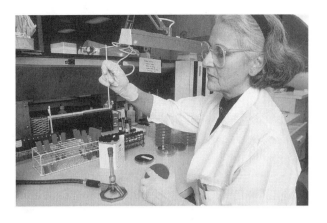

Medical laboratory technologists perform a variety of tests on body fluids and tissues to help physicians determine diagnoses and evaluate therapies. *(Custom Medical Stock Photo. Reproduced by permission.)*

Education and training

The Clinical Laboratory Improvement Act of 1988 (CLIA '88) sets minimum standards for testing personnel who work in clinical laboratories. For labs performing high complexity tests, the minimum requirement for testing personnel is an associate's degree in laboratory science. Persons who hold an associate degree from an accredited training program and certification are referred to as technicians. Persons who hold a bachelor's degree and certification in a clinical laboratory field are referred to as technologists. Certification is a prerequisite for most jobs, and some states require laboratory scientists to be licensed. Those holding a bachelor's degree with a major in medical technology or in one of the life sciences typically earn more money and receive more opportunities for advancement. While both technicians and technologists perform laboratory procedures, the technologist has greater knowledge of scientific principles and problem solving skills, and is responsible for oversight of quality assurance, method evaluation, and laboratory management.

Both bachelor and associate degree programs include courses in general and organic chemistry, general biology, microbiology, and anatomy and physiology. Specialized training includes courses in the specific laboratory disciplines. Baccalaureate programs also include courses in statistics, biochemistry, and immunology. Many four-year programs also offer courses in management, business, and computer technology.

There are several certifications available for laboratory personnel. The two most prominent organizations that certify lab personnel in the United States are the American Society of Clinical Pathologists board of Registry and the National Certification Agency for

KEY TERMS

Blood banking tests—Typing, antibody screening, and cross matching that are used to identify and prepare blood components that are compatible for transfusion.

Chemistry tests—Those tests for the measurement of electrolytes, glucose, lipids, proteins, hormones, enzymes, trace metals, drugs, and toxins.

Cytogenetic procedures—Techniques for chromosome counting and identification of abnormal chromosomes and disease genes.

Cytology procedures—Staining and examination of tissue samples in order to identify cancerous changes within cells.

Hematology tests—Tests to count and classify blood cells, diagnose blood diseases including coagulation disorders.

Histology procedures—Cutting, staining, and mounting of specimens for microscopic examination by pathologists.

Immunology tests—Tests which are used to determine a person's ability to resist infections, diagnose autoimmune diseases, allergies, and infectious diseases, and determine tissue compatibility for organ transplantation.

Medical laboratory technician—A clinical laboratory worker who may perform all levels of testing including quality control monitoring, specimen processing, and other laboratory operations.

Medical technologist—A clinical laboratory worker who performs all levels of testing, evaluates laboratory methods, verifies results, detects and resolves analytical problems, performs quality assurance, and consults with physicians and allied health professionals regarding laboratory services.

Microbiology tests—Those tests for the isolation and identification of pathogenic bacteria, yeast, fungi, parasites, and viruses and antibiotic sensitivity testing.

Medical Laboratory Personnel. Technicians with general certification by the American Society of Clinical Pathologists Board of Registry are denoted by the letters MLT (ASCP) and technologists with general certification by MT (ASCP). Technicians with general certification by the National Certification Agency for Medical Laboratory Personnel are denoted by the letters CLT (NCA) and technologists with general certification by CLS (NCA).

Advanced education and training

Technicians can become technologists through additional education and experience, which may be covered, partially or fully, by a tuition reimbursement program offered by their current employer. Specialist certification is also available in blood banking, chemistry, cytotechnology, hematology, hemapheresis, immunology, and microbiology. For those desiring supervisor and management responsibilities the U.S. Department of Labor's *Occupational Outlook Handbook* suggests that a "graduate education in medical technology, one of the biological sciences, chemistry, management, or education usually speeds advancement." CLIA '88 mandates that a laboratory director hold an M.D. or Ph.D. with board certification or prior laboratory experience. Laboratory managers usually hold a bachelor's degree or higher.

Future outlook

According to the *2000 Wage and Vacancy Survey of Medical Laboratories* conducted by the American Society of Clinical Pathologists, "the year 2000 marked the highest vacancy rates reported per position over the 12-year comparison period." With 87% of the responding laboratories reporting vacancies in medical technologist and manager positions, it is easy to see why the U.S. Department of Labor expects employment opportunities for laboratory scientists to grow through the year 2008.

These shortages are most profound in the Northeast and East North Central regions of the United States, though no region seems unaffected. While over 65% of all laboratories with a vacancy were having trouble filling at least one shift for a staff medical technologist; cytotechnologists, histological technicians, histotechnologists and phlebotomists vacancies pose the greatest concern. The breadth of the problem is clear as over 70% of laboratories are using some combination of salary, benefits, sign-on bonuses, and tuition reimbursement to attract personnel to their facility.

For those laboratory scientists seeking something new, there are also numerous opportunities outside the laboratory in corporations and other businesses. As previously mentioned, manufacturers of home diagnostic testing kits and laboratory equipment and supplies seek experienced technologists to work in product development, marketing, and sales. In addition, the highly computerized laboratory of today is preparing many laboratory scientists for positions in information technology for the laboratory, the hospital, or any other business. Positions involving quality assurance or performance improvement, remote site testing, safety compliance or **infection control**, accrediting organizations, employee education, and laboratory consulting represent other avenues of opportunity for laboratory scientists. Better still, an article in the July 1999 issue of *Clinical Laboratory News* entitled "Where Will You Be Working in 2010?" predicts that "One of the major changes in how laboratorians are employed is that many will be self-employed, performing services for multiple companies and organizations. Furthermore, these changes will allow many laboratorians to work from home."

Regardless of the career path chosen, the key to remaining employable is to continuously strive to gain new skills and to develop a network of contacts from a variety of sources, including co-workers, associations, and vendors.

Resources

PERIODICALS

Frings, C. S. "Answering your questions on alternative careers for laboratorians and necessary credentials for managing a high-complexity POL." *Medical Laboratory Observer* (Nov. 1999) 31: 20.

Frings, C. S. "Where will you be working in 2010? Novel opportunities for future laboratorians." *Clinical Laboratory News* 25, no.7 (July 1999): 28-30.

Ward-Cook, K., and S. Tunnar. "2000 Wage and Vacancy Survey of Medical Laboratories." *Laboratory Medicine* 3, no. 32 (March 2001): 124-138.

ORGANIZATIONS

American Medical Technologists. 710 Higgins Rd., Park Ridge, IL 60068. <http://www.amt1.com>.

American Society for Clinical Laboratory Science. 7910 Woodmont Ave., Suite 530, Bethesda, MD 20814.

American Society of Clinical Pathologists, Board of Registry. P.O. Box 12277, Chicago, IL 60612. <http://www.ascp.org/bor>.

International Society for Clinical Laboratory Technology. 917 Locust St., Suite 1100, St. Louis, MO 63101-1413.

OTHER

Occupational Handbook Outlook. U.S. Department of Labor, Bureau of Labor Statistics. <http://stats.bls.gov/oco/ocos096.htm>.

Victoria E. DeMoranville

Medical lasers

Definition

A laser is a device that transforms one type of energy, usually electrical, into optical energy. The light waves in the beam produced by a laser are nearly parallel (collimated), nearly monochromatic, and coherent. The light beam is produced by exciting atoms and causing them to radiate their energy in phase. The word *laser* is an acronym that stands for Lightwave Amplification by Stimulated Emission of Radiation.

Purpose

Lasers have proven useful in all medical specialties to vaporize or coagulate tissue. Surgeons use lasers to perform controlled linear vaporization in order to to cut tissue. Lasers can be used for surgery on all parts of the body, but are used most extensively in eye surgery and cosmetic skin procedures. An additional function of lasers is the sensing of physiological parameters.

Description

Lasers affect human tissue by transferring radiant energy to the target cells. The radiant energy turns into heat when the cells absorb it. As the target cells are heated, all their **proteins** are destroyed and their internal pressure rises rapidly. The cells then explode, giving off smoke-like steam called a laser plume. The major effects of most lasers on tissue are coagulation of **blood** and protein, and vaporization. Vaporization is the removal of tissue through its conversion from a solid to a gas.

Laser types

In general, there are two types of medical laser systems, contact and non-contact. Contact systems work by sending laser light through a fiber or sapphire crystal tip. The tip absorbs the radiant energy and becomes hot. Direct contact between the tissue and the heated tip causes conduction of the heat energy from the tip to the tissue, resulting in the vaporization of the target cells. In contrast, non-contact laser systems do not directly touch the tissue. Instead, the laser light transfers radiant energy to the tissue. Heat results when the cell absorbs the radiant energy and the molecules in the tissue begin to move. In both types of system, the laser light itself is not hot. Heat is created only after the laser's radiant energy is absorbed, either by the tip or by the tissue.

Laser components

All lasers, regardless of size, style, or application, have four main components: the active medium, the excitation mechanism, the feedback mechanism (high reflectance mirror), and the output coupler (partially transmissive mirror). Active media may be solid, liquid, gas, or electronic. Lasers are named for the medium that is used to produce the light. Some solid medium lasers commonly used in medical applications are erbium:yttrium aluminum garnet (Er:YAG); holium:yttrium aluminum garnet (Ho:YAG); neodymium:yttrium aluminum garnet (Nd:YAG); and alexandrite, ruby, and potassium titanyl phosphate (KTP). Carbon dioxide (CO_2), argon, copper vapor, and excimer lasers are examples of medical lasers with gas media. Dye lasers have liquid media and diode lasers have electronic media.

When energy is applied to the active medium of a laser, its electrons are raised to an unstable level of energy, from which they return spontaneously to a lower but relatively long-lived metastable (chemically unstable but not liable to spontaneous transformation) condition. These electrons will not return to their ground energy level. It is therefore possible to pump large amounts of energy into the active medium, to the point that most of its atoms are in a metastable state. The lasing action begins with an electron that returns to its ground state, producing a photon. If the photon has exactly the right wavelength, it will stimulate a metastable atom to emit another photon of the same wavelength. This process is called stimulated emission. If enough stimulated photons travel parallel to the long axis of the laser tube they will continue to stimulate the emissions of photons of the same wavelength. These photons combine coherently until they reach the mirrored ends of the laser tube. When the light beam strikes the reflecting mirror, it is reversed and continues to stimulate the emission of more photons. The beam increases in intensity until it reaches the partially reflecting mirror. A portion of the light is released while the rest is reflected back through the active medium to continue stimulating photon emission.

Medical lasers have three types of excitation mechanisms. In most gas lasers, high-voltage direct current electricity is used. With some CO_2 lasers, radiofrequency electricity excites the gas. This type of excitation is needed to produce an ultrapulsed output, which is the delivery of very fast, extremely powerful bursts of light. Media that do not conduct electricity, such as solid and liquid media, are excited with light produced by flashlamps or other lasers.

Specific medical applications

Certain lasers tend to be used for particular procedures to take advantage of the quality of the light and amount of absorption by different types of tissue. The CO_2 laser is quite versatile, able to perform both cutting and bulk vaporization. It is often used to perform gynecological procedures involving **colposcopy** as well as ear-nose-and throat (ENT) procedures using microlaryngoscopy, such as the treatment of snoring. The CO_2 laser is also useful for cosmetic skin resurfacing and in neurosurgery.

The Nd:YAG laser is a contact laser. It is used in abdominal, gynecological, or urological surgeries performed through laparoscopes, endoscopes, or hysteroscopes. The Er:YAG laser is used for bone cutting, hard tissue drilling in dentistry, and skin resurfacing. The Ho:YAG laser is useful for such orthopedic procedures as joint arthroscopies, as well as for urologic **lithotripsy** and ophthalmologic procedures.

Cosmetic laser hair removal is a very popular procedure that can be performed by diode, alexandrite, and ruby lasers. Ruby lasers can be used to remove tattoos. Argon and excimer lasers are used primarily to reshape the cornea in laser eye surgeries, although **heart** surgeons also use excimer lasers to perform angioplasties. Copper vapor or dye lasers are used to treat port-wine birthmarks. Tunable dye lasers and argon lasers are often used to repair such cosmetic vascular problems as varicose or spider veins.

Pulmonary and esophageal tumors are treated by a laser technique called photodynamic therapy (PDT). This technique has potential applications for treating many other types of tumors. In PDT, a photoreactive drug called dihematoporphyrin is administered systemically. The drug collects in tumor cells at a significantly higher concentration than in normal cells. Laser light from red dye lasers is then applied to the tumor site. The drug preferentially absorbs the light, causing the tumor cells to be vaporized and leaving the normal cells intact.

Operation

When a laser is used in surgery, there are three central control parameters—power in watts (set by the laser nurse); time of exposure (dependent on the speed of movement of the beam or tip); and spot size (an increase or decrease in the area contacted by the laser light, controlled by the surgeon in the field). In general, cutting is done with the smallest possible spot; that is, the beam is kept in tight focus. A change in power level changes the speed of incision. If the surgeon is vaporizing or debulking tissue, the key consideration is power density. Thus, the spot size can be increased but the power is increased proportionately. Rather than continuous use of a lower level of power that can cause thermal damage to surrounding tissue, the surgeon may use a higher level of power on a pulsed setting. Superpulsing and ultrapulsing are the two levels of pulsing available.

Setting tests

Laser settings can be tested on a wet tongue depressor blade before they are used to vaporize tissue. Ideally, a 0.1-second test shot will leave a scoop-shaped depression in the wood shaped like a golf ball cut in half, with no point. A point indicates that the power density is too high. Rather than vaporizing the tissue cleanly, the laser will carve ridges and furrows in the tissue that might cause bleeding. If the depression is too shallow, the laser will be in use too long and cause charring.

The spatial quality of a laser beam can also be tested on a piece of thermal paper.

Safety issues and precautions

The use of lasers raises important safety issues. Categorized as Class IV devices by the Bureau of Radiological Health (BRH), all medical laser systems are fire hazards. They are also chemical hazards because of the compressed gases required to operate them and the fumes produced from lasing of the active medium. In addition, the laser dyes or solvents may be toxic. Lasers can produce skin or eye **burns**, and can cause retinal damage from direct or reflected beams. Lastly, lasers are explosion hazards; lasing of the active medium may cause flying fragments that can injure nearby personnel. Accordingly, a significant number of safety precautions are recommended. The American National Standards Institute (ANSI) standard Z136.3 addresses the safe use of lasers in health care settings and is an excellent resource for laser safety concerns. The ANSI directive establishes both engineering and administrative/procedural controls for four classes of lasers.

The following are among the recommended precautions:

- warning signs posted outside procedure room entrances
- all windows protected from transmission of laser light (not required for CO_2 lasers because it does not transmit through glass)
- protective eyewear rated for the wavelength being used for all personnel within the nominal hazard zone (which may be the entire procedure room)
- protection of the patient's eyes

> ## KEY TERMS
>
> **Active medium**—The solid, liquid, gas, or electronic substance used to produce the laser light. It contains atoms whose electrons can be excited to a metastable level of energy.
>
> **Excitation**—The use of energy to move electrons present in the laser medium to a higher orbit around the atom nucleus.
>
> **Feedback**—The use of mirrors in a laser tube to reflectively increase the intensity of the produced light.
>
> **Metastable**—Chemically unstable but not liable to spontaneous transformation. Most of the atoms in the active medium of a laser must be raised to a metastable state before the lasing action can begin.
>
> **Output coupler**—A mirror in the laser tube that part of the light beam can flow through because it is both reflective and transmissive.
>
> **Photodynamic therapy**—The use of a photosensitive drug to selectively target tumor cells during laser treatment.
>
> **Pulsed laser**—A laser that delivers energy in single or multiple pulses less than or equal to 0.25 second.

- lasers operated only by those who have received formal training in laser theory, control techniques, and operation
- the presence of a trained laser nurse or laser safety operator during the procedure
- the proper use of a laser smoke evacuator, equipped with a 0.3-micron filter if viral contamination is a concern
- judicious use of dulled (anodized) **surgical instruments** to reduce beam reflection
- careful packing of tissue surrounding beam area to avoid accidental exposure
- availability of water within the procedure room and a nearby fire extinguisher

Despite the numerous safety concerns associated with lasers, the light is not an ionizing radiation risk. Precautions such as those used with x-ray equipment are not necessary.

Maintenance

The maintenance of lasers requires specially trained laser technicians, often members of the hospital **biomedical engineering** department or an outsource company. Power calibrations are required every six months. Routine maintenance includes changing the laser's filters and deionizer water, replacing flashlamps, checking alignments, power outputs and fail-safe shields, and cleaning optics.

It is important to store lasers away from high-traffic areas to avoid miscalibration and damage to their internal mechanisms.

Health care team roles

Physicians who have received special training in the use of lasers are the only personnel who actually use the laser and control the foot pedal. Laser nurses aid in setting the controls of the device and are often responsible for filling out the laser log documenting the procedure. Laser technicians are responsible for the maintenance of the equipment and, if they are specially trained, laser repair.

The ANSI guidelines recommend the appointment of a laser safety officer (LSO) for the hospital. This person is responsible for ensuring that the safety procedures are followed for every laser procedure performed in the facility. Trained laser nurses or technicians may act under the LSO's authority. In many hospitals, the LSO is a senior laser nurse, a senior laser technician, or even a physician. This person has the authority to turn off the laser if he or she determines that its use would be hazardous to the patient or other personnel.

Training

Although there are no national accreditation standards for laser use, most hospitals have set up a laser committee that reviews applications from physicians who wish to perform laser procedures within the facility. In order to obtain operating privileges, many hospitals require training of at least eight hours with the particular type of laser that is to be used.

Some hospitals run their own training programs, while others rely on outside medical education companies. In either case, the training programs will cover the principles of laser use and safety; have a clinical practicum taught by specialists in the area of the physician's practice, and hands-on sessions with the laser. Many hospitals require practice with both inanimate and animal specimens.

Training for laser nurses is also run internally by each individual hospital. Course work includes basic information about laser function, operation, and safety as well as specific training with the lasers used in the different procedures. Because laser nurses are often the LSO's eyes and hands in the operating room, it is essential for them to understand and implement the procedures required for safe laser use.

Resources

BOOKS

Absten, Gregory T., ed. *Laser Medicine and Surgery.* Marathon Shores, FL: Professional Medical Education Association, Inc., 2000.

Fitzpatrick, Richard E., MD, and Mitchel P. Goldman, MD, eds. *Cosmetic Laser Surgery.* St. Louis: Mosby, 2000.

PERIODICALS

Loesel, Frieder H. "Ultrafast surgical lasers provide vision correction." *Laser Focus World* (January 2001): 143-148.

ORGANIZATIONS

American Society for Laser Medicine and Surgery (ASLMS). 2404 Stewart Square, Wausau, WI 54401. (715) 845-9283. <http://www.aslms.org>.

The Laser Institute of America. 12424 Research Parkway, Orlando, FL 32826.

Michelle L. Johnson, M.S., J.D.

Medical malpractice *see* **Malpractice**

Medical nutrition therapy

Definition

Medical **nutrition** therapy (MNT) refers to the assessment of the nutritional status of patients with an illness, diet-related condition, or injury, in order to benefit the patient's own health and reduce health-care costs. MNT includes setting goals for the patient's treatment and developing a specialized nutrition prescription that includes **patient education** and self-management training. MNT, which is also called therapeutic nutrition, has become an increasingly important component of integrated health-care systems.

Purpose

The purpose of MNT is to identify patients at risk for major nutrition-related health problems and recommend dietary adjustments leading to better health outcomes and improved quality of life. Eight of the 10 leading causes of death in the American population—including coronary **heart** disease, stroke, **diabetes mellitus**, and some cancers—are related to food and alcohol consumption patterns. Other important patient populations who benefit from MNT include the obese, the elderly, and infants of low birth weight. **Obesity** increases the risk of **gout**, **osteoarthritis**, sleep apnea, and **hypertension** as well as stroke and cardiovascular disease; while many of the elderly suffer from malnutrition. Low birth rate is the greatest single health risk in newborns.

MNT is also used to treat such disorders as anorexia and bulimia nervosa, **cystic fibrosis**, irritable bowel syndrome, hyperlipidemia, difficulty with lactose digestion, gastric ulcers, sprue (a **malabsorption syndrome**), and (in children) failure to thrive. Adequate nutrition is essential to reduce morbidity and mortality from these and other acute or chronic conditions. MNT helps to contain health-care costs while benefiting patients directly by offering alternatives to more expensive drug treatments and minimizing the need for surgery or lengthy hospital stays.

Description

Medical nutritional therapy is used in a variety of treatment settings, including **home care** and outpatient care as well as acute or long-term care facilities. In most of these settings, medical nutrition therapy includes a comprehensive review of the patient's medical history and a **dietary assessment** with laboratory values and anthropometric measurements.

Intake assessment

A key part of MNT includes an assessment of the patient's current and past diet history. A dietary assessment is often conducted to determine the macronutrient (energy or caloric, protein, and fat) content and the micronutrient (vitamin and mineral) content of the patient's food intake. Some of the most common dietary assessment tools include food records, dietary recalls, food frequency questionnaires, diet histories, and several other methods of data collection, including biochemical indices. A scientific assessment of nutritional status may be compiled from the information collected from clinical evaluations, biochemical tests, and dietary information. The clinical evaluation includes measurements of the patient's height, weight, and percentage of body fat (determined by skinfolds or hydrostatic weighing). In addition, a clinical evaluation may also include observation for signs of nutrient deficiencies in the mouth, skin, eyes, and nails. The information collected from a clinical evaluation is added to the results of the dietary assessment and biochemical tests to provide a comprehensive picture of the patient's current nutritional status and relative risk factors for diet-related illnesses. MNT can then

be designed to treat the patient's specific illness or diet-related condition.

In addition to the patient's overall medical history and specific evaluation of any diet-related illnesses or conditions, an intitial evaluation may include an assessment of his or her:

- psychosocial data, including food-related attitudes and behaviors
- sociological data, including cultural practices, housing, cooking facilities, financial resources, and support of family and friends.
- general understanding of nutrition, including the relationship of diet to his or her disease or condition.
- learning style, together with his or her readiness to modify or change behavior.
- current **exercise** and activity level

Dietary modification

Dietary modification may include implementation of specialized diets for chronic conditions and diseases. Specialized diets in medical nutrition therapy may include:

- supplemental nutrition for patients who cannot obtain adequate nutrients through food intake alone
- enteral nutrition delivered via tube feeding into the gastrointestinal tract for those unable to eat normally or digest food
- parenteral nutrition delivered via intravenous infusion (IV) for those who cannot absorb nutrients

Patient education

Patient education is a critical dimension of medical nutrition therapy, in that patient compliance is essential to the success of any preventive or therapeutic nutritional program. Patient education in MNT may include task, guideline, and meal planning exercises. These exercises help to educate patients regarding proper food choices in the treatment or control of their specific illness or condition. Tasks are usually simple and objective responsibilities agreed upon by the dietitian, nutritionist, or doctor and the patient. An example of a task might include the patient's reviewing an itemized grocery receipt with the dietitian to determine if the foods that were purchased were appropriate to the nutrition plan.

A guideline approach provides the patient with nutrition information related to their specific illness, to be applied to their current eating habits. The patient can learn to plan and prepare appropriate meals with the

KEY TERMS

Dietary assessment—An estimation of food and nutrients eaten over a particular time point. Some of the most common dietary assessment methods are food records, dietary recalls, food frequency questionnaires, and diet histories.

Dietary counseling—Nutritional advice provided to an individual patient by a registered dietitian, nutritionist, or doctor for encouraging modification of eating habits.

Dietitian—A health professional with expertise in the field of nutrition and dietetics. Most have a bachelor's degree, followed by a period of clinical training.

Enteral nutrition—Feedings administered through a nose tube (or surgically placed tubes) for patients with eating difficulties.

Parenteral nutrition—Feeding administered most often by an infusion into a vein. It can be used if the gut is not functioning properly or due to other reasons that prevent normal or enteral feeding.

Therapeutic nutrition—Another term for medical nutrition therapy.

dietitian's help, and eventually become able to manage their nutritional regimen on their own.

Preventive care at all points along the spectrum of illness—primary (preventing disease), secondary (early diagnosis), and tertiary (preventing or slowing deterioration)—requires active patient participation as well as guidance from the dietitian and physician or nurse. Education, motivation, and counseling contribute to effective patient participation.

Preparation

There are many nonmedical issues that must be factored into planning appropriate **dietary counseling** and MNT. Due attention must be given to the patient's usual food choices, food likes and dislikes, cultural values, and the patient's ability to implement the dietary changes. In particular, the attitudes of other family members often influence the patient's compliance. Family members who are embarrassed by a patient's eating disorder, for example, may make her or his eating patterns and weight fluctuations the focus of most of the family's interactions. This focus will tend to reinforce the eating disorder rather than the medical nutrition therapy.

Aftercare

Nutrition therapy will be effective only if the patient is willing to implement the suggested recommmendations. If a patient does not follow the recommended dietary guidance, then they will not receive a health benefit from MNT.

Patients who require continued MNT (parenteral or enteral nutrition) after leaving a hospital should receive frequent follow-up and monitoring by a registered dietitian.

Results

The large-scale results of MNT have been impressive enough in terms of cost-effectiveness to capture the attention of many large companies. A number of registered dietitians are now conducting on-site nutrition classes in corporate workplaces, participating in health and wellness fairs, and working with corporation food services to design more healthful menus, in addition to offering MNT to the firm's employees.

On the individual level, the effectiveness of MNT depends on the commitment of all members of the health-care team—but especially on the patient who has the nutrition-related illness. Prioritized goals are critical when developing the nutrition treatment plan, together with ongoing assessment by the patient and health care team members. Physicians must understand the patient's dietary plan and reinforce the nutrition therapy when interacting with the patient.

The American Dietetic Association maintains as its official position that MNT is an essential and cost-effective part of comprehensive health care services. Medical nutrition therapy is also effective in treating disease and preventing disease complications.

Health care team roles

In general, only registered dietitians (R.D.) have sufficient training and knowledge to accurately assess the nutritional adequacy of a patient's diet. Nutrition support teams, however, include registered dietitians as team members, often as team leaders. Because food and nutrition services span both medical and social contexts, medical nutrition therapy should be an interdisciplinary task in patient care. Physicians should learn the indications for special diets in order to facilitate referrals to dietitians and to reinforce patient compliance. Dietitians are needed to monitor patient populations receiving enteral, parenteral, and specialized oral therapies in conjunction with other health care team members (physicians, nurses/aids, home care workers, etc).

Some insurance plans cover fees for nutritional counseling by physicians and nurse practitioners as well as by registered dietitians directly supervised by physicians or employed by a participating institution. This inclusiveness reflects the growing significance of MNT in health care as well as the importance of coordinating the work of different health professionals in the area of nutrition.

Resources

BOOKS

Baron, Robert B., MD, MS. "Nutrition." *Current Medical Diagnosis & Treatment 2001*. Edited by Lawrence M. Tierney Jr., MD, et al. New York: Lange Medical Books/McGraw-Hill, 2001.

Institute of Medicine. *Dietary Reference Intakes: Risk Assessment (Compass Series)*. Washington, DC: National Academy Press, 1999.

Larson-Duyff, Roberta. *The American Dietetic Association's Complete Food & Nutrition Guide*. New York: John Wiley & Sons, 1998.

National Academy Press Food and Nutrition Board. *Recommended Dietary Allowances*. 10th ed. Washington, DC: National Academy Press, 1989.

Netzer, Corinne T. *The Complete Book of Food Counts*. New York: Dell Publishing Company, 2000.

PERIODICALS

Baranoski, Cynthia L. N., and Sondra L. King. "Insurance companies are reimbursing for medical nutrition therapy." *Journal of the American Dietetic Association* 100, no. 12 (December 2000): 1530-1532.

"Cost-effectiveness of medical nutrition therapy—Position of ADA." *Journal of the American Dietetic Association* 95, no. 1 (January 1995): 88-91.

Dixon, L. B. and N. D. Ernst. "Choose a diet that is low in saturated fat and cholesterol and moderate in total fat: Subtle changes to a familiar message." *Journal of Nutrition* 131(February 2001; 2S-1): 510S-526S.

Kant, A. K. "Consumption of energy-dense, nutrient-poor foods by adult Americans: Nutritional and health implications. The third National Health and Nutrition Examination Survey, 1988-1994." *American Journal of Clinical Nutrition* 72, no. 4 (October 2000): 929-936.

Larson, Eric. "MNT: An innovative employee-friendly benefit that saves." *Journal of the American Dietetic Association* 101, no. 1 (January 2001): 24-26.

ORGANIZATIONS

American Dietetic Association. 216 W. Jackson Blvd. Chicago, IL 60606-6995. (312) 899-0040. <http://www.eatright.org>.

Food and Nutrition Information Center Agricultural Research Service, USDA. National Agricultural Library, Room 304, 10301 Baltimore Avenue, Beltsville, MD 20705-2351. (301) 504-5719. Fax: (301) 504-6409. <http://www.nal.usda.gov/fnic>. fnic@nal.usda.gov.

OTHER

Food and Nutrition Professionals Network. <http://nutrition.cos.com>.

Crystal Heather Kaczkowski, MSc.

Medical physics

Definition

Medical physics is the use of physics principles in the practice of medicine. It is most often used to describe physics applications related to the use of radiation in medicine—for example, the physics of diagnostic radiology, radiation oncology, and nuclear medicine. More broadly defined, medical physics may include the physics of other electromagnetic waveforms used in medical procedures such as **electrocardiography** (the study of electrical impulses in the **heart**) and **laser surgery**.

Description

Medical physics refers to the application of physics in medical diagnosis and treatment. The bulk of medical physics is encompassed by four subfields: diagnostic radiological physics, therapeutic radiological physics, medical nuclear physics, and medical health physics.

Diagnostic radiological physics

Diagnostic radiological physics is the branch of physics associated with diagnostic procedures that use x-rays, gamma rays, ultrasound, radio frequency radiation, and magnetic sources (**magnetic resonance imaging**). In this subfield, physicists advise on the protocols and technology used for the creation of images that are generated by these diagnostic methods. Responsibilities of the medical physicist include establishing, monitoring, and evaluating procedures related to equipment use; reporting to regulatory agencies on compliance matters; evaluating and monitoring equipment; and acting as consultant on matters related to instrumentation, equipment, and use of these radiological imaging systems.

Therapeutic radiological physics

Therapeutic radiological physics concerns itself with the physics of therapeutic procedures that use x rays, gamma rays, neutrons, charged particles, and radionuclides from sealed sources (radioactive material that is sealed permanently in a container). These therapeutic procedures are often used in the treatment of **cancer** and include external beam therapy (where ionizing radiation is directed at the cancer site) and brachytherapy (where containers with radioactive material are placed near or in the tumor). Duties of the therapeutic radiological physicist include providing consultation on matters related to appropriate radiation dose and risks to patients; managing procedures and equipment related to dose and delivery of therapeutic radiation; reporting to regulatory agencies on compliance matters; and designing, evaluating, and monitoring radiation safety program related to therapeutic radiological procedures.

Medical nuclear physics

Also known as nuclear medicine physics, medical nuclear physics is the study of physics related to medical procedures requiring the use of radionuclides (except those radionuclides from sealed sources). These procedures may be diagnostic or therapeutic, and include such procedures as single photon emission computed tomography (SPECT), **positron emission tomography (PET)**, and radioimmunotherapy (radioisotopes attached to molecules that can be targeted to cancer cells). The medical nuclear physicist acts as consultant on matters related to appropriate radionuclide dose and risks; manages procedures and equipment related to dose and delivery of radionuclide imaging equipment; reports to regulatory agencies on compliance matters; and designs, evaluates, and monitors radiation safety program related to the nuclear medicine facility.

Medical health physics

The medical health physicist specializes in issues related to radiation safety in medical procedures. There is some overlap between medical health physics and the three other subfields since the use of radiation for medical purposes always requires some safety safeguards. The medical health physicist takes part in designing and specifying the radiation shielding required to protect patients, health care workers, and the general public; conducts risk assessment of procedures and protective equipment used in radiological and nuclear medicine; acts as consultant on issues related to radiation safety in a medical context; and evaluates and monitors compliance with regulatory radiation guidelines.

Work settings

Medical physicists and medical physics technologists work in clinical settings. Most medical physicists and technologists are employed by hospitals because the equipment used for the radiation-based medical procedures is located in these advanced medical facilities.

At teaching hospitals, medical physicists may, in addition to their role as physicists, be academic faculty at affiliated medical schools and/or clinical residency programs. At larger teaching hospitals, medical physicists may be organized into a medical physics department that provides services to other clinical departments. At non-teaching hospitals, medical physicists are members of individual clinical departments and are part of the hospital staff.

Education and training

The minimum education requirements for a medical physicist are an undergraduate degree—in physics, engineering, mathematics, or a related field—and a master's degree in medical physics. Graduate training should be done in a medical physics program that is accredited by the Commission on Accreditation of Medical Physics Educational Programs, Inc. Graduate work covers the physics principles and technologies associated with the relevant medical procedures and allow for specialization in a medical physics subfield. After the master's degree program, a medical physicist must attend a clinical residency program that lasts one to two years. Medical physicists with master's degrees who have completed residency and have obtained appropriate certification typically provide consultation services in hospitals.

The requirements for a technologist working in medical physics areas are a certificate, associate's degree, or a bachelor's degree in the appropriate subfield (e.g., nuclear medicine, radiography, radiation therapy) from an accredited program.

The requirements for a technologist working in medical physics areas are a certificate, associate's degree, or a bachelor's degree in the appropriate subfield (e.g., nuclear medicine, radiography, radiation therapy) from an accredited program.

Advanced education and training

After formal education, certification in a subfield of medical physics is required for medical physicists but is voluntary for technologists. Certification for United States medical physicists is obtained through one of three organizations: the American Board of Medical Physics, the American Board of Radiology, and the American Board of Science in Nuclear Medicine. Certification to become a qualified medical physicist through the American Board of Medical Physics consists of completing three steps. Part one of the process requires having obtained a graduate degree in physics, medical physics, or other relevant field, and having passed a written exam in general medical physics. The second part requires passing the first part and having finished a clinical residency program, as well as having passed a written exam in a medical physics subfield. The third part requires having passed the first and second parts, having practiced independently as a medical physicist for a specified number of years, and having passed an oral exam in a medical physics subfield.

If a medical physicist wishes to pursue an academic career of teaching and research, a master's degree is generally not sufficient; he or she will need to have completed a PhD program in medical physics to be seriously considered for academic positions. Other requirements for an academic career include a post-doctoral fellowship of one to two years, certification as described above, and licensure if required by the state.

For technologists working in the areas related to medical physics, certification is voluntary and can be obtained through the American Registry of Radiologic Technologists or, if the specialty is nuclear medicine, the **Nuclear Medicine Technology** Certification Board. Certification may be obtained solely through finishing a specified medical technology program, or through a combination of formal education, clinical experience, and additional Board coursework. Some states also require licensure of their medical technologists.

Future outlook

The demand for medical physicists is expected to grow at a rate of 7% per year, which is about the average rate of job growth. The specialty of radiation therapy is expected to be the source of most new jobs, but developments in nuclear medicine and diagnostic techniques may provide a boost to labor demand in these fields. The average salary of a medical physicist (master's and PhD degree holders combined) in 2000–2001 is estimated to be $57,060.

The demand for nuclear medicine technologists and radiologic technologists is expected to also grow at the same rate as the average rate for all jobs. There is a shift towards the merging of nuclear medicine and radiology departments, so that demand will be greatest for those technologists who have both nuclear medicine and radiologic skills. In 1998, the average salary of a nuclear medicine technologist was $40,000; the average salary of a radiologic technician was $33,000.

Resources

BOOKS

Bushberg, Jerrold T., et al. *Essential Physics of Medical Imaging.* 2nd ed. Philadelphia: Lippincott, Williams, and Wilkins, 2001.

Stanton, Robert, and Donna Stinson. *Applied Physics for Radiation Oncology.* Madison, WI: Medical Physics Publishing, 1996.

ORGANIZATIONS

American Association of Physicists in Medicine. One Physics Ellipse, College Park, MD 20740. (301) 209-3350. <http://aapm.org>.

American College of Medical Physics. 11250 Roger Bacon Drive, Suite 8, Reston, VA 20190-5202. (703) 481-5001. <http://www.acmp.org>.

American Registry of Radiologic Technologists. 1255 Northland Drive, St. Paul, MN 55120-1155. (651) 687-0048. <http://www.arrt.org>.

Genevieve Pham-Kanter

Medical records

Definition

Medical records are physical collections of patient-related materials that include written notes and materials, graphs, test results, x rays, and other data.

Purpose

Medical records have different purposes for the health care practitioner and the patient. The practitioner maintains records to document individual contacts with the patient, to monitor the individual patient's health status, to comply with legal requirements, and to monitor the practitioner's own professional behaviors.

The patient uses his or her medical record to provide information to various health care providers and to maintain a knowledge of his or her own health care.

Description

Medical records are created and maintained by health care professionals to supply medical practitioners with a sequential history of a patient's medical care and conditions affecting it. An individual's medical record is the collection of information that pertains solely to that person. It contains the information health care practitioners need to evaluate and treat the patient's health care needs. The record provides the patient's history of health care, past illnesses, test results, and other specific data.

Individual medical records are confidential, except in cases where disclosure of its contents are required by law. Information contained in a patient's medical record cannot be released without the patient's written consent.

KEY TERMS

Apprenticeship—Training a person who is new to the particular work being done, can also be on-the-job training.

Confidential—In medicine, implies a mutual trust between the patient and health care practitioner.

Medical history—Information about the patient's past medical services, procedures, illnesses, and needs.

Practitioner—Someone who engages in the science of medicine.

Social history—Information about the patient's past social needs and services utilized.

Operation

Medical records are created by health care professionals and are an aid in the care of their patients. Specific information regarding a patient is contained in the records. Contents of medical records include health care professionals' notes about the patient, medical and social histories, physicians' assessments, x ray reports, the results of tests, and other materials specific to the treatment of the patient. Materials may be provided to other health care professionals or hospitals only with the patient's written consent.

Maintenance

Medical records are maintained by physicians, physician assistants, nurses, and medical records clerks. Only authorized personnel can make entries in the record.

Health care team roles

Health care professionals are required to keep accurate records. Information is recorded every time the patient is seen by a health care practitioner. Findings of each practitioner who treats the patient records are recorded in the appropriate section of the record.

Training

Health care practitioners receive training in keeping accurate medical records in several different ways, including:

- training during medical or nursing school
- classes at a vocational or business school

- apprenticeship or on-the-job training

Resources

BOOKS

Clayton, Paul D. M.D. *For the Record: Protecting Electronic Health Information.* Washington, DC: National Academy Press, 2000.

PERIODICALS

Applebaum, Paul S., M.D. "Threats to the Confidentiality of Medical Records-No Place to Hide." *Journal of the AMA* 283, no. 6 (February 9, 2000).

ORGANIZATIONS

U.S. House of Representatives Committee on Commerce. Washington, DC (202) 225-5735. <http://com-notes.house.gov>.

Peggy Elaine Browning

Medical terminology

Definition

Medical terminology is a system of words that are used to describe specific medical aspects and diseases. It is based on standard root words, prefixes, and suffixes.

Description

Medical terminology has evolved in great measure from the Latin and Greek languages. During the Renaissance period, the science of anatomy was begun. Many early anatomists were faculty members in Italian schools of medicine. These early anatomists assigned Latin names to structures that they discovered. This tradition has continued. For this reason, Latin accounts for the majority of root words in the English language.

Some names for conditions were retained from the teachings of Galen (A.D. 130–200), a Greek physician who wrote texts on medicine in the later part of his life. These remained influential for almost 1,500 years. Many of the disease and condition names first used by Galen have been retained. This accounts for the fact that the second most common source of medical root words is the Greek language.

Other older roots have their origins in Arabic. This is due to the fact that Arabic scholars were important teachers of medicine through the middle ages. Some modern roots are taken from the English language. This reflects the pre-eminence of the English language in medicine and biomedical sciences for the past half century.

The Latin language adds suffixes to nouns to denote different syntax constructions. Since suffixes were commonly used by Italian scientists, their use in medical settings were also retained. Some prefixes are adaptations of Latin words. In medical descriptions and terminology, they were attached to root words rather than being separate from the word that they were modifying. Prefixes are often used to indicate locations on the body or directions relative to planes or structures in the body.

Some words in modern medical terminology have been borrowed from biology. Many of these are names of genus and species of pathogens. The use of Latin for these names dates to Carl Linnaeus (1707–1778) who founded the modern system of taxonomy.

Finally, from approximately 1650 through to 1850—while the system of medical terminology currently in use was being developed—Latin was the language of educated persons. This is another reason for the inclusion of so many linguistic elements (prefixes, roots, and suffixes) from the Latin language.

An example will illustrate how the system works. Consider that task of describing the movement of a finger and its associated structures. Two sets of muscles are involved. Extensors move a structure away form the body while flexors bring the same structure back towards the body. The fingers are called digits. A problem arises with realization that there are three bones in the fingers. Structures that are nearer to the center of the body are referred to as being proximal, whole structures that are farther away are distal. A muscle that move the smallest bone in a finger towards the palm is called a flexor digiti minimus. Thus, an accurate description of a person curling the small finger is action by the flexor digiti minimus on the distal phalanx of the fourth finger. Uncurling the same finger requires action by the extensor digiti minimus on the distal phalanx. While this system may seem cumbersome, it is precise and unambiguous.

Consider another example: an adenocarcinoma of the left superior lobe of the lung. The root (carcin-) indicates tissue that is cancerous. The suffix (-oma) indicates a tumor or abnormal growth. The prefix (adeno-) pertains to a gland. Thus, there is a abnormal or cancerous growth that has its origins in a glandular cell. The remainder of the description indicates the location of the growth. The designation (left) is in reference to the person who has the growth or is being examined, not the person who is performing the examination. Superior indicates the upper of the two lobes of the left lung.

Medical terminology is also employed when describing diseases or procedures. As an example, review acute **pancreatitis** in the posterior portion of the organ. The root (pancrea-) indicates the organ of involvement,

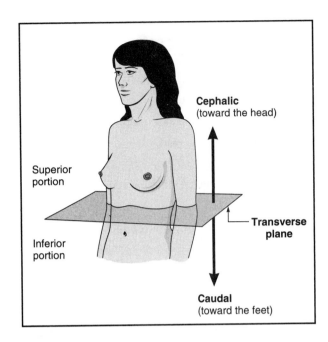

The transverse plane, also known as the horizontal plane, divides the body into superior (upper) and inferior (lower) portions. This division can be at the waist or any other level across the body. *(Delmar Publishers, Inc. Reproduced by permission.)*

the **pancreas**. The suffix (-itis) indicates an inflammation. Acute denotes a rapid onset, as contrasted to chronic which is of long duration. Posterior refers to the portion of the pancreas that is to the rear of the body. This portion of the organ is also called the head of the pancreas. This illustrates another important aspect of medical terminology, that there is frequently more than one way to accurately describe a location or structure.

An example of a procedure is a choledocholithotomy. This is a surgical operation to remove (-otomy) a stone (-litho-) that originated in the gall bladder (chole-) but is currently located in the common bile duct (-docho-). An hysterosalpingogram is an x-ray image (-gram) of the uterus (hystero-) and Fallopian tubes (-salpingo-).

The rules for combining prefixes, roots, and suffixes are generally based on Latin. In the Latin language, nouns have five different cases and can be singular or plural. Different endings indicate the form and meaning of the word. To make things more confusing for individuals who have not studied Latin, there may also be different forms of a word. The nominative singular form of the word for Fallopian tube is salpinx. The combining root is salpingo-. There are examples of combining forms in English. The plural of index is indices, the plural of apex is apices. As in Latin, English has different forms. Indexes is an acceptable plural form. The rules for words

KEY TERMS

Ab-—Prefix meaning away from.

Ad-—Prefix meaning to or toward.

Caudal—Toward the tail or rump.

Cranial—Toward the head.

Distal—Toward the periphery of the body.

-itis—Suffix meaning inflammation of.

Myo-—Root word meaning muscle.

Ophthalmo-—A root meaning eye.

-osis—Suffix meaning an increase when referring to a pathogenic condition.

Proximal—Toward the center of the body.

that come from Greek are quite similar although the endings may vary.

Viewpoints

One of the keys to medical terminology is learning a list of common prefixes, root words, and suffixes. Once that task is accomplished, constructing and understanding previously unseen words becomes possible. The system does not eliminate a medical dictionary but it does facilitate learning and communication.

In many respects, medical terms form a language that must be memorized and mastered. A second key to acquiring proficiency in medical terminology is practice with applications. This task is not fundamentally different than developing skill in a sport or learning to play a musical instrument.

Early anatomists and modern surgeons both share a need for precision in description. The system of medical terminology currently in use provides such details. Taken together, the system of prefixes and suffixes provides great precision and specificity.

Professional implications

A working knowledge of medical terminology is an absolute necessity for success in any of the medical sciences. It is highly useful for individuals who interact with medical professionals. Although knowledge of classical Latin or Greek is no longer the prerequisite for medical training as it was 50 years ago, knowledge of Latin eases the burden of learning much modern medical terminology.

Resources

BOOKS

Anderson, Kenneth N. *Mosby's Medical, Nursing, & Allied Health Dictionary.* 6th ed. St. Louis: Mosby Yearbook, 2001.

Austrin, Miriam G., and Harvey R. Austrin. *Learning Medical Terminology.* St. Louis: Mosby-Yearbook, 2000.

Birmingham, J. J. *Medical Terminology: A Self-Learning Text.* St. Louis: Mosby-Yearbook, 2000.

Brooks, Myrna L. *Exploring Medical Language.* 4th ed. St. Louis: Mosby, 2001.

Chabner, Davi-Ellen. *Medical Terminology.* Philadelphia: Saunders, 2000.

Ehrlich, Ann, and Carol L. Schroeder. *Medical Terminology for Health Professions.* 4th ed. Albany, NY: Delmar, 2000.

Miosio, Marie A. *Medical Terminology: A Student-Centered Approach.* Albany, NY: Delmar, 2001.

Venes, Donald, Clayton L. Thomas, and Clarence Wilbur Taber. *Tabers Cyclopedic Medical Dictionary.* 19th ed. Philadelphia: F. A. Davis Co, 2001.

PERIODICALS

Angelillo, V. A. "'Wet' Label Can Be Dangerously Misleading." *Postgraduate Medicine* 109, no. 5 (2001): 23-24.

Beeler Jr., G. W. "The Crucial Role of Standards. *Healthcare Informatics* 18, no. 2 (2001): 98-104.

Cimino, J. J., V. L. Patel, and A. W. Kushniruk. "Studying the Human-Computer-Terminology Interface." *Journal of the American Medical Informatics Association* 8, no. 2 (2001): 163-173.

Elfrink, V., et al. "Standardized Nursing Vocabularies: A Foundation for Quality Care." *Seminars in Oncology Nursing* 17, no. 1 (2001): 18-23.

Gordon, B. M. "Medical Errors: Creating the Tension for Change." *American Journal of Health System Pharmacy* 58, no. 10 (2001): 908-912.

Mareckova, E., F. Simon, and L. Cerveny. *Annals of Anatomy* 183, no. 3 (2001): 201-207.

Reid, C., and L. Chan. "Emergency Medicine Terminology in the United Kingdom—Time to Follow the Trend?" *Emergency Medicine Journal* 18, no. 2 (2001): 79-80.

Rosse, C. "Terminologia Anatomica: Considered from the Perspective of Next-Generation Knowledge Sources." *Clinical Anatomy* 14, no. 2 (2001): 120-133.

Rubin, G. "Medical Errors. Terminology of 'Error' is Important." *British Medical Journal* 322, no. 7299 (2001): 1422.

Sharp, D. "Resuscitating Dead Languages." *Lancet* 357, no. 9265 (2001): 1310-1312.

ORGANIZATIONS

American Academy of Family Physicians. 11400 Tomahawk Creek Parkway, Leawood, KS 66211-2672. (913) 906-6000. <http://www.aafp.org>.

American Medical Informatics Association. 4915 St. Elmo Avenue, Suite 401, Bethesda, MD 20814. (301) 657-1291. <http://www.amia.org>.

College of American Pathologists. 325 Waukegan Road, Northfield, IL 60093. (800) 323-4040. <http://www.cap.org>.

OTHER

British Medical Informatics Society. <http://www.bmis.org>.

English Centre. <http://ec.hku.hk/mt/>.

International Medical Informatics Association. <http://www.imia.org>.

University of Minnesota. <http://www.gen.umn.edu/faculty_staff/jensen/1135/med_term_activites/default.html>.

L. Fleming Fallon, Jr., MD, DrPH

Medicare

Definition

Medicare is a national health insurance program created and administered by the federal government in the United States to address the medical needs of older American citizens. Medicare is available to U.S. citizens 65 years of age and older and some people with disabilities under age 65.

Description

Medicare is the largest health insurance program in the United States. The program was created as part of the Social Security Act in 1965 and was put into effect in 1966. At the end of 1966, Medicare served approximately 3.9 million individuals; today it serves about 39 million people.

In 1973, the Medicare program was expanded to include people who have permanent kidney failure and need dialysis or transplants and people under the age of 65 who have specific types of disabilities. Medicare was originally administered by the Social Security Administration, but in 1977, the program was transferred to the Health Care Financing Administration (HCFA), which is a part of the United States Department of Health and Human Services (DHHS). HCFA also administers **Medicaid** and the State Children's Heath Insurance Program.

Medicare is an entitlement program similar to Social Security and is not based on financial need. Medicare benefits are available to all American citizens over the age of 65 because they or their spouses have paid Social Security taxes through their working years. Since Medicare is a federal program, the rules for eligibility remain constant throughout the nation and coverage remains constant regardless of where the person receives treatment in the United States.

Medicare benefits are divided into two different types referred to as Part A or B. Medicare Part A is hospital insurance and it provides basic coverage for hospital stays and post-hospital nursing facilities, home health care, and hospice care for terminally ill patients. Most people automatically receive Part A when they turn 65 and do not have to pay a premium because they or their spouse paid Medicare taxes while they were working.

Medicare Part B is medical insurance. It covers most fees associated with basic doctor visits and laboratory testing. It also pays for some outpatient medical services such as medical equipment, supplies, and home health care and **physical therapy**. However, these services and supplies are only covered by Part B when medically necessary and prescribed by a doctor. Enrollment in Part B is optional and the Medicare recipient pays a premium of approximately $50 per month for these added benefits. Not every person who receives Medicare Part A enrolls in Part B.

Although Medicare provides fairly broad coverage of medical treatment, neither Part A or B pays for the cost of prescription drugs or other medications.

Medicare is funded solely by the federal government. States do not make matching contributions to the Medicare fund. Social Security contributions, monthly premiums paid by program participants, and general government revenues generate the money used to support the Medicare program. Insurance coverage provided by Medicare is similar to that provided by private health insurance. Medicare usually pays 50–80% of the medical bill, while the recipient pays the remaining balance for services provided.

Viewpoints

As the population of the United States ages, concerns about health care and the financing of quality health care for all members of the elderly population grow. One concern is that health insurance provided by the Medicare program will become obsolete or will be cut from the federal budget in an attempt to save money. Another concern is that money provided by the Social Security Administration for Medicare will be depleted before the aging population of the United States can actually benefit from the taxes they are now paying.

KEY TERMS

DHHS—Department of Health and Human Service. The federal agency that distributes funds for Medicare.

HCFA—Health Care Financing Administration. The federal agency that provides guidelines for the Medicare program.

Medicare Part A—Hospital insurance provided by Medicare, provided free to persons aged 65 and older.

Medicare Part B—Medical insurance provided by Medicare that requires recipients pay a monthly premium. Part B pays for some medical services Part A does not.

Professional implications

During the Clinton administration, several initiatives were started that saved funds for Medicare. The DHHS also supports several initiatives to save and improve the program. However, continuance of the federal health insurance program is still a problem U.S citizens expect legislation to resolve.

Some of the successful initiatives include:

• Fighting fraud and abuse: A great amount of attention has focused on Medicare abuse, fraud, and waste. As a result, over-payments were stopped, fraud was decreased, and abuse was investigated. This saved the Medicare program $500 million in just one year.

• Preserving the Medicare benefit: Due to aggressive action by the HCFA and the Balanced Budget Act, it is estimated that funds have been appropriated to keep Medicare viable through 2026.

• Prescription drug benefit proposal: Health care reformers suggest that prescription drugs be made available through the Medicare program due to the high cost of prescription medication.

• Supporting Preventive Medicine and the Healthy Aging Project: Medicare programs are supporting preventive medicine and diagnostic treatments in anticipation that preventive measures will improve the health of older Americans and thereby reduce health care costs.

Medicare benefits and health care financing are major issues in the United States. Legislators and federal agencies continue to work on initiatives that will keep health care programs in place and working for the good of American citizens.

Resources

ORGANIZATIONS

Health Care Financing Administration. United States Department of Health and Human Services. 200 Independence Avenue SW, Washington, DC 20201. <http://www.hcfa.gov>.

United States Department of Health and Human Services. 200 Independence Avenue SW, Washington, DC 20201. <http://www.hhs.gov>.

Peggy Elaine Browning

Medication administration *see*
Administering medication

Medication preparation from a vial

Definition

Medical preparation from a vial is the method of preparing a drug contained in a vial into a usable form that is safe and effective for human delivery.

Purpose

• To facilitate safe and effective delivery of medications.

• To transform the medication from solid form to fluid form where appropriate.

• To prepare and transport the medication to equipment more suitable for final delivery.

Precautions

There are several precautions that health care providers need to keep in mind when preparing medications. These precautions protect both the practitioner and the patient. Risks most common to the health care provider include needlestick injuries from the equipment used to prepare the medication and the risk of splashing harmful drugs onto the skin, eyes and other mucous membranes, by which the body may uptake all or part of the drug. These are generally caused by incorrect methods of medication preparation. Failure to maintain sterility and contamination of the medication are the largest possible risks for the patient during this procedure. Strict adherence to guidelines set out by the health institution as well as those guidelines recommended for preparing particular medications provided by the manufacturers are vital to ensure safe preparation of any medication.

Description

Nearly all medications used for injections are distributed by manufacturers in sterile containers called vials. Some medications in these vials are in liquid form, whereas others are in solid form. Those in solid form usually break down readily in liquid form, losing their effectiveness. The solid (often powder) medication is then prepared by the health care provider shortly before use. Liquid medications are usually stable at room temperature and retain their quality. Many do not require further preparation or dilution to use, depending of course, on the route of administration chosen. It is considered safe practice to first read the manufacturer's documentation before preparing any drug for the first time or in cases where there is difference of opinion between health care providers in how the medication should be prepared from the vial. Workplace policy for delivery of particular drugs should also consult, as these can vary from institution to institution.

Preparation

Preparation of solid/powder medication from a vial:

- Check the medication order to ensure the right drug, the right dosage, the right medication chart for your patient, the correct time, the correct date, and the correct route of administration.

- Ensure familiarity with the correct dilution or mixing fluid to be used for the drug, for example, sterile water or normal saline.

- Gather the items to be used to prepare the medication from the vial. Usually for basic drug delivery, this requires a syringe, needle, dilution fluid, an alcohol swab, and the medication vial.

- Remove the protective cover from the vial and rub the penetrable surface with an alcohol swab. (This procedure is not standard at all institutions.)

- Wash the hands and don protective clothing (gloves, gowns, face mask, etc.) if you are drawing up hazardous drugs such as those used in chemotherapy.

- Maintain an **aseptic technique** throughout the preparation. While gloves are not always necessary, do not touch any parts of the equipment that deliver the medication directly to the patient.

- Draw up the dilution fluid into the syringe.

- Attach a needle to the same syringe (if not attached already) and insert directly into the vial.

- Inject all or a portion of the dilution fluid (depending on the manufacturer's recommendations) into the vial. Do not withdraw the syringe or needle from the vial.

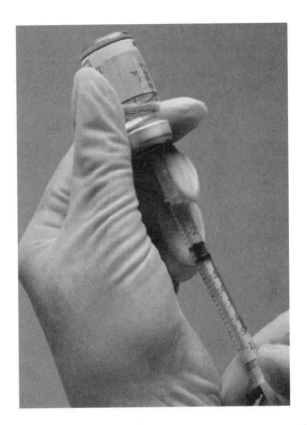

Gloved hands should be used to take medication from a vial into a syringe. *(Delmar Publishers, Inc. Reproduced by permission.)*

- While holding the vial, **syringe and needle** (still inserted into the vial) in one hand, shake the vial vigorously to allow the dilution fluid and solid form medication to mix. Keep shaking the vial vigorously until all solid elements of the medication have been fully dissolved.

- Withdraw the contents of the vial back into the syringe. Remove all the fluid content of the vial to ensure the patient receives the full dose.

- Remove the needle and syringe from the vial.

- Remove the needle used for preparing your medication and attach a new sterile needle for delivery of the drug.

- Check the drug vial and medication order again for the correct drug and dosage requirements. The prepared medication should then be verified by a second health care provider (if required by the institution) for accuracy.

- Dispose of the used needle and vial safely and according to institution policy. Your prepared medication should now be safe for patient delivery.

Aftercare

It is essential to correctly dispose of items used during medication preparation. Needles should be disposed of in needles or sharps containers, and vials should be disposed of in the appropriate manner. If hazardous chemicals are spilled, these should be cleaned according to protocol before any other staff member enters the area.

Complications

Needlestick injuries and splashing of medication onto the health care provider are common risks. Complications for the patient may arise if the medication was contaminated through improper preparation on behalf of the health care provider.

Results

Correct methods result in a medication successfully prepared for safe and effective delivery.

Health care team roles

Medication may be prescribed by a physician or advanced practice nurse. Medication may be prepared from the vial by a variety of health care professionals, including doctors, nurses, and emergency medical personnel. Medication preparation usually takes place in a professional health care environment, such as a hospital, clinic, or physician's office.

Resources

BOOKS

Elkin, M. K., A. G. Perry and P. A. Potter. *Nursing Interventions and Clinical Skills.* St. Louis: Mosby-Year Book, Inc., 1996.

Kozier, B., G. Erb, K. Blais, et al. *Techniques in Clinical Nursing.* Canada: Addison-Wesley Nursing, 1993.

Dean Andrew Bielanowski, R.N.

Meditation

Definition

Meditation is a practice of concentrated focus upon a sound, object, visualization, the breath, movement, or attention itself in order to increase awareness of the present moment, reduce **stress**, promote **relaxation**, and enhance personal and spiritual growth.

Origins

Meditation techniques have been practiced for millennia. Originally, they were intended to develop spiritual understanding, awareness, and direct experience of ultimate reality. The many different religious traditions in the world have given rise to a rich variety of meditative practices. These include the contemplative practices of Christian religious orders, the Buddhist practice of sitting meditation, and the whirling movements of the Sufi dervishes. Although meditation is an important spiritual practice in many religious and spiritual traditions, it can be practiced by anyone regardless of their religious or cultural background to relieve stress and **pain**.

As Western medical practitioners begin to understand the mind's role in health and disease, there has been more interest in the use of meditation in medicine. Meditative practices are increasingly offered in medical clinics and hospitals as a tool for improving health and quality of life. Meditation has been used as the primary therapy for treating certain diseases; as an additional therapy in a comprehensive treatment plan; and as a means of improving the quality of life of people with debilitating, chronic, or terminal illnesses.

Benefits

Meditation benefits people with or without acute medical illness or stress. People who meditate regularly have been shown to feel less **anxiety** and depression. They also report that they experience more enjoyment and appreciation of life and that their relationships with others are improved. Meditation produces a state of deep relaxation and a sense of balance or equanimity. According to Michael J. Baime, "Meditation cultivates an emotional stability that allows the meditator to experience intense emotions fully while simultaneously maintaining perspective on them." Out of this experience of emotional stability, one may gain greater insight and understanding about one's thoughts, feelings, and actions. This insight in turn offers the possibility to feel more confident and in control of life. Meditation facilitates a greater sense of calmness, empathy, and acceptance of self and others.

Meditation can be used with other forms of medical treatment and is an important complementary therapy for both the treatment and prevention of many stress-related conditions. Regular meditation can reduce the number of symptoms experienced by patients with a wide range of illnesses and disorders. Based upon clinical evidence as well as theoretical understanding, meditation is considered to be one of the better therapies for panic disorder, generalized anxiety disorder, substance dependence and abuse, ulcers, colitis, chronic pain, psoriasis, and dysthymic disorder. It is considered to be a valuable adjunctive therapy for moderate **hypertension** (high **blood pressure**), prevention of cardiac arrest (**heart** attack), prevention of atherosclerosis (hardening of arteries), arthritis (including **fibromyalgia**), **cancer**, insomnia, migraine, and prevention of stroke. Meditation may also be a valuable complementary therapy for **allergies** and **asthma** because of the role stress plays in these conditions. Meditative practices have been reported to improve function or reduce symptoms in patients with some neurological disorders as well. These include people with **Parkinson's disease**, people who experience fatigue with **multiple sclerosis**, and people with epilepsy who are resistant to standard treatment.

Overall, a 1995 report to the National Institutes of Health on alternative medicine concluded that, "More than 30 years of research, as well as the experience of a large and growing number of individuals and health care providers, suggests that meditation and similar forms of relaxation can lead to better health, higher quality of life, and lowered health care costs..."

Description

Sitting meditation is generally done in an upright seated position, either in a chair or cross-legged on a cushion on the floor. The spine is straight yet relaxed. Sometimes the eyes are closed. Other times the eyes are open and gazing softly into the distance or at an object. Depending on the type of meditation, the meditator may be concentrating on the sensation of the movement of the breath, counting the breath, silently repeating a sound, chanting, visualizing an image, focusing awareness on the center of the body, opening to all sensory experiences including thoughts, or performing stylized ritual movements with the hands.

Movement meditation can be spontaneous and freeform or involve highly structured, choreographed, repetitive patterns. Movement meditation is particularly helpful for those people who find it difficult to remain still.

Generally speaking, there are two main types of meditation. These types are concentration meditation and mindfulness meditation. Concentration meditation practices involve focusing attention on a single object. Objects of meditation can include the breath, an inner or external image, a movement pattern (as in tai chi or **yoga**), or a sound, word, or phrase that is repeated silently (mantra). The purpose of concentrative practices is to learn to focus one's attention or develop concentration. When thoughts or emotions arise, the meditator gently directs the mind back to the original object of concentration.

Mindfulness meditation practices involve becoming aware of the entire field of attention. The meditator is instructed to be aware of all thoughts, feelings, perceptions or sensations as they arise in each moment. Mindfulness meditation practices are enhanced by the meditator's ability to focus and quiet the mind. Many meditation practices are a blend of these two forms.

The study and application of meditation to health care has focused on three specific approaches: transcendental meditation (TM); the "relaxation response," a general approach to meditation developed by Dr. Herbert Benson; and mindfulness meditation, specifically the program of mindfulness-based stress reduction (MBSR) developed by Jon Kabat-Zinn.

Transcendental meditation

TM has its origins in the Vedic tradition of India and was introduced to the West by Maharishi Mahesh Yogi. TM has been taught to somewhere between two and four million people. It is one of the most widely practiced forms of meditation in the West. TM has been studied many times; these studies have produced much of the information about the physiology of meditation. In TM, the meditator sits with closed eyes and concentrates on a single syllable or word (mantra) for 20 minutes at a time, twice a day. When thoughts or feelings arise, the attention is brought back to the mantra. According to Charles Alexander, an important TM researcher, "During TM, ordinary waking mental activity is said to settle down, until even the subtlest thought is transcended and a completely unified wholeness of awareness...is experienced. In this silent, self-referential state of pure wakefulness, consciousness is fully awake to itself alone..." TM supporters believe that TM practices are more beneficial than other meditation practices.

The relaxation response

The relaxation response involves a similar form of mental focusing. Dr. Herbert Benson, one of the first Western doctors to conduct research on the effects of meditation, developed this approach after observing the profound health benefits of a state of bodily calm he calls "the relaxation response." In order to elicit this response in the body, he teaches patients to focus upon the repetition of a word, sound, prayer, phrase, or movement activity (including swimming, jogging, yoga, and even knitting) for 10–20 minutes at a time, twice a day. Patients are also taught not to pay attention to distracting thoughts and to return their focus to the original repetition. The choice of the focused repetition is up to the individual. Instead of Sanskrit terms, the meditator can choose what

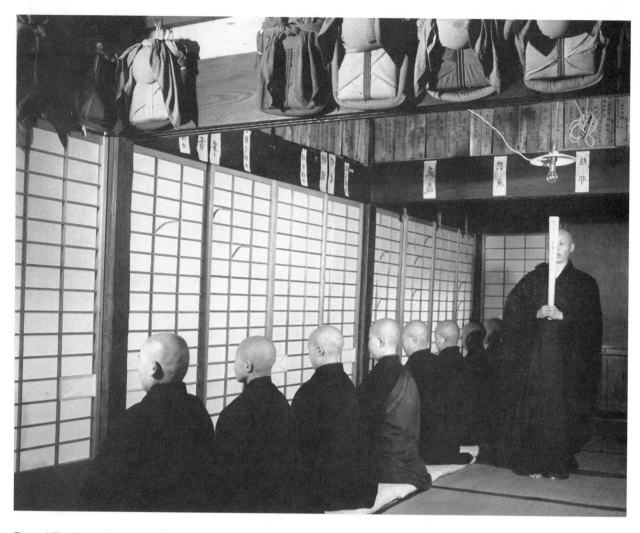

Row of Zen Buddhist nuns with shaved heads and dark robes.. *(Horace Bristol/Corbis. Reproduced by permission.)*

is personally meaningful, such as a phrase from a Christian or Jewish prayer.

Mindfulness meditation

Mindfulness meditation comes out of traditional Buddhist meditation practices. Psychologist Jon Kabat-Zinn has been instrumental in bringing this form of meditation into medical settings. In formal mindfulness practice, the meditator sits with eyes closed, focusing the attention on the sensations and movement of the breath for approximately 45–60 minutes at a time, at least once a day. Informal mindfulness practice involves bringing awareness to every activity in daily life. Wandering thoughts or distracting feelings are simply noticed without resisting or reacting to them. The essence of mindfulness meditation is not what one focuses on but rather the quality of awareness the meditator brings to each moment. According to Kabat-Zinn, "It is this investiga-

tive, discerning observation of whatever comes up in the present moment that is the hallmark of mindfulness and differentiates it most from other forms of meditation. The goal of mindfulness is for you to be more aware, more in touch with life and whatever is happening in your own body and mind at the time it is happening—that is, the present moment." The MBSR program consists of a series of classes involving meditation, movement, and group process. There are over 240 MBSR programs offered in health care settings around the world.

Meditation is not considered a medical procedure or intervention by most insurers. Many patients pay for meditation training themselves. Frequently, religious groups or meditation centers offer meditation instruction free of charge or for a nominal donation. Hospitals may offer MBSR classes at a reduced rate for their patients and a slightly higher rate for the general public.

Precautions

Meditation appears to be safe for most people. There are, however, case reports and studies noting some adverse effects. Thirty-three to 50% of the people participating in long silent meditation retreats (two weeks to three months) reported increased tension, anxiety, confusion, and depression. On the other hand, most of these same people also reported very positive effects from their meditation practice. Kabat-Zinn notes that these studies fail to differentiate between serious psychiatric disturbances and normal emotional mood swings. These studies do suggest, however, that meditation may not be recommended for people with psychotic disorders, severe depression, and other severe **personality disorders** unless they are also receiving psychological or medical treatment.

Side effects

There are no reported side effects from meditation except for positive benefits.

Research and general acceptance

The scientific study of the physiological effects of meditation began in the early 1960s. These studies prove that meditation affects **metabolism**, the **endocrine system**, the **central nervous system**, and the **autonomic nervous system**. In one study, three advanced practitioners of Tibetan Buddhist meditation practices demonstrated the ability to increase "inner heat" as much as 61%. During a different meditative practice they were able to dramatically slow down the rate at which their bodies consumed oxygen. Preliminary research shows that mindfulness meditation is associated with increased levels of melatonin. These findings suggest a potential role for meditation in the treatment and prevention of breast and prostrate cancer.

Despite the inherent difficulties in designing research studies, there is a large amount of evidence of the medical benefits of meditation. Meditation is particularly effective as a treatment for chronic pain. Studies have shown meditation reduces symptoms of pain and pain-related drug use. In a four-year follow-up study, the majority of patients in a MBSR program reported "moderate to great improvement" in pain as a result of participation in the program.

Meditation has long been recommended as a treatment for high **blood** pressure; however, there is a debate over the amount of benefit that meditation offers. Although most studies show a reduction in blood pressure with meditation, medication is still more effective at lowering high blood pressure.

Meditation may also be an effective treatment for **coronary artery disease**. A study of 21 patients practicing TM for eight months showed increases in their amount of **exercise** tolerance, amount of workload, and a delay in the onset of ST-segment depression. Meditation is also an important part of Dean Ornish's program, which has been proven to reverse coronary artery disease.

Research also suggests that meditation is effective in the treatment of chemical dependency. Gelderloos and others reviewed 24 studies and reported that all of them showed that TM is helpful in programs to stop smoking and also in programs for drug and alcohol abuse.

Studies also imply that meditation is helpful in reducing symptoms of anxiety and in treating anxiety-related disorders. Furthermore, a study in 1998 of 37 psoriasis patients showed that those practicing mindfulness meditation had more rapid clearing of their skin condition, with standard UV light treatment, than the control subjects. Another study found that meditation decreased the symptoms of fibromyalgia; over half of the patients reported significant improvement. Meditation was one of several stress management techniques used in a small study of HIV-positive men. The study showed improvements in the T-cell counts of the men, as well as in several psychological measures of well-being.

Training and certification

There is no program of certification or licensure for instructors who wish to teach meditation as a medical therapy. Meditation teachers within a particular religious tradition usually have extensive experience and expertise with faith questions and religious practices but may not have been trained to work with medical patients. Different programs have varied requirements for someone to teach meditation. In order to be recognized as an instructor of TM, one must receive extensive training. The Center for Mindfulness in Medicine, Health Care and Society at the University of Massachusetts Medical Center offers training and workshops for health professionals and others interested in teaching mindfulness-based stress reduction. The Center does not, however, certify that someone is qualified to teach meditation. The University of Pennsylvania program for Stress Management suggests that a person have at least ten years of personal experience with the practice of mindfulness meditation before receiving additional instruction to teach meditation. Teachers are also expected to spend at least two weeks each year in intensive meditation retreats.

Resources

BOOKS

Astin, John A., et al. "Meditation." In *Clinician's Complete Reference to Complementary and Alternative Medicine.* Edited by Donald Novey. St. Louis: Mosby, 2000.

Baime, Michael J. "Meditation and Mindfulness." In *Essentials of Complementary and Alternative Medicine*, ed. Wayne B. Jonas and Jeffrey S. Levin. New York: Lippencott, Williams and Wilkins, 1999.

Benson, Herbert, M.D. *The Relaxation Response.* New York: William Morrow, 1975.

Kabat-Zinn, John. *Full Catastrophe Living: Using the Wisdom of Your Body and Mind to Face Stress, Pain, and Illness.* New York: Dell, 1990.

Roth, Robert. *TM Transcendental Meditation: A New Introduction to Maharishi's Easy, Effective and Scientifically Proven Technique for Promoting Better Health.* Donald I Fine, 1994.

ORGANIZATIONS

The Center for Mindfulness in Medicine, Health Care and Society. Stress Reduction Clinic. University of Massachusetts Memorial Health Care. 55 Lake Avenue North, Worcester, MA 01655. (508) 856-2656. Fax (508) 856-1977. jon.kabat-zinn@banyan@ummed.edu. <http://www.mbst.com>.

Insight Meditation Society. 1230 Pleasant, St. Barre, MA 01005. (978) 355-4378. FAX: (978) 355-6398. <http://www.dharma.org>.

Mind-Body Medical Institute. Beth Israel Deaconess Medical Center. One Deaconess Road, Boston, MA 02215. (617) 632-9525. <http://www.mindbody.harvard.edu.>.

OTHER

Videos are available from the organizations listed above.

Linda Chrisman

Meiosis *see* **Cell division**

Melanoma *see* **Malignant melanoma**

Membranes *see* **Cell membranes**

▌Memory

Definition

Memory is the ability to recall information in the form of past events, ideas, and feelings. People have different types of memories, including short-term and long-term memory, and auditory and visual memory.

Description

A brief history

The study of memory can be traced all the way back to Plato and Aristotle. Plato's metaphor for memory likened it to the impression made by a seal on wax and has been sustained throughout the history of Psychology. Aristotle's differentiation between memory and recollection closely parallels what we now refer to as short- and long-term memory. Although many other explanations of memory have been offered throughout history it would be another 1500 years before scientific methods were used in the study of memory.

The first use of the scientific method (i.e., rigorous experimental controls and statistical analyses) in the study of memory is credited to the German psychologist Hermann Ebbinghaus (1850–1909). Prior to the publication of his book *On Memory* in 1885, very little had been written about memory utilizing scientific methods and precise terminology. Ebbinghaus began by memorizing lists of unrelated words and later tested his memory for these words. He soon realized that some words were more familiar than others and were easier to recall. Consequently, he constructed lists of nonsense syllables, consisting of a consonant, a vowel, and a consonant. They are often referred to as CVCs, or trigrams (e.g., BIJ, VUN, PIB). Ebbinghaus wanted to know how much he could remember after various delay intervals, from 20 minutes to 30 days. It quickly became obvious that much of what he learned was quickly forgotten. But he also noticed that the more frequently he rehearsed (i.e., repeated) the list on day 1, the more quickly he could relearn it on day 2. He thus established a basic principle, namely that the time spent on learning affects the subsequent recall of the material. Ebbinghaus's approach has been referred to as a quantity-orientated approach. This perspective treats memory as a storehouse in which items are deposited and are later retrieved. It continues to be used to produce much of the data found in scientific journals today.

Ebbinghaus laid the foundation for the study of memory but he had little to say about the causes of forgetting. Georg Elias Muller (1850–1934) was the pioneer of what we now call the interference theory of forgetting. The interference theory, simplified, suggests that forgetting is not a consequence of material dying away but rather is due to other memories interfering at the time of retrieval. Two types of interference are retroactive interference and proactive interference. Retroactive interference refers to recently learned material interfering with the ability to remember previously stored information. Proactive interference refers to just the opposite phenomenon, when previously learned material interferes with the remembering of similar newly learned material.

Decay theory refers to the notion that the passage of time will cause memory traces to erode if they are not accessed from time to time. Generally speaking the longer the interval between learning and recall the less information will be recalled. The decay theory more effectively accounts for forgetting in the short term (e.g., remembering a phone number), whereas interference theory better accounts for long term forgetting.

The three-box model of memory

There are several existing models of memory but we will focus our attention on the three-box model because it is effective in organizing and accounting for many of the major research findings, and is the most widely used model you will encounter.

The three-box approach was originally termed the separate storage model by its developers, Atkinson and Shiffrin, in 1971. They proposed three separate but interacting systems that are used to gather, store, maintain, and retrieve information. The three systems are: sensory memory which acquires and holds incoming information for a second or two; short-term memory (STM) which holds information for approximately 30 seconds, unless an effort is made to keep it there longer; and long-term memory (LTM) which can hold information from a few minutes to decades.

Information from the environment enters the sensory memory store and remains there for half a second for visual stimuli and approximately two seconds for auditory stimuli. We also receive information from our sense of **smell** and from our sense of touch. These are referred to respectively as olfactory memory and tactile memory. Research in these latter two areas is relatively limited. The sensory memory store has been studied most extensively in regard to **vision** or iconic memory. A flash of lightening lasts only a fraction of a second but we can see the impression of the countryside for a moment after it occurs. This persisting impression is what is referred to as iconic sensory memory store.

We have all had the experience of performing a task while people are speaking in the background. In such situations you are not attending to the conversation but are instead focussed on the task at hand. Now suppose you hear your own name come up in the ongoing conversation. You suddenly become aware of it. This is an example of auditory sensory memory. Obviously, some portion of the speech stream is being stored in memory, otherwise you would not be able to recognize your name when it occurs.

One important thing to remember about both visual and auditory sensory memory is that the information is maintained for, at the very most, a few seconds before it is lost forever unless you pay attention to it and place it in your short term memory. Information that has been attended to is transferred from the sensory system to the short term memory (STM) store and remains there for thirty seconds or so unless the information is rehearsed, in which case it may remain for a longer period of time. STM is sometimes referred to as working memory or immediate memory because we have easy access to its contents. We have all experienced dialing the operator to obtain a phone number. Typically, we rehearse (i.e., repeat) the number to commit it to memory, hang up the receiver, and then dial the number. Should we need to use the same number later that day we most will likely have to look it up again. This illustrates the fact that information in STM will disappear unless we make a concerted effort to maintain it. Moreover, the capacity of STM is limited. If phone numbers were any longer than seven digits, dialing errors would increase substantially. Push button phones lowered the frequency of dialing errors because the time required to maintain the phone number in memory was reduced. With the old rotary phones, we used to have to wait until the disk returned to its original position before dialing the next number. With the higher digits (0, 9, 8, etc.) this could take a couple of seconds, thus putting an extra burden on our short term memory.

If information is transferred from STM to the LTM store it's retention may last from minutes to decades and in some cases its storage is permanent. It is here, in LTM, that information is organized and indexed. You know your name, what you did last Saturday night, how to ride a bicycle, and who the president of the United States is. These are all examples of information that resides in LTM. There are three different types of information in LTM: episodic memory; procedural memory; and semantic memory.

Episodic memory refers to the memory of events or activities (e.g., summer vacation or graduation day). What these memories have in common is that they refer to specific experiences. Some episodic memories are readily recalled while others may need prompting. Generally speaking the more significant the experience the more readily it can be recalled. Some insignificant events may need considerable prompting if they are to be remembered and some may not be remembered at all.

Procedural memory contains stored physical skills and behavioral operations. For example you may have learned how to roller-blade or skateboard. You have learned how to write a letter or an essay. Procedural memories are "how-to" memories. These memories are readily available even after years of disuse. The expression "It's like riding a bike, you never forget" captures this sense of permanency.

Semantic memory refers to general knowledge (e.g., the capital of France; what a zebra looks like). Semantic memory involves the meaning of words and objects. For example, most people know what an igloo is, but not as a result of having built one or being inside one.

WHAT GETS STORED AND WHAT GETS LOST? If we stop to consider the sheer volume of sensory input with which we are bombarded each day, it would be inconceivable that all of it passes into STM let alone LTM. What determines what gets saved and what gets lost? As mentioned earlier what we attend to in the sensory memory gets transferred to STM store. But how does this occur?

Encoding is the process by which information is added to our memory stores. Encoding changes the information we receive from our senses into a format that our brains can process and store. We do not encode into memory all that we see, hear, smell, touch, or feel. Sensory memory not only acts a holding tank from which items are selected for encoding and storage in STM, but it also acts as a filter, keeping out unimportant bits of information.

Information that is rehearsed in STM is accessible for immediate use, and can also be transferred to LTM. Other than acting as a retaining center for new information, the STM store also holds information for immediate use that has been recovered from the LTM store. It is for this reason that it is often referred to as working memory. When you spell a word the letters themselves and their appropriate arrangements enter the STM system as a result of having been retrieved from LTM.

When we make a deliberate effort to remember material we not only use rehearsal strategies, but other processes as well. Two of these processes are deep processing and mnemonics. Deep processing refers to the degree or "depth" to which we analyze or deal with the information. It can be contrasted with rote memorization, which can occur without our having any real understanding of the material. For example, it is possible (with considerable effort), to memorize passages of Latin without having any knowledge whatsoever of what the sentences mean. With deep processing however, the material to be remembered is not simply rehearsed but understood, elaborated upon, and thought about. It is its meaning that is encoded, not merely its initial form of expression. For example suppose you are trying to remember that an erythrocyte is a red **blood** cell. If you also appreciate that that the protein hemoglobin produces the red color, and the unique biconcave shape of the erythrocyte increases its surface area and thus facilitates the exchange of O_2 and CO_2 into or out of the cells of our bodies, you are using deep processing. On the other hand if you simply memorize the spelling of erythrocyte and repeat to yourself that it is a red blood cell you are using rehearsal.

To increase the chances of retrieving information from LTM, mnemonics may help. A mnemonics is a trick or device that we can use when encoding information that will help us retrieve it later on. Using our above example of erythrocytes, if you were to use the mnemonic "Red Engines Haul Oil to Boston" you could use that simple sentence to recall a fair amount of information about erythrocytes. In this example, the first letter of each word corresponds to some aspect of the to-be-remembered material (red blood cells, erythrocytes, hemoglobin, oxygen, and body) and the sentence describes what the red blood cells do—carry oxygen to the bodies cells. A good mnemonic is one that is simple, uses concrete nouns, and permits the formation of a clear visual image. If the mnemonic itself is difficult to remember, its usefulness is nullified.

Resources

BOOKS

Anderson, J. R. *Learning and memory: An integrated approach*. New York: Wiley, 1995.

Wade, C., and C. Tavris. *Psychology, Sixth ed*. New York: Addison Wesley Longham, Inc., 2000.

PERIODICALS

Koriat, A. Toward a psychology of memory accuracy." *Annual Review of Psychology* 51 (May 2001): 481-537.

Timothy E. Moore

Meningioma *see* **Brain tumor**

Meningitis

Definition

Meningitis is a potentially fatal inflammation of the meninges, the thin, membranous covering of the **brain** and the **spinal cord**. Meningitis is most commonly caused by **infection** (**bacteria**, **viruses**, or **fungi**), although it can also be caused by bleeding into the meninges, **cancer**, diseases of the **immune system**, and an inflammatory response to certain types of **chemotherapy** or other chemical agents. The most serious and difficult-to-treat types of meningitis tend to be those caused by bacteria.

Description

Meningitis is a particularly dangerous infection because of the very delicate nature of the brain. Brain cells are among a very small number of cells in the body that, once killed, will not regenerate. Therefore, if enough brain tissue is damaged, serious, life-long handicaps may remain.

To understand meningitis, it is important to have a basic understanding of the anatomy of the brain. The meninges are three separate membranes layered together that encase the brain and spinal cord:

- The dura is the toughest, outermost layer, and is closely attached to the inside of the **skull**.

- The arachnoid, the middle layer, is important because of its involvement in the normal flow of the cerebrospinal fluid (CSF), a lubricating and nutritive fluid that bathes both the brain and the spinal cord.

- The pia, the innermost layer, helps direct **blood vessels** into the brain.

The space between the arachnoid and the pia contains CSF, which helps insulate the brain from trauma. Many **blood** vessels course through this space.

CSF, produced within specialized chambers deep inside the brain, flows over the surface of the brain and spinal cord. This fluid serves to cushion these relatively delicate structures, as well as to supply important nutrients for brain cells. CSF is reabsorbed by blood vessels located within the meninges. A careful balance between CSF production and reabsorption is important to avoid the accumulation of too much CSF.

Because the brain is enclosed in the hard, bony case of the skull, any disease that produces swelling of the brain will be damaging. The skull cannot expand at all; so, when any swollen brain tissue pushes up against the skull's hard bone, brain tissue may become damaged and ultimately die. Swelling on one side of the brain will not only cause pressure and damage to that side of the brain, but, because it takes up precious space within the tight confines of the skull, the opposite side of the brain will also be pushed against the skull, causing damage to that side also.

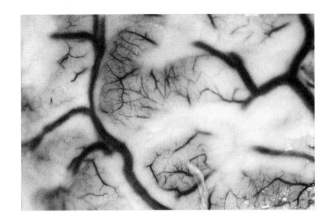
Brain tissue covered with thick white exudate from acute meningitis. *(Custom Medical Stock Photo. Reproduced by permission.)*

Another way that infections injure the brain involves the way the chemical environment of the brain changes in response to that infection. Brain cells require a very well-regulated environment. Careful balance of oxygen, carbon dioxide, sugar (glucose), sodium, **calcium**, potassium, and other substances must be maintained to avoid damage to brain tissue. An infection upsets this balance. Brain damage can occur when cells are either deprived of important nutrients or exposed to toxic levels of particular substances.

The cells lining the brain's tiny blood vessels (capillaries) are specifically designed to prevent many substances from passing into brain tissue. This is commonly referred to as the blood-brain barrier. The blood-brain barrier prevents various substances that could be harmful to brain tissue (toxins), as well as many agents of infection, from crossing from the blood stream into the brain tissue. While this barrier is obviously an important protective feature for the brain, it also serves to complicate treatment in the case of an infection by making it difficult for medications to pass out of the blood and into the brain tissue where an infection is located.

Causes and symptoms

The most common infectious causes of meningitis vary according to an individual's age, habits, living environment, and health status. While nonbacterial types of meningitis are most common, bacterial meningitis is the more potentially life threatening. Three bacterial agents are responsible for about 80% of all bacterial meningitis cases. These bacteria are *Haemophilus influenzae* type b, *Neisseria meningitidis* (causing meningococcal meningitis), and *Streptococcus pneumoniae* (causing pneumococcal meningitis).

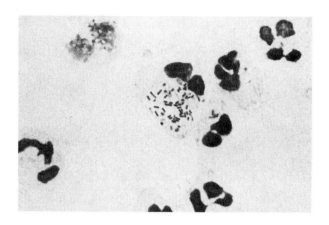

Gram stain of *Haemophilus influenzae* (causes bacterial meningitis) in cerebrospinal fluid (CSF). *(Delmar Publishers, Inc. Reproduced by permission.)*

In newborns, the most common agents of meningitis are those contracted from the newborn's mother, including Group B streptococci (which is becoming an increasingly common infecting organism in the newborn period), *Escherichia coli*, and *Listeria monocytogenes*. The highest incidence of meningitis occurs in babies younger than a month old, with an increased risk of meningitis continuing through about two years of age.

Older children are more frequently infected by the bacteria *Haemophilus influenzae*, *Neisseria meningitidis*, and *Streptococci pneumoniae*.

Adults are most commonly infected by either *S. pneumoniae* or *N. meningitidis*, with pneumococcal meningitis the most common. Certain conditions predispose an individual to this type of meningitis, including **alcoholism** and chronic upper respiratory tract infections (especially of the middle ear, sinuses, and mastoids).

N. meningitidis is the only organism that can cause epidemics of meningitis. In particular, these appear to occur when a child in a crowded day-care situation, or a military recruit in a crowded training camp, has fallen ill with meningococcal meningitis.

Viral causes of meningitis include the herpes simplex virus, the mumps and measles viruses (against which most children are protected due to mass immunization programs), the virus that causes chicken pox, the rabies virus, and a number of viruses that are acquired through the bites of infected mosquitoes.

A number of medical conditions predispose individuals to meningitis caused by specific organisms. People with **AIDS** (acquired **immunodeficiency** syndrome) are more prone to getting meningitis from fungi, as well as from the agent that causes **tuberculosis**. Persons who have had their spleens removed, or whose spleens are no longer functional (as in the case of individuals with **sick-**le cell disease) are more susceptible to meningococcal and pneumococcal meningitis.

The majority of meningitis infections are acquired by blood-borne spread. A person may have another type of infection (of the **lungs**, throat, or tissues of the **heart**) caused by an organism that can also cause meningitis. If this initial infection is not properly treated, the organism will continue to multiply, find its way into the blood stream, and be delivered in sufficient quantities to pass the blood brain barrier. Direct spread occurs when an organism spreads to the meninges from infected tissue next to or very near the meninges. This can occur, for example, with a severe, poorly treated ear or sinus infection.

Persons who suffer from skull **fractures** possess abnormal openings to the sinuses, nasal passages, and middle ears. Organisms that usually live in the human **respiratory system** without causing disease can pass through such openings, reach the meninges, and cause infection. Similarly, people who undergo surgical procedures or who have had **foreign bodies** surgically placed within their skulls (such as tubes to drain abnormal amounts of accumulated CSF) have an increased risk of meningitis.

Organisms can also reach the meninges via an uncommon but interesting method called intraneural spread. This involves an organism invading the body at a considerable distance away from the head, spreading along a nerve, and using that nerve as a ladder into the skull where the organism can multiply and cause meningitis. Herpes simplex virus is known to use this type of spread, as is the rabies virus.

The most classic symptoms of meningitis (particularly of bacterial meningitis) include **fever**, headache, vomiting, sensitivity to light (photophobia), irritability, severe fatigue (lethargy), stiff neck, and a reddish purple rash on the skin. Untreated, the disease progresses with seizures, confusion, and eventually **coma**.

A very young infant may not show the classic signs of meningitis. Early in infancy, a baby's immune system is not yet developed enough to mount a fever in response to infection, so fever may be absent. In some infants with meningitis, seizures are the only identifiable symptom. Similarly, debilitated elderly people may not have fever or other identifiable symptoms of meningitis.

Brain damage due to meningitis occurs from a variety of phenomena. The action of infectious agents on the brain tissue is one direct cause of damage. Other types of damage may be due to the mechanical effects of swelling and compression of brain tissue against the skull. Swelling of the meninges may interfere with the normal absorption of CSF by blood vessels, causing accumulation of CSF and damage from the resulting pressure on the brain. Interference with the brain's carefully regulated chemical environment may cause abnormal and damaging amounts of normally present substances (carbon dioxide, potassium) to accumulate. Inflammation may cause the blood-brain barrier to become less effective at preventing the passage of toxic substances into brain tissue.

Diagnosis

A number of techniques are used when examining a person suspected of having meningitis to verify the diagnosis. Certain manipulations of the head (lowering the head, chin towards chest, for example) are difficult to perform and painful for a person with meningitis.

The most important test used to diagnose meningitis is the lumbar puncture (commonly called a spinal tap). Lumbar puncture (LP) involves the insertion of a thin needle into a space between the vertebrae in the lower back and the withdrawal of a small amount of CSF. The CSF is then examined under a **microscope** to look for bacteria or fungi. Normal CSF contains set percentages of glucose and protein. These percentages will vary with bacterial, viral, or other causes of meningitis. For example, bacterial meningitis causes a greatly decreased percentage of glucose in the CSF because the bacteria are essentially consuming or "eating" that glucose and using it for their own **nutrition** and energy production. Normal CSF should contain no infection-fighting cells (white blood cells), so the presence of white blood cells in CSF is another indication of meningitis. Some of the withdrawn CSF is put into special lab dishes to allow growth of the infecting organism, which can then be identified more easily. Special immunologic and serologic tests may also be used to help identify the infectious agent.

In rare instances a lumbar puncture cannot be performed because of the amount of swelling and pressure within the skull (intracranial pressure). This pressure is measured immediately upon insertion of an LP needle. If it is found to be high, no fluid is withdrawn because doing so could cause herniation of the brain stem. Herniation of the brain stem occurs when the part of the brain connecting to the spinal cord is thrust through the opening at the base of the skull into the spinal canal. Such herniation will cause compression of those structures within the brain stem that control the most vital functions of the body (breathing, heart beat, consciousness). Death or permanent debilitation follows herniation of the brain stem.

Treatment

Antibiotic medications (forms of penicillin and cephalosporins, for example) are the most important ele-

ments of treatment against bacterial meningitis. Because of the effectiveness of the blood-brain barrier in preventing passage of substances into the brain, medications must be delivered directly into an affected person's veins (intravenously, or IV), at very high doses. **Antiviral drugs** (acyclovir) may be helpful in shortening the duration of viral meningitis, and antifungal medications are also available.

Other treatments involve decreasing inflammation (with steroid preparations) and paying careful attention to the balance of fluids, glucose, sodium, potassium, oxygen, and carbon dioxide in a person's system. People who develop seizures will require medications to halt the seizures and prevent their return.

Prognosis

Viral meningitis is the least severe type, and persons usually recover with no long-term effects from the infection. Bacterial infections, however, are much more severe, and rapidly progress. Without very rapid treatment with the appropriate antibiotic, an infection can swiftly lead to coma and death, often in less than 24 hours. While death rates from meningitis vary depending upon the specific infecting organism, the overall death rate is just under 20%.

The most frequent long-term effects of meningitis include deafness and blindness, which may be caused by the compression of specific nerves and brain areas responsible for the senses of **hearing** and sight. Some people develop permanent seizure disorders, requiring life-long treatment with antiseizure medications. Scarring of the meninges may result in obstruction of the normal flow of CSF, causing abnormal accumulation of CSF. This may be a chronic problem for some people, requiring the installation of shunt tubes to drain the accumulation on a regular basis.

Health care team roles

Family physicians, pediatricians, emergency physicians, or internists usually make the initial diagnosis of meningitis. Laboratory technicians identify organisms that cause meningitis. Nurses and other hospital staff provide supportive care, and patient and family education. Occasionally, physical therapists are needed to help the patient recover lost muscle functioning.

Prevention

Prevention of meningitis primarily involves the appropriate treatment of other infections an individual may acquire, particularly those known to seed to the

KEY TERMS

Arachnoid mater—The middle layer of the meninges.

Blood-brain barrier—An arrangement of cells within the blood vessels of the brain that prevents toxic substances, infectious agents, and many medications, from passing from the blood into the brain.

Cerebrospinal fluid (CSF)—Fluid made in chambers within the brain which then flows over the surface of the brain and spinal cord. CSF provides nutrition to cells of the nervous system, as well as providing a cushion for the nervous system structures.

Dura mater—The outermost layer of the meninges.

Lumbar puncture (LP)—A medical test in which a very narrow needle is inserted into a specific space between the vertebrae of the lower back in order to obtain a sample of CSF for examination.

Meninges—The three-layer membranous covering of the brain and spinal cord, composed of the dura, arachnoid, and pia. It provides protection for the brain and spinal cord, as well as housing many blood vessels and participating in the appropriate flow of CSF.

Photophobia—Abnormal sensitivity to light.

Pia mater—The innermost layer of the meninges.

meninges (such as ear and sinus infections). Preventive treatment with **antibiotics** is sometimes recommended for those in close contacts with an individual who is ill with meningococcal or *H. influenzae* type b meningitis. A meningococcal vaccine is sometimes recommended to individuals traveling to very high risk areas. A vaccine for *H. influenzae* type b is now given to babies as part of the standard array of childhood immunizations.

Resources

BOOKS

Adams, Raymond D, Maurice Victor, and Allan H. Ropper. *Adam's & Victor's Principles of Neurology.* 6th ed. New York: McGraw Hill, 1997.

Koroshetz, Walter J, and Morton N. Swartz. "Chronic and Rrecurrent Meniingitis." In *Harrison's Principles of Internal Medicine.* 14th ed. Ed. Anthony S. Fauci, et al. New York: McGraw-Hill, 1998, 2434-2439.

Nath, Avindra, and Joseph R. Berger. "Acute Viral Meningitis and Encephalitis." In *Cecil Textbook of Medicine.* 21st ed. Ed. Lee Goldman and J. Claude Bennett. Philadelphia: W.B. Saunders, 2000, 2123-2126.

Pollard, Andrew J., and Martin C. J. Maiden. *Meningococcal Disease: Methods and Protocols.* Totowa: Humana Press, 2001.

Prober, Charles G. "Acute Bacterial Meningitis Beyond the Neonatal Period." In *Nelson Textbook of Pediatrics.* 16th ed. Ed. Richard E. Behrman et al., Philadelphia: Saunders, 2000, 751-757.

Prober, Charles G. "Eosinophilic Meningitis." In *Nelson Textbook of Pediatrics.* 16th ed. Ed. Richard E. Behrman et al., Philadelphia: Saunders, 2000, 760-761.

Prober, Charles G. "Viral Meningoencephalitis." In *Nelson Textbook of Pediatrics.* 16th ed. Ed. Richard E. Behrman et al., Philadelphia: Saunders, 2000, 757-760.

Scheld, W. Michael. "Bacterial Meningitis, Brain Abscess, and Other Suppurative Intracranial Infections." In *Harrison's Principles of Internal Medicine.* 14th ed. Ed. Anthony S. Fauci, et al. New York: McGraw-Hill, 1998, 2419-2434.

Tyler, Kenneth L. "Aseptic Meningitis, Viral Encephalitis, and Prion Diseases." In *Harrison's Principles of Internal Medicine.* 14th ed. Ed. Anthony S. Fauci, et al. New York: McGraw-Hill, 1998, 2451-2457.

PERIODICALS

Agarwal, R., and A. J. Emmerson. "Should Repeat Lumbar Punctures be Routinely Done in Neonates with Bacterial Meningitis? Results of a Survey into Clinical Practice." *Archives of Diseases of Children* 84, no. 5 (2001): 451-452.

Colby, C. E., W. J. Steinbach, and A. K. Haiman. "A 10-week Old Infant with Meningitis." *Clinics in Pediatrics* 40, no. 3 (2001): 155-158.

Glennie, L. "Meningitis: A Rash Diagnosis." *Nursing Times* 96, no. 12 (2000): 44-45.

Kerr, C. "Meningitis Hits West Africa." *Trends in Microbiology* 9, no. 5 (2001): 203-205.

van den Berg, H., M. van der Flier, and M. D. van de Wetering. "Cytarabine-Induced Aseptic Meningitis." *Leukemia* 15, no. 4 (2001): 697-699.

von Vigier, R. O., S. M. Colombo, P. B. Stoffel, P. Meregalli, A. C. Truttmann, and M. G. Bianchetti. "Circulating Sodium in Acute Meningitis." *American Journal of Nephrology* 21, no. 2 (2001): 87-90.

ORGANIZATIONS

American Academy of Emergency Medicine. 611 East Wells Street, Milwaukee, WI 53202. (800) 884-2236. <http://www.aaem.org>.

Meningitis Foundation of America Inc. 7155 Shadeland Station, Suite 190, Indianapolis, Indiana 46256-3922. (800) 668-1129 or (317) 595-6383. <http://www.musa.org/default.htm>.

OTHER

American Academy of Family Practice. <http://www.aafp.org/afp/990515ap/2761.html> and <http://www.aafp.org/afp/971001ap/tunkel.html>.

Association of State and Territorial Directors of Health Promotion and Public Health Education. <http://www.astdhpphe.org/infect/bacmeningitis.html>.

Centers for Disease Control and Prevention. <http://www.cdc.gov/od/oc/media/pressrel/r991021.htm> and <http://www.cdc.gov/ncidod/dbmd/diseaseinfo/meningococcal_g.htm>.

Meningitis Research Foundation of UK. <http://www.meningitis.org.uk>.

National Institute for Medical Research (UK). <http://www.nimr.mrc.ac.uk/MillHillEssays/1999/meningitis.htm>.

National Institute of Neurological Disorders and Stroke. <http://www.ninds.nih.gov/health_and_medical/disorders/encmenin_doc.htm>.

National Library of Medicine. <http://www.nlm.nih.gov/medlineplus/meningitis.html>.

National Meningitis Trust of UK. <http://www.meningitis-trust.org.uk/frame.htm>.

University of Illinois School of Medicine. <http://www.mckinley.uiuc.edu/health-info/dis-cond/commdis/meningit.html>.

University of Maryland College of Medicine. <http://umm.drkoop.com/conditions/ency/article/000680.htm>.

L. Fleming Fallon, Jr., M.D., Dr.P.H.

Menkes' syndrome *see* **Mineral deficiency**

Menopause

Definition

Medically, menopause is the cessation of menstruation and signifies the inability to bear children. It is determined as one year from the last menstrual cycle. Menopause is a natural life-stage transition. Medical events, like surgery or **chemotherapy**, however, can also produce menopause.

Description

Menopause is a natural transition that will affect every woman. By the year 2020, it is estimated that there will be 62 million American women reaching menopause.

Most of these women will spend one-third to one-half of their lives postmenopause.

No changes in life expectancy or general health have affected the age at which menopause occurs. The average age of onset of natural menopause is 51, with a normal range between 48 and 58. There are women who experience it as early as 35 and as late as 60. Eight percent of women stop menstruating before age 40, and 5% continue to have periods until they are near 60. Usually, there is an underlying factor to extremely early or late menopause.

Attempts at defining factors that can predict age of onset have not been successful. It is clear that heredity and smoking seem to be linked to the timing of menopause. A mother's age at menopause may indicate when her daughter will cease menstruation, though this is not a hard- and-fast rule. If a mother entered **puberty** late and her daughter had her first period at an early age, there may be no correlation. The mother may have experienced poor **nutrition** as a child or had an hormonal deficiency or some other medical condition to delay puberty.

Smokers enter menopause as much as 1.5 years earlier than non-smokers. Other determinants can be number of pregnancies, body mass, depression, chemical exposure, and exposure to pelvic radiation as a child. Women who have had children, have larger body mass, and who had higher cognitive scores as children may enter menopause later. Conversely, women who never had children, are depressed, were exposed to toxic chemicals, or had pelvic radiation usually have an earlier menopause.

There are four types of menopause. The most prevalent is natural, spontaneous menopause. Premature (spontaneous), surgical, and induced menopause occur because of a medical condition, a surgical procedure, or other outside cause.

Natural (spontaneous) menopause

Most menopause is natural and occurs as part of the aging cycle for women. Technically, it refers to a state in a woman's menstrual cycle which happens a year from the date of her last menstrual period. Indications that the process is starting may occur in a woman's 40's with the lengthening and irregularity of menstrual cycles. The process can take as long as eight years, or may be over in two. Only 10% of women report that menstruation ceases suddenly, with no cycle irregularity prior.

There are four stages that a woman experiences when she experiences natural menopause.

MENSTRUATION. When a woman enters puberty, each month her body releases one of the more than 400,000 eggs that are stored in her ovaries, and the lining of the womb (uterus) thickens in anticipation of receiving a fertilized egg. If the egg is not fertilized, progesterone levels drop and the uterine lining sheds. This is a normal menstrual cycle.

By the time a woman reaches her late 30s or 40s, her ovaries begin to produce less estrogen and progesterone, releasing eggs less often. The gradual decline of estrogen causes a wide variety of changes in tissues that respond to estrogen—including the vagina, vulva, uterus, bladder, urethra, breasts, bones, **heart**, **blood vessels**, **brain**, skin, hair, and mucous membranes.

As the levels of hormones fluctuate, the menstrual cycle begins to change. Some women may have longer periods with heavy flow followed by shorter cycles and hardly any bleeding, beginning as much as two to eight years before menopause. Others will begin to miss periods completely. During this time, a woman also becomes less able to get pregnant (although **contraception** should be continued until the postmenopausal state is established). This is the stage of premenopause which represents the very beginning of the process. Typically, it begins when a woman is in her mid-to-late forties.

PERIMENOPAUSAL TRANSITION. Perimenopause is the stage most women consider as going through menopause. Here a woman's cycles become very erratic. She may experience more hot flashes and other symptoms. Only about 15% of women report severe symptoms. This stage lasts about four years, the two years prior to the last cycle and the two years following it. For 95% of women, the age of onset ranges from 39 to 51 years. The average age for perimenopause is 47.5 years, with completion at 51.

MENOPAUSE. This is the permanent cessation of menstruation following the loss of ovarian activity. It often is not officially noted until a year with no cycles has passed.

POSTMENOPAUSE. This stage represents the last years of a woman's life. She may well spend a third to half of her life in this stage. During the first years after menopause, a woman may still experience some perimenopausal symptoms. Here, a woman will begin to deal with some of the effects of aging. In 2001, a woman at 50 or 51 may truly be at mid-life, according to the calendar, since many women will live to be a hundred.

Premature (spontaneous) menopause

Premature menopause occurs spontaneously, without any outside interventions or stresses, and affects about 0.3% of women. It is generally due to ovarian failure and occurs before age 40. Because hormonal levels plummet dramatically, these women experience severe vasomotor symptoms that can last as long as 8.5 years. Fertility may end over several months or immediately.

Surgical menopause

What a woman would normal experience between a two to eight-year period during normal menopause, women with surgical or premature menopause experience immediately and at a very young age. Some of these women are as young as 15. Fertility ends immediately.

Bilateral oophorectomy, or the surgical removal of both ovaries, can be the result of several different procedures. A complete hysterectomy, or the removal of the uterus and the ovaries, results in menopause. It is performed to remove cancerous growths in the ovaries, uterus, or cervix, and may be done in some types of colon **cancer** surgery. It can also be done to remove non-malignant fibroid tumors in the uterus or to mitigate the effects of endometriosis (although these procedures do not always require the removal of the ovaries). If surgery leaves one or both ovaries, often menopause is avoided. However, in some cases, menopause occurs regardless of whether the ovaries are left intact.

Induced menopause

Induced menopause occurs when a woman has been exposed to pelvic radiation or chemotherapy. The drugs in chemotherapy used to combat cancer can seriously damage the ovaries. This condition may be temporary, lasting only a few months or years. Permanent menopause is more likely if a combination of drugs are used or the woman is close to perimenopause. Pelvic radiation therapy usually produces permanent menopause. Other types of radiation therapy, away from the ovaries, may not affect ovarian hormones at all, thus avoiding induced menopause.

Causes and symptoms

Causes

The cause of most menopausal symptoms has been attributed in part to low estrogen levels in the body. Increased amounts of follicle-stimulating hormone (FSH) and luteinizing hormone (LH) are also involved. If a woman is overweight, she may experience milder symptoms because the fat stored in her body is converted to estrogen when the hormone levels fall. Also, women who endure premenstrual syndrome (PMS) are more apt to report mood swings. This may be due to differences in hormone levels. New research is beginning to tie psychological factors to these symptoms as well. For example, women who are depressed and angry, especially if they are unhappy in their relationships, often report more pronounced symptoms.

Ethnicity may also be a factor in the development of symptoms. Since most of the menopausal research has been conducted on white women, cross-ethnic studies in 2000 were conducted to discover any racial or ethnic variables. The frequency and type of symptoms reported varied widely between ethnic groups. Japanese American and Chinese American women reported fewer symptoms than the other women. African-American women experienced more hot flashes and vaginal dryness. Hispanic women had more vaginal dryness, urine leakage, and heart palpitations. Non-Hispanic white women reported more sleep difficulties.

It is unclear whether cultural or biological factors are involved in these differences. As for causal agents, that may be too early to tell. In any case, the health care team should be aware that ethnic differences in symptom manifestation do exist in menopause.

Symptoms

About 20% of women in the United States experience menopause with few symptoms. All others report a variety of complaints throughout perimenopause; some mild, some severe enough to interfere with work or daily activities.

There are a variety of symptoms a woman may experience in perimenopause:

- changes in the menstrual cycle, resulting in long cycles and missed periods
- hot flashes
- night sweats
- insomnia
- mood swings/irritability
- **memory** or concentration problems
- vaginal dryness
- heavy bleeding
- fatigue
- depression
- hair changes
- headaches
- heart palpitations
- sexual disinterest
- urinary changes
- weight gain

Diagnosis

The clearest indication of menopause is the absence of a period for one year. It is also possible to diagnose menopause by testing hormone levels. One important test measures the levels of follicle-stimulating hormone (FSH), which rise steadily as a woman ages.

Treatment of specific symptoms should be handled as they manifest and are reported.

Treatment

Hormone replacement therapy

The standard treatment for menopause has been hormone replacement therapy, primarily with estrogen. Hormone replacement therapy can treat menopausal symptoms by boosting the estrogen levels enough to suppress symptoms while also providing protection against heart disease and **osteoporosis**, which causes the bones to weaken. Experts disagree on whether HRT increases or decreases the risk of developing **breast cancer**.

There are two types of hormone treatments: hormone replacement therapy (HRT) and estrogen replacement therapy (ERT). HRT is the administration of estrogen and progesterone; ERT is the administration of estrogen alone. Only women who have had a hysterectomy (removal of the uterus) can take estrogen alone, since taking this "unopposed" estrogen can cause uterine cancer. The combination of progesterone and estrogen in HRT eliminates the risk of uterine cancer.

Most physicians do not recommend HRT until a woman's periods have stopped completely for one year. This is because women in early menopause who still have an occasional period are still producing estrogen; HRT would then provide far too much estrogen. One way of determining if HRT may be necessary is to measure FSH levels yearly beginning at age 50. When these levels are at or greater than 20 U/l, a postmenopausal hormone program may be recommended.

Many doctors believe that every woman (except those with certain cancers) should take hormones as they approach menopause because of the protection against heart disease, osteoporosis, and uterine cancer and the relatively low risk of breast cancer. Heart disease and osteoporosis are two of the leading causes of disability and death among post-menopausal women. Research in 2000 and 2001 has been challenging the effectiveness of estrogen in preventing heart disease, as well as **colorectal cancer** and **Alzheimer's disease**. No substantial study has proven that estrogen is a sound preventative.

Women are poor candidates for hormone replacement therapy if they:

- have ever had breast or endometrial cancer

- have a close relative (mother, sister, grandmother) who died of breast cancer or have two relatives who got breast cancer before age 40

- have had endometrial cancer

- have had **gallbladder** or **liver** disease

- have **blood** clots or phlebitis

Some women with liver or gall bladder disease, or who have clotting problems, may be able to go on HRT if they use a patch to administer the hormones through the skin, bypassing the liver.

Women would make good candidates for HRT if they:

- need to prevent osteoporosis

- have had their ovaries removed

- have significant symptoms

In some women, taking hormones can eliminate hot flashes, vaginal dryness, urinary incontinence (depending on the cause), insomnia, moodiness, memory problems, heavy irregular periods, and concentration problems. But side effects of treatment include bloating, breakthrough bleeding, headaches, vaginal discharge, fluid retention, swollen breasts, and nausea. There can also be an increased risk of gall bladder disease and blood clots. Up to 20% of women who try hormone replacement stop within nine months because of these side effects. However, some side effects can be lessened or prevented by changing the HRT regimen.

The decision should be made by a woman and her doctor after taking into consideration her medical history and situation. Women who choose to take hormones should have an annual mammogram, breast exam, and pelvic exam and should report any unusual vaginal bleeding or spotting (a sign of possible uterine cancer).

Designer estrogen

A new type of hormone therapy offers some of the same protection against degenerative diseases and bone loss as estrogen, but without the increased risk of breast cancer. This new class of drugs, known as designer estrogens. Under development for nearly a decade, new drugs like Evista are being approved to prevent and treat osteoporosis in 2001. Unfortunately, these drugs have not been effective in combating hot flashes.

Male hormones

The ovaries also produce a small amount of male hormones, which decreases slightly as a woman enters menopause. The vast majority of women never need testosterone replacement, but it can be important if a woman has declining interest in sex. Testosterone can improve the libido, and decrease **anxiety** and depression; adding testosterone especially helps women who have had hysterectomies. Testosterone also eases breast tenderness and helps prevent bone loss.

However, testosterone does have side effects. Some women experience mild acne and some facial hair growth, but because only small amounts of testosterone are prescribed, most women do not appear to have extreme masculine changes.

Birth control pills

Women who are still having periods but who have annoying menopausal symptoms may take low-dose birth control pills to ease the problems; this treatment has been approved by the FDA for perimenopausal symptoms in women under age 55. HRT is the preferred treatment for menopause, however, because it uses lower doses of estrogen.

Alternative treatment

Some women also report success in using natural remedies to treat unpleasant symptoms of menopause. Not all women need estrogen, and some women cannot take it. Many doctors do not want to give hormones to women who are still having their periods, however erratically. Indeed, only a third of menopausal women in the United States try HRT and of those who do, eventually half of them drop the therapy. Some are worried about breast cancer, some cannot tolerate the side effects, some do not want to medicate what they consider to be a natural occurrence.

HERBS. Herbs have been used to relieve menopausal symptoms for centuries. In general, most herbs are considered safe, and there is no substantial evidence that herbal products are a major source of toxic reactions. But because herbal products are not regulated in the United States, contamination or accidental **overdose** is possible. Herbs should be bought from a recognized company or through a qualified herbal practitioner.

Women who choose to take herbs for menopausal symptoms should learn as much as possible about herbal products and work with a qualified practitioner (an herbalist, a specialist in Chinese medicine, or a naturopathic physician). Pregnant women should avoid herbs because of unknown effects on a developing fetus.

The following list of herbs include those that herbalists most often prescribe to treat menstrual complaints:

- Black cohosh (*Cimicifuga racemosa*): hot flashes and other menstrual complaints.
- Black currant: breast tenderness.
- Chaste tree/chasteberry (*Vitex agnus-castus*): hot flashes, excessive menstrual bleeding, fibroids, and moodiness.
- Evening primrose oil (*Oenothera biennis*): mood swings, irritability, and breast tenderness.
- Fennel (*Foeniculum vulgare*): hot flashes, digestive gas, and bloating.
- Flaxseed (linseed): excessive menstrual bleeding, breast tenderness, and other symptoms, including dry skin and vaginal dryness.
- Gingko (*Gingko biloba*): memory problems.
- Ginseng (*Panax ginseng*): hot flashes, fatigue and vaginal thinning.
- Hawthorne (*Crataegus laevigata*): memory problems, fuzzy thinking.
- Lady's mantle: excessive menstrual bleeding.
- Mexican wild yam (*Dioscorea villosa*) root: vaginal dryness, hot flashes and general menopause symptoms.
- Motherwort (*Leonurus cardiaca*): night sweats, hot flashes.
- Oat (*Avena sativa*) straw: mood swings, anxiety.
- Red clover (*Trifolium pratense*): hot flashes.
- Sage (*Salvia officinalis*): mood swings, headaches, night sweats.
- Valerian (*Valeriana officinalis*): insomnia.

NATURAL ESTROGENS (PHYTOESTROGENS). Research in the efficacy of phytoestrogens, particularly soy products, have been mixed. Some trials suggest that the estrogen compounds in soy products can indeed relieve the severity of hot flashes and lower cholesterol. Others do not.

It is true that people in Asian countries who eat foods high in plant estrogens (especially soy products) have lower rates of breast cancer and report fewer "symptoms" of menopause. While up to 80% of menopausal women in the United States complain of hot flashes, night sweats, and vaginal dryness, only 15% of Japanese women have similar complaints. It is unclear whether this statistic is due to eating phytoestrogens alone or is a factor of genetics or culture.

The study of phytoestrogens is so new that there are not very many recommendations on how much a woman can consume. Herbal practitioners recommend a dose based on a woman's history, body size, lifestyle, diet, and reported symptoms. In one study at Bowman-Gray Medical School in North Carolina, women were able to ease their symptoms by eating a large amount of fruits, vegetables, and whole grains, together with 4 oz (113g) of tofu four times a week.

What concerns some critics of other alternative remedies is that many women think that "natural" or "plant-based" means "harmless." In large doses, phytoestrogens can promote the abnormal growth of cells in the uterine lining. Unopposed estrogen of any type can lead to endometrial cancer, which is why women on conventional estrogen-replacement therapy usually take progesterone (progestin) along with their estrogen. However, a plant-based progesterone product can sometimes be effective alone, without estrogen, in assisting the menopausal woman in rebalancing her hormonal action throughout this transition time.

YOGA. Some women find that **yoga** (the ancient meditation/exercise developed in India 5,000 years ago) can ease menopausal symptoms. Yoga focuses on helping women unite the mind, body, and spirit to create balance. Studies have found that yoga can reduce **stress**, improve mood, boost a sluggish **metabolism**, and slow the heart rate. Specific yoga positions deal with particular problems, such as hot flashes, mood swings, vaginal and urinary problems, and other pains.

EXERCISE. **Exercise** helps ease hot flashes by lowering the amount of circulating FSH and LH and by raising endorphin levels (which drop when having a hot flash). Even exercising 20 minutes three times a week can significantly reduce hot flashes.

ACUPUNCTURE. This ancient Asian art involves placing very thin needles into different parts of the body to stimulate the system and unblock energy. It is usually painless and has been used for many menopausal symptoms, including insomnia, hot flashes, and irregular periods. Practitioners believe that acupuncture can facilitate the opening of blocked energy channels, allowing the life force energy (chi) to flow freely. Blocked energy, they report, increases the symptoms of menopause.

ACUPRESSURE AND MASSAGE. Therapeutic massage involving **acupressure** can bring relief from a wide range of menopause symptoms by placing finger pressure at the same meridian points on the body that are used in acupuncture. There are more than 80 different types of massage, including foot reflexology, **Shiatsu** massage, or Swedish massage, but they are all based on the idea that boosting the circulation of blood and lymph benefits health, and relaxing the body and mind.

KEY TERMS

Amenorrhea—The cessation of menstrual cycles.

Bilateral oophorectomy—The surgical removal of both ovaries.

Endometrium—The lining of the uterus, which is shed with each menstrual period.

Estrogen—Female hormone produced by the ovaries and released by the follicles as they mature. Responsible for female sexual characteristics, estrogen stimulates and triggers a response from at least 300 tissues, and may help some types of breast cancer to grow. After menopause, the production of the hormone gradually stops.

Estrogen replacement therapy (ERT)—A treatment for menopause in which estrogen is given in pill, patch, or cream form.

Follicle-stimulating hormone (FSH)—The pituitary hormone that stimulates the ovary to mature egg capsules (follicles). It is linked with rising estrogen production throughout the cycle. An elevated FSH (above 40) indicates menopause.

Hormone—A chemical messenger secreted by a gland that is released into the blood, and that travels to distant cells where it exerts an effect.

Hormone replacement therapy (HRT)—The use of estrogen and progesterone to replace hormones that the ovary no longer supplies.

Hot flash—A wave of heat that is one of the most common perimenopausal symptoms, triggered by the hypothalamus' response to estrogen withdrawal.

Hysterectomy—Surgical removal of the uterus.

Ovary—One of the two almond-shaped glands in the female reproductive system responsible for producing eggs and the hormones estrogen and progesterone.

Ovulation—The monthly release of an egg from the ovary.

Pituitary gland—The "master gland" at the base of the brain that secretes a number of hormones responsible for growth, reproduction, and other activities. Pituitary hormones stimulate the ovaries to release estrogen and progesterone.

Progesterone—The hormone that is produced by the ovary after ovulation to prepare the uterine lining for a fertilized egg.

Testosterone—Male hormone produced by the testes and (in small amounts) in the ovaries. Testosterone is responsible for some masculine secondary sex characteristics such as growth of body hair and deepening voice.

Uterus—The female reproductive organ that contains and nourishes a fetus from implantation until birth. Also known as the womb.

Vagina—The tube-like passage from the vulva (a woman's external genital structures) to the cervix (the portion of the uterus that projects into the vagina).

BIOFEEDBACK. Some women have been able to control hot flashes through biofeedback, a painless technique that helps a person train her mind to control her body. A biofeedback machine provides information about body processes (such as heart rate) as the woman relaxes her body. Using this technique, it is possible to control the body's temperature, heart rate, and breathing.

Prognosis

Menopause is a natural condition of aging. Some women have no problems at all with menopause, while others notice significant unpleasant symptoms. A wide array of treatments, from natural products to hormone replacement, mean that no woman needs to suffer through this time of her life.

Health care team roles

Physicians, nurses, physician assistants, and alternative/complimentary health care practitioners assume important roles in a woman's successful transition into postmenopause. Since new research in menopause treatment is occurring every year, it will be the health care team's obligation to provide the woman with accurate options that are specific to her individual case. Referrals for counseling and other psychological services may be necessary if depression or anxiety about aging is a problem. Since the symptoms of perimenopause are not life-threatening, the health care team may be more willing to suggest alternative methods like herbal remedies, yoga, and acupressure, as well as lifestyle changes like exercise and a healthy diet. The goal of the health care team should be to normalize this transition as much as possible and not stigmatize it as a medical condition.

Prevention

Menopause is a natural part of the aging process and not a disease that needs to be prevented. A variety of treatments are available to treat uncomfortable perimenopausal symptoms. Hormone replacement therapy is often used to combat serious symptoms and prevent a number of degenerative diseases such as heart disease and osteoporosis.

Resources

BOOKS

Corio, Laura E., and Linda G. Kahn. *The Change Before the Change: Everything You Need to Know to Stay Healthy in the Decade before Menopause.* New York: Bantam Books, 2000.

Lieberman, Shari. *Get Off the Menopause Roller Coaster: Natural Solutions for Mood Swings, Hot Flashes, Fatigue, Anxiety, Depression, and Other Symptoms* New York: Penguin Putnam, 2000.

Moore, Michele. *The Only Menopause Guide You'll Need.* Baltimore: John Hopkins University Press, 2000.

Posner, Trisha. *This Is Not Your Mother's Menopause: One Woman's Natural Journey Through Change.* New York: Villard, 2000.

PERIODICALS

"Alternatives for the Menopause." *Chemist & Druggist* (January 27, 2001): 23.

Minkin, Mary Jane, and Toby Hanlon. "Answers to Your Top Five Menopause Questions." *Prevention* 53, no. 1 (January 2001): 89.

Morris, Kelly. "U.S. Survey Finds that Race Matters." *The Lancet* 356, no. 9233 (September 9, 2000): 916.

Speroff, Leon. "Management of the Perimenopausal Transition." *Contemporary OB/GYN* 45, no. 10 (October 2000): 14.

ORGANIZATIONS

American Menopause Foundation, Inc., Empire State Bldg., 350 Fifth Ave., Ste. 2822, New York, NY 10118. (212) 714-2398.

Federation of Feminist Women's Health Centers. 633 East 11th Ave., Eugene, OR 97401. (503) 344-0966.

Hysterectomy Educational Resources and Services Foundation (HERS). 422 Bryn Mawr Ave., Bala Cynwyd, PA 19004. (215) 667-7757.

National Women's Health Network. 1325 G St. NW, Washington, DC 20005. (202) 347-1140.

North American Menopause Society. PO Box 94527, Cleveland, OH 44101. (440) 442-7550, (800) 774-5342. <http:www.menopause.org/>.

Resources for Midlife and Older Women. 226 E. 70 St., Ste. 1C, New York, NY 10021. (212) 439-1913.

OTHER

Menopause. <http://www.howdyneighbor.com/menopaus/>.

Menopause Online. <http://www.menopause-online.com/links.htm>.

Meno Times. <http://www.aimnet.com/~hyperion/meno/menotimes.index.html>.

Power Surge Reading Room. <http://members.aol.com/dearest/news.htm>.

Women's Health. <http://women.shn.net/index.html>.

Women's Health Initiative. <http://www.nih.gov/od/odp/whi>.

Janie F. Franz

Mercury hygiene

Definition

Proper handling and use of mercury in the oral health care setting is referred to as mercury hygiene. Designated as a hazardous substance by the National Occupational Health and Safety Commission, mercury is considered a health risk in the workplace and must be handled according to specific guidelines.

Precautions

Permissible exposure limits in the United States are 0.1 and 0.05 mg/cubic meters. Dental offices, which use liquid mercury on a regular basis in amalgam restorations, are required to follow appropriate measures to manage and reduce the risk of mercury spills and vapor release.

Description

Pure mercury in the dental workplace is found in predosed amalgam capsules that include separate compartments for alloy powder and mercury. Amalgam has been used to fill teeth for thousands of years and has been available in its present formulation since the late nineteenth century. Amalgam contains 50% metallic mercury, 35% silver, 9% tin, 6% **copper**, and a trace of **zinc**. United States dentists place more than 100 million amalgam fillings each year. Dental mercury, supplied in the form of an odorless, silvery liquid with a metallic luster, is considered harmful at concentrations greater than 3%, and toxic at concentrations greater than 25%.

KEY TERMS

Amalgam—As applied to dentistry, a filling material composed of mercury, silver, tin, copper, and zinc.

Erethism—Morbid excitability, characterized by abnormal shyness, depression, despondency, and irritability.

Mercurialism—Chronic poisoning from mercury.

Preparation

Dental employers are required to conduct a risk assessment for mercury hygiene that includes the following documentation:

- date of the assessment
- the product name for mercury-containing substances
- a statement that the material safety data sheet (MSDS) and other relevant information have been reviewed
- a statement on the significance of the degree of risk
- a list of control measures in place
- a decision on the need for health surveillance

Amalgam that is mixed but unused during restoration care is normally collected and sold for reprocessing. Minor particles, plus amalgam dust formed during the removal of old restorations, is removed by rinsing or by high speed suction. Significantly lower amounts of mercury are found in dental operatory waste water when amalgam separators are used. Use of a rubber dam and high-speed evacuation are also appropriate control measures.

The American Dental Association reports that amalgamators, the mixing machines used to produce amalgam, may become contaminated with mercury and emit minute amounts of mercury vapor. Old amalgamators may need to be classified as hazardous waste for disposal.

Disposable monitoring discs are available that measure any hazard from mercury vapor in dental offices. Discs are assessed by an appropriate agency, and the office is given a report and advice on mercury hygiene.

Aftercare

First aid

Following mercury exposure, **first aid** procedures are as follows:

- Eye contact: Flush under upper and lower lids for 15 minutes, and seek medical attention.

- Skin contact: Wash contaminated clothing thoroughly with soap and water. Seek medical attention.

- Inhalation: Move victim to fresh air, give artificial respiration if necessary. Seek medical attention.

- Ingestion: Give a conscious victim water and induce vomiting. Seek medical attention. For a person who is unconscious or convulsing, do not give anything by mouth or induce vomiting.

Spill management

Since spilled mercury gives off a toxic, odorless vapor, spills must be cleaned up immediately if predosed capsules break. Persons handling cleanup should wear gloves and collect mercury with a suction pump and aspirator bottle. A regular vacuum cleaner is not appropriate since a vacuum cleaner can spread mercury vapor. No mercury should enter drains. Fine droplets may be covered with **calcium** polysulphide, powdered sulfur, or a 20% solution of sodium thiosulphate. Droplets are to be put in a closed container.

Complications

Inhalation of mercury vapor is toxic, and there is danger of cumulative effects of exposure. Possible complications include difficulty breathing, cough, **fever**, nausea, vomiting, headache, excessive salivation and metallic **taste**, cardiac abnormalities, pulmonary irritation and pneumonitis, **edema**, fibrosis, kidney and **brain** damage, and death.

Effects of accidental ingestion are burning of the mouth and throat, thirst, nausea, and vomiting. Mercury is not usually absorbed well enough through ingestion to cause acute effects.

Eye contact with mercury in liquid form may cause irritation and redness. Skin contact may result in allergic reactions and irritation. Enough mercury can be absorbed through the skin for toxicity.

The chronic health effects of mercury exposure are termed mercurialism. Mercurialism includes fine tremors and erethism, a syndrome of psychological effects including abnormal shyness, depression, despondency, irritability, or excitability. With severe mercury exposure, hallucinations, loss of **memory**, and mental deterioration may occur. Other possible chronic health effects are kidney damage, **stomatitis**, increased tooth mobility, blue pigmentation of the gum tissue, **diarrhea**, and weight loss. Individuals with pre-existing conditions affecting the **respiratory system**, **kidneys**, and nervous system may find their conditions aggravated by mercury exposure.

Results

Proper mercury hygiene results in a safe working environment for dental personnel. With control measures in place, dental amalgam does not appear to represent an environmental problem. Organized dentistry claims that mercury combined into amalgam forms a biologically inactive substance. Its widespread and long-term use have not brought to light any adverse side effects in dental patients.

Health care team roles

An employer is required to identify staff members who may be exposed to mercury, such as dentists and chair-side assistants, then conduct and document appropriate training. Issues to be addressed include any factors that may affect the level of exposure, such as working hours and preventive measures used in the practice. Safe work practices in handling mercury overlap with dental workplace safety in general. They include:

- avoiding contact and inhalation of vapor during handling of mercury
- wearing gloves and protective eyewear
- storing capsules in a cool area in labeled containers and protected from breakage
- never disassembling capsules
- salvaging amalgam waste and residue for recycling
- separating clinical clothing from street wear

Dental employers must re-evaluate mercury risk when work practices are modified with new or improved control measures, when new information becomes available, or every five years.

Resources

PERIODICALS

Roberts, Howard W., D.M.D.; Daniel Leonard, D.D.S.; and John Osborne, D.D.S., M.S.D. "Potential Health and Environmental Issues of Mercury-contaminated Amalgamators." *Journal of the American Dental Association* (January 2001): 58.

ORGANIZATIONS

American Dental Association. 211 East Chicago Ave., Chicago, IL 60611. (312) 440-2500. <http://www.ada.org>.

Consumers for Dental Choice. National Institute for Science, Law and Public Policy, 1424 16th St., NW Suite 105, Washington, DC 20036. <http://www.amalgam.org>.

United States Environmental Protection Agency. Office of Emergency and Remedial Response, 1200 Pennsylvania Ave. NW, Washington, DC 20460. <http://www.epa.gov/superfund/tools/merc/index.htm>.

OTHER

"The Dental Amalgam Issue." *DAMS Inc., Consumers for Dental Choice website.* <http://www.www.amalgam.org>.

"Mercury—Emergency Spill and Release Facts." *EPA Office of Emergency and Remedial Response website* March 1997. <http://www.epa.gov/superfund/tools/merc/index.htm>.

"Potential Biological Consequences of Mercury Released from Dental Amalgam." *Swedish Medical Research Council, Appendix VIII.* <http://www.health.gov/environment/amalgam/appendixVIII.htm>.

Walsh, L. J. "Hazardous Substance Assessment for Mercury in Dentistry." *WHSO Dental School website* <http://www.www.members.nbci.com/_XMCM/dnl-walsh/mercury.htm>.

Cathy Hester Seckman, R.D.H.

Mercy killing *see* **Euthanasia**

Metabolism

Definition

Metabolism refers to the highly integrated network of chemical reactions by which living cells grow and sustain themselves.

Description

The metabolism's network of chemical reactions are composed of two major types of pathways: anabolism and catabolism. Anabolism uses energy stored in the form of adenosine triphosphate (ATP) to build larger molecules from smaller molecules. Catabolic reactions degrade larger molecules in order to produce ATP and raw materials for anabolic reactions.

Function

Together, the body's anabolic and catabolic networks have three major functions:

- to extract energy from nutrients
- to synthesize the building blocks that make up the large molecules of life: **proteins**, **fats**, **carbohydrates**, nucleic acids, and combinations of these substances
- to synthesize and degrade molecules required for special functions in the cell

These reactions are controlled by *enzymes*, protein catalysts that increase the speed of chemical reactions in the cell without themselves being changed. Each enzyme catalyzes a specific chemical reaction by acting on a specific substrate, or raw material. Each reaction is just one in a sequence of catalytic steps in a metabolic pathway(s). These sequences may be composed of up to 20 enzymes, each one creating a product that becomes the substrate or raw material for the subsequent enzyme. Often, an additional molecule called a *coenzyme*, is required for the enzyme to function. For example, some coenzymes accept an electron that is released from the substrate during the enzymatic reaction. Most of the water-soluble **vitamins** of the B complex serve as coenzymes; **riboflavin** (vitamin B_2) for example, is a precursor of the coenzyme flavine adenine dinucleotide, while pantothenate is a component of coenzyme A, an important intermediate metabolite.

The series of products created by the sequential enzymatic steps of anabolism or catabolism are called metabolic intermediates, or metabolites. Each step represents a small change in the molecule, usually the removal, transfer, or addition of a specific atom, molecule or group of atoms that serves as a functional group, such as the amino groups ($-NH_2$) of proteins.

Typically, these metabolic pathways are linear. That is, they begin with a specific substrate and end with a specific product. Some pathways, such as the Krebs cycle, are cyclic. Often, metabolic pathways also have branches that feed into or out of them. The specific sequences of intermediates in the pathways of cell metabolism are called intermediary metabolism.

There are thousands of chemical reactions in the body and many of these pathways are identical in most forms of life.

According to the first law of thermodynamics, in any physical or chemical change, the total amount of energy in the universe remains constant, that is, energy cannot be created or destroyed. Thus, when the energy stored in nutrient molecules is released and captured in the form of ATP, some energy is lost as heat but the total amount of energy is unchanged.

The second law of thermodynamics states that physical and chemical changes proceed in such a direction that useful energy undergoes irreversible degradation into a randomized form—entropy. The dissipation of energy during metabolism represents an increase in the randomness, or disorder, of the organism's environment. Because this disorder is irreversible, it provides the driving force and direction to all metabolic enzymatic reactions.

Even in the simplest cells, such as **bacteria**, there are at least a thousand such reactions. Regardless of the

number, all cellular reactions can be classified as one of two types of metabolism: anabolism and catabolism. These reactions, while opposite in nature, are linked through the common bond of energy. Anabolism, or biosynthesis, is the synthetic phase of metabolism during which small building block molecules, or precursors, are built into large molecular components of cells, such as carbohydrates and proteins.

Catabolic reactions are used to capture and save energy from nutrients, as well as to degrade larger molecules into smaller, molecular raw materials for reuse by the cell. The energy is stored in the form of energy-rich ATP, which powers the reactions of anabolism. The useful energy of ATP is stored in the form of a high-energy bond between the second and third phosphate groups of ATP. The cell makes ATP by adding a phosphate group to the molecule adenosine diphosphate (ADP). Therefore, ATP is the major chemical link between the energy-yielding reactions of catabolism, and the energy-requiring reactions of anabolism.

In some cases, energy is also conserved as energy-rich hydrogen atoms in the coenzyme nicotinamide adenine dinucleotide phosphate (NADPH) in the reduced form of NADPH. The NADPH can then be used as a source of high-energy hydrogen atoms during certain biosynthetic reactions of anabolism.

In addition to the obvious difference in the direction of their metabolic goals, anabolism and catabolism differ in other significant ways. For example, the various degradative pathways of catabolism are convergent. That is, many hundreds of different proteins, polysaccharides and **lipids** are broken down into relatively few catabolic end products. The hundreds of anabolic pathways, however, are divergent. That is, the cell uses relatively few biosynthetic precursor molecules to synthesize a vast number of different proteins, polysaccharides and lipids.

The opposing pathways of anabolism and catabolism may also use different reaction intermediates or different enzymatic reactions in some of the steps. For example, there are 11 enzymatic steps in the breakdown of glucose into pyruvic acid in the **liver**. But the liver uses only nine of those same steps in the synthesis of glucose, replacing the other two steps with a different set of enzyme-catalyzed reactions. This occurs because the pathway to degradation of glucose releases energy, while the anabolic process of glucose synthesis requires energy. The two different reactions of anabolism are required to overcome the energy barrier that would otherwise prevent the synthesis of glucose.

Another reason for having slightly different pathways is that the corresponding anabolic and catabolic routes must be independently regulated. Otherwise, if the two phases of metabolism shared the exact pathway (only in reverse) a slowdown in the anabolic pathway would slow catabolism, and vice versa.

In addition to regulating the direction of metabolic pathways, cells, especially those in multicellular organisms, also exert control at three different levels: allosteric enzymes, hormones, and enzyme concentration.

Allosteric enzymes in metabolic pathways change their activity in response to molecules that either stimulate or inhibit their catalytic activity. While the end product of an enzyme cascade is used up, the cascade continues to synthesize that product. The result is a steady-state condition in which the product is used up as it is produced and there is no significant accumulation of product. However, when the product accumulates above the steady-state level for any reason, in excess of the cell's needs, the end product acts as an inhibitor of the first enzyme of the sequence. This process is called allosteric inhibition, and is a type of feedback inhibition.

A classic example of allosteric inhibition is the case of the enzymatic conversion of the amino acids: L-threonine into L-isoleucine by bacteria. The first of five enzymes, threonine dehydratase is inhibited by the end product, isoleucine. This inhibition is very specific, and is accomplished only by isoleucine, which binds to a site on the enzyme molecule called the regulatory, or allosteric, site. This site is different from the active site of the enzyme, which is the site of the catalytic action of the enzyme on the substrate, or molecule being acted on by the enzyme.

Some allosteric enzymes may be stimulated by modulator molecules. These molecules are not the end product of a series of reactions, but rather may be the substrate molecule itself. These enzymes have two or more substrate binding sites, which serve a dual function as both catalytic sites and regulatory sites. Such allosteric enzymes respond to excessive concentrations of substrates that must be removed. Also, some enzymes have two or more modulators with opposite effects and possess their own specific allosteric site. When occupied, one site may speed up the catalytic reaction, while the other may slow it down. ADP and AMP (adenosine monophosphate) stimulate certain metabolic pathway enzymes, for example, while ATP inhibits the same allosteric enzymes.

The activity of allosteric enzymes in one pathway may also be modulated by intermediate or final products from other pathways. Such cross-reaction is an important way in which the rates of different enzyme systems can be coordinated with each other.

Hormonal control of metabolism is regulated by chemical messengers secreted into the **blood** by different endocrine glands. These messengers, called hormones, travel to other tissues or organs, where they may stimulate or inhibit specific metabolic pathways.

A classic example of hormonal control of metabolism is the hormone adrenaline, which is secreted by the medulla of the adrenal gland and carried by the blood to the liver. In the liver, adrenaline stimulates the breakdown of glycogen to glucose, increasing the blood sugar level. In the **skeletal muscles**, adrenaline stimulates the breakdown of glycogen to lactate ATP.

Adrenaline exerts its effect by binding to a receptor site on the cell surfaces of liver and muscle cells. From there, adrenaline initiates a series of signals that ultimately causes an inactive form of the enzyme glycogen phosphorylase to become active. This enzyme is the first in a sequence that leads to the breakdown of glycogen to glucose and other products.

Finally, the concentration of the enzymes themselves exert a profound influence on the rate of metabolic activity. For example, the ability of the liver to turn enzymes on and off—a process called enzyme induction—assures that adequate amounts of needed enzymes are available, while inhibiting the cell from wasting its energy and other resources on making enzymes that are not needed.

For example, in the presence of a high-carbohydrate, low-protein diet, the liver enzymes that degrade amino acids are present in low concentrations. In the presence of a high-protein diet, however, the liver produces increased amounts of enzymes needed for degrading these molecules.

The basis of both anabolic and catabolic pathways is the reactions of reduction and oxidation. Oxidation refers to the combination of an atom or molecule with oxygen, or the loss from it of hydrogen or of one or more electrons. Reduction, the opposite of oxidation, is the gain of one or more electrons by an atom or molecule. The nature of these reactions requires them to occur together; i.e., oxidation always occurs in conjunction with reduction. The term "redox" refers to this coupling of reduction and oxidation.

Redox reactions form the basis of metabolism and are the basis of oxidative phosphorylation, the process by which electrons from organic substances such as glucose are transferred from organic compounds such as glucose to electron carriers (usually coenzymes), and then are passed through a series of different electron carriers to molecules of oxygen molecules. The transfer of electrons in oxidative phosphorylation occurs along the electron transport chain. During this process, called aerobic respiration, energy is released, some of which is used to make ATP from ADP. The major electron carriers are the coenzymes nicotinamide adenine dinucleotide (NADH) or flavin adenine dinucleotide ($FADH_2$). Oxidative phosphorylation is the major source of ATP in aerobic organisms, from bacteria to humans.

Some anaerobic bacteria, however, also carry out respiration, but use other inorganic molecules, such as nitrate (NO_3^-) or sulfate (SO_4^{2-}) ions as the final electron acceptors. In this form of respiration, called anaerobic respiration, nitrate is reduced to nitrite ion (NO_2^-), **nitrous oxide** (N_2O) or nitrogen gas (N_2), and sulfate is reduced to form hydrogen sulfide (H_2S).

Much of the metabolic activity of cells consists largely of central metabolic pathways that transform large amounts of proteins, fats and carbohydrates. Foremost among these pathways are glycolysis, which can occur in either aerobic or anaerobic conditions, and the Krebs cycle, which is coupled to the electron transport chain, which accepts electrons removed from reduced coenzymes of glycolysis and the Krebs cycle. The final electron acceptor of the chain is usually oxygen, but some bacteria use specific, oxidized ions as the final acceptor in anaerobic conditions.

As vital as these reactions are, there are other metabolic pathways in which the flow of substrates and products is much smaller, yet the products quite important. These pathways constitute secondary metabolism, which produces specialized molecules needed by the cell or by tissues or organs in small quantities. Such molecules may be coenzymes, hormones, nucleotides, toxins, or **antibiotics**.

The process of extracting energy by the central metabolic pathways that break down fats, polysaccharides and proteins, and conserving it as ATP, occurs in three stages in aerobic organisms. In anaerobic organisms, only one stage is present. In each case, the first step is glycolysis.

Metabolic pathways

Glycolysis is a ubiquitous central pathway of glucose metabolism among living things, from bacteria to plants and humans. The glycolytic series of reactions converts glucose into the molecule pyruvate, with the production of ATP. This pathway is controlled by both the concentration of substrates entering glycolysis as well as by feedback inhibition of the pathway's allosteric enzymes.

Glucose, a hexose (6-carbon) sugar, enters the pathway through phosphorylation of the number six carbon by the enzyme hexokinase. In this reaction, ATP relinquishes one of its phosphates, becoming ADP, while glucose is converted to glucose-6-phosphate. When the need for further oxidation of glucose-6-phosphate by the cell decreases, the concentration of this metabolite increases, as serves as a feedback inhibitor of the allosteric enzyme hexokinase. In the liver, however, glucose-6-phosphate is converted to glycogen, a storage form of glucose. Thus a buildup of glucose-6-phosphate is normal for liver, and feedback inhibition would interfere with this vital pathway. To produce glucose-6-phosphate, the liver must use the enzyme glucokinase, which is not inhibited by an increase in the concentration of glucose-6-phosphate.

In the liver and muscle cells, another enzyme, glycogen phosphorylase, breaks down glycogen into glucose molecules, which then enter glycolysis.

Two other allosteric enzyme regulatory reactions also help to regulate glycolysis: the conversion of fructose 6-phosphate to fructose 1,6-diphosphate by phosphofructokinase and the conversion of phosphoenolpyruvate to pyruvate by pyruvate kinase.

The first stage of glycolysis prepares the glucose molecule for the second stage, during which energy is conserved in the form of ATP. As part of the preparatory state, however, two ATP molecules are consumed.

At the fourth step of glycolysis, the doubly phosphorylated molecule (fructose 1,6-diphosphate) is cleaved into two 3-carbon molecules, dihyroxyacetone phosphate and glyceraldehyde 3-phosphate. These 3-carbon molecules are readily converted from one to another, however it is only glyceraldehyde 3-phosphate that undergoes five further changes during the energy conserving stage. In the first step of this second stage, a molecule of the coenzyme NAD^+ is reduced to NADH. During oxidative phosphorylation, the NADH will be oxidized, giving up its electrons to the electron transport system.

At steps seven and 10 of glycolysis, ADP is phosphorylated to ATP, using phosphate groups added to the original 6-carbon molecule in the preparatory stage. Since this phosphorylation of ADP occurs by enzymatic removal of a phosphate group from each of two substrates of glycolysis, this process is called substrate level phosphorylation of ADP. It differs markedly from the phosphorylation of ADP that occurs in the more complex oxidative phosphorylation processes in the electron transport chain. Since two three-carbon molecules derived from the original six-carbon hexose undergo this process, two molecules of ATP are formed from glucose during this stage, for a net overall gain of two ATP (two ATP having been used in the preparatory stage).

Aerobic organisms use glycolysis as the first stage in the complete degradation of glucose to carbon dioxide and water. During this process, the pyruvate formed by glycolysis is oxidized to acetyl-Coenzyme A (acetyl-CoA), with the loss of its carboxyl group as carbon dioxide.

The fate of pyruvate formed by glycolysis differs among species, and within the same species depending on the level of oxygen available for further oxidation of the products of glycolysis.

Under aerobic conditions, or in the case of bacteria using a non-oxygen final electron acceptor, acetyl-CoA, enters the Krebs cycle by combining with citric acid. The Krebs cycle continues the oxidation process, extracting electrons as it proceeds. The electrons are carried by coenzymes (NADH and FADH) to the electron transport chain, where the final reactions of oxidation produce ATP.

During these reactions, the acetyl group is oxidized completely to carbon dioxide and water by the citric acid cycle. This final oxidative degradation requires oxygen as the final electron acceptor in the electron transport chain.

Organisms that lack the enzyme systems necessary for oxidative phosphorylation also use glycolysis to produce pyruvate and a small amount of ATP. But pyruvate is then converted into lactate, ethanol or other organic alcohols or acids. This process is called fermentation, and oes not produce more ATP. The NADH produced during the energy-conserving stage of fermentation is used during the synthesis of other molecules. Thus, glycolysis is the major central pathway of glucose catabolism in virtually all organisms.

While the main function of glycolysis is to produce ATP, there are minor catabolic pathways that produce specialized products for cells. One, the pentose phosphate pathway, produces NADPH and the sugar ribose 5-phosphate. NADPH is used to reduce substrates in the synthesis of fatty acids, and ribose 5-phosphate is used in the synthesis of nucleic acids.

Another secondary pathway for glucose in animal tissues produces D-glucuronate, which is important in detoxifying and excreting foreign organic compounds and in synthesizing **vitamin C**.

Most of the energy conservation achieved by the oxidative phosphorylation of glucose occurs during the Krebs cycle. Pyruvate is first converted to acetyl-CoA, in an enzymatic step that converts one of its carbons into carbon dioxide, and NAD^+ is reduced to NADH. Acetyl-CoA enters the 8-step Krebs cycle by combining with the

4-carbon oxaloacetic acid to form the 6-carbon citric acid. During the next seven steps, three molecules of NAD^+ and one molecule of FAD^+ are reduced, one ATP is formed by substrate level phosphorylation, and two carbons are oxidized to CO_2.

The reduced coenzymes produced during conversion of pyruvic acid to acetyl-CoA and the Krebs cycle are oxidized along the electron transport chain. As the electrons released by the coenzymes pass through the stepwise chain of redox reactions, there is a stepwise release of energy that is ultimately used to phosphorylate molecules of ADP to ATP. The energy is converted into a gradient of protons established across the membrane of the bacterial cell or of the organelle of the eucaryotic cells. The energy of the proton flow back into the cell or organelle is used by the enzyme ATP synthetase to phosphorylate ADP molecules.

$FADH_2$ releases its electrons at a lower level along the chain than does NADH. The electrons of the former coenzyme thus pass along fewer electron acceptors than NADH, and this difference is reflected in the number of ATP molecules produced by the sequential transfer of each coenzymes electrons along the chain. The oxidation of each NADH produces three ATP, while the oxidation of $FADH_2$ produces two.

The total number of ATP produced by glycolysis and metabolism is 38, which includes a net of two from glycolysis (substrate level phosphorylation), 30 from the oxidation of 10 NADH molecules, four from oxidation of two $FADH_2$ molecules, and two from substrate level phosphorylation in the Krebs cycle.

In addition to their role in the catabolism of glucose, glycolysis and the Krebs cycle also participate in the breakdown of proteins and fats. Proteins are initially degraded into constituent amino acids, which may be converted to pyruvic acid or acetyl-CoA before being passed into the Krebs cycle; or they may enter the Krebs cycle directly after being converted into one of the metabolites of this metabolic pathway.

Lipids are first hydrolyzed into glycerol and fatty acids, glycerol being converted to the glyceraldehyde 3-phosphate metabolite of glycolysis, while fatty acids are degraded to acetyl-CoA, which then enters the Krebs cycle.

Although metabolic pathways in both single-celled and multicellular organisms have much in common, especially in the case of certain central metabolic pathways, they may occur in different locations.

In the simplest organisms, the prokaryotes, metabolic pathways are not contained in compartments separated by internal membranes. Rather, glycolysis takes place in

KEY TERMS

Coenzyme—A coenzyme is required for the enzyme to function.

Enzymes—Enzymes are protein catalysts that increase the speed of chemical reactions in the cell without themselves being changed.

Glycolysis—The major central pathway of glucose catabolism in virtually all organisms. The main function of glycolysis is to produce ATP.

Hormones—Hormones are messengers that travel to tissues or organs, where they may stimulate or inhibit specific metabolic pathways.

Oxidation—Oxidation refers to the combination of an atom or molecule with oxygen, or the loss from it of hydrogen or of one or more electrons.

Phenylketonuria (PKU)—A rare hereditary condition in which phenylalanine (an amino acid) is not properly metabolized. PKU may cause severe mental retardation.

Reduction—Reduction, the opposite of oxidation, is the gain of one or more electrons by an atom or molecule. The nature of these reactions requires them to occur together; i.e., oxidation always occurs in conjunction with reduction. The term "redox" refers to this coupling of reduction and oxidation.

the cytosol, while the electron transport chain and lipid synthesis occurs in the cell membrane. Proteins are made on ribosomes in the cytosol.

In eucaryotic cells, glycolysis, gluconeogenesis and fatty acid synthesis takes place in the cytosol, while the Krebs cycle is isolated within mitochondria; glycogen is made in glycogen granules, lipid is synthesized in the endoplasmic reticulum and lysosomes carry on a variety of hydrolytic activities. As in procaryotic cells, ribosomes in the cytosol are the site of protein synthesis.

Role in human health

All reactions of metabolism are part of the overall goal of the organism to maintain its internal order; whether the organism is a single celled protozoan or a human. Organisms maintain this order by removing energy from nutrients or sunlight and returning to their environment an equal amount of energy in a less useful form, mostly heat. This heat becomes dissipated throughout the rest of the organism's environment.

The metabolic pathways discussed oxidize organic matter to produce ATP in order to supply the body with the energy and nutrients it needs for maintenance of body functions, growth, tissue repair, and other processes.

Common diseases and disorders

There are a number of disorders affecting the metabolism. Inborn errors of metabolism (or human hereditary biochemical disorders) have genetic origins; these errors interfere with the synthesis including proteins, carbohydrates, fats enzymes, and many other substances in the body. If the abnormality with synthesis is severe, clinical and chemical consequences may result. Abnormalities in the breakdown, storage, or production of proteins, fats and carbohydrates or in the energy cycles of cells are typically the manifestation of this disorder. Disease and death may result from the absence or excess of normal or abnormal metabolites. Some examples of these inborn errors of metabolism are: galactosemia, phenylketonuria, lactose intolerance, and maple syrup urine disease. Many of these inborn errors of metabolism are untreatable. Some inborn errors of metabolism require dietary and/or nutrient modification depending on the specific metabolic error. Registered dietitians and physicians can assist the patient with the diet modifications needed for each disease.

A disorder with the **thyroid gland** may have an effect on metabolism. Thyroid hormones have an impact on growth, use of energy, and heat production as well as affecting the use of vitamins, proteins, carbohydrates, fats, electrolytes, and water. They can also alter the effect of other hormones and drugs. Hypothyroidism may result if there is a temporary or permanent reduction in thyroid hormone secretion. Treatment for this condition is most often successful and allows patients to live normally.

Resources

BOOKS

Greenspan, Francis S., and David G. Gardner, eds. *Basic & Clinical Endocrinology.* 6th ed. Stamford, CT: Appleton & Lange, 2000.

Salway, J. G. *Metabolism at a Glance.* 2nd ed. Oxford: Blackwell Science Inc., 1999.

PERIODICALS

Academic Press. *Molecular Genetics and Metabolism.* San Diego, CA: Harcourt Science and Technology Company. <http://www.apnet.com/www/journal/gm.htm>.

The Endocrine Society. *The Journal of Clinical Endocrinology & Metabolism* <http://jcem.endojournals.org/>.

ORGANIZATIONS

Center for Inherited Disorders of Energy Metabolism, Case Western Reserve University School of Medicine,

Cleveland, OH. <http://www.cwru.edu/2352896/med/CIDEM/cidem.htm>.

Metabolism Foundation, 622 Leatherwood Circle, Edmond, OK 73003. <http://www.metabolism.net>.

Society for Inherited Metabolic Disorders, incorporated through the State of Oregon, non-profit society. <http://www.simd.org>.

Society for the Study of Inborn Errors of Metabolism, Cardiff, Wales. <http://www.ssiem.org/uk/ssiemj.html>.

Crystal Heather Kaczkowski, MSc.

Methylcobalamin *see* **Vitamin B₁₂**

Microalbumin test *see* **Urinalysis**

Microscope

Definition

A microscope is an optical instrument consisting of a lens or combination of lenses for enlarging images of objects. It is typically used in a laboratory to view objects that are not visible to the naked eye.

Purpose

In health care, a microscope is used in a laboratory to determine the amount or number of analytes (measured substances) present in a specimen, such as **blood**, urine, or stool. Laboratory tests may be ordered for various reasons:

• to detect disease or to quantify the risk of future disease

• to establish or exclude a diagnosis

• to assess the severity of a disease

• to direct the selection of interventions

• to monitor the progress of a disorder

• to monitor the effectiveness of a treatment

Description

In health care, the most commonly used microscope to evaluate laboratory specimens is the compound microscope, a kind of light microscope (also known as an optical microscope). The compound microscope contains several lenses that magnify the image of a specimen. The lens located directly over the object is called the objective lens, and the lens closest to the eye is called the eyepiece. The total magnification is a product of the magnification of these two lenses-if the objective lens

magnifies 100-fold, and the eyepiece magnifies 10-fold, then the final magnification will be 1,000-fold. But enlarging the image of a specimen is not the only consideration for selection of a microscope. A key property of a microscope is its power of resolution—its ability to distinguish between two objects, such as two cells, positioned closely together. The resolving power of a microscope is denoted by the numerical aperature value (NA). The larger the number, the greater the resolution of the lens.

In addition to the eyepiece and objective there are several other components of a compound microscope that require adjustment by the user. The condenser is a lens that is located below the stage. Its purpose is to focus the light on the specimen. The iris diaphragm is located beneath the condenser. It can be closed to reduce the amount of peripheral light passing through the specimen. This is useful when viewing unstained cells because a narrow diaphragm adds contrast; however, if closed too much the brightness and resolution are reduced significantly. For most applications the iris diaphragm can be positioned correctly by closing it all the way, and then opening it until the black diaphragm is just beyond the field of view. The type of illumination used by most microscopes is called Koehler illumination. To use Koehler illumination the filament of the microscope lamp should be focused on the iris diaphram by moving the condenser lens. This will evenly distribute the light through the specimen.

In addition to the light microscope, there are several other types that are used for specific purposes. A brief description of those used in a clincial laboratory follows:

• Darkfield microscope. A darkfield microscope uses a special condenser that directs the light away from the objective unless it passes through the cell or object from the side. The background appears dark and the object light. The darkfield scope is used when examining unstained cells or objects. The most frequent clincial application is the examination of fluid from a genital chancre for the characteristic corkscrew shaped organism that causes **syphilis**, *Treponema pallidum*.

• The fluorescence microscope. Fluorescence is the emission of long wavelength light (visible light of a specific color) by compounds when excited by short wavelength (higher energy) light. Fluorescence microscopes are used to examine cells or objects stained with fluorescent dyes. They use an ultraviolet light source (mercury vapor lamp) to transmit short wavelength light through the specimen. The light passes through a darkfield condenser that blocks all light from the objective except rays that pass through the object. A barrier filter above the objective removes any residual ultravi-

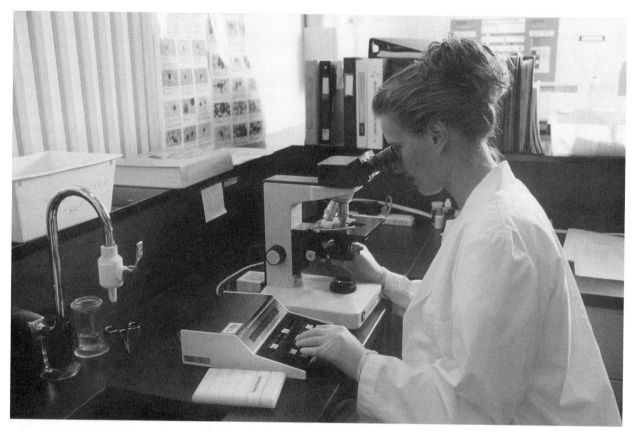

A lab technologist uses a microscope to examine blood films. *(Photograph by Carolyn A. McKeone. Science Source/Photo Researchers. Reproduced by permission.)*

olet light and transmits the wavelength emitted by the fluorochrome. This technique is used to identify antibodies attached to cell components. Because the background is dark and fluorescence dyes are more sensitive than other stains, it permits the detection of extremely low concentrations of antibody.

- An inverted microscope is one in which the light source is above the stage and the objectives are beneath the specimen rather than above it. This type of microscope is ideal for examining cells in tissue culture and for manipulating cells as is done in artificial reproductive procedures. The cell culture can be placed on the stage and the technologist can manipulate the cells because access to them is unobstructed.

- Phase contrast microscope. This type of microscope uses a condenser with a diaphragm inside that contains an annulus (ring cutout) in the center. The objective is constructed so that it diffracts the light transmitted through the annulus. When this light passes through the specimen, dense objects such as nuclei enhance this effect. Light from dense objects seem to reach the eye a fraction of a second later and the objects appears darker. Phase contrast makes it easier to distinguish dif-

ferent types of unstained cells and is preferred for **urinalysis**.

- Interference-contrast microscope. One disadvantage of phase contrast is that light is refracted from the edge of objects giving cells a halo. Interference-contrast microscopy uses polarizing filters and prisms to achieve the same effect as the annulus without the halo effect.

- Polarizing microscope. Some objects, such as certain crystals or minerals are able to change the direction (rotate) of light. This property is called birefringence and the object is said to be anisotropic. The polarizing microscope uses a polarizing filter beneath the stage. This transmits all the light from the lamp through the specimen in the same plane. A second polarizing filter called the analyzer is placed before the eyepiece so that it is out of phase with the substage polarizing filter. The analyzer blocks all of the light causing a dark background unless the object on the slide is anisotropic. Birefringent objects rotate the light so that it passes through the analyzer lens and the object appears light (white) against a dark background. This technique is used to identify uric acid needles in joint fluid from a patient with **gout**, since uric crystals are birefringent.

- The transmission electron microscope uses electromagnetic lenses, not optical lenses, that focus a high-velocity electron beam instead of visible light. A transmission electron microscope directs a beam of electrons through a specimen. Only a small piece of a cell can be observed in any one section. Generally, an electron microscope cannot be used to study live cells because they are too vulnerable to the required conditions and preparatory techniques. However, magnification can be achieved on the order of one thousand fold higher than a compound microscope.

Many medical tests require the use of a compound microscope for evaluation. These include:

- Biopsy. Tissue examined for **cancer** or other abnormalities.

- Blood cells. Identification of abnormal red and white blood cells, immature cells, and the different types of white cells.

- Bone marrow aspiration. Examination of marrow from hipbone or breastbone under a microscope for abnormalities of blood cell precursors and bone marrow tissue.

- Chorionic villus sampling. Examination of chromosomes of fetal cells under the microscope to determine if an abnormal number are present of if there is structural damage.

- Papanicolaou (Pap) test. Microscopic examination of cells scraped from the cervix to detect cancer.

- Microbiological exam. Microscopic examination of specimens (some normally sterile) for the presence of **bacteria**, parasites, yeast, and **fungi**. Most often this involves use of the **Gram stain** or acid-fast stain.

- Cytological exam of body fluids. Examination of urine, cerebrospinal fluid, pleural, pericardial, and synovial fluid for blood cells, malignant cells, crystals, bacteria, and other cells.

- Seminal fluid exam. The determination of sperm concentration, viability, and morphology (appearance).

Operation

After a specimen is prepared and placed on the microscope, the microscope is adjusted to change the magnification and focus the image. Precise mechanical adjustments are necessary to manipulate the objective and eyepiece, the substage condenser, iris diaphragm, and the object.

KEY TERMS

Condenser—A lens or system of lenses to collect light rays and converge them to a focus.

Electron microscope.—A device which beams electrons instead of light beams at and through an object. A powerful magnet is used to bend the electron beam (instead of a glass lens). This type of microscope provides the greatest resolution of extremely small details, such as individual atoms in an object or substance.

Eyepiece—The lens system nearest the eye which magnifies the primary image produced by the objective so as to form a secondary, virtual image 10 in (25 cm) away from the eyepoint.

Light microscope—A device that works by passing visible light through a condenser and an objective lens.

Objective—The lens system near the object which forms the primary inverted image.

Magnification—The apparent increase in size under the microscope.

Resolution—Degree of detail, ranging from low to high, determining the ability to distinguish between two objects positioned closely together.

Maintenance

The microscope should be kept covered when not in use. It should be cleaned, lubricated, and adjusted by a microscope technician at least once a year to conserve the life of the instrument. Lenses should be cleaned after each use taking care to remove any oil from the lens surface. When cleaning the lenses, use only lens paper to avoid scratching the lenses.

Health care team roles

Collection of a specimen for laboratory evaluation is typically done by a nurse or other health care practitioner. For example, venipuncture (puncture of a vein for the withdrawal of blood) may be performed by various members of the health care team. Although labs employ phlebotomists (individuals who perform venipuncture) to collect blood specimens, nurses must know how to perform this procedure because they routinely perform it in the home, in long-term care settings, and in hospital critical care units.

The nurse may inform the client about the reasons for the test, what to expect during the test, and any associated side effects or risks. The nurse should notify the practitioner of any client or family concerns not alleviated by discussions.

Assessment of the client for symptoms such as postpuncture bleeding or occlusion is the responsibility of a nurse or other allied health professional.

Training

Microscopes are usually used by pathologists, laboratory technologists, and technicians who evaluate specimens. Proper use of a microscope is part of training for nurses and other allied health care professionals.

Resources

BOOKS

Berkow, R., M. H. Beers, A. J. Fletcher and R. M. Bogin, eds. *The Merck Manual of Medical Information—Home Edition*. Whitehouse Station, NJ: Merck & Co, 2001.

White, Lois, ed. *Foundations of Nursing: Caring for the Whole Person*. Albany, NY: Delmar Thomson Learning, 2001.

ORGANIZATIONS

American Society of Clinical Pathologists. 2100 West Harrison Street, Chicago, IL 60612. (312) 738-1336. <http://www.ascp.org>.

Jennifer F. Wilson

Migraine headache

Definition

Migraine is a type of headache marked by severe head **pain** lasting several hours or more.

Description

A migraine is an intense, often debilitating type of headache. Migraines affect as many as 24 million people in the United States, and are responsible for approximately $17 billion in lost work, poor job performance, and direct medical costs. Approximately 18% of women and 6% of men experience at least one migraine attack per year. More than three million women and one million men have one or more severe headaches every month. Migraines often begin in adolescence, and are uncommon after age 60.

Two types of migraine are recognized. Eighty percent of migraine sufferers experience migraine without aura, formerly called common migraine. In migraine with aura, formerly called classic migraine, pain is preceded or accompanied by visual or other sensory disturbances, including hallucinations, partial obstruction of the visual field, numbness or tingling, or a feeling of heaviness. Symptoms are often more prominent on one side of the body, and may begin as early as 72 hours before the onset of pain.

Causes and symptoms

Causes

The physiological basis of migraine has proved difficult to uncover. Genetics appear to play a part for many, but not all, people with migraine. There are many potential triggers for a migraine attack, and discovering one's own set of triggers is often the key to prevention.

PHYSIOLOGY. The most widely accepted hypothesis suggests that a migraine attack is precipitated when pain-sensing nerve cells in the **brain** (called nociceptors) release chemicals called neuropeptides. Another brain chemical, a neurotransmitter called substance P, increases the pain sensitivity of nearby nociceptors. Neuropeptides act on the smooth muscle that surrounds cranial **blood vessels**. This smooth muscle regulates **blood** flow in the brain by relaxing or contracting, which dilates (enlarges) or constricts (narrows) the enclosed blood vessels.

At the onset of a migraine headache, neuropeptides are thought to cause muscle **relaxation**, which allows vessel dilation and increased blood flow. Other neuropeptides increase the leakiness of cranial vessels, allowing fluid leak, and promote inflammation and tissue swelling. The pain of migraine is thought to result from this combination of increased pain sensitivity, tissue and vessel swelling, and inflammation. The aura seen during a migraine may be related to constriction in the blood vessels that dilate in the headache phase.

GENETICS. Susceptibility to migraine may be inherited. A child of a migraine sufferer has as much as a 50% chance of developing migraine. If both parents are affected, the probability rises to 70%. However, the gene or genes responsible have not been identified, and many cases of migraine have no obvious familial basis. It is likely that whatever genes are involved set the stage for migraine, and that full development requires environmental influences as well.

TRIGGERS. A wide variety of foods, drugs, environmental cues, and personal events are known to trigger migraines. It is not known how most triggers set off the events of migraine, nor why individual migraine sufferers are affected by particular triggers but not others.

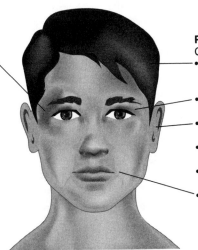

Phase 1 (The Prodrome): up to 24 hours prior to the headache
Roughly half of all migraine sufferers experience this stage, which is characterized by symptoms of heightened or dulled perception, irritability or withdrawal, and food cravings.

Phase 2 (The Aura): up to 1 hour prior to the headache
One out of five migraine sufferers experience this stage of visual disturbances. There may be flashing lights, shimmering zig-zag lines, and luminous blind spots, as well as non-visual sensations like numbness and pins and needles in the hands.

Phase 3 (The Headache): 4-72 hours long
Characterized by:
• Severe aching, often pulsating or throbbing pain on one or both sides of the head
• Intolerance of light (photophobia)
• Intolerance of noise (phonophobia)
• Nausea and vomiting
• Sensitivity to movement
• And less commonly, speech difficulties

Phase 4 (The Postdrome): up to 24 hours after the headache
Most migraine sufferers experience aching muscles and feel tired and drained after the headache, although some few go through a period of euphoria.

The phases of a typical migraine headache. *(Illustration by Hans & Cassidy.)*

Common food triggers include:
• aged cheese
• alcohol, especially red wine
• **caffeine** and caffeine withdrawal
• chocolate
• intensely sweet foods
• dairy products
• fermented or pickled foods
• citrus fruits
• nuts
• aspartame
• processed foods, especially those containing nitrites, sulfites, or monosodium glutamate (MSG)

Environmental and event-related triggers include:
• **stress** or time pressure
• menstrual periods, menopause
• sleep changes or disturbances, oversleeping
• prolonged overexertion or uncomfortable posture
• hunger or fasting
• odors, smoke, or perfume
• strong glare or flashing lights

Drugs that may trigger migraine include:
• oral contraceptives
• estrogen replacement therapy
• nitrates, often found in cured meats such as bacon and ham
• theophylline, an **asthma** drug
• reserpine, a tranquilizer
• nifedipine, a **calcium** channel blocker
• indomethacin, an NSAID
• cimetidine, a histamine H_2 antagonist
• decongestant overuse
• analgesic overuse
• benzodiazepine (a type of tranquilizer) withdrawal

Symptoms

Migraine without aura may be preceded by elevations in mood or energy level for up to 24 hours before the attack. Other premigraine symptoms may include fatigue, depression, and excessive yawning.

Aura most often begins with shimmering, jagged arcs of white or colored light progressing through the visual field over the course of 10–20 minutes. This may be preceded or replaced by dark areas or other visual disturbances. Numbness and tingling is common, especially of the face and hands. These sensations may spread, and may be accompanied by a sensation of weakness or heaviness in the affected limb.

The pain of migraine is often present only on one side of the head, although it may involve both, or switch sides during attacks. The pain is usually throbbing, and may range from mild to incapacitating. It is often accompanied by nausea or vomiting, painful sensitivity to light (photophobia) and sound (phonophobia), and intolerance of food or odors. Blurred **vision** is common.

Migraine pain tends to intensify over the first 30 minutes to several hours, and may last from several hours to a day or longer. Afterward, the affected person is usually weary, and sensitive to sudden head movements.

Diagnosis

Migraine is diagnosed by a careful medical history. Lab tests and imaging studies such as computed tomography (CT) or **magnetic resonance imaging** (MRI) scans have not been useful for identifying migraine. However, for some patients, those tests may be needed to rule out a **brain tumor** or other structural causes of migraine headache.

Treatment

Once a migraine begins, the person will usually seek out a dark, quiet room to lessen painful stimuli. Several drugs may be used to reduce the pain and severity of the attack, and many people with migraines learn to prevent attacks altogether by recognizing and avoiding their triggers.

Nonsteroidal anti-inflammatory drugs (NSAIDs) are helpful for early and mild headache. NSAIDs include acetaminophen, ibuprofen, naproxen, and others. A recent study concluded that a combination of acetaminophen, aspirin, and caffeine could effectively relieve symptoms for many migraine patients. One such over-the-counter preparation is Excedrin Migraine.

More severe or unresponsive attacks may be treated with drugs that act on serotonin receptors in the smooth muscle surrounding cranial blood vessels. Serotonin, also known as 5-hydroxytryptamine, constricts these vessels, relieving migraine pain. Drugs that mimic serotonin and

bind to these receptors have the same effect. The oldest of them is ergotamine, a derivative of a common grain fungus. Ergotamine and dihydroergotamine are used for both acute relief and preventive treatment. Derivatives with fewer side effects have come onto the market in the past decade, including sumatriptan (Imitrex). Some of these drugs are available as nasal sprays, intramuscular injections, or rectal suppositories for patients in whom vomiting precludes oral administration. Other drugs used for acute attacks include meperidine (Demerol) and metoclopramide (Reglan).

Continued use of some antimigraine drugs can lead to "rebound headache," marked by frequent or chronic headaches, especially in the early morning hours. This can be avoided by using antimigraine drugs under a health care provider's supervision, with the minimum dose necessary to treat symptoms. Patients with frequent migraines may need preventive therapy.

Alternative treatments are aimed at prevention. Since migraines are often linked with food **allergies** or intolerances, identifying and eliminating the offending food or foods can decrease the frequency of migraines and/or alleviate these headaches altogether. Herbal therapy with feverfew (Chrysanthemum parthenium) may lessen the frequency of attacks. Learning to increase the flow of blood to the extremities through biofeedback training may allow a patient to prevent some of the vascular changes once a migraine begins. Relaxation using focused breathing techniques can also be useful. During a migraine, keep the lights low; put the feet in a tub of hot water and place a cold cloth on the occipital region (the back of the head). This draws the blood to the feet and decreases the pressure in the head.

Prognosis

Most people with migraines can bring their attacks under control by recognizing and avoiding their triggers, and by using the appropriate drugs when migraines occur. There are, unfortunately, some people with severe migraines that do not respond to either preventive or drug therapy. Migraines usually wane in intensity after age 60.

Health care team roles

The advanced practice nurse (APN) can play a pivotal role in helping patients control migraine symptoms. One of the most important screening questions for a patient with a headache is "Do you think that this is the worst headache you have ever had?" If the answer is yes, a more thorough diagnostic work up is justified in order to rule out any tumor or brain bleed. Imaging studies, like

CT and/or MRI scanning, which are performed by a radiologist technician, should be considered.

The APN must recognize that many people with migraines are underdiagnosed and unhappy with the practitioner's treatment plan. Knowing this will help the APN focus on both quick pain relief methods and complementary therapies.

The **registered nurse** (RN) and **licensed practical nurse** (LPN) can also contribute to a patient's successful migraine management by reinforcing the concept of rapid medication administration at the initial onset of migraine symptoms.

Patient education

The importance of teaching patients about their migraine medications and any potential side effects cannot be overstated. Explaining the expected time frame for relief before administering the next medication is helpful. Nurses can also advise patients about nonpharmacological interventions that may also be beneficial for migraine sufferers. Finally, the RN or LPN can demonstrate breathing relaxation techniques for patient to reinforce their proper use and understanding.

Prevention

The frequency of migraine may be lessened by avoiding triggers. It is useful to keep a headache journal, recording the particulars and noting possible triggers for each attack. Specific measures which may help include:

- eating at regular times, and not skipping meals
- reducing the use of caffeine and pain relievers
- restricting physical exertion, especially on hot days
- keeping regular sleep hours, but not oversleeping
- managing time to avoid stress at work and home

Some drugs can be used for migraine prevention, including specific members of these drug classes:

- beta blockers
- tricyclicantidepressants
- calcium channel blockers
- anticonvulsants
- fluoxetine (Prozac)
- monoamine oxidase inhibitors (MAOIs)
- serotonin antagonists

For most patients, preventive drug therapy is not an appropriate option, since it requires continued use of powerful drugs. However, for women whose migraines coincide with their menstrual periods, limited preventive

---

KEY TERMS

Migraine—A type of headache marked by severe head pain lasting several hours or more.

Neuropeptide—A peptide (chemical derived from protein) that affects nerves and their functions. Endorphins and enkephalins are neuropeptides.

Neurotransmitter—Chemical produced by nerve cells that sends an impulse across a synapse to a muscle, organ, or another nerve cell. Norepinephrine and acetylcholine are types of neurotransmitters.

Nociceptors—Nerve cells in the brain that are responsible for the sensation of pain.

Photophobia—Sensitivity to light.

Phonophobia—Sensitivity to sound.

---

treatment may be effective. Since these drugs are appropriate for patients with other medical conditions, the decision to prescribe them for migraine may be influenced by expected benefit elsewhere.

Resources

PERIODICALS

Clinch, C. Randall. "Evaluation of Acute Headaches in Adults." *American Family Physician* 63 (February, 2001): 685–692.

Kunkel, Robert. "Managing Primary Headache Syndromes." *Patient Care* 34 (January, 2000): 100 ff.

Lipton, Richard B. "Sumatriptan for the Range of Headaches in Migraine Sufferers: Results of the Spectrum Study." *Headache* 40 (2000): 783–791.

Scholz, Mary. "Treatment Options for Acute Migraine." *RN* 63 (October, 2000): 99.

OTHER

American Medical Association. Journal of the American Medical Association: Migraine Information Center. <http://www.ama-assn.org/special/migraine/>.

Matchar, David B., Douglas C. McCrory, and Rebecca N. Gray. "Toward Evidence-Based Management of Migraines." <http://jama.ama-assn.org/issues/v284n20/ffull/jed00081.html>. (April 27, 2001).

Lori Beck

Milk of magnesia *see* **Antacids**

Mineral deficiency

Definition

Mineral deficiency describes a condition in which the concentration of any one of the **minerals** essential to human health is abnormally low in the body. In some cases, an abnormally low mineral concentration is defined as that which leads to an impairment in a function dependent on the mineral. In other cases, an abnormally low mineral concentration signifies a lower level than that found in a specific healthy population.

Mineral nutrients are the inorganic elements or inorganic molecules required for life. As far as human **nutrition** is concerned, the inorganic nutrients include water, sodium, potassium, chloride, **calcium**, phosphate, sulfate, magnesium, **iron**, **copper**, **zinc**, manganese, iodine, selenium, and molybdenum. Some of the inorganic nutrients, such as water, do not occur as single atoms, but occur as molecules. Other inorganic nutrients that are molecules include phosphate, sulfate, and selenite. Phosphate contains an atom of **phosphorus**. Sulfate contains an atom of sulfur. Humans do not need to eat sulfate, since the body can acquire all the sulfate it needs from protein. Selenium occurs in foods as selenite and selenate.

The mineral content of the body can be measured by testing samples of **blood** plasma, red blood cells, or urine. In the case of calcium and phosphate deficiency, the diagnosis may also involve taking x rays of the skeleton. In the case of iodine deficiency, the diagnosis may include examining the patient's neck with the eyes and hands. In the case of iron deficiency, the diagnosis may include the performance of a stair-stepping test by the patient. Since all the minerals serve strikingly different functions in the body, the tests for the corresponding deficiency are markedly different from each other.

Description

Laboratory studies with animals have revealed that severe deficiencies in any one of the inorganic nutrients can result in very specific symptoms, and finally in death, due to the failure of functions associated with that nutrient. In humans, deficiency in one nutrient may occur less often than deficiency in several nutrients. A patient suffering from malnutrition is deficient in a variety of nutrients. In the United States, malnutrition is most often found among severe alcoholics. In part, this is because the alcohol consumption may supply half of the energy requirement, resulting in a mineral and vitamin intake of half the expected level. Deficiencies in one nutrient do occur, for example, in human populations living in iodine-poor regions of the world, and in iron deficient persons who lose excess iron by bleeding.

Inorganic nutrients have a great variety of functions in the body. Water, sodium, and potassium deficiencies are most closely associated with abnormal nerve action and cardiac arrhythmias. Deficiencies in these nutrients tend to result not from a lack of content in the diet, but from excessive fluid and electrolyte losses due to severe **diarrhea** and other causes. Iodine deficiency is a global **public health** problem. It occurs in parts of the world with iodine-deficient soils, and results in goiter, which involves a relatively harmless swelling of the neck, and cretinism, a severe birth defect. The only use of iodine in the body is for making thyroid hormone. However, since thyroid hormone has a variety of roles in development of the embryo, iodine deficiency during **pregnancy** results in a number of birth defects.

Calcium from the diet is absorbed in the gastrointestinal tract while the excess is excreted in the urine. A minimum of 500–1000 mg of calcium is required daily in order to maintain a normal calcium concentration. Normally, the body transfers calcium to the blood from the bones to maintain calcium homeostasis. If calcium intake falls short of requirement, too much calcium will be mobilized from the bones, weakening the bones and contributing to **osteoporosis**.

Dietary phosphate deficiency is rare because phosphate is plentiful in plant and animal foods, but also because phosphate is efficiently absorbed from the diet into the body.

Iron deficiency causes anemia (lack of red blood cells), which results in tiredness and shortness of breath.

Dietary deficiencies in the remaining inorganic nutrients tend to be rare. Magnesium deficiency is uncommon, but when it occurs it tends to occur in chronic alcoholics, in persons taking diuretic drugs, and in those suffering from severe and prolonged diarrhea. Magnesium deficiency tends to occur with the same conditions that provoke deficiencies in sodium and potassium. Zinc deficiency is found primarily in impoverished populations in the Middle East, who rely on unleavened whole wheat bread as a major food source. Copper deficiency is rare but dramatic, and health-threatening changes in copper **metabolism** occur in two genetic diseases, Wilson's disease and Menkes' disease.

Selenium deficiency may occur in regions of the world where the soils are poor in selenium. Low-selenium soils can produce foods that are also low in selenium. **Premature infants** may also be at risk for selenium deficiency.

Causes and symptoms

Sodium deficiency

Sodium deficiency (hyponatremia) and water imbalances (**dehydration**) are the most serious and widespread deficiencies in the world. These electrolyte deficiencies tend to arise from excessive losses from the body, as during prolonged and severe diarrhea or vomiting. Diarrheal diseases are a major world health problem, and are responsible for about a quarter of the 10 million infant deaths that occur each year. Nearly all of these deaths occur in impoverished parts of Africa and Asia, where they result from contamination of the water supply by animal and human feces.

The main concern in treating diarrheal diseases is dehydration, that is, the losses of sodium and water which deplete the fluids of the circulatory system (the **heart**, veins, arteries, and capillaries). Severe losses of the fluids of the circulatory system result in **shock**. Shock nearly always occurs when dehydration is severe enough to produce a 10% reduction in body weight. Shock, which is defined as inadequate supply of blood to the various tissues of the body, results in a lack of oxygen to all the cells of the body. Although diarrheal fluids contain a number of electrolytes, the main concern in avoiding shock is the replacement of sodium and water.

Sodium deficiency also frequently results during treatment with drugs called diuretics. Diuretics cause a loss of sodium from the body. These drugs are used to treat high **blood pressure** (**hypertension**), where the resulting decline in blood pressure reduces the risk for cardiovascular disease. However, diuretics can lead to sodium deficiency, resulting in low plasma sodium levels. Hyponatremia occurs in approximately 1% of all hospital admissions and is especially problematic in the elderly.

Potassium deficiency

Potassium plays a major part in cell metabolism and in nerve and muscle cell function. Most of the body's potassium is located in the cells. Too high or low concentrations of blood potassium can have serious effects such as an abnormal heart rhythm or cardiac arrest. Like other electrolytes, potassium balance is regulated through gastrointestinal tract absorption of food, while excretion is controlled by the kidney.

A low potassium blood level is referred to as hypokalemia. Hypokalemia is common in the elderly. Common causes include decreased intake of potassium during acute illness, nausea and vomiting, and treatment with diuretics. Since several foods contain potassium, hypokalemia is not typically due to a low intake. It is usually due to malfunction of the **kidneys** or abnormal loss through the gastrointestinal tract. People with heart disease have to be especially cautious regarding hypokalemia (particularly when taking digoxin), because they are prone to developing abnormal rhythms. A side effect of some diuretics is excessive loss of potassium, therefore, hypokalemia may result.

High sources of potassium are:

- bananas
- melons
- tomatoes
- oranges
- potatoes and sweet potatoes
- green leafy vegetables such as spinach, turnip greens, collard greens, kale, etc.
- most peas and beans
- potassium supplements
- salt substitutes (potassium chloride)

Calcium and phosphate deficiency

Calcium and phosphate are closely related nutrients. About 99% of the calcium and 85% of the phosphate in the body occur in the skeleton, where they exist as crystals of solid calcium phosphate. Conditions such as growth, pregnancy, and **lactation** are associated with increased phosphate requirements.

The body's calcium reserves are predominantly stored in bones although the blood and cells also contain calcium. Calcium is necessary for proper functioning in many areas of the body including nerve conduction, **muscle contraction**, and enzyme functions. Like other electrolytes, calcium levels are controlled both in blood and cells. A low calcium blood level is referred to as hypocalcemia. Hypocalcemia can result from a number of problems. The most common reason is an inability to mobilize calcium from the bones or a chronic loss of calcium in the urine.

Other causes of hypocalcemia include:

- low blood albumin concentration
- hypoparathyroidism
- **vitamin D** deficiency
- renal failure
- magnesium depletion
- acute pancreatitis
- hypoproteinemia (low blood protein)
- septic shock

- hyperphosphatemia (high blood phosphate levels)
- drugs such as those used to treat hypercalcemia or anti-convulsants
- excessive secretion of calcitonin

An abnormally low blood calcium concentration may not produce any symptoms. However, over time, the lack of calcium in the blood can affect **brain** function, causing neurologic symptoms such as **memory** loss, depression, confusion, delirium, and hallucinations. Once calcium levels return to normal, these symptoms are reversible. Very severe cases of hypocalcemia can lead to seizures, tetany, and muscle spasms in the throat, affecting breathing.

Calcium deficiency due to vitamin D deficiency can be found among certain populations. Vitamin D is required for the efficient absorption of calcium from the diet, and hence vitamin D deficiency in growing infants and children can result in calcium deficiency. The body can produce Vitamin D with sun exposure. Vitamin D deficiency can be found among young infants, the elderly, and others who may be shielded from sunshine for prolonged periods of time. Vitamin D deficiency impairs the absorption of calcium from the diet, and in this way can provoke calcium deficiency even when the diet contains adequate calcium.

Both calcium and phosphate occur in a great variety of foods, but many men, and women in particular, consume less than the required amount of calcium daily. Men over 65 years, postmenopausal women, and women who are lactating tend to be in negative calcium balance, and thus calcium is drawn from the bones to maintain calcium homeostatis. Milk, eggs, and green, leafy vegetables are rich in calcium and phosphate. Whole cow milk, for example, contains about 1.2 g calcium and 0.95 g phosphorus per 2.2 lbs (1 kg) of food. Broccoli contains 1.0 g calcium and 0.67 g phosphorus per 2.2 lbs (1 kg) of food. Meat, poultry, and fish are also high in phosphorus (phosphate).

Iodine deficiency

Iodine deficiency tends to occur in regions of the world where the soil is poor in iodine. Where soil used in agriculture is low in iodine, the foods grown in the soil will also be iodine poor. An iodine intake of 0.10–0.15 mg/day is considered to be nutritionally adequate, while iodine deficiency occurs at below 0.05 mg/day. Goiter, an enlargement of the **thyroid gland** (located in the neck), results from iodine deficiency. Goiter continues to be a problem in eastern Europe, parts of India and South America, and in Southeast Asia. Goiter has been eradicated in the United States because of the fortification of foods with iodine. Iodine deficiency during pregnancy results in cretinism in the newborn. Cretinism involves mental retardation, a large tongue, and sometimes deafness, muteness, and lameness.

Iron deficiency

Iron deficiency occurs due to periods of dietary deficiency, rapid growth, and excessive loss of the body's iron. Human milk and cow milk both contain low levels of iron. Infants are at risk for iron deficiency because their rapid rate of growth needs a corresponding increased supply of dietary iron, for use in making blood and muscles. Human milk is a better source of iron than cow milk, since about half of the iron in human breast milk is absorbed by the infant's digestive tract. In contrast, only 10% of the iron in cow milk is absorbed by the infant. Surveys of lower-income families in the United States have revealed that about 6% of the infants are anemic indicating a deficiency of iron in their diets. Blood loss that occurs with menstruation in women, as well as with a variety of causes of intestinal bleeding, is a major cause of iron deficiency. The symptoms of iron deficiency are generally limited to anemia, and the resulting tiredness, weakness, and a reduced ability to perform physical work.

Magnesium deficiency

Magnesium influences the function of many enzymes. Dietary intake is essential to maintain normal levels. The body's magnesium stores are predominately found in bone with little appearing in the blood. Excess is excreted in the urine or stool.

Magnesium deficiency results in hypomagnesemia, which is defined as serum magnesium levels below 0.8 mmol/L. Normal blood serum magnesium levels are 1.2–2.0 mmol/L. Some of the symptoms of hypomagnesemia, which include twitching and convulsions, actually result from hypocalcemia. Other symptoms of hypomagnesemia, such as cardiac arrhythmias, result from low potassium levels. Metabolic and nutritional disorders are usually the culprit of hypomagnesemia, most often when intake of magnesium is decreased during starvation or intestinal malabsorption compounded with greater kidney excretion. Magnesium levels below 0.5 mmol/L provoke a decline in serum calcium levels. Hypomagnesemia can also result in low serum potassium.

Zinc deficiency

Zinc deficiency has been found among peasant populations in rural areas of the Middle East. Unleavened whole wheat bread can account for 75% of the energy intake in these areas. This diet, which does not contain meat, does contain zinc, but it also contains phytic acid at a level of about 3 g/day. The phytic acid, which naturally occurs in wheat, inhibits zinc absorption. The yeast used to leaven bread produces enzymes that inactivate the phytic acid. Unleavened bread does not contain yeast, and therefore, contains intact phytic acid. The symptoms of zinc deficiency include lack of sexual maturation, lack of pubic hair, and small stature. The amount of phytic acid in a typical American diet cannot provoke zinc deficiency.

Zinc deficiency is relatively uncommon in healthy adults in the United States, but often occurs in adults with **alcoholism** or intestinal malabsorption problems. Zinc levels also may be problematic in the elderly, pregnant women, diabetics, **AIDS** patients, and those with chronic infections and/or trauma. Low plasma zinc has been found in patients with alcoholic cirrhosis, **Crohn's disease**, and celiac disease. Experimental studies with humans have shown that the signs of zinc deficiency are detectable after two to five weeks of consumption of the zinc-free diet. The signs include a rash and diarrhea. The rash occurs on the face, groin, hands, and feet. These symptoms can easily be reversed by administering zinc. Absorption of zinc is largely dependent on the presence or absence of other foods that affect zinc absorption. Meats, **liver**, eggs, and seafoods are good choices of zinc because these foods do not contain many other components which interfere with zinc absorption. An emerging concern is that increased calcium intake can interfere with zinc absorption or retention. Hence, there is some interest in the question of whether persons taking calcium to prevent osteoporosis should also take zinc supplements.

Copper deficiency

Copper deficiency is relatively uncommon but severe alterations in copper metabolism occur in two genetic diseases, Wilson's disease and Menkes' disease. Both of these diseases are rare. Menkes' disease occurs in about one in 50,000 to 100,000 births while Wilson's disease occurs in approximately one in 200,000 births in the United States. Both diseases involve mutations in copper transport **proteins**, that is, in special channels that allow the passage of copper ions through **cell membranes**. Menkes' disease is a genetic disease involving mental retardation and death before the age of three years. The disease also results in steely or kinky hair. The hair is tangled, grayish, and easily broken. Menkes' disease involves a decrease in copper levels in the serum, liver, and brain, and increases in copper in the cells of the intestines and kidney.

The richest sources of copper are shellfish, nuts, seeds, cocoa powder, liver, organ meats, legumes, and the germ and bran portions of grains.

Selenium deficiency

Selenium deficiency may occur in premature infants, since this population naturally tends to have low levels of plasma selenium. Full term infants have plasma selenium levels of about 0.001–0.002 mmol/L, while premature infants may have levels about one third this amount. Whether these lower levels result in adverse consequences is not clear. Total parental nutrition often leads to selenium deficiency if it is not administered in the fluids. Selenium deficiency occurs in regions of the world containing low-selenium soils. These regions include Keshan Province in China, New Zealand, and Finland. In Keshan Province, a disease (Keshan disease) occurs which results in deterioration of regions of the heart and the development of fibers in these regions. Keshan disease, which may be fatal, is thought to result from a combination of selenium deficiency and a virus.

The richest sources of selenium are organ meats and seafood. In addition, muscle meats, cereals and grains, dairy products, and fruits and vegetables provide good sources of selenium.

Other ultratrace mineral deficiencies

Manganese deficiency is very rare. Experimental studies with humans fed a manganese deficient diet have revealed that the deficiency produces a scaly, red rash on the skin of the upper torso. The importance of manganese in human nutrition still needs to be established. It is thought that the possibility in becoming manganese deficient is increased in alcohol abusers. Molybdenum deficiency has probably never occurred, but indirect evidence suggests that if molybdenum deficiency could occur, it would result in mental retardation and death

There is some evidence that other inorganic nutrients, such as chromium and boron, play a part in human health, but their role is not well established. Chromium has a function related to insulin and thus influences carbohydrate, lipid, and protein metabolism. Boron is believed to affect macromineral metabolism in humans. Fluoride has been proven to increase the strength of bones and teeth, but there is little or no reason to believe that is needed for human life.

Diagnosis

The diagnosis of deficiencies in water, sodium, potassium, iron, calcium, and phosphate involve chemical testing of the blood plasma, urine, and red blood cells.

KEY TERMS

Dehydration—A deficit of body water that results when the output of water exceeds intake.

Diuretic—An agent or drug that eliminates excessive water in the body by increasing the flow of urine.

Electrolyte—A substance such as an acid, bases, or salt. An electrolyte's water solution will conduct an electric current and ionizes. Calcium, potassium, magnesium, and sodium are electrolytes.

Homeostatis—An organism's regulation of body processes to maintain internal equilibrium in temperature and fluid content.

Recommended Dietary Allowance—The Recommended Dietary Allowances (RDAs) are quantities of nutrients that are required each day to maintain human health. RDAs are established by the Food and Nutrition Board of the National Academy of Sciences and may be revised every few years. A separate RDA value exists for each nutrient. In 2001, the RDA will be replaced by the Dietary Reference Intakes (DRI) and will apply to Americans and Canadians.

Hypocalcemia is usually first discovered during routine blood tests because often there are no symptoms evident.

Iodine deficiency can be diagnosed by measuring the concentration of iodine in the urine. A urinary level greater than 0.05 mg iodine per gram creatinine means adequate iodine status. Levels under 0.025 mg iodine/g creatinine indicate a serious risk.

There is no reliable test for zinc deficiency. When humans eat diets containing normal levels of zinc (16 mg/day), the level of urinary zinc is about 0.45 mg/day, while humans consuming low-zinc diets (0.3 mg/day) may have urinary levels of about 0.150 mg/day. Plasma zinc levels tend to be maintained during a dietary deficiency in zinc. Plasma and urinary zinc levels can be influenced by a variety of factors, and for this reason cannot provide a clear picture of zinc status.

Selenium deficiency may be diagnosed by measuring the selenium in plasma (70 ng/mL) or red blood cells (90 ng/mL), where the normal values are indicated. There is also some interest in measuring the activity of an enzyme in blood platelets, in order to assess selenium status. This enzyme is glutathione peroxidase. Platelets are small cells of the bloodstream which are used mainly to allow the clotting of blood after an injury.

Treatment

The treatment of deficiencies in sodium, potassium, calcium, phosphate, and iron often involves intravenous injections of the deficient mineral. Potassium, however, usually can be replaced relatively easily by eating foods rich in potassium or by taking potassium salts (potassium chloride) orally.

Iodine deficiency can be easily prevented and treated by fortifying foods with iodine. Table salt is fortified with 100 mg potassium iodide per kg sodium chloride. Goiter was once common in the United States in areas from Washington State to the Great Lakes region, but this problem has been eliminated by iodized salt. Public health programs in impoverished countries have administered injections of synthetic oils containing iodine. Goiter is reversible, but cretinism is not.

Magnesium deficiency can be treated with a magnesium rich diet. If magnesium deficiency is due to a prolonged period of depletion, treatment may include injections of magnesium sulfate (2.0 mL of 50% $MgSO_4$). Where magnesium deficiency is severe enough to provoke convulsions, magnesium needs to be administered by injections or infusions. For infusion, 500 mL of a 1% solution (1 gram/100 mL) of magnesium sulfate is gradually introduced into a vein over the course of about five hours. When hypomagnesemia occurs along with hypocalcemia, the magnesium must be replaced before successful treatment of the calcium disorder.

Zinc deficiency and copper deficiency are quite uncommon, but when they are detected or suspected, they can be treated by consuming zinc or copper, on a daily basis, at levels defined by the RDA.

Selenium deficiency in adults can be treated by eating 100 mg selenium per day for a week, where the selenium is supplied as selenomethionine. The incidence of Keshan disease in China has been reduced by supplementing children with 1.0 mg sodium selenite per week.

Prognosis

In iodine deficiency, the prognosis for treating goiter is excellent, however cretinism cannot be reversed. The effects of iron deficiency are not life-threatening and can be easily treated. The prognosis for treating magnesium deficiency is excellent. The symptoms may be relieved promptly or, at most, within two days of starting treatment. In cases of zinc deficiency in Iran and other parts of the Middle East, supplementation of affected young adults with zinc has been found to provoke the growth of pubic hair and enlargement of genitalia to a normal size within a few months.

Health care team roles

Mineral deficiencies are normally diagnosed and treated by physicians. Dieticians may be employed in efforts of **patient education**. For example, the dietetician may counsel a patient about a healthy diet to prevent further deficiencies, or be involved in community programs to educate the public at large.

Prevention

In the healthy population, all mineral deficiencies can be prevented by the consumption of inorganic nutrients at levels defined by the Recommended Dietary Allowances (RDA) or Dietary Reference Intakes (DRI). Where a balanced diet is not available, government programs for treating individuals, or for fortifying the food supply, may be used. Government sponsored programs for the prevention of iron deficiency and iodine deficiency are widespread throughout the world. Selenium treatment programs have been used in parts of the world where selenium deficiency exists. Attention to potassium status, and to the prevention of potassium deficiency, is an issue mainly in patients taking diuretic drugs. In many cases of mineral deficiency, the deficiency occurs because of disease, and individual medical attention, rather than preventative measures, is used. Calcium supplements are widely used with the hope of preventing osteoporosis. The prevention of deficiencies in magnesium, copper, manganese, or molybdenum are not major health issues in the United States. Ensuring an adequate intake of these minerals, by eating a balanced diet or by taking mineral supplements, is the best way to prevent deficiencies.

Resources

BOOKS

Brody, Tom. *Nutritional Biochemistry*. San Diego: Academic Press, 1998.

Institute of Medicine, ed. *Dietary Reference Intakes: Risk Assessment (Compass Series)*. Washington: National Academy Press, 1999.

Larson-Duyff, Roberta. *The American Dietetic Association's Complete Food & Nutrition Guide*. New York: John Wiley & Sons, 1998.

Murray, Michael T. *Encyclopedia of Nutritional Supplements: The Essential Guide for Improving Your Health Naturally*. Rocklin, CA: Prima Publishing, 2001.

National Academy Press Food and Nutrition Board *Recommended Dietary Allowances, 10th edition*. Washington: National Academy Press, 1989.

PERIODICALS

Foote, J. A., A. R. Giuliano, and R. B. Harris. "Older adults need guidance to meet nutritional recommendations." *Journal of the American College of Nutrition* 19, no. 5 (Oct. 2000): 628-40.

Fryer, M. J. "Selenium and human health." *Lancet* 356, no. 9233 (Sept. 9, 2000): 943.

Lonnerdal, B. "Dietary factors influencing zinc absorption." *Journal of Nutrition* 130, no. 5S Suppl (May 2000): 1378S-83S.

Rayman, M. P. "The importance of selenium to human health." *Lancet* 356, no. 9225 (Jul 15, 2000): 233-41.

ORGANIZATIONS

American Dietetic Association. 216 W. Jackson Blvd. Chicago, IL 60606-6995. (312) 899-0040. <http://www.eatright.org/>.

Food and Nutrition Information Center Agricultural Research Service, USDA. National Agricultural Library, Room 304, 10301 Baltimore Avenue, Beltsville, MD 20705-2351. (301) 504-5719. Fax (301) 504-6409. <http://www.nal.usda.gov/fnic/>. fnic@nal.usda.gov.

OTHER

Food and Nutrition Professionals Network. <http://nutrition.cos.com/>.

Crystal Heather Kaczkowski, MSc.

Minerals

Definition

Minerals are naturally occurring inorganic substances that are obtained from food and perform a range of important functions in the body. Minerals are categorized as major minerals, or macronutrients, which are present in the body in amounts greater than five grams; and trace minerals, which are present in amounts below five grams. Trace minerals are sometimes called micronutrients.

Description

Major minerals

The major minerals consist of **calcium, phosphorus**, potassium, sulfur, sodium, chloride, and magnesium. Sodium, potassium, and chloride are sometimes grouped together as electrolytes. An electrolyte is a substance that breaks down into ions when it is dissolved in a suitable medium and thus becomes a conductor of electricity. Each of the major minerals aids in maintaining the body's fluid, electrolyte, and **acid-base balance** as well as having specific functions.

CALCIUM. Calcium is the most abundant mineral in the human body; 99% of it is stored in the bones and teeth. Calcium maintains bone structure and helps regulate **blood** calcium levels. This mineral is also necessary for the transport of electrical ions across **cell membranes**. Inadequate calcium intake during childhood and adulthood can result in **osteoporosis**, in which there is loss of bone substance. Many Americans do not get enough calcium in their diets. Good dietary sources of calcium include milk, broccoli, mustard greens, kale, cheese, and sardines. The recommended dietary allowance (RDA) of calcium for adults is about 800 mg.

PHOSPHORUS. Phosphorus is also an abundant mineral. Most of the phosphorus—about 80%—that occurs in the body is combined with calcium in the bones and teeth. Phosphorus plays a role in the energy **metabolism** of cells; helps maintain the body's acid-base balance; and is needed for tissue growth and renewal. Animal products that are high in protein, such as milk, cottage cheese, and steak, are excellent sources of phosphorus. Deficiencies of phosphorus are rare except in patients taking **antacids** for long periods of time. The RDA of phosphorus for adults is 800 mg.

MAGNESIUM. About 50% of the body's magnesium is in the bones, with the remainder in the cells of the muscles and soft tissues. Magnesium functions in the operation of enzymes and aids in the metabolism of calcium, potassium, and **vitamin D**. Magnesium deficiency can result from a low intake of the mineral, from **diarrhea**, and from **alcoholism**. Magnesium deficiency can cause hallucinations and has been associated with **heart** problems. Good dietary sources of magnesium include spinach, oysters, baked potatoes, and sunflower seeds.

Magnesium is used in a number of over-the-counter preparations as an antacid and laxative. The most common uses of magnesium in clinical medicine include treatment of tachycardia (excessively rapid heartbeat), and depletion of electrolytes (chloride, potassium, and sodium). It is also used to manage premature labor. The RDA of magnesium is 350 mg for men, 280 mg for women.

SODIUM. Sodium is a mineral that plays an important role in the proper functioning of nerves and muscles. It is also an important component of intracellular fluid. Sodium deficiency does not occur with a normal diet, but may result from illness or injury. Too much sodium in the diet may raise **blood pressure** and cause **hypertension**. Salt is the main source of sodium in the diet, but table salt is not the most significant source of sodium. Most sodium in the average American's diet comes from processed and fast foods. The RDA of sodium is between 100 and 3300 mg.

POTASSIUM. Potassium helps maintain fluid and **electrolyte balance** in the body. Potassium is found in a variety of foods; however, potassium deficiency can result from illness, injury, or treatment with diuretics. The best sources of dietary potassium are fresh fruits and vegetables, especially bananas, potatoes, and raisins. The RDA of potassium is between 1875 and 5625 mg.

CHLORIDE. Chloride helps maintain **fluid balance** in the body. It is an essential component of the hydrochloric acid in the gastric fluid required for digestion. Chloride deficiency can result from repeated vomiting, diuretic therapy, or kidney disease. The RDA of chloride is between 1700 and 5100 mg.

SULFUR. Sulfur occurs in the body in such other compounds as **thiamine** and **proteins**. It helps to maintain the structure of skin, hair, and nails, and functions in oxidation/reduction reactions. Sulfur deficiency is a relatively unusual condition, because the body's need for sulfur is satisfied by the amino acids contained in foods high in protein.

Trace minerals

The trace minerals, or micronutrients, include **iron**, iodine, **zinc**, fluoride, selenium, chromium, and **copper**. Even though these elements are present in very small amounts in the human body, they serve many important functions.

IRON. Iron is a component of hemoglobin in red blood cells and myoglobin in muscle cells. It helps these compounds to hold and carry oxygen throughout the blood and the muscles. Iron also aids in enzyme activity and cell synthesis. Lack of iron in the diet can cause iron-deficiency anemia, which is the most common nutrient deficiency in the world. Symptoms include tiredness, weakness, and a tendency to feel cold. Animal foods such as meat, poultry, and fish are excellent sources of iron. **Vitamin C** also helps promote the absorption of iron. The RDA of iron is 10 mg for men, 18 mg for women.

IODINE. Iodine is a mineral that is needed for the hormone thyroxine, which plays a part in energy metabolism. Iodine deficiency causes an enlargement of the **thyroid gland** in the neck, which is known as a goiter. A deficiency in pregnant women can also result in mental and physical retardation known as cretinism. Iodine can be found in seafood, foods grown on land, and bakery products. The RDA of iodine is 150 micrograms.

ZINC. Zinc is needed in only very small amounts, but it functions in nearly every organ of the body. It plays a role in the **immune system**, sperm production, **taste**

perception, and wound healing. Inadequate intakes of zinc can result in poor growth and appetite as well as poor taste acuity. Too much zinc can impair the absorption of iron and copper in the body. Sources of zinc include meat, shellfish, poultry, legumes, and whole grains. The RDA of zinc is 15 mg.

SELENIUM. Selenium is a relatively rare nonmetallic trace element; there is less than 1 milligram of selenium in the average human body. The selenium is concentrated in the **liver**, **kidneys**, and **pancreas**; and in males, in the testes and seminal vesicles. It also activates thyroid hormone, which regulates the body's metabolism. Selenium can be found in a variety of foods; good sources of it include brewer's yeast, wheat germ, wheat bran, kelp (seaweed), shellfish, brazil nuts, barley, and oats. Selenium is most widely recognized as a substance that speeds up the metabolism of fatty acids and works together with **Vitamin E** (tocopherol) as an antioxidant. Antioxidants are organic substances that are able to counteract the damage done by oxidation to human tissue. The RDA of selenium is between 0.05 and 0.2 micrograms.

FLUORIDE. Fluoride has not been proven to be an essential mineral, but it does play a role in forming bones and teeth. Fluoride is most readily available from fluoridated drinking water. Too much of this element can cause a discoloration of the teeth known as **fluorosis**, but adequate fluoride consumption throughout life will help protect against **dental caries**. The RDA of fluoride is between 1.5 and 4.0 mg.

CHROMIUM. Chromium is closely associated with the hormone insulin, which regulates blood glucose levels. Chromium is usually depleted during food processing, which increases the chance for a deficiency if fast foods are eaten very often. Good sources of chromium include liver, whole grains, cheese, and nuts. The RDA of chromium is between 0.05 and 0.2 mg.

COPPER. Copper helps to form hemoglobin and collagen in the body as well as enzymes. Copper deficiency can impair growth and development, but is rarely encountered. Copper toxicity is also rare, but can occur from too much supplementation. Copper can be found in cherries, legumes, whole grains, seafood, nuts, and organ meats. The RDA of copper is 2–3 mg.

OTHER MICRONUTRIENTS. There are other trace minerals found in the body including boron, molybdenum, cobalt, and nickel. These minerals are all important to the body's health, but they are readily available in a normal diet. Deficiencies of these micronutrients are extremely rare.

KEY TERMS

Acid-base balance—The balance between the acidity and alkalinity of body fluids.

Antioxidant—A substance that works to counteract the damage done by oxidation to human tissue. Dietary antioxidants include the trace mineral selenium.

Electrolyte—An element or compound that dissociates in water and acts as a conductor of electricity.

Hemoglobin—A protein found in red blood cells that carries oxygen from the lungs to the tissues of the body.

Inorganic—Pertaining to chemical compounds that are not hydrocarbons or their derivatives.

Myoglobin—A form of hemoglobin found in muscle tissue.

Trace element—An element that is required in only minute quantities for the maintenance of good health. Trace elements are also called micronutrients.

Complications

Vitamin and mineral supplementation has become a very common practice in the general population, due in part to aggressive advertising and marketing of dietary supplements. While vitamin and mineral supplements are beneficial to those whose diets are lacking in certain nutrients, extremely high doses of some minerals can have toxic effects. For example, too much iron can cause tissue damage and **infection**. High levels of magnesium can cause depressed deep tendon **reflexes**, fatigue, and sleepiness. High levels of selenium have been associated with tooth decay.

On the other hand, care should be taken to meet the body's needs for higher levels of mineral intake during **pregnancy** and periods of high physical or emotional **stress** (surgery, trauma, etc.).

Health care team roles

Professional dietitians and other **nutrition** experts are primarily responsible for recommending mineral supplementation when it is necessary and for educating consumers on the dangers of excess supplementation. They also play a role in educating the public on the benefits of eating a well-balanced diet in order to receive adequate amounts of the various minerals.

Dentists and dental hygienists should instruct patients about the importance of dietary calcium and fluoridated water to healthy teeth.

Physicians, registered nurses, and pharmacists should instruct patients about the possible side effects of certain medications— particularly diuretics, antihypertensives, and some types of laxatives— that may cause electrolyte imbalance. Emergency room personnel should be knowledgeable about mineral deficiencies and mineral toxicities in the differential diagnosis of such symptoms as cardiac arrhythmias, seizures, disorientation, muscle twitching, and muscle weakness.

Resources

BOOKS

Baron, Robert B., MD, MS. "Nutrition." *Current Medical Diagnosis & Treatment 2001*. Edited by Lawrence M. Tierney, Jr., MD, et al. New York: Lange Medical Books/McGraw-Hill, 2001.

Mahan, Kathleen L., and Sylvia Escott-Stump. *Krause's Food, Nutrition, and Diet Therapy*. 10th ed. Philadelphia: W. B. Saunders Company, 2000.

The Merck Manual of Diagnosis and Therapy. Edited by Mark H. Beers, MD, and Robert Berkow, MD. Whitehouse Station, NJ: Merck Research Laboratories, 1999.

Russell, Percy J., and Anita Williams. *The Nutrition and Health Dictionary*.New York: Chapman & Hall, 1995.

Sizer, Frances S., and Eleanor N. Whitney. *Nutrition: Concepts and Controversies*, 7th ed. Belmont, CA: Wadsworth Publishing Company, 1997.

ORGANIZATIONS

Committee on the Scientific Evaluation of Dietary Reference Intakes. *Institute of Medicine (1997) Dietary Reference Intakes for Calcium, Phosphorus, Magnesium, Vitamin D, and Fluoride*. Washington, DC: National Academy Press, 1997.

Nutrition Hotline, American Dietetic Association. 216 West Jackson Blvd., Suite 800, Chicago, IL 60606. (800) 366-1655.

Lisa M. Gourley

Miscarriage

Definition

A miscarriage is the loss of an embryo or fetus before the twentieth week of **pregnancy**. A pregnancy loss after the twentieth week is called a stillbirth.

Description

According to the December 1999 news release from the U.S. government's National Center for Health Statistics, about 16% of recognized pregnancies end in miscarriage (i.e., prior to 20 weeks' gestation) or stillbirth (after 20 weeks' gestation). The medical term used for a miscarriage is spontaneous abortion, or early pregnancy loss. Most miscarriages occur during the first trimester of pregnancy. However, the statistics are unclear for the total number of recognized and unrecognized miscarriages in the United States. This is because a number of recognized miscarriages go undetected. When the pregnancy loss occurs early, the woman may not have missed her period yet. In this instance, she would not be aware of the pregnancy loss. Medical attention would not have been sought, and no statistic would have been generated.

Causes and symptoms

Causes of miscarriage may be genetic, anatomic, endocrinologic, infectious, immunologic, or exposure to a toxin. About 50–60% of first-trimester miscarriages occur as a result of a chromosomal abnormality, which renders the fetus non-viable. A definitive cause for the loss of a pregnancy cannot always be determined, as the products of conception (POC) are often passed by the woman at home or at work; they have not been collected for pathologic examination. The chromosomal abnormality is usually of spontaneous origin, a mutation that is not repeated in a subsequent pregnancy that continues to term.

A woman with a malformed uterus (e.g., bicornate) or cervix is also at increased risk for miscarriage. Women whose mothers took the medication diethylstilbestrol (DES) while they were *in utero* are especially likely to have suffered reproductive tract anomalies. The presence of fibroids can compete with the fetus for space and **blood** supply, and may result in miscarriage.

In about 17% of cases, a miscarriage is hormonal in nature, such as with insufficient secretion of progesterone, which results in a luteal phase insufficiency. Polycystic ovarian syndrome (PCOS), thyroid dysfunction, and poorly controlled **diabetes mellitus** are other hormonal causes of miscarriage.

Bacterial vaginosis, which may be present in as many as 31% of pregnant women, has been shown to increase the risk of miscarriage two fold, although it does not appear to affect a woman's ability to conceive. Individuals with a compromised **immune system**, causing them to be more susceptible to infectious organisms, are at increased risk of miscarriage. Toxoplasmosis can also cause miscarriages. The age of the egg at the time of fertilization may also be a factor. The older the egg, relative to ovulation, may be at greater risk of pregnancy loss.

Toxins and other workplace hazards that may increase the risk of miscarriage include:

- smoking, where the risk increases with each 10 cigarettes smoked daily
- caffeine, as in coffee, when four or more cups are consumed daily
- alcohol
- exposure to arsenic, lead, formaldehyde, benzene, and ethylene oxide
- multiple pregnancy, as in the case of carrying twins
- treatment with **anticancer drugs**, such as methotrexate
- exposure to ionizing radiation

The most common sign that a pregnancy is in danger is vaginal bleeding. The amount can vary from very light to heavy. The color of the blood varies as well, from brown to bright red. However, bleeding in early pregnancy is relatively common, and does not necessarily indicate impending miscarriage. One in four or five pregnant women experience bleeding in early pregnancy. Many women have some bleeding at the time of implantation, which occurs seven to 10 days after conception. Because of the possibility of pregnancy loss, any bleeding during pregnancy should be immediately reported to a woman's health care provider. The blood may be clotted, containing visible pieces of tissue. Bleeding may also be a sign of ectopic pregnancy, where the egg implants in a location other than the uterus, 95% of the time in a fallopian tube. Growth of the fertilized egg can lead to rupture of the tube, and can be life-threatening to the mother if untreated.

Cramping is another sign of a possible miscarriage. Cramping occurs as the uterus tries to expel the POC. The woman may also experience **pain**, dull and unrelenting, or sharp and intermittent, in the lower abdomen or back. When pain and bleeding persist, miscarriage is most likely to occur.

Diagnosis

If a woman experiences any sign of potential miscarriage, she should be examined by her health care provider. The physician, nurse midwife or nurse practitioner will usually perform a pelvic examination to check whether the cervix is closed or open. The cervix should remain closed throughout the pregnancy, opening only at the time of labor and delivery. If the cervix is open, the miscarriage has either already taken place or is inevitable. The size, firmness, and tenderness of the uterus will be checked by the practitioner. Blood tests may be ordered to determine if the level of beta-hCG, which should have been rising as the pregnancy continued, has begun to decline. If bleeding has been heavy, blood work may be ordered to check the woman's hemoglobin (oxygen-carrying red blood cells; how much hemoglobin is in the blood) and **hematocrit** (volume of packed blood cells) levels. An ultrasound may also be conducted to see if miscarriage has already occurred, if the fetus is alive or dead, and to check for intrauterine versus extrauterine implantation. An ultrasound can also detect the presence of any uterine abnormalities.

The further into the gestation period, the more likely it is that the fetus and placenta may be expelled separately. If some of the POC has been retained, the miscarriage is referred to as an incomplete abortion. An incomplete abortion presents the risk of **infection**, which, left untreated and unpassed, can lead to a potential life-threatening sepsis. A missed abortion is defined by the death of the fetus that has remained *in utero* for several weeks. Most missed abortions terminate spontaneously.

Treatment

Most miscarriages require no treatment. However, if infection has set in (i.e., indicated by **fever** and/or chills), or the POC have been retained, a D & C (i.e., prior to 16 weeks) or a D & E (i.e., after 16 weeks) may be required to remove any remaining tissue or blood clots from inside the uterus. An IV solution containing oxytocin may be used to induce uterine contractions to assist in complete expulsion of the POC, although this is not done in some practices. In early gestation (prior to six weeks), oral mifepristone (antiprogesterone RU 486) may be used to effect abortion. Two clinical studies, one in 1992 and another in 1993, demonstrated that the drug was effective as an abortifacient. In the earlier investigation, RU 486 administration to pregnant women was followed by a prostaglandin analogue; the success rate was 95%. In 1993, when a single 600-mg dose of RU 486 was given to women prior to six weeks' gestation, an 85% abortion rate was achieved.

Antibiotics will be prescribed in the event of infection, and may be ordered prophylactically. The woman is usually told to avoid the use of tampons and to abstain from sexual intercourse until the cervix has had a chance to close and heal. Rh-negative women will be given an injection of RhoGAM by the nurse. The purpose of this is to prevent Rh incompatibility between the mother and her baby in a future pregnancy.

KEY TERMS

Abortifacient—An agent that induces abortion.

Diethylstilbestrol (DES)—A synthetic estrogen drug used to treat several hormonal conditions. DES was used from 1938 until 1971, when it was found to cause reproductive tract defects in the children of women who took the drug while pregnant.

Dilation and curettage (D & C)—An obstetrical or gynecologic procedure in which the cervix is dilated and the contents of the uterus scraped and suctioned out. During pregnancy it is the term used until 16 weeks gestation.

Dilatation and evacuation (D & E)—An obstetrical procedure performed after 16 weeks gestation in which the cervix is dilated and the contents evacuated.

Embryo—The unborn child in the first eight weeks after conception. After the eighth week, the unborn child is called a fetus.

Mifepristone—A drug used to induce abortion. Also called RU-486.

Prostaglandin analogue—Any of a group of naturally occurring, chemically related hydroxy fatty acids that stimulate contractility of the uterine and other smooth muscle. These compounds have structures similar to those of others, but they differ in terms of a particular component.

Prognosis

Most miscarriages are uncomplicated and do not affect the woman's future ability to carry to term. About 90% of women who had one miscarriage have a successful pregnancy in the future. About 75% of women experiencing two miscarriages will carry to term in the future. Even women who have three consecutive miscarriages have a 50% chance of a successful fourth pregnancy. However, women who have had three or more miscarriages (repeated pregnancy loss [RPL]) may pursue further medical evaluation—earlier, if the woman is 35 or older. Following a miscarriage a woman should wait at least until she has had her next period before attempting to become pregnant again.

While the woman is able to recover physically from a miscarriage from within a few days to a couple of months, an emotional recovery may take much longer. Grieving the loss of the pregnancy may take some time

for the woman, her partner, other family members, and even close friends. Some women may develop major depression, acute **stress** disorder, or even **post-traumatic stress disorder** (PTSD). Feelings of loss, of self-blame, of anger at a body that has "failed" them are all common.

Health care team roles

A nurse may be the first contact for the woman experiencing a miscarriage, either by telephone, at the clinic or doctor's office, or in the emergency department. The nurse's ability to create a calm environment, and to be supportive of the woman's grieving can enable the woman to move forward after the experience. The nurse should be able to supply the woman with information about miscarriage and community resources, such as support groups.

The ultrasound technologist may perform the ultrasound on the woman undergoing a miscarriage. Usually the technologist will give the report of the findings to the woman's practitioner, not to the woman directly. However, **anxiety** and fear can affect how information is heard and processed. The technologist's use of a soft, soothing voice can help calm the woman, better enabling her to hear the outcome of the ultrasound from her practitioner.

Prevention

Because the majority of miscarriages are spontaneous chromosomal abnormalities, little prevention is available. However, regular screening for sexually transmitted diseases (STDs) and bacterial vaginosis can decrease the risks to a future pregnancy. If the miscarriage was due to a luteal phase deficiency, supplemental progesterone may be prescribed for future pregnancies.

If the nurse has telephone contact with the woman during the miscarriage, the nurse should request that the woman collect any tissue that is expelled—and collected, perhaps, on a sanitary pad. The nurse should ask the patient to bring it along with her to her next examination, so that it may be analyzed. While this may place an emotional burden on the woman, it can allow for the possible determination of the cause of the miscarriage. This information can help the woman and her practitioner prepare for a subsequent pregnancy. In addition, studies have shown that determining the cause can often assist the woman in overcoming her feelings of self-blame.

Resources

BOOKS

Creasy, Robert K., and Robert Resnik. *Maternal-Fetal Medicine*. Philadelphia: W.B. Saunders Company, 1999.

Fumia, Molly. *A Piece of My Heart*. Berkeley, CA: Conari, 2000.

Hinton, Clara H. *Silent Grief; Miscarriage—Finding Your Way Through the Darkness*. Green Forest, AK: New Leaf Press, 1998.

Kohn, Ingrid, and Perry-Lynn Moffitt. *A Silent Sorrow. Pregnancy Loss: Guidance and Support for You and Your Family*. New York: Routledge, 2000.

Pasquariello, Patrick S. *Children's Hospital of Philadelphia: Book of Pregnancy and Child Care*. New York: John Wiley & Sons, 1999.

Scott, James R., Philip J. Di Saia, Charles B. Hammond, and William N. Spellacy, eds. *Danforth's Obstetrics and Gynecology*. Philadelphia: Lippincott Williams & Wilkins, 1999.

PERIODICALS

"The Effects of Workplace Hazards on Female Reproductive Health." <http://www.cdc.gov/niosh>.

ORGANIZATIONS

Hygeia. <http://www.hygeia.org>.

March of Dimes Birth Defects Foundation. 1275 Mamaroneck Avenue, White Plains, NY 10605. (888) 663-4637. <http://www.modimes.org>.

Resolve: The National Infertility Association.1310 Broadway, Somerville, MA 02144. (617) 623-0744. resolveinc@aol.com. <http://www.resolve.org>.

Esther Csapo Rastegari, R.N., B.S.N., Ed.M.

Mitosis *see* **Cell division**

Mongolism *see* **Down syndrome**

Mouth cancer *see* **Oral cancer**

Mouthwash *see* **Oral hygiene aids**

Movement disorders

Definition

Movement disorders are a group of neurological diseases and syndromes that involve the motor and movement systems' ability to produce and control movement.

Description

Though it seems simple and effortless, normal movement actually requires an astonishingly complex system of control. Disruption of any portion of this system can cause a person to produce movements that are too weak, too forceful, too uncoordinated, or too poorly controlled for the task at hand. Unwanted movements may occur at rest. Intentional movement may become impossible. These conditions are examples of movement disorders.

Abnormal movements themselves are symptoms of underlying disorders. In some cases, the abnormal movements are the only symptoms. The more common diseases causing motor disorders include:

- **spinal cord injury** (SCI)
- stroke
- **multiple sclerosis** (MS)
- **muscular dystrophy** (MD)
- huntington's chorea (HC)
- **cerebral palsy** (CP)
- dystonias
- tremor
- myasthenia gravis (MG)
- parkinsonism (PD)
- Tourette syndrome

Other causes of motor disorders are Wilson's disease (WD), inherited ataxias (Friedreich's ataxia, Machado-Joseph disease, and spinocerebellar ataxias), and encephalopathies.

Causes and symptoms

Causes

Movement is produced and coordinated by several interacting **brain** centers, including the motor cortex, the cerebellum, and a group of structures in the inner potions of the brain called the basal ganglia. Sensory information provides critical input on the current position and velocity of body parts, and spinal nerve cells (**neurons**) help prevent opposing muscle groups from contracting simultaneously.

To understand how movement disorders occur, it is helpful to consider a normal volunteer movements, such as reaching to touch a nearby object with the right index finger. To accomplish the desired movement, the arm must be lifted and extended. The hand must be held out to align with the forearm, and the forefinger must be extended while the other fingers remain flexed.

THE MOTOR CORTEX. Voluntary motor commands begin in the motor cortex located on the outer, wrinkled surface of the brain. Movement of the right arm is begun by the left motor cortex, which generates a large volley of signals to the involved muscles. These electrical signals pass along upper motor neurons, through the midbrain, to the **spinal cord** (SC). Within the SC, these signals connect to lower motor neurons, which convey the signals from the SC to the surface of the muscles involved. Neural activation of the muscles causes contraction, and the force of contraction pulling on the skeleton causes movement of the arm, hand, and fingers.

Damage to, or death of any of the neurons along this path, can cause weakness or **paralysis** of the affected muscles.

THE CEREBELLUM. Once the movement of the arm is initiated, sensory information is needed to guide the finger to its precise destination. In addition to sight, the most important source of information comes from the "position sense," provided by the many sensory receptors located within the limbs (proprioception). Proprioception allows a person to touch his or her nose with a finger even with the eyes closed. The balance organs in the ears provide important information about posture. Both postural and proprioceptive information are processed by a structure at the rear of the brain, called the cerebellum. The cerebellum sends out electrical signals to modify movements as they progress, "sculpting" the barrage of voluntary commands into a tightly controlled, constantly evolving pattern. Cerebellar disorders cause inability to control the force, fine positioning, and speed of movements (ataxia). Disorders of the cerebellum may also impair the ability to judge distance, so that a person under- or overreaches the target (dysmetria). Tremor during voluntary movements can also result from cerebellar damage.

THE BASAL GANGLIA. Both the cerebellum and the motor cortex send information to a set of structures deep within the brain that helps control involuntary components of movement (basal ganglia). The basal ganglia send output messages to the motor cortex, helping to initiate movements, regulate repetitive or patterned movements, and control muscle tone.

Circuits within the basal ganglia are complex. Within this structure, some groups of cells begin the action of other basal ganglia components, and some groups of cells block the action. These complicated feedback circuits are not entirely understood. Disruptions of these circuits are known to cause several distinct movement disorders. A portion of the basal ganglia, called the *substantia nigra,* sends electrical signals that block output from another structure, the subthalamic nucleus. The subthalamic nucleus sends signals to the globus pallidus, which in turn blocks the thalamic nuclei. Finally, the thalamic nuclei send signals to the motor cortex. The *sub-*

stantia nigra, then begins movement, and the globus pallidus blocks it.

This complicated circuit can be disrupted at several points. Loss of *substantia nigra,* cells increases blocking of the thalamic nuclei and prevents them from sending signals to the motor cortex. Degeneration of these nerve cells, as in PD, results in lower production of dopamine and fewer connections with other nerve cells and muscles, leading to a loss of movement (motor activity).

In contrast, cell loss in early HD decreases the blocking of signals from the thalamic nuclei, causing more cortex stimulation and stronger, but uncontrolled, movements.

Disruptions in other portions of the basal ganglia are thought to cause tics, tremors, dystonia, and a variety of other movement disorders, although the exact mechanisms are not well understood.

Some movement disorders, including HD, are caused by inherited genetic defects and inherited ataxias. Some diseases that cause sustained **muscle contraction** limited to a particular muscle group (focal dystonia) are inherited, but others are caused by trauma. The cause of most cases of PD is unknown, although genes have been identified for some familial forms.

ANTAGONISTIC MUSCLE PAIRS. This picture of movement, however, is too simple. One important refinement to it comes from considering the role of opposing, or antagonistic, muscle pairs. Contraction of the bicep muscle, located on the top of the upper arm, pulls on the forearm to flex the elbow and bend the arm. Contraction of the triceps, located on the opposite side, extends the elbow and straightens the arm. Within the spine, these muscles are normally wired so that willed (voluntary) contraction of one is automatically accompanied by blocking of the other. In other words, the command to contract the biceps provokes another command within the spine to prevent contraction of the triceps. In this way, these antagonist muscles are kept from resisting one another. Spinal cord or brain injury, can damage this control system and cause involuntary simultaneous contraction and spasticity, an increase in resistance to movement during motion.

While the peripheral mechanism, antagonistic muscle pairs, is certainly important, it is not the only one of concern with regard to movement disorders. Central pattern generators (CPGs) in the spinal cord are especially relevant because of their role in sensory processing. Filtration and processing of sensory input is accomplished locally, where the response of spinal pattern generator circuitry fits into continual movement, as necessary. Thus, although the brain receives much of the sensory input, the responses to spinal inputs are first the responsibility of the local spinal circuitry. Multi-segmental **reflexes** and anticipatory postural adjustments are as critical in the etiology of these syndromes.

Common conditions causing motor disorders

SPINAL CORD INJURY (SCI). Spinal cord injury (SCI) is very complex and can be very serious. An injury can affect the body in a multitude of ways depending on where the spinal cord (SC) is damaged. It is the largest nerve in the body and is composed of nerve fibers. These nerve fibers that manage the body's communication systems are responsible for its motor, sensory, and autonomic functions. They act as messenger between the brain and the rest of the body. The vertebral column—protective bone segments—surrounds the SC, perhaps because of its important in the nervous system. Approximately 18 inches (39 cm) long, the SC runs from the base of the brain, down the middle of the back, to the waist. Nerve fibers in the upper SC are upper motor neurons (UMNs). Spinal nerves branching off the SC that run up and down the neck and back are lower motor neurons (LMNs), and branch off between each vertebrae and go out to all parts of the body. The lower spinal nerve fibers continue down through the spinal canal to the sacram (tailbone) at the end of the SC.

Divided into four sections at the top of the spinal column is the cervical spine. It is composed of eight cervical nerves and seven cervical vertebrae. Further down is the thoracic sine, which includes the chest and twelve thoracic vertebrae. The lumbar spine is below that, and comprises five lumbar vertebrae. The bottom section is the sacral area, and there the bones fuse together into one bone.

When the SC is damaged by either a traumatic injury or from a disease, all nerves above the injury level still function normally. Those from the point of injury and below, however, are damaged, and messages between the brain and parts of the body that could once be sent are no longer are no longer possible. The patient must undergo **physical examination** by the doctor to earn the exact location of injury to the spinal cord. Frequently, the physician will use a "pin-prick" test," which evaluates the patient's level of feeling (sensory level). X rays are also frequently used to image the affected vertebrae. The patient's input is critical; he or she will be asked what parts of the body can be moved, and all major muscle groups will be tested (motor level) for strength. All of these tests are important, as they reveal what nerves and muscles are functioning. Each SCI is unique, and is defined by its type and level. Its level will be judged by the lowest level on the SC after which there is absence of feeling and/or movement (motor level).

Loss of feeling and/or movement in the head, neck, shoulder, arms, and/or upper chest is termed "tetraplegia," and is injury at level C1 to T1. The cervical spine is the highest part of the spinal cord and is designated by the letter "C." The thoracic spine is next to the highest, and is designated by the letter "T." T2 to S5 is paraplegia. The higher on the **vertebral column**, the closer the SCI is to the brain. Therefore, someone with a T-8 (thoracic spine; eight of 12 thoracic vertebrae) level injury would have more feeling and movement than someone with a C-5 (cervical spine; five of seven cervical vertebrae) level of injury.

STROKE. During a stroke, brain tissue is destroyed. This is cause by some malfunction of the brain's **blood vessels**. There are two major classifications of stroke: hemorrhagic and ischemic. The most common type of stroke is ischemic, caused by the same kind of vascular disease as **heart** attack. By "ischemic" it is meant that the **blood** flow to an area is insufficient; there is not enough oxygen to support the cells. The brain cells will cease to function if blood circulation is not restored quickly enough after a stroke. Cell death by lack of oxygen is termed "infarction." To be more specific, physicians often refer to this type of infarction as "cerebral." As of 2001, stroke is the third leading cause of disability and the fifth leading cause of death in the United States. Annually, 500,000 people suffer strokes; 150,000 die of them.

A hemorrhagic stroke happens with the rupture of a blood vessel. Bleeding occurs inside the **skull**. Usually, the cause is **hypertension**, or high blood pressure—but it can also be caused by trauma. An aneurysm (a sac formed by localized dilatation of the wall of an artery, a vein or the heart) may also cause a hemorrhagic stroke. Whatever the origin of the stroke, bleeding can rip through the tender connections within the brain, and ultimately compress brain cells until they die.

The extent of damage due to stroke depends on the severity of the stroke and where in the brain the blood supply was suspended. Each area of the brain is served by specific blood vessels; if a blood vessel in the area that controls muscle movements became blocked, those muscles will be weak, or paralyzed. The loss of function is greatest immediately after a stroke, but some usually some function is regained. Some brain cells do die, while some injured cells may recover. Bleeding on the brain, such as from a **head injury** or brain aneurysm, can also cause brain cell death from lack of oxygen. Symptoms may resemble those of a stroke. The best prevention for a stroke is for the patient to discuss risk factors with a physician.

MULTIPLE SCLEROSIS (MS). Multiple sclerosis (MS) is a demyelinating disease that is related to the inflammatory process. One feature of MS is multiple, separate, and harmful neurologic episodes caused by **central nervous system** (CNS) lesions. The result is multiple, clearly defined areas (plaque) of myelin (the protective sheath around nerves) in the brain's white matter SC known as perivenous distribution (i.e., not in the peripheral nervous system).

MS occurs early in the inflammatory phase, and disrupts the messages that are being transmitted within the body. The disease is called MS because the scar tissue (sclerosis) forms at various locations. Some of the diseased areas of the myelin may cause no obvious symptoms, while other areas may interfere with functions or sensations controlled by the brain or SC. For this reason, the symptoms and the severity of the disability varies greatly among persons with MS.

The cause of MS remains unknown, but many think that it may be an autoimmune disease. Normally, the **immune system** works by recognizing foreign invaders and producing its own cells to counteract or defend against attacks. In MS, the immune system is disrupted as the body incorrectly identifies itself as an invader and begins to attack its own cells. The body no longer recognizes myelin as its own and declares war on this nerve tissue. Further, linkage studies have noted significant genetic factors. A common first symptom is visual impairment, due to optic neuritis (inflammation of the optic nerve).

MUSCULAR DYSTROPHY (MD). The name "muscular dystrophy" (MD) encompasses a number of progressive hereditary diseases that makes muscles weaken and degenerate. Not a contagious disease, there are a multitude of variations. Each type has its own pattern of heredity, onset age, and speed with which muscle is lost. Alterations in specific genes causes different types of disease. There was no prevention or cure for MD as of 2001. However, because of research being done at this time, there is reason for hope for a cure.

HUNTINGTON'S CHOREA (HC). A genetically inherited disease, Huntington's chorea (HC) has neurological and psychotic characteristics. The forties or fifties are the usual ages of onset, but early and late onset are also possible. Either neurological or psychotic changes can mark the beginning of the disease. Symptoms of neurological changes may vary, but can begin with chorea—a series of movements that resemble dancing, with jerkiness and one part of the body moving to another. One might display clumsiness, jumpiness, and become fidgety. There may be movement in the face, particularly around the jaw, and walking may become difficult. It may be diffi-cult to maintain posture. Paranoia, personality changes, and confusion may present, as well. It is also possible for **dementia** to occur.

Diagnosis of HC is dependent upon clinical symtomatology and MRI (magnetic brain imaging), as well as discovering family history of the disease. An MRI that reveals atrophy (shrinkage) of part of the basal ganglia, which is involved in movement and known as the caudate nucleus, is characteristic of HC.

CEREBRAL PALSY. In cerebral palsy (CP), abnormal development of or damage to motor areas in the brain disrupts the brain's ability to control movement and posture. The term CP is a term used to describe a group of chronic disorders impairing control of movement that appear in the first few years of life and generally do not worsen over time. Symptoms differ from person to person, and may change over time. Individuals with the disease may have difficulty with fine motor tasks (e.g., writing), and balance or walking. They may have involuntary movements. Cerebral palsy, which may be congenital (present at birth) or acquired after birth, results from brain injury that does not worsen over time. Possible causes of CP include developmental abnormalities of the brain, brain injury caused by low oxygen levels (asphyxia) or poor circulation, **infection**, and trauma to the fetus or newborn. Doctors encourage pregnant women to follow a program of regular **prenatal care** beginning early in **pregnancy** to help prevent CP.

DYSTONIAS. Dystonias are sustained muscle contractions that often cause twisting or repetitive movements and abnormal postures. Dystonias may be limited to one area (focal) or may affect the entire body (general). Focal dystonias may affect the neck (cervical dystonia or torticollis), the face (one-sided, or hemifacial spasm), contraction of the eyelid (blepharospasm), contraction of the mouth and jaw (oromandibular dystonia), simultaneous spasm of the chin and eyelid (Meige syndrome), the vocal cords (laryngeal dystonia), or the arms and legs (writer's and occupational cramps). Dystonia may be painful and incapacitating.

TREMORS. Uncontrollable (involuntary) shaking of body parts are known as tremors. Tremors may occur only when muscles are relaxed, during actions, or when holding active postures.

MYASTHENIA GRAVIS (MG). Myasthenia gravis (MG), a chronic autoimmune disease, is characterized by fluctuating degrees of weakness of the skeletal, or voluntary muscles. Muscle weakness of increasing severity is the key symptom of this disorder; it worsens with activity, and improves after periods of rest. It does not always include muscles that control facial expression, such as muscles of the eyes, talking, chewing, and swallowing, but can affect the muscles involved with breathing, the neck, and limb movements. A defect in the transmission of nerve impulses to muscles is responsible for MG. The symptoms of MG range in type and degree. It is not directly genetic, and it is not infectious. It can be controlled through medications that improve neuromuscular transmission, thereby improving muscle strength, or through medications that suppress the manufacture by the body of abnormal antibodies. Because of unpleasant, major side effects, these drugs must be used with caution and monitored carefully. Myasthenia gravis is caused by an autoimmune response attack on acetylcholine (neurotransmitter) receptors at muscular junctions.

PARKINSON'S DISEASE (PD). The possibility of developing **Parkinson's disease**, or parkinsonism, increases with age, with age of onset usually not less than 40 years of age. Approximately 500,000 people in the United States suffer from the disease, which affects both sexes equally. The cause of its most common form, PD (as well as related disorders) is not known—though genetic risk has been identified as a probable factor by the National Institutes of Health. Interestingly, the disorder is observed at the same rate in almost part of the globe, and is as common today as it was in late 1800s.

The two terms, Parkinson's disease (PD) and parkinsonism, are used interchangeably, as they both describe patients with the same symptoms. The four primary symptoms of PD are tremor or trembling, rigidity or stiffness of the limbs and trunk, bradykinesia (slowness of movement), and impaired balance and coordination.

There are a number of causes of parkinsonism, including degenerative neurologic disease, metabolic conditions, toxins, drugs, viral encephalitis (von Economo's disease), and related disorders result from the loss of dopamine, a chemical messenger responsible for transmitting signals within the brain. When certain nerve cells (neurons) that produce dopamine die or become impaired, dopamine is depleted. The result is nerve cells that fire out of control. Individuals with PD are then unable to direct or control their movements in a normal manner. The disease, which is usually not inherited, is both chronic and progressive, with subtle early symptoms and gradual progression.

Management of a movement disorder begins with determining its cause. Physical and **occupational therapy** may help to compensate for lost control and strength. Pharmacologic therapy can help to compensate for some imbalances of the basal ganglionic circuit. For instance, levodopa (L-dopa), or related compounds, can substitute for the loss of dopamine-producing cells in PD. Conversely, blocking normal dopamine action may be used to treat some hyperkinetic disorders, including tics.

Oral medications can also help to reduce overall muscle tone. Local injections of botulinum toxin (BOTOX) can selectively weaken overactive muscles in dystonia and spasticity. Destruction of peripheral nerves through injection of phenol can reduce spasticity. It should be noted, however, that all of these treatments have some side effects.

Other movement disorders

Tic disorders are very quick, involuntary, rapid, non-rhythmic, and short-lived movements or sounds; tics can sometimes be controlled briefly. Tics are usually repeated movements. They commonly involve the motor systems and often involve the facial muscles, such as the eyelids or eyebrows. The most well-known tic disorder is Tourette syndrome. Tourette syndrome (TS) is an abnormal condition that causes uncontrollable facial grimaces and tics, and arm and shoulder movements. Tourette syndrome is best known, perhaps, for uncontrollable vocal tics that include grunts, shouts, and use of obscene language (coprolalia). It is also known as Gilles de la Tourette syndrome. Tics are more common among males than females. As with Tourette syndrome, tics may be associated with head injury, stroke, **carbon monoxide poisoning**, and mental retardation.

Myoclonus is a sudden, shock-like muscle contraction. Myoclonic jerks may occur singly or repetitively. Unlike tics, myoclonus cannot be controlled even briefly.

Postural instability is the loss of ability to maintain upright posture, caused by slow or absent righting reflexes (those that help to maintain balance).

Spasticity is a condition in which certain muscles are continuously contracted, causing stiffness or tightness of the muscles.

Flaccid paralysis is the loss of muscle tone of the paralyzed part and an accompanying absence of reflexes.

Diagnosis

A complete and thorough clinical examination should be performed. Diagnosis of movement disorders requires a careful medical history and a thorough physical and neurological examination. A thorough orthopedic exam may be important because patients with increased muscle tone may develop curvature of the spine (**scoliosis**), hip dislocation, and tendon shortening. During the neurologic exam, the doctor will observe the individual's posture, tone, symmetry, and reflexes.

Certain symptoms may indicate a movement disorder disease. Doctors will pay special attention to the rate of development of children with CP, particularly with

KEY TERMS

Botulinum toxin (botox)—Any of a group of potent bacterial toxins or poisons produced by different strains of the bacterium *Clostridium botulinum*. The toxins cause muscle paralysis, and thus force the relaxation of a muscle in spasm.

Cerebral palsy (CJP)—A movement disorder caused by a permanent brain defect or an injury present at birth, or shortly after. It is frequently associated with premature birth. Cerebral palsy is not progressive.

Computed tomography (CT)—An imaging technique in which cross-sectional x rays of the body are compiled to create a three-dimensional image of the body's internal structures.

Encephalopathy—An abnormality in the structure or function of tissues of the brain.

Fetal tissue transplantation (FTT)—A method of treating PD and other neurological diseases by grafting brain cells from human fetuses onto the basal ganglia. Human adults cannot grow new brain cells, but developing fetuses can. Grafting fetal tissue stimulates the growth of new brain cells in affected adult brains.

Huntington's chorea (HC) disease (HD)—A rare, genetically inherited condition with both neurological and psychiatric manifestations that begins with either type of change. The chorea is progressive, and presents as jerky muscle movements and mental deterioration that ends in dementia. The symptoms of HC usually appear in patients in their 40s or 50s; however, early- or late-onset is possible. Huntington's chorea may also cause clumsiness, jumpiness, and fidgetiness, and facial movements—particularly around the jaw—may occur. It may become difficult to walk, and can affect posture. Paranoia, confusion, or personality changes may noted. A significant dementia develops as the disease progresses. There is no cure or effective treatment for the condition.

Levodopa (L-dopa)—A substance used in the treatment of PD. Levodopa can cross the blood-brain barrier that protects the brain. Once in the brain, it is converted to dopamine, and thus can replace the dopamine lost in PD.

Magnetic resonance imaging (MRI)—An imaging technique that uses a large circular magnet and radio waves to generate signals from atoms in the body. These signals are used to construct images of internal structures.

Paraplegia—Paralysis of the lower half of the body involving both legs and usually due to disease or injury to the spinal cord.

Parkinson's disease (PD)—A slowly progressive disease that destroys nerve cells in the basal ganglia and thus causes loss of dopamine, a chemical that aids in transmission of nerve signals (neurotransmitter). Parkinsonism is characterized by shaking in resting muscles, a stooping posture, slurred speech, muscular stiffness, and weakness.

Positron emission tomography (PET)—A diagnostic technique in which computer-assisted x rays are used to track a radioactive substance inside a patient's body. Biochemical activity of the brain can be studied using PET.

Progressive supranuclear palsy—A rare disease that shows some of the same features of PD, but differs in several ways. They usually do not develop tremors, but they have rigidity, bradykniesia (slow movements), and falls. The disorder gradually destroys nerve cells in the parts of the brain that control eye movements, breathing, and muscle coordination. The loss of nerve cells causes palsy (paralysis) that slowly gets worse as the disease progresses. The palsy affects the ability to move the eyes vertically (up and down) at first. Their eye movements then become even more restrictive (ophthalmoplegia). The ability to relax the muscles is lost, as is control over balance.

Tourette syndrome (TS)—An abnormal condition that causes uncontrollable facial grimaces and tics, and arm and shoulder movements. Tourette syndrome is best known, perhaps, for uncontrollable vocal tics that include grunts, shouts, and use of obscene language (coprolalia). Also known as Gilles de la Tourette syndrome.

Wilson's disease (WD)—An inborn defect of copper metabolism in which free copper may be deposited in a variety of areas of the body. Deposits in the brain can cause tremor and other symptoms of PD.

regard to head size and head growth, since abnormalities in these areas may point to a brain problem. Eye problems, such as blurred or double **vision**, red-green color distortion, or blindness in one eye, may occur. When combined with muscle weakness in extremities and paresthesias (transitory abnormal sensory feeling such as numbness or prickling), MS may be suspected.

Diagnostic tests should be conducted. These include brain imaging studies, such as computed tomography (CT) scan, **positron emission tomography (PET)**, or **magnetic resonance imaging** (MRI) scans. Routine blood and urine analyses are performed. A lumbar puncture (spinal tap) may be necessary. Video recording of the abnormal movement is often used to analyze movement patterns and to track progress of the disorder and its management. **Genetic testing** is available for some forms of movement disorders. If MS is suspected, physicians may study the patient's cerebrospinal fluid and the antibody, immunoglobulin G.

Treatment

Ongoing clinical studies indicate that estrogen may have beneficial effects on controlling movement disorders, such as PD, chorea, dystonia, tics, and myoclonus.

Deep brain stimulation, which inactivates the thalamus or globus pallidus through electrical shocks, may be useful to ease tremor of the arm in individuals with ET and tremor due to MS. In PD, the procedure may improve arm speed and dexterity, reduce tremor, and block the involuntary movements (dyskinesia) associated with the medications used to treat the disease.

Surgical destruction, or inactivation of basal ganglionic circuits, has proven effective for PD, and as of 2001 is being tested for other movement disorders. Transplantation of fetal cells into the basal ganglia has produced mixed results in PD.

Health care team roles

Nursing and allied health professionals play a key role in educating individuals with movement disorders about their conditions and appropriate treatment options. Physical, speech, and occupational therapy are often essential to the rehabilitation of individuals with movement disorders. Psychological counseling may be helpful to the individual and to family members and close friends.

The patient who has had a stroke may be treated by doctors, therapists, and nurses who work to keep the patient's muscles strong, prevent muscular contractions, avoid the bedsores that can result from being in one position for too long, and teach the patient to walk and talk

again. With SCI, expert nursing care is important to prevent complications from weakness and paralysis, including bedsores. Physical and occupational therapy help to preserve muscle function and teach techniques to help the patient function despite lost functionality.

Prognosis

The prognosis for a patient with a movement disorder depends on the nature of the disorder. The age of onset has major implications in prognosis.

Prevention

Prevention depends on the specific disorder. With some diseases, certain preventive strategies can be particularly helpful. In the case of MS and stroke, for example, smoking cessation would drastically reduce the number of cases. Longtime smokers may face a much higher risk of both MS and stroke, according to researchers at Harvard University. In the case of MS, women who smoked at least one pack per day for at least 25 years had a greater chance of developing the disorder than nonsmokers.

A number of permanent cases of parkinsonism that presented in the early 1980s were caused by a contaminant found in some illicit street drugs. For the most part, cases of the disease induced by legal, prescribed drugs were only temporary: when the drug was stopped, the symptoms stopped, too. Permanent parkinsonism had only been the result of the contaminant found in the street drug.

In 1996, clinicians at the University of Hawaii found that patients with high blood levels of uric acid, a natural antioxidant, have a lower chance of developing Parkinsonism and **gout** (acute inflammatory arthritis) than people with lower levels. The study concluded that people with high levels of the antioxidant, uric acid, may be more resistant to developing parkinsonism. This was also shown in a pilot student in 1991, when investigator Stanley Fahn of Columbia University found that parkinsonism patients who were administered large doses of oral **vitamin C** and synthetic **vitamin E** supplements (3000 mg and 3200 iu daily, respectively) delayed the progression of the disease. He concluded that it was likely that it was the vitamin C alone, or in combination with vitamin E that actively worked.

- Parkinsonism (PD). Deprenyl (selegiline), administered early in the onset of the disorder, can slow progression of the disease. Antioxidants such as vitamin E and selenium may be of some benefit, as well.

- Spinal cord injury (SCI). Attention to following safety precautions may help to reduce the risk of SCI. The most frequent causes of SCI are motor vehicle crashes, **falls**, violence, and sports and recreation, especially diving. Proper protective equipment should be used if an injury is possible, and appropriate safety measures should be practiced. Depth of water should be checked and obstructions should be noted before diving. When in an automobile, seat belts should always be used.

- Stroke. Major risk factors include high **blood pressure**, high cholesterol level, smoking, and diabetes. Drugs, such as aspirin (half of an adult tablet or one children's tablet daily), can be taken to reduce the tendency of blood platelets (responsible for the clotting of blood) to form dangerous blood clots, a major cause of stroke. When stronger drugs are needed, a doctor may prescribe anticoagulants, such as heparin or warfarin (Coumadin). Research in the year 2001 suggests that paralysis and other symptoms may be prevented or reversed if certain drugs that break up clots are given within three hours of the onset of a stroke.

Resources

BOOKS

Adler, Charles H. and J. Eric Ahlskog, eds. *Parkinson's Disease and Movement Disorders: Diagnosis and Treatment Guidelines for the Practicing Physician.* Totowa, N.J.: Humana Press, 2000.

Cicala MD, Roger S. *Brain Disorders Sourcebook.* Lincolnwood, IL: Lowell House; NTC/Contemporary Publishing Group, Inc., 1999.

Floyd, R.T. and Clem W. Thompton. *Manual of Structural Kinesiology.* Dubuque, IA: McGraw-Hill, 2001.

Jankovic, Joseph and Eduardo Tolosa, ed. *Parkinson's Disease and Movement Disorders.* Baltimore: Williams & Wilkins, 1998.

Sawle, Guy, ed. *Movement Disorders in Clinical Practice.* Oxford: Isis Medical Media, 1999.

Vander, Arthur, James Sherman, and Dorothy Luciano. *Human Physiology: The Mechanisms of Body Function.* Boston: McGraw-Hill, 2001.

ORGANIZATIONS

American Association of Neuroscience Nurses, 4700 W. Lake Avenue, Glenview, IL 60025. (888) 557-2266. <http://www.aann.org>.

American Spinal Injury Association. 345 E. Superior Street, Chicago, IL 60611. (312)238-1242. <http://www.asia-spinalinjury.org>.

Muscular Dystophy Association, 3300 East Sunrise Drive, Tucson, AZ 85718-3208, (520) 529-2000 or (800) 572-1717. <http://www.mdausa.org/>.

Myasthenia Gravis Foundation of America, Inc., 5841 Cedar Lake Road, Suite 204, Minneapolis, MN 55416, (952) 545-9438 or (800)541-5454. <http://www.myasthenia.org>.

National Institute of Neurological Disorders and Stroke. P.O. Box 5801, Bethesda, MD 20824, (800) 352-9424. <http://www.ninds.nih.gov>.

National Spinal Cord Injury Association, The Zalco Building, 8701 Georgia Avenue, Suite 500, 8701 Georgia Avenue, Silver Springs, MD 20910, (800) 962-9629 or (301) 588-6959. <http://www.spinalcord.org>.

National Spinal Cord Injury Statistical Center, UAB-Spain Rehabilitation Center, Rm 544, 619 19th Street South, SRC 544, Birmingham, AL 35249-7330, (205) 934-5359.

Paralyzed Veterans of America. 801 18th Street NW, Washington, DC 20006, (800) 424-8288 or infor@pva.org, <http://www.pva.org>.

The Movement Disorder Society. 611 East Wells Street, Milwaukee, WI 53202, (414) 276-2145. <http://www.movementdisorders.org>.

WE MOVE. 204 West 84th Street, New York, NY 10024. (800) 437- MOV2 or (212) 875-8389. <http://www.wemove.org>.

OTHER

"Smoking Risk Factor for Multiple Sclerosis: Study." National Library of Medicine. National Institutes of Health. Medline Plus. <http://www.nlm.nih.gov/medlineplus/news/fullstory_2440.html>.

"Spinal Cord Injury Information Network: Understanding Spinal Cord Injury and Functional Goals." University of Alabama at Birmingham. <http://www.spinalcord.uab.edu>.

Randi B. Jenkins

Movement therapy

Definition

Movement therapy refers to a broad range of Eastern and Western movement approaches used to promote physical, mental, emotional, and spiritual well-being.

Origins

Movement is fundamental to human life. In fact movement is life. Contemporary physics tells us that the universe and everything in it is in constant motion. We can move our body and at the most basic level our body is movement. According to the somatic educator Thomas Hanna, "The living body is a moving body—indeed, it is a constantly moving body." The poet and philosopher Alan Watts eloquently states a similar view, "A living body is not a fixed thing but a flowing event, like a flame or a whirlpool." Centuries earlier, the great Western philosopher Socrates understood what modern physics has proven, "The universe is motion and nothing else."

Since the beginning of time, indigenous societies around the world have used movement and dance for individual and community healing. Movement and song were used for personal healing, to create community, to ensure successful crops, and to promote fertility. Movement is still an essential part of many healing traditions and practices throughout the world.

Western movement therapies generally developed out of the realm of dance. Many of these movement approaches were created by former dancers or choreographers who were searching for a way to prevent injury, attempting to recover from an injury, or who were curious about the effects of new ways of moving. Some movement therapies arose out of the fields of **physical therapy**, psychology, and bodywork. Other movement therapies were developed as way to treat an incurable disease or condition.

Eastern movement therapies, such as **yoga**, **qigong**, and **t'ai chi** began as a spiritual or self-defense practices and evolved into healing therapies. In China, for example, Taoist monks learned to use specific breathing and movement patterns in order to promote mental clarity, physical strength, and support their practice of **meditation**. These practices, later known as qigong and t'ai chi, eventually became recognized as ways to increase health and prolong life.

Benefits

The physical benefits of movement therapy include greater ease and range of movement, increased balance, strength and flexibility, improved muscle tone and coordination, joint resiliency, cardiovascular conditioning, enhanced athletic performance, stimulation of circulation, prevention of injuries, greater longevity, **pain** relief, and relief of rheumatic, neurological, spinal, **stress**, and respiratory disorders. Movement therapy can also be used as a meditation practice to quiet the mind, foster self-knowledge, and increase awareness. In addition, movement therapy is beneficial in alleviating emotional distress that is expressed through the body. These conditions include eating disorders, excessive clinging, and **anxiety** attacks. Since movements are related to thoughts and feelings, movement therapy can also bring about changes in attitude and emotions. People report an increase in self-esteem and self-image. Communication skills can be enhanced and tolerance of others increased. The physical openness facilitated by movement therapy leads to greater emotional openness and creativity.

Description

There are countless approaches to movement therapy. Some approaches emphasize awareness and attention to inner sensations. Other approaches use movement as a form of **psychotherapy**, expressing and working through deep emotional issues. Some approaches emphasize alignment with gravity and specific movement sequences, while other approaches encourage spontaneous movement. Some approaches are primarily concerned with increasing the ease and efficiency of bodily movement. Other approaches address the reality of the body "as movement" instead of the body as only something that runs or walks through space.

The term movement therapy is often associated with **dance therapy**. Some dance therapists work privately with people who are interested in personal growth. Others work in mental health settings with autistic, **brain** injured and learning disabled children, the elderly, and disabled adults.

Laban movement analysis (LMA), formerly known as Effort-Shape, is a comprehensive system for discriminating, describing, analyzing, and categorizing movements. LMA can be applied to dance, athletic coaching, fitness, acting, psychotherapy, and a variety of other professions. Certified movement analysts can "observe recurring patterns, note movement preferences, assess physical blocks and dysfunctional movement patterns, and suggest new movement patterns." As a student of Rudolf Laban, Irmgard Bartenieff developed his form of movement analysis into a system of body training or reeducation called Bartenieff fundamentals (BF). The basic premise of this work is that once the student experiences a physical foundation, emotional and intellectual expression becomes richer. BF uses specific exercises that are practiced on the floor, sitting, or standing to engage the deeper muscles of the body and enable a greater range of movement.

Authentic movement (AM) is based upon Mary Starks Whitehouse's understanding of dance, movement, and depth psychology. There is no movement instruction in AM, simply a mover and a witness. The mover waits and listens for an impulse to move and then follows or "moves with" the spontaneous movements that arise. These movements may or may not be visible to the witness. The movements may be in response to an emotion, a dream, a thought, pain, joy, or whatever is being experienced in the moment. The witness serves as a compassionate, non judgmental mirror and brings a "special quality of attention or presence." At the end of the session the mover and witness speak about their experiences together. AM is a powerful approach for self development and awareness and provides access to preverbal memories, creative ideas, and unconscious movement patterns that limit growth.

Gabrielle Roth (5 Rhythms movement) and Anna Halprin have both developed dynamic movement practices that emphasize personal growth, awareness, expression, and community. Although fundamentally different forms, each of these movement/dance approaches recognize and encourage our inherent desire for movement.

Several forms of movement therapy grew out of specific bodywork modalities. Rolfing movement integration (RMI) and Rolfing rhythms are movement forms which reinforce and help to integrate the structural body changes brought about by the hands-on work of Rolfing (structural integration). RMI uses a combination of touch and verbal directions to help develop greater awareness of one's vertical alignment and habitual movement patterns. RMI teacher Mary Bond says, "The premise of Rolfing Movement Integration... is that you can restore your structure to balance by changing the movement habits that perpetuate imbalance." Rolfing rhythms are a series of lively exercises designed to encourage awareness of the Rolfing principles of ease, length, balance, and harmony with gravity.

The movement education component of Aston-Patterning bodywork is called neurokinetics. This movement therapy teaches ways of moving with greater ease throughout everyday activities. These movement patterns can also be used to release tension in the body. Aston fitness is an **exercise** program which includes warm-up techniques, exercises to increase muscle tone and stability, stretching, and cardiovascular fitness.

Rosen method movement (an adjunct to Rosen method bodywork) consists of simple fun movement exercises done to music in a group setting. Through gentle swinging, bouncing, and stretching, every joint in the body experiences a full range of movement. The movements help to increase balance and rhythm and create more space for effortless breathing.

The movement form of Trager psychophysical integration bodywork, Mentastics, consists of fun, easy swinging, shaking, and stretching movements. These movements, developed by Dr. Milton Trager, create an experience of lightness and freedom in the body, allowing for greater ease in movement. Trager also worked successfully with polio patients.

Awareness through movement, the movement therapy form of the Feldenkrais method, consists of specific structured movement experiences taught as a group lesson. These lessons reeducate the brain without tiring the muscles. Most lessons are done lying down on the floor or sitting. Moshe Feldenkrais designed the lessons to

"improve ability... turn the impossible into the possible, the difficult into the easy, and the easy into the pleasant."

Ideokinesis is another movement approach emphasizing neuromuscular reeducation. Lulu Sweigart based her work on the pioneering approach of her teacher Mabel Elsworth Todd. Ideokinesis uses imagery to train the nervous system to stimulate the right muscles for the intended movement. If one continues to give the nervous system a clear mental picture of the movement intended, it will automatically select the best way to perform the movement. For example, to enhance balance in standing, Sweigart taught people to visualize "lines of movement" traveling through their bodies. Sweigart did not train teachers in ideokinesis but some individuals use ideokinetic imagery in the process of teaching movement.

The Mensendieck system of functional movement techniques is both corrective and preventative. Bess Mensendieck, a medical doctor, developed a series of exercises to reshape, rebuild, and revitalize the body. A student of this approach learns to use the conscious will to relax muscles and release tension. There are more than 200 exercises that emphasize correct and graceful body movement through everyday activities. Unlike other movement therapy approaches this work is done undressed or in a bikini bottom, in front of mirrors. This allows the student to observe and feel where a movement originates. Success has been reported with many conditions including **Parkinson's disease**, muscle and joint injuries, and repetitive strain injuries.

The Alexander technique is another functional approach to movement therapy. In this approach a teacher gently uses hands and verbal directions to subtly guide the student through movements such as sitting, standing up, bending and walking. The Alexander technique emphasizes balance in the neck-head relationship. A teacher lightly steers the students head into the proper balance on the tip of the spine while the student is moving in ordinary ways. The student learns to respond to movement demands with the whole body, in a light integrated way. This approach to movement is particularly popular with actors and other performers.

Pilates or physical mind method is also popular with actors, dancers, athletes, and a broad range of other people. Pilates consists of over 500 exercises done on the floor or primarily with customized exercise equipment. The exercises combine sensory awareness and physical training. Students learn to move from a stable, central core. The exercises promote strength, flexibility, and balance. Pilates training is increasingly available in sports medicine clinics, fitness centers, dance schools, spas, and physical therapy offices.

Many approaches to movement therapy emphasize awareness of internal sensations. Charlotte Selver, a student of somatic pioneer Elsa Gindler, calls her style of teaching sensory awareness (SA). This approach has influenced the thinking of many innovators, including Fritz Perls, who developed gestalt therapy. Rather than suggesting a series of structured movements, visualizations, or body positions, in SA the teacher outlines experiments in which one can become aware of the sensations involved in any movement. A teacher might ask the student to feel the movement of her breathing while running, sitting, picking up a book, etc. This close attunement to inner sensory experience encourages an experience of body-mind unity in which breathing becomes less restricted and posture, coordination, flexibility, and balance are improved. There may also be the experience of increased energy and aliveness.

Gerda Alexander Eutony (GAE) is another movement therapy approach that is based upon internal awareness. Through GAE one becomes a master of self-sensing and knowing which includes becoming sensitive to the external environment, as well. For example, while lying on the floor sensing the breath, skin or form of the body, one also senses the connection with the ground. GAE is taught in group classes or private lessons which also include hands-on therapy. In 1987, after two years of observation in clinics throughout the world, GAE became the first mind-body discipline accepted by the World Health Organization (WHO) as an alternative health-care technique.

Kinetic awareness developed by dancer-choreographer Elaine Summers, emphasizes emotional and physical inquiry. Privately or in a group, a teacher sets up situations for the student to explore the possible causes of pain and movement restrictions within the body. Rubber balls of various sizes are used as props to focus attention inward, support the body in a stretched position and massage a specific area of the body. The work helps one to deal with chronic pain, move easily again after injuries and increase energy, flexibility, coordination, and comfort.

Body-mind centering (BMC) was developed by Bonnie Bainbridge Cohen and is a comprehensive educational and therapeutic approach to movement. BMC practitioners use movement, touch, guided imagery, developmental repatterning, dialogue, music, large balls, and other props in an individual session to meet the needs of each person. BMC encourages people to develop a sensate awareness and experience of the ligaments, nerves, muscles, skin, fluids, organs, glands, fat, and fascia that make up one's body. It has been effective in preventing and rehabilitating from chronic injuries and in improving neuromuscular response in children with **cerebral palsy** and other neurological disorders.

Continuum movement has also been shown to be effective in treating neurological disorders including spinal chord injury. Developed by Emilie Conrad and Susan Harper, continuum movement is an inquiry into the creative flux of our body and all of life. Sound, breath, subtle and dynamic movements are explored that stimulate the brain and increase resonance with the fluid world of movement. The emphasis is upon unpredictable, spontaneous or spiral movements rather than a linear movement pattern. According to Conrad, "Awareness changes how we physically move. As we become more fluid and resilient so do the mental, emotional, and spiritual movements of our lives."

Eastern movement therapies such as yoga, t'ai chi, and qigong are also effective in healing and preventing a wide range of physical disorders, encouraging emotional stability, and enhancing spiritual awareness. There are a number of different approaches to yoga. Some emphasize the development of physical strength, flexibility, and alignment. Other forms of yoga emphasize inner awareness, opening, and meditation.

Precautions

People with acute injuries and chronic physical and mental conditions need to be careful when choosing a form of movement therapy. It is best to consult with a knowledgeable physician, physical therapist, or mental health therapist.

Research and general acceptance

Although research has documented the effects of dance therapy, qigong, t'ai chi, yoga, Alexander technique, awareness through movement (Feldenkrais), and Rolfing movement, other forms of movement therapy have not been as thoroughly researched.

Training and certification

Training and certification varies widely with each form of movement therapy. Many approaches require several years of extensive training and experience with the particular movement form.

Resources

BOOKS

Halprin, Anna. *Dance as a Healing Art: Returning to Health Through Movement and Imagery.* Life Rhythm, 1999.

Hartley, Linda. *Wisdom of the Body Moving: An Introduction to Body-Mind Centering.* Berkeley, CA: North Atlantic Press, 1995.

Knaster, Mirka. *Discovering the Body's Wisdom.* New York, NY: Bantam Books, 1996.

PERIODICALS

Cottingham, John T., and Jeffrey Maitland. "Integrating Manual and Movement Therapy With Philosophical Counseling for Treatment of a Patient With Amyotrophic Lateral Sclerosis: A Case Study That Explores the Principles of Holistic Intervention." *Alternative Therapies Journal* (March 2000): 120-128.

Linda Chrisman

MR *see* **Magnetic resonance imaging**

MRA *see* **Magnetic resonance imaging**

MRI *see* **Magnetic resonance imaging**

MRI unit *see* **Magnetic resonance imaging unit**

MRS *see* **Magnetic resonance imaging**

MS *see* **Multiple sclerosis**

Mucoviscidosis *see* **Cystic fibrosis**

MUGA scan *see* **Multiple-gated acquisition (MUGA) scan**

Multiple-gated acquisition (MUGA) scan

Definition

The **multiple-gated acquisition (MUGA) scan**, also called a cardiac **blood** pool study, is a non-invasive nuclear medicine test that displays the distribution of a radioactive tracer in the **heart**. The images of the heart are obtained at intervals throughout the **cardiac cycle** and are used to calculate ejection fraction and evaluate regional myocardial wall motion.

Purpose

A MUGA scan may be done at rest and with **stress**. The resting study is primarily performed to obtain the ejection fraction of the right and left ventricles, to evaluate the left ventricular regional wall motion, to assess the effects of cardiotoxic drugs (i.e., **chemotherapy**), and to differentiate the cause of shortness of breath (pulmonary vs. cardiac). Ejection fraction and wall motion are also important measurements made during a stress study, but the stress study is performed primarily to detect **coronary artery disease** and to evaluate angina.

Precautions

The use of a radioactive material is required to perform this study, so pregnant women should not have this test unless absolutely necessary. Women who are breast feeding are asked to stop for a specified period of time, typically 24 hours. Patients who have had other recent nuclear medicine studies may need to wait until residual radioactivity in the body has cleared before having this test.

Description

The MUGA scan is a series of images that demonstrate the flow of blood through the heart, enabling clinicians to obtain information about heart muscle activity. Before images are taken, a radionuclide is injected into the bloodstream, a process that requires two injections in most institutions. The first contains a chemical that adheres to red blood cells, and the second contains a radioactive tracer (Tc99m) that attaches to that chemical. Alternatively, the two chemicals can be mixed together first and then injected, but the material then tends to accumulate in bone and may obscure the heart.

A gamma camera takes the pictures, which is driven by a computer program that times the pictures, processes the information, and performs the mathematical calculations to provide ejection fraction and demonstrate wall motion. Images are obtained at various intervals during the cardiac cycle. Electrodes are placed on the patient so that a time frame can be established, for example, the time period between each "R" wave. The time frame is divided into several intervals, or "multiple gates." The result is a series of pictures showing the left and right ventricles at end-diastole and end-systole, and a number of stages in between.

A MUGA scan is performed in a hospital nuclear medicine department or in an out-patient facility and takes approximately 30 minutes to one hour. The patient lies down on a bed alongside the gamma camera and receives the radionuclide injections, then multiple images are taken. If a stress study is indicated, the rest study is performed first. For stress, the patient usually lies on a special bed fitted with a bicycle apparatus. While an image is being recorded, the patient is asked to cycle for about two minutes, then the resistance of the wheels are increased. After another two minutes of **exercise**, another image is obtained and the resistance is increased again.

Blood pressure and ECG are also monitored. After the stress portion is finished, one more resting, or recovery, study is obtained.

Preparation

Standard preparation an ECG for is required. In addition, special handling of nuclear materials may be required for the injections.

Aftercare

The patient can resume normal activities immediately after the test.

Results

A normal MUGA scan should not demonstrate areas of akinesis (lack of movement), or hypokinesis (decreased movement) of the walls. Abnormal motion, especially in the left ventricle, is suggestive of an infarct or other myocardial defect. The ejection fraction is a measure of heart function and should be within the normal limits established by the testing facility.

Health care team roles

A MUGA scan is performed by a nuclear medicine technologist, who is trained to handle radioactive materials, give injections, operate the equipment, take blood pressures, and process the data. The data is interpreted by a radiologist, nuclear medicine specialist, or cardiologist. The stress portion of the test may be monitored by a doctor. Patients receive results from their personal physician or the doctor who ordered the test.

Resources

BOOKS

DeBakey, Michael E. and Antonio M. Gotto, Jr. "Noninvasive Diagnostic Procedures." In *The New Living Heart.* Holbrook, MA: Adams Media Corporation, 1997, pp. 59-70.

Klingensmith III, M.D., Wm. C., Dennis Eshima, Ph.D., John Goddard, Ph.D. *Nuclear Medicine Procedure Manual 2000-2001.*

"Radionuclide Angiography." In *Cardiac Stress Testing & Imaging,* edited by Thomas H. Marwick. New York: Churchill Livingstone, 1996, pp. 517-521.

Raizner, Albert E. "Nuclear Cardiology Testing." In *Indications for Diagnostic Procedures: Topics in Clinical Cardiology.* New York, Tokyo: Igaku-Shon, 1997, pp. 44-47.

Texas Heart Institute. "Diagnosing Heart Diseases." In *Texas Heart Institute Heart Owner's Handbook.* New York: John Wiley & Sons, 1996, p. 333.

ORGANIZATIONS

American Heart Association. National Center. 7272 Greenville Avenue, Dallas, TX 75231-4596. (214) 373-6300. <http://www.medsearch.com/pf/profiles/amerh/>.

Texas Heart Institute Heart Information Service. P.O. Box 20345, Houston, TX 77225-0345. (800) 292-2221. <http://www.tmc.edu/thi/his.html>.

Christine Miner Minderovic, B.S., R.T., R.D.M.S.

Multiple pregnancy

Definition

A multiple **pregnancy** is a pregnancy in which more than one fetus develops in the uterus at the same time. Multiple pregnancies occur in 1–2% of pregnancies. The rate of twinning (the bearing of twins) is believed to be underestimated, as twin pregnancies with a singleton (an offspring born singly) birth are usually not recorded as twins.

Description

A multiple pregnancy may be the result of the natural process of twinning, or it may be the result of the woman having taken fertility drugs. Because of the increase in artificial reproductive technology (ART), the incidence of multiple pregnancies has increased. An April 1999 National Vital Statistics report from the Centers for Disease Control and Prevention (CDC) states that since

1980 the number of twins has risen by 52% and the number of triplets and high order multiples (more than three) has increased by 404%. An older maternal age and the use of fertility techniques are seen as the two major factors in these increases. While singletons have a 10% risk of being born preterm, multiple births have a 57% chance of being born prematurely. Premature birth places a neonate at higher risk for morbidity and mortality.

There are two categories of twins: monozygotic and dizygotic. Monozygotic twins are twins that have developed from a single fertilized ovum that split during embryonic development. These twins have the same genetic makeup and are always the same sex. They may be surrounded by one chorion (the outer embryonic membrane of the developing fetus), or may each have their own chorion. They may be surrounded by one amniotic sac (innermost of the membranes surrounding the embryo) or may each have their own amniotic sac. They may share a placenta or may each have their own placenta. These different possibilities depend on the time of the embryonic development at which the division took place. About two to 5% of monozygotic twins will share one amniotic sac. This rare occurrence puts the twins at risk for umbilical cord entanglement, cessation of **blood** flow, and death.

Double survival of monoamniotic twins is rare. Monozygotic twins may be referred to as identical. Dizygotic twins have developed from two fertilized ova. Their genetic makeup is different, and they are no more similar as any two siblings in a family. They may be the same or different sex. Each have their own chorion, amniotic sac, and placenta. While each twin has its own placenta, the placental implantations may be close enough that they fuse into one. Dizygotic twins may be referred to as fraternal. Multiple pregnancies of three or more fetuses may be the result of a single fertilized egg that splits, of multiple egg fertilizations, or a combination of the two processes.

Twins may not grow at the same rate. When there is 25% or more disparity between them, this is referred to as discordance, which occurs in about 10% of twin pregnancies. An extreme case of discordance occurs in the condition called twin-to-twin transfusion, also known as twin oligohydramnios polyhydramnios sequence. In this situation, one twin becomes the donor twin (receives too little blood from vessels in the fetuses' shared placenta that connect their blood circulations) and the other twin is the recipient (receives too much blood). The donor twin becomes small, pale, hypotensive, and anemic, with very little amniotic fluid. The recipient twin is large, polycythemic, hypertensive, with an excess of amniotic fluid. Both are at risk for **heart failure** and death.

At the time of delivery twins may be in any of the following combinations: vertex-vertex, breech-vertex, vertex-breech, breech-breech, vertex-transverse, or breech-transverse.

Causes and symptoms

In a woman's menstrual cycle, one egg, or ovum, is released every month. If more than one egg is released, it is possible for each egg to be fertilized separately by different spermatozoans. Fertility drugs encourage the release of more than one egg during the monthly menstrual cycle. In the case of monozygotic twins, only one egg was released and fertilized; but after fertilization it split, and separate fetuses developed. If the split is not complete, conjoined twins develop. Conjoined twins share certain body parts and organs. They may be referred to as Siamese twins. The chance of multiple pregnancy increases with an increase in parity and in maternal age up to about 35 years old, and then the incidence begins to decline. Genetics and racial background also play a role.

Diagnosis

A multiple pregnancy is suspected if the woman's uterus is growing too quickly for the gestational age, with excessive maternal weight gain, elevated levels of alphafetoprotein (a fetal protein that increases in the mother's blood during pregnancy) levels, unexplained severe maternal anemia, or with the auscultation (listening to sound to aid in diagnosis and treatment) of more than one fetal heartbeat. If undiagnosed at the time of quickening, the mother may feel movement in different parts of the uterus at the same time. Ultrasound can confirm or deny the presence of a multiple pregnancy. Once the multiple pregnancy is confirmed, ultrasonography may be used to check fetal growth over time, and the presence of any anomalies. There is a condition referred to as vanishing twin that occurs in up to 50% of twin pregnancies diagnosed very early by ultrasound. While twin sacs were seen on early sonography, a singleton is born. In these cases, there may have been early pregnancy vaginal bleeding and a lower human chorionic gonadotropin (hCG; a type of hormone) level than would be expected. The placenta often shows a whitish area and the remnant of a gestational sac. The mother and surviving twin (born singly) are both healthy.

Treatment

The diagnosis of a multiple pregnancy will result in it being treated as a **high-risk pregnancy** because of associated maternal and fetal risks. In a triplet pregnancy

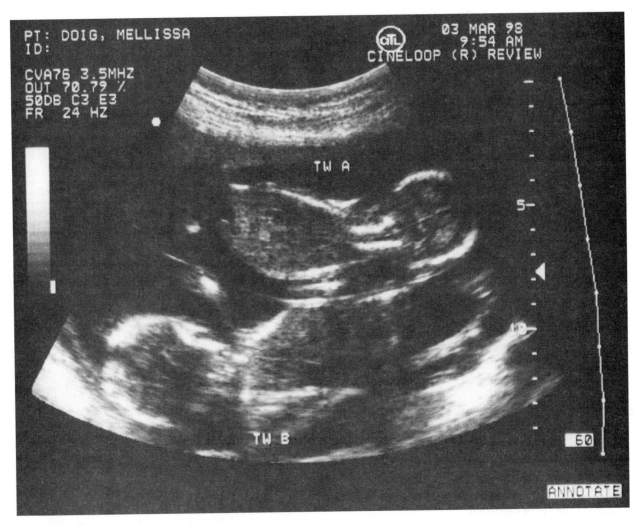

An ultrasound image of identical twin male fetuses. The distortion is due to "twin B" being closer to the monitor. *(Courtesy of Melissa Doig.)*

the mother may be offered the choice of selective reduction to twins. However, the literature is unclear as to the overall value of reduction from three to two fetuses. In high order multiples, to decrease the risk of very early preterm birth and potential loss of fetal viability, selective reduction may take place. In selective reduction high order multiples are reduced to triplets or twins. The procedure is usually completed prior to the end of the third month of gestation and involves a chemical injection into one or more developing embryos. A fetus that shows chromosomal damage is usually targeted first. While this process increases the chances of the viability of the remaining fetuses, it carries a significant emotional burden for the mother and partner. It also raises ethical issues concerning the "right-to-life" of a fetus. Efforts are being made in the field of ART to prevent the development of high order multiples in order to avoid this particular situation.

Prognosis

Prognosis for a multiple pregnancy depends on many factors. The higher the number of fetuses, the greater the risks. A twin pregnancy carries significantly more risks than a singleton pregnancy. The risks for triplets are similar to that of twins. The risks increase significantly with multiples of four or higher. Twins have a ten-fold risk of perinatal mortality over singletons.

While many multiple pregnancies have an excellent outcome, it is still considered a high-risk pregnancy. The average gestation for a singleton is 38 to 42 weeks. For twins gestation averages 37 weeks; for triplets, 33 weeks; and for quadruplets, 31 weeks. The mother carrying a multiple pregnancy has an increased risk of:

- premature birth

- pregnancy-related **hypertension** and preeclampsia

KEY TERMS

Breech—The buttocks or hind end of the body.

Chorion—The outer embryonic membrane of the developing fetus that gives rise to the placenta. Inside the chorion is the amniotic sac or sacs, inside of which are the fetuses.

Morbidity—Morbidity refers to an illness or disease condition. In statistics it refers to the rate at which a disease occurs.

Mortality—Mortality means death. In statistics it refers to the rate at which death occurs in a population for a particular disease condition.

Parity—The number of pregnancies with a fetus reaching viable gestation.

Singleton—A singleton is a fetus that develops alone in the uterus.

Transverse—At right angles to the anterior-posterior body axis.

Vertex—The top of the head or highest point of the skull.

- hydramnios (excess amniotic fluid)
- placenta previa (placenta covering the mouth of the womb-cervix)
- folic acid and **iron** deficiency
- gestational diabetes
- urinary tract infection
- placental abruption after the vaginal delivery of the first twin (separation of the placenta from the uterus before the baby is born)
- uterine atony (failure of the uterus to contract after birth) and postpartal hemorrhage due to exaggerated stretching of the uterus
- fatigue and backache
- cesarian delivery

The risks to fetuses in a multiple pregnancy are greater than that for a singleton and include:

- premature birth (**Preterm labor** for twins is seven to ten times more likely than for singletons and is a significant factor in perinatal morbidity and mortality.)
- intrauterine growth restriction
- congenital anomalies

- cerebral palsy with increased risk often due to preterm delivery
- discordance; more common with triplets than with twins
- dead fetus syndrome
- combined pregnancy, in which one twin develops in the uterus while the other is ectopic (other than in the uterus, such as the fallopian tube or peritoneal cavity)
- delayed delivery of second twin
- placental abruption

Health care team roles

While a mother carrying a singleton may have one ultrasound done during the pregnancy, the mother of a multiple pregnancy is much more likely to have several ultrasounds done. The experience, skill, and ability of the ultrasound technician to provide a calm environment can be a great help to the mother and her partner. The nurse working in a high-risk obstetric practice can provide a great deal of teaching both to inform the mother about what to expect and to decrease **anxiety** through knowledge.

Prevention

Twinning is a naturally occurring phenomenon and cannot be completely prevented. It occurs more often in older mothers. Multiple births due to ART are a concern because a multiple pregnancy represents a complication of pregnancy. Efforts within the ART community are being made to minimize the incidence of high order multiples. Efforts to prevent or minimize maternal and fetal complications will result in closer monitoring. More frequent ultrasounds, biophysical profile, and/or nonstress tests may be ordered. Cervical length and change may be monitored as an indicator of preterm delivery. If both twins are vertex and vaginal delivery is attempted, both fetal **heart** rates will be monitored. Caesarian deliveries of twins are more common than for singletons. This is especially true in high order multiples. The overall cesarian delivery rate tends to be about 75%.

Resources

BOOKS

Creasy, Robert K. and Robert Resnik. *Maternal-Fetal Medicine,* 4th ed. Philadelphia, PA: W.B. Saunders Company, 1999.

Pillitteri, Adele. *Maternal & Child Health Nursing: Care of the Childbearing and Childrearing Family.* Philadelphia, PA: Lippincott, 1999.

Scott, James. *Danforth's Obstetrics and Gynecology*, 8th ed. Philadelphia, PA: Lippincott Williams & Wilkins, 1999.

ORGANIZATIONS

The National Organization of Mothers of Twins Clubs, Inc. (NOMOTC). Executive Office, P.O. BOX 438, Thompson Station, TN 37179-0438. (615) 595-0936. (877) 540-2200. <http://www.nomotc.org/>.

Esther Csapo Rastegari, R.N., B.S.N., Ed.M.

Multiple sclerosis

Definition

Multiple sclerosis (MS) is a chronic autoimmune disorder affecting movement, sensation, and bodily functions. It is caused by destruction of the myelin sheath (insulation) covering nerve fibers (**neurons**) in the **central nervous system** (**brain** and **spinal cord**).

Description

MS is a nerve disorder caused by destruction of the insulating layer surrounding neurons in the brain and spinal cord. This insulation, called myelin, helps electrical signals pass quickly and smoothly between the brain and the rest of the body. When the myelin is destroyed neuronal messages are sent more slowly and less efficiently. Patches of scar tissue, called plaque, form over the affected areas, further disrupting neuronal communication. The symptoms of MS occur when the brain and spinal cord nerves no longer communicate properly with other parts of the body. MS causes a wide variety of symptoms and can affect **vision**, balance, strength, sensation, coordination, and bodily functions.

Multiple sclerosis affects more than a quarter of a million people in the United States. Most people have their first symptoms between the ages of 20 and 40 years; symptoms rarely begin before 15 years or after 60 years of age. Women are almost twice as likely as men to get MS, especially in their early years. People of northern European heritage are more likely to be affected than people of other racial backgrounds, and MS rates are higher in the United States, Canada, and Northern Europe than in other parts of the world. MS is very rare among Asians, North and South American natives, and Eskimos. Between 10% and 20% of people with MS have a benign type, meaning their symptoms progress very little over the course of their lives.

Causes and symptoms

Causes

Multiple sclerosis is an autoimmune disease, meaning its cause is due to an attack by the body's own **immune system**. For unknown reasons immune cells attack and destroy the myelin sheath that insulates neurons in the brain and spinal cord. This myelin sheath, created by other brain cells called glia, speeds transmission and prevents electrical activity in one cell from short-circuiting to another cell. Disruption of communication between the brain and other parts of the body prevents normal passage of sensations and control messages, leading to the symptoms of MS. The demyelinated areas appear as plaques, small round areas of gray neurons without the white myelin covering. The progression of symptoms is correlated with development of new plaques in the portion of the brain or spinal cord controlling the affected areas. Because there appears to be no pattern in the appearance of new plaques, the progression of MS is unpredictable.

Despite considerable research the trigger for this autoimmune destruction is still unknown. At various times evidence has pointed to genes, environmental factors, **viruses**, or a combination of these factors.

The risk of developing MS is higher if another family member is affected, suggesting the influence of genetic factors. In addition, the higher prevalence of MS among people of northern European ancestry suggests some genetic susceptibility.

The role of an environmental factor is suggested by studies of the effect of migration on the risk of developing MS. Age plays an important role in determining this change in risk. Young people in low-risk groups who move into countries with higher MS rates display the risk rates of their new surroundings, while older migrants retain the risk of their original home country. One interpretation of these studies is that an environmental factor, either protective or harmful, is acquired in early life. The risk of disease later in life reflects the effects of the early environment.

These same data can be used to support the involvement of a slow-acting virus, one that is acquired early on but begins its destructive effects much later. Slow viruses are known to cause other diseases, including **Creutzfeldt-Jakob disease** and bovine spongiform encephalopathy ("mad cow" disease). In addition, viruses have been implicated in other autoimmune diseases. Many claims have been made for the role of viruses, slow or otherwise, as the trigger for MS; however, as of 2001, no strong candidate has emerged.

How a virus could trigger the autoimmune reaction is also unclear. There are two main models of virally induced autoimmunity. The first suggests the immune system is actually attacking a virus (one too well hidden for detection in the laboratory), and the myelin damage is an unintentional consequence of fighting the **infection**. The second model suggests the immune system mistakes myelin for a viral protein encountered during a prior infection. Primed for the attack, the immune system destroys myelin because it resembles the previously recognized viral invader.

Either of these models allows a role for genetic factors, since certain genes can increase the likelihood of autoimmunity. Environmental factors, as well, might change the sensitivity of the immune system or interact with myelin to provide the trigger for the secondary **immune response**. Possible environmental triggers that have been invoked in MS include viral infection, trauma, electrical injury, and chemical exposure—although controlled studies have not supported a causative role.

Symptoms

The symptoms of multiple sclerosis may occur in one of three patterns:

• The most common pattern is the "relapsing-remitting" pattern, in which there are clearly defined symptomatic attacks lasting 24 hours or more, followed by complete or almost complete improvement. The period between attacks may be a year or more at the beginning of the disease, but may shrink to several months as the disease progresses. This pattern is especially common among younger people who develop MS.

• In the "primary progressive" pattern, the disease progresses without remission, or with occasional plateaus or slight improvements. This pattern is more common among older people.

• In the "secondary progressive" pattern, the person with MS begins with relapses and remissions, followed by more steady progression of symptoms.

Because plaques may form in any part of the central nervous system, the symptoms of MS vary widely from person-to-person and from stage-to-stage of the disease. Initial symptoms often include:

• muscle weakness causing difficulty walking

• loss of coordination or balance

• numbness, "pins and needles," or other abnormal sensations

• visual disturbances, including blurred or double vision

Later symptoms may include:

• fatigue

• muscle spasticity and stiffness

• tremors

• paralysis

• **pain**

• vertigo

• speech or swallowing difficulty

• loss of bowel and bladder control

• sexual dysfunction

• changes in cognitive ability

Weakness in one or both legs is common, and may be the first symptom noticed by a person with MS. Muscle spasticity, or excessive tightness, is also common and may be more disabling than weakness.

Double vision (diplopia) or eye tremor (nystagmus) may result from involvement of the nerve pathways controlling movement of the eye muscles. Visual disturbances result from involvement of the optic nerves (optic neuritis) and may include development of blind spots in one or both eyes, changes in color vision, or blindness. Optic neuritis usually involves only one eye at a time and is often associated with movement of the effected eye.

More than half of all people affected by MS have pain during the course of their disease. Many experience chronic pain, including pain from spasticity. Acute pain occurs in about 10% of cases. This pain may be a sharp, stabbing pain especially in the face, neck, or down the back. Facial numbness and weakness are also common.

Cognitive changes, including **memory** disturbances, depression, and personality changes, are found in people affected by MS, though it is not entirely clear whether these changes are due primarily to the disease or to the psychological reaction to it. Depression may be severe enough to require treatment in up to 25% of those with MS. A smaller number of people experience disease-related euphoria, or abnormally elevated mood, usually after a long disease duration and in combination with other psychological changes.

Symptoms of MS may be worsened by heat or increased body temperature including **fever**; intense physical activity; or exposure to sun, hot baths, or showers.

Diagnosis

There is no single test that confirms the diagnosis of multiple sclerosis and there are a number of other diseases with similar symptoms. While one person's diagnosis may be immediately suggested by symptoms and history, another's may not be confirmed without multiple

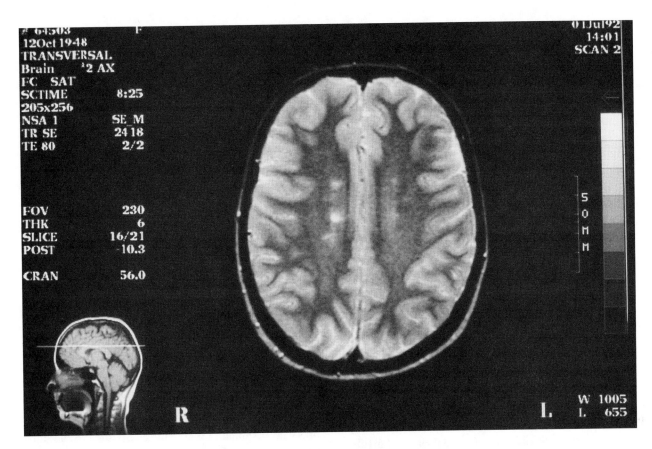

This image, made using magnetic resonance imaging (MRI), shows lesions on the left lobe of the brain of a multiple sclerosis patient. *(Comp-Unique/Custom Medical Stock Photo. Reproduced by permission.)*

tests and prolonged observation. The distribution of symptoms is important, as MS affects multiple areas of the body over time. The pattern of symptoms is also critical, especially evidence of the relapsing-remitting pattern. Thus, a detailed medical history is one of the most important parts of the diagnostic process. A thorough search to exclude other causes of a person's symptoms is especially important if the following features are present: 1) family history of neurologic disease, 2) symptoms and findings attributable to a single anatomic location, 3) persistent back pain, 4) age of onset over 60 or under 15 years of age, or 5) progressively worsening disease.

In addition to a medical history and a standard neurological exam, several lab tests are used to help confirm or rule out a diagnosis of MS:

• **Magnetic resonance imaging** (MRI) can reveal plaques on the brain and spinal cord. Gadolinium enhancement can distinguish between old and new plaques, allowing a correlation of new plaques with new symptoms. Plaques may be seen in several other diseases as well, including encephalomyelitis, neurosarcoidosis, and cerebral lupus. Plaques seen on an MRI may, however, be difficult to distinguish from

damage caused by small strokes, areas of decreased **blood** flow, or changes seen with trauma or normal aging.

• A lumbar puncture, or spinal tap, is done to measure levels of immune **proteins**, which are usually elevated in the cerebrospinal fluid of a person with MS. This test may not be necessary if other diagnostic tests are positive.

• Evoked potential tests, electrical tests of conduction speed in the neurons, can reveal reduced speeds consistent with the damage caused by plaques. These tests may be done with small electrical charges applied to the skin (somatosensory evoked potential), with light patterns flashed on the eyes (visual evoked potential), or with sounds presented to the ears (auditory evoked potential).

A clinician making the diagnosis, usually a neurologist, may classify the disease in one of three ways:

• "Definite MS" means that the symptoms and test results all point toward MS as the cause.

• "Probable MS" and "Possible MS" reflect less certainty and may require more time for observing the progression of the disease and the distribution of symptoms.

Treatment

As of 2001 three drugs shown to affect the course of the disease have been approved for the treatment of MS. None of these drugs is a cure, but they can slow disease progression in many cases.

Avonex and Betaseron are forms of the immune system protein beta interferon, while Copaxone is glatiramer acetate (formerly called copolymer-1). All three have been shown to reduce the rate of relapse in the relapsing-remitting form of MS. Different measurements from tests of each drug have demonstrated other benefits as well. Avonex may slow the progress of physical impairment, Betaseron may reduce the severity of symptoms, and Copaxone may decrease disability. All three drugs are administered by injection. Copaxone is given daily, Betaseron every other day, and Avonex weekly. Betaseron, however, is know to lead to the development of neutralizing antibodies, which reduce the effectiveness of treatment.

Immunosuppressant drugs have been used for many years to treat acute exacerbations (relapses). These drugs include **corticosteroids** such as prednisone and methylprednisolone, the hormone adrenocorticotropic hormone (ACTH), and azathioprine. Recent studies indicate that several days of intravenous methylprednisolone may be more effective than other immunosuppressant treatments for acute symptoms. This treatment may require hospitalization.

MS causes a large variety of symptoms, and the treatments for these are equally diverse. Most symptoms can be treated and complications avoided with good care and attention from medical professionals. Good health and **nutrition** remain important preventive measures. **Vaccination** against **influenza** can prevent respiratory complications and, contrary to earlier concerns, is not associated with worsening of symptoms. Preventing complications such as **pneumonia**, bed sores, injuries from **falls**, or urinary infection requires attention to the primary problems that may cause them. Shortened life spans with MS are almost always due to complications rather than primary symptoms themselves.

Physical therapy helps a person with MS to strengthen and retrain affected muscles; to maintain range of motion to prevent muscle stiffening; to learn to use assistive devices such as canes and walkers; and to learn safer and more energy-efficient ways of moving, sitting, and transferring. **Exercise** and stretching programs are usually designed by a physical therapist and taught to patients and their caregivers for use at home. Exercise is an important part of maintaining function for a person with MS. Swimming is often recommended, not only because it is a low-impact workout, but also because it allows strenuous activity without overheating.

Occupational therapy helps a person with MS adapt to the local environment and adapt the environment. An occupational therapist may suggest alternate strategies and assistive devices for activities of daily living, such as dressing, feeding, and washing, and may evaluate both home and work environments for safety and efficiency improvements.

Training in bowel and bladder care may be needed to prevent or compensate for incontinence. If the urge to urinate becomes great before the bladder is full, some drugs may be helpful, including propantheline bromide (Probanthine), oxybutynin chloride (Ditropan), or imipramine (Tofranil). Baclofen (Lioresal) may relax the sphincter muscle, allowing full emptying. Intermittent catheterization is effective in controlling bladder dysfunction. In this technique, a catheter is used to periodically empty the bladder.

Spasticity can be treated with oral medications, including baclofen and diazepam (Valium), or by injection with botulinum toxin (Botox). Spasticity relief may also bring relief from chronic pain. Other more acute types of pain may respond to carbamazepine (Tegretol) or diphenylhydantoin (Dilantin). Low back pain is common from increased use of the back muscles to compensate for weakened legs. Physical therapy and over-the-counter pain relievers may be helpful.

Fatigue may be partially avoidable with changes in the daily routine to allow more frequent rests. Amantadine (Symmetrel) and pemoline (Cylert) may improve alertness and lessen fatigue. Visual disturbances often respond to corticosteroids. Other symptoms that may be treated with drugs include seizures, vertigo, and tremor.

Myloral, an oral preparation of bovine myelin, has recently been tested in clinical trials for its effectiveness in reducing the frequency and severity of relapses. Preliminary data indicate no difference between it and placebo.

Alternative treatment

Bee venom has been suggested as a treatment for MS, but no studies or objective reports support this claim.

In British studies **marijuana** has been shown to have variable effects on the symptoms of MS. Improvements have been documented for tremor, pain, and spasticity, and worsening for posture and balance. Side effects have included weakness, dizziness, **relaxation**, and lack of coordination, as well as euphoria. As a result marijuana is not recommended as an alternative treatment. As of 2001 the use of marijuana for medical purposes was still illegal in most states of the United States.

Some studies support the value of high doses of **vitamins**, **minerals**, and other dietary supplements for controlling disease progression or improving symptoms. Alpha-linoleic and linoleic acids, as well as selenium and **vitamin E**, have shown effectiveness in the treatment of MS. Selenium and vitamin E act as antioxidants. In addition, the Swank diet (low in saturated **fats**), maintained over a long period of time, may retard the disease process.

Removal of mercury fillings has been touted as a possible cure, but is of no proven benefit.

Prognosis

It is difficult to predict how multiple sclerosis will progress in any one person. Most people with MS will be able to continue to walk and function at their work for many years after their initial diagnosis. The factors associated with the mildest course of MS are being female, having the relapsing-remitting form, having the first symptoms at a younger age, having longer periods of remission between relapses, and initial symptoms of decreased sensation or vision rather than of weakness or lack of coordination.

Approximately 5% of people with MS have the severe progressive form that leads to death from complications within five years. At the other extreme, 10-20% have a benign form, with very slow or no progression of their symptoms. The most recent studies show that about seven out of 10 people with MS are still alive 25 years after their diagnosis, compared to about nine out of 10 people of similar age without the disease. On average, MS shortens the lives of affected women by about six years and men by about 11 years. Suicide is a significant cause of death in MS, especially in younger persons.

The degree of disability a person experiences five years after onset is, on average, about three-quarters of the expected disability at 10-15 years. A benign course for the first five years usually indicates the disease will not cause marked disability.

Health care team roles

Physicians provide initial diagnoses. Neurologists may support diagnoses and monitor disease progression. Physical and occupational therapists provide exercise and environmental support for relief from muscle strains

KEY TERMS

Evoked potentials—Tests that measure the brain's electrical response to stimulation of sensory organs (eyes or ears) or peripheral nerves (skin).

Myelin—A layer of fatty cells that surrounds many nerve fibers in the brain and spinal cord. The myelin sheath acts as insulation that channels electrical impulses.

Nystagmus—Uncontrollable movements of the eye.

Plaque—Patches of scar tissue that form where a layer of myelin covering the nerve fibers is destroyed by the multiple sclerosis disease process.

Primary progressive—A pattern of symptoms of multiple sclerosis in which the disease progresses without remission, or with occasional plateaus or slight improvements.

Relapsing-remitting—A pattern of symptoms of multiple sclerosis in which symptomatic attacks last 24 hours or more, followed by complete or almost complete improvement.

Secondary progressive—A pattern of symptoms of multiple sclerosis in which there are relapses and remissions, followed by more steady progression of symptoms.

and weakness. Radiologists are important in documenting disease progression. Psychiatrists, psychologists, and other therapists may be helpful in treating depression that may accompany MS. Nurses provide bedside care, education for the patient and caregiver, preparation for home management of the disease, and home safety assessment.

Prevention

There is no known way to prevent MS. Until its cause is discovered, this situation is unlikely to change. Good nutrition; adequate rest; avoidance of **stress**, heat, and extreme physical exertion; and good bladder hygiene may improve quality of life and reduce symptoms for those who are affected by the disease.

Resources

BOOKS

Adams, Raymond D., Maurice Victor, and Allan H. Ropper. *Adam's & Victor's Principles of Neurology,* 6th ed. New York: McGraw Hill, 1997.

Burks, Jack S. and Kenneth P. Johnson. *Multiple Sclerosis: Diagnosis, Medical Management, and Rehabilitation.* New York: Demos Medical Publishing, 2000.

Cook, Stuart D. *Handbook of Multiple Sclerosis,* 3rd ed. New York: Marcel Dekker, 2001.

Hauser, Stephen L., and Donald E. Goodkin. "Multiple Sclerosis and Other Demyelinating Diseases." In *Harrison's Principles of Internal Medicine,* 14th ed. Ed. Anthony S. Fauci, et al. New York: McGraw-Hill, 1998, 2409-2419.

Hawkins, Clive, and Jerry S. Wolinsky. *Principles of Treatments in Multiple Sclerosis.* Woburn: Butterworth-Heinemann, 2000.

Joy, Janet E., and Richard B. Johnston. *Multiple Sclerosis: Current Status and Strategies for the Future.* Washington: National Academy Press, 2001.

Nichols, Judith L., and Lily Jung. *Living Beyond Multiple Sclerosis: A Woman's Guide.* Alameda: Hunter House, 2000.

Rudick, Richard A. "Multiple Sclerosis and Related Conditions." In *Cecil Textbook of Medicine,* 21st ed. Ed. Goldman, Lee, and J. Claude Bennett. Philadelphia: W.B. Saunders, 2000, 2141-2149.

PERIODICALS

Arnold, D.L., N. De Stefano, S. Narayanan, and P.M. Matthews. "Proton Magnetic Resonance Spectroscopy in Multiple Sclerosis." *Neuroimaging Clinics of North America* 10, no. 4 (2000): 789-798.

Bjartmar, C., and B.D. Trapp. "Axonal and Neuronal Degeneration in Multiple Sclerosis: Mechanisms and Functional Consequences." *Current Opinion in Neurology* 14, no. 3 (2001): 271-278.

Frank, J.A., and H.F. McFarland. "How to Participate in a Multiple Sclerosis Clinical Trial." *Neuroimaging Clinics of North America* 10, no. 4 (2000): 817-830.

Freeman, J.A. "Improving Mobility and Functional Independence in Persons with Multiple Sclerosis." *Journal of Neurology* 248, no. 4 (2001): 255-259.

Hickman, S.J. and D.H., Miller. "Imaging of the Spine in Multiple Sclerosis." *Neuroimaging Clinics of North America* 10, no. 4 (2000): 689-704.

Hohlfeld, R., and H. Wekerle. "Immunological Update on Multiple Sclerosis." *Current Opinion in Neurology* 14, no. 3 (2001): 299-304

Lucchinetti, C., W. Bruck, and J. Noseworthy. "Multiple Sclerosis: Recent Developments in Neuropathology, Pathogenesis, Magnetic Resonance Imaging Studies and Treatment." *Current Opinion in Neurology* 14, no. 3 (2001): 259-269.

Matthews, P.M., and D.L. Arnold. "Magnetic Resonance Imaging of Multiple Sclerosis: New Insights Linking Pathology to Clinical Evolution." *Current Opinion in Neurology* 14, no. 3 (2001): 279-287.

Nyul, L.G., and J.K. Udupa. "Magnetic Resonance Image Analysis in Multiple Sclerosis." *Neuroimaging Clinics of North America* 10, no. 4 (2000): 799-816.

Rovaris, M., and M. Filippi. "Contrast Enhancement and the Acute Lesion in Multiple Sclerosis." *Neuroimaging Clinics of North America* 10, no. 4 (2000): 705-716.

Simon, J.H. "Brain and Spinal Cord Atrophy in Multiple Sclerosis." *Neuroimaging Clinics of North America* 10, no. 4: 753-770.

ORGANIZATIONS

American Academy of Neurology. 1080 Montreal Avenue, St. Paul, Minnesota 55116, (651) 695-1940. <http://www.aan.com>.

Multiple Sclerosis Foundation. 6350 North Andrews Ave., Fort Lauderdale, Fl 33309-2130, (800) 441-7055. <http://www.msfacts.org>.

National Multiple Sclerosis Society. 733 Third Avenue, New York, NY 10017, (800) 344-4867. <http://www.nmss.org>.

OTHER

Computer Literate Advocates for Multiple Sclerosis. <http://www.clams.org>.

International Multiple Sclerosis Support Foundation. <http://www.msnews.org>.

MS World. <http://www.msworld.org>.

Multiple Sclerosis International Federation. <http://www.ifmss.org.uk>.

Multiple Sclerosis Society of UK. <http://www.mssociety.org.uk>.

Multiple Sclerosis Society of Canada. <http://www.mssociety.ca>.

National Institute of Neurological Disorders and Stroke. <http://ninds.nih.gov/health_and_medical/disorders/multiple_sclerosis.htm>.

L. Fleming Fallon, Jr., M.D., Dr.P.H.

Muscle contraction

Definition

Muscle contraction is the response a muscle has to any kind of stimuli where the result is shortening in length and development of force.

Description

There are three general types of muscle in our bodies. They are skeletal (striated), cardiac, and smooth (visceral) muscle. When **skeletal muscles** contract, they help the body move and breathe. Skeletal muscles are attached to bones and function in a fashion similar to a lever. Skeletal muscle responds to stimuli that are both voluntary and involuntary.

Although similar to skeletal muscle, cardiac muscle is unique to the **heart**. Cardiac cells are smaller and contain more mitochondria than skeletal muscle. The mitochondria produce high-energy molecules in the form of ATP to supply cardiac muscles with the fuel they need to continuously contract, pumping **blood** through the circulatory system. The heart is an involuntary muscle and does not need any input from the nervous system to initiate and maintain a contraction.

Myofibrils within the muscle fibers (muscle cells) of skeletal and cardiac muscle have thick and thin filaments that overlap to create patterns called I-bands, H-zones, A-bands, Z-discs, and M-line. Thin filaments contain two strands of protein called actin that is wound into a helical structure with a strand of two other **proteins** called troponin and tropomyosin. Thick filaments contain many small filaments of protein called myosin filaments, which consist of a head and a tail. These patterns give skeletal and cardiac muscle a "striated" appearance. During skeletal and cardiac muscle contraction, the I-band shortens, while the other bands and zones remain the same length.

Smooth muscle lines the walls of the body's viscera (organs), particularly the **blood vessels** and **digestive system**. It lacks striations found in skeletal muscle. When smooth muscles contract, they control the passage of substances through the tubular structures of the blood vessels and intestines. Smooth muscle is controlled involuntarily.

Function

The nature of the contraction

Muscle contractions generally involve the shortening of a muscle while exerting a force and performing work. However, there are many different types of contractions, and some do not strictly follow that definition. Isometric contraction occurs when the muscle does not shorten, but it does exert force (e.g. pushing or pulling an immovable object). Isotonic contractions take place when the muscle length shortens and the force remains the same (e.g. lifting a weight at the gym). In an auxotonic contraction the force gradually increases while the muscle length is shortening (e.g. pulling on a rubber band). Conversely, a meiotonic contraction occurs when the force decreases as the muscle length shortens (e.g. depressing a key on a computer keyboard). Most muscle contractions involve a combination of two or more of the above contractions and are called mixed contractions.

For example, when lifting a large bucket filled with water, there is first an isometric contraction, followed by isotonic shortening.

While skeletal muscle is resting, there is still a force exerted due to the tension created from the muscle's connection to the bone on each end of the muscle. This force is called the resting force and is similar to the force of a rubber band that is stretched. Tests performed in the laboratory demonstrate that muscles have an optimal length where contraction produces a maximum active force. Maximum force usually occurs at the natural length of the muscle and is termed optimal length (L_0).

Since cardiac muscle is not connected to bones like skeletal muscle, it functions over a greater range of lengths. Additionally, its maximum force ability is observed at a lower L_0, giving it a "reserve" length. This allows cardiac muscle to contract more forcefully when necessary. The muscle is re-lengthened when the chamber of the heart fills with blood.

Smooth muscle does not make the typical isotonic contractions seen in skeletal and cardiac muscle. Most smooth muscle contractions of the digestive tract occur as a substance passes through the hollow tube that smooth muscle comprises; therefore, smooth muscle shortens against a decreasing load. On the other hand, smooth muscle in blood vessels maintains a partially isometric contraction where the force is held constant for an extended period of time, resulting in a particular **blood pressure**.

The nature of the biochemistry of the contraction

Muscle contraction involves the sliding of thick filaments of myosin past thin filaments of actin. The interaction of myosin and actin begins when a high-energy molecule of ATP located in the head of the myosin filament is hydrolyzed into an inorganic phosphate (P_i) molecule and ADP. The myosin head subsequently attaches to an actin filament forming a crossbridge. The ADP and P_i are then released, and the myosin head undergoes a conformational change that causes the actin filament to move relative to the myosin filament. Then, ATP once again binds to the myosin head and causes myosin to dissociate from the actin filament. These steps are repeated very rapidly, causing the myosin head to "walk" along the actin filament, resulting in a muscle contraction. Only when ATP is present can the myosin head detach from the actin filament to continue the process. If ATP is not present, then the muscle will become stiff and unable to relax as is seen in rigor mortis.

The nature of control of the contraction

Muscle cells contain a highly excitable membrane called the sarcoplasmic reticulum, which can be excited to release **calcium** ions and produce an action potential. Most stimulation occurs through motor **neurons** that originate in the somatic portion of the **central nervous system** and innervate the muscles at the myoneural junction. When the motor neuron nears the muscle it branches to innervate several different muscle fibers. Many different nerves innervate muscles responsible for fine and precise motor movements, each nerve innervating only a couple muscle fibers. Conversely, only a few nerves innervate muscles responsible for large, imprecise movements, each nerve branching many times to innervate many muscle fibers.

The nerve side of the myoneural junction makes up the presynaptic portion. Muscle is located on the other side of the junction, forming the postsynaptic portion. As an action potential travels down the nerve and reaches the axon terminal, extracellular calcium ions enter the terminal. Neurotransmitter vesicles in the axon terminal migrate to the axon membrane, fusing with it to release acetylcholine into the synaptic cleft. Molecules of acetylcholine diffuse across the cleft and bind to receptors on the postsynaptic membrane of the muscle. Then, ion channels in the postsynaptic membrane open, allowing potassium and sodium ions to enter. This creates an electrical potential (end-plate potential) and depolarization of the postsynaptic membrane, which then travels down the entire muscle membrane, resulting in a muscle action potential. As an action potential travels down the muscle fiber, a membrane system located within the muscle called the sarcoplasmic reticulum releases calcium ions, which are stored within the membrane system. The calcium ions diffuse into an area of actin and myosin filaments where they bind to troponin molecules associated with the actin filaments. Then the actin filaments are enabled to interact with the myosin filaments and the result is a muscle contraction.

In order to halt a contraction after the initial action potential is fired, acetylcholine diffuses away from the receptor in the postsynaptic cleft, and an enzyme called cholinesterase hydrolyzes acetylcholine into choline and acetate. Choline is taken back into the presynaptic cleft and recycled into more acetylcholine in the neurotransmitter vesicles.

Role in human health

The coordination between the nervous system and muscles permits many actions such as walking, talking, eating, digesting food, breathing, and giving birth. Muscle contractions have several roles. When a muscle functions as a motor it consumes fuel and does work (e.g. walking, lifting, etc.). This produces heat, which helps to warm the body (e.g. shivering). Muscles also function as regulators. They control the passage of substances through the digestive system, and control the beating of the heart muscle and the diameter of blood vessels, resulting in specific blood pressures.

If the body develops any one of a number of problems that affect muscle contraction, both the motor and regulatory properties of muscles can be injured. Anything from walking, breathing, talking, or digesting food can be damaged, depending on the problem encountered.

Common diseases and disorders

Muscle contraction can be affected on a multitude of levels. Neurological problems, autoimmune diseases, infectious diseases and **spinal cord** injuries can all contribute to impaired muscle contraction.

Muscle cramping is a common disorder. Cramping occurs when the muscle contracts involuntarily at a rate of about 300 contractions per second, a much higher rate than the maximum voluntary contraction. It is not known why cramping occurs. Researchers think that it may be a result of electrolyte imbalance in the extracellular fluid surrounding the muscle fiber and nerves. Drinking a sports beverage or eating a banana can replace electrolytes. This is especially important after strenuous **exercise**.

About 12,000 Americans suffer from myasthenia gravis. Myasthenia gravis is an autoimmune disease in which the body's **immune system** has a reaction to acetylcholine receptors, reducing the number of receptors on the postsynaptic membrane. As a result, not enough acetylcholine binds to receptors, and not enough sodium and potassium ion channels open. Therefore, end-plate potentials may not be high enough to create an action potential, resulting in muscle weakness. Myasthenia gravis can be treated with administration of cholinesterase inhibitors, which allow acetylcholine to remain in the cleft for a longer period of time. Thus, the receptors present can be stimulated over and over to permit sufficient ion flow to create an end-plate potential.

Microorganisms can cause some muscle disorders. Tetanus, also called "lock jaw," is a neurological disorder caused by tetanospasmin, a powerful toxin produced by the **bacteria** *Clostridium tetani*. The toxin blocks inhibitory neurotransmitters that normally stop the release of acetylcholine. A build-up of acetylcholine occurs in the space between the pre- and postsynaptic cleft, resulting in a summation of muscle contractions. Summation of muscle contractions produces muscle rigidity. Tetanus is treated with **antibiotics** and antitoxins.

Resources

BOOKS

Braunwald, Eugene et. al. *Harrison's Principles of Internal Medicine,* 15th ed. McGraw-Hill, 2001.

Guyton, Arthur C., M.D. and John E. Hall, Ph.D. *Textbook of Medical Physiology,* 10th ed. W.B. Saunders Company, 2000.

Vander, Arthur. *Human Physiology: The Mechanisms of Body Function,* 7th ed. WBC McGraw-Hill, 1998.

PERIODICALS

Sieck G.C., and M. Regnier. "Invited Review: Plasticity and Energetic Demands of Contraction in Skeletal and Cardiac Muscle." *Journal of Applied Physiology* 90, no. 3 (March 2001): 1158-64.

OTHER

Holmes, K.C. *Muscle Contraction.* Expanded from "The Limits of Reductionism in Biology" Wiley, Chichester (Novartis Foundation Symposium 213, pp 76-92). <http://lala.mpimf-heidelberg.mpg.de/~holmes/muscle/muscle1.html>.

Sally C. McFarlane-Parrott

Muscle relaxants

Definition

Skeletal muscle relaxants are drugs that relax striated muscles (those that control the skeleton). They are a separate class of drugs from the muscle relaxant drugs used during intubations and surgery to reduce the need for anesthesia and facilitate intubation.

Purpose

Skeletal muscle relaxants may be used for relief of spasticity in neuromuscular diseases, such as **multiple sclerosis**, as well as for **spinal cord injury** and stroke. They may also be used for **pain** relief in minor strain injuries and control of the muscle symptoms of tetanus. Dantrolene (Dantrium) has been used to prevent or treat malignant hyperthermia in surgery.

Description

Although the muscle relaxants may be divided into only two groups, centrally acting and peripherally acting, the centrally acting group, which appears to act on the **central nervous system**, contains 10 drugs which are chemically different, while only dantrolene has a direct action at the level of the nerve-muscle connection.

Baclofen (Lioresal) may be administered orally or intrathecally for control of spasticity due to neuromuscular disease.

Carisoprodol (Soma), chlorphenesin (Maolate), chlorzoxazone (Paraflex), cyclobenzaprine (Flexeril), diazepam (Valium), metaxalone (Skelaxin), methocarbamol (Robaxin), and orphenadrine (Norflex) are used primarily as an adjunct for rest in management of acute muscle spasms associated with sprains. Muscle relaxation may also be an adjunct to **physical therapy** in rehabilitation following stroke, **spinal cord** injury, or other musculoskeletal conditions.

Diazepam and methocarbamol are also used by injection for relief of tetanus.

Recommended dosage

Dose varies with the drug, route of administration, and purpose. There may be individual variations in absorption that require doses higher than those usually recommended, particularly with methocarbamol. Consult specific references for further information.

Precautions

All drugs in this class may cause sedation. Baclofen, when administered intrathecally, may cause severe central nervous system (CNS) depression with cardiovascular collapse and **respiratory failure**.

Diazepam may be addictive. It is a controlled substance under federal law.

Dantrolene has a potential for hepatotoxicity. The incidence of symptomatic hepatitis is dose related, but may occur even with a short period of doses at or above. Even short periods of doses at or above 800 mg per day

KEY TERMS

Central nervous system—The brain and spinal cord.

Intrathecal—Introduced into or occurring in the space under the arachnoid membrane which covers the brain and spinal cord.

Pregnancy category—A system of classifying drugs according to their established risks for use during pregnancy. Category A: Controlled human studies have demonstrated no fetal risk. Category B: Animal studies indicate no fetal risk, but no human studies, or adverse effects in animals, but not in well-controlled human studies. Category C: No adequate human or animal studies, or adverse fetal effects in animal studies, but no available human data. Category D: Evidence of fetal risk, but benefits outweigh risks. Category X: Evidence of fetal risk. Risks outweigh any benefits.

Sedative—Medicine used to treat nervousness or restlessness.

Spasm—Sudden, involuntary tensing of a muscle or a group of muscles.

Tranquilizer (minor)—A drug that has a calming effect and is used to treat anxiety and emotional tension.

greatly increases the risk of serious **liver** injury. Overt hepatitis has been most frequently observed between the third and twelfth months of therapy. Risk of hepatic injury appears to be greater in women, in patients over 35 years of age and in patients taking other medications in addition to dantrolene.

Tizanidine may cause low **blood pressure**, but this may be controlled by starting with a low dose and increasing it gradually. The drug may rarely cause liver damage.

Methocarbamol and chlorzoxazone may cause harmless color changes in urine—orange or reddish-purple with chlorzoxazone and purple, brown, or green with methocarbamol. The urine will return to its normal color when the patient stops taking the medicine.

Most drugs in this class are well tolerated.

Not all drugs in this group have been evaluated for safety in **pregnancy** and breast feeding.

Baclofen is pregnancy category C. It has caused fetal abnormalities in rats at doses 13 times above the human dose. Baclofen passes into breast milk, and breast feeding while taking baclofen is not recommended.

Diazepam is category D. All benzodiazepines cross the placenta. Although the drugs appear to be safe for use during the first trimester of pregnancy, use later in pregnancy may be associated with cleft lip and palate. Diazepam should not be taken while breast feeding. Infants who were breast fed while their mothers took diazepam were excessively sleepy and lethargic.

Dantrolene is category C. In animal studies it has reduced the rate of survival of the newborn when given in doses seven times the normal human dose. Mothers should not breast feed while receiving dantrolene.

Interactions

Skeletal muscle relaxants have many potential **drug interactions**. Individual references should be consulted.

Because these drugs cause sedation, they should be used with caution with other drugs that may also cause drowsiness.

The activity of diazepam may be increased by drugs that inhibit its **metabolism** in the liver. These include: cimetidine, oral contraceptives, disulfiram, fluoxetine, isoniazid, ketoconazole, metoprolol, propoxyphene, propranolol, and valproic acid.

Dantrolene may have an interaction with estrogens. Although no interaction has been demonstrated, the rate of liver damage in women over the age of 35 who were taking estrogens is higher than in other groups.

Samuel D. Uretsky, PharmD

Muscle strain *see* **Sprains and strains**

Muscle testing

Definition

Muscle testing is the evaluation of contractile units, including muscles and tendons, and their ability to generate forces.

Purpose

Muscle testing is indicated in any individual with suspected or actual impaired muscle performance, including strength, power, or endurance. Impairments in muscle function may result from cardiovascular, pulmonary, musculoskeletal or neuromuscular disease or disorders. Identification of specific muscles or muscle groups with impaired function provides information for appropriate intervention, which may include strengthening exercises, functional drills, bracing, or compensatory muscle use.

Precautions

It is important to determine the patient's ability to withstand the force to be applied. The patient should have good cardiovascular function, be instructed against using the Valsalva maneuver, and be positioned appropriately. Care should be taken with any body part that is under movement restriction due to fracture, post-surgical, or other tissue healing.

Description

Forms of muscle testing include manual strength testing, functional tests, and dynamometry.

Manual muscle testing

Manual muscle strength testing is a widely used form of muscle testing in the clinic. In this form of testing, the individual is asked to hold a limb or other body part at the end of its available range or at another point in its range of motion while the clinician provides manual resistance. General procedures include the following:

- The patient should be placed in a position that provides overall support to the body so that he or she can concentrate his or her effort on the part being tested.

- The part to be tested initially is placed in an antigravity position. If muscles are too weak to function against gravity, they are then tested in the horizontal plane.

- The proximal part of the area being tested should be stabilized to reduce the opportunity for compensatory action by muscles other than those being tested.

- Resistance needs to be applied directly opposite the "line of pull" of the muscles being tested.

- Gradual, not sudden, application of pressure should take place, using a long lever arm in most cases.

- Both sides should be assessed to provide a comparison, especially when one side is affected by pathology and the other is not.

Grading of muscle tests is used to determine a patient's **physical therapy** diagnosis and in assessing progress over time. Objective observation includes determining the patient's ability to hold a test position, move through a full range of motion, or to overcome gravity. Care must be taken in grading, however, due to the inevitable subjectivity of muscle testing. Subjective factors include the clinician's impression of how much resistance to apply and how much is tolerated. Consistent testing procedures, including accurate joint placement and prohibition of compensatory movements, allow for increased reliability in using manual muscle testing as an evaluation tool. In studies comparing manual testing and dynamometry, results show positive correlation; however, manual muscle testing is less sensitive than dynamometry.

Traditional grading has been described using either the terms "zero," "trace," "poor," "fair," "good," and "normal," or using a numerical scale from 0 through 5. When determining a grade, first determine whether or not the patient can move the body part through its full range against gravity and hold the body part in the test position. This ability results in a grade of fair, or 3, and is the most objective observation made during testing due to the consistency of gravity. A poor grade, or 2, is given when a patient is able to move the body part through its complete range of motion in the horizontal plane, that is, with the effect of gravity eliminated. A trace grade, or 1, is given when there is no visible movement through a part's range, but a slight contraction can be palpated. When there is no evidence of even a slight contraction, a grade of zero is given.

Grades above fair are assessed with the body part in the specified test position. A grade of good, or 4, denotes the ability of the patient to hold the body part in the test position against moderate pressure. A normal grade, or 5, denotes that the patient holds the body part against strong pressure by the clinician.

Pluses and minuses can be added to the above grades to further describe muscle ability, but some discourage their use because it introduces even more subjectivity to grading. In some cases, however, the use of a plus or minus grade provides important information. For example, a patient with a fair grade (3) for a muscle group may not be able to use an orthosis effectively, but if that patient achieves a fair plus (3+), he or she can withstand minimal resistance against gravity and therefore may be able to tolerate the additional weight of an orthosis. Descriptors for plus and minus grades are included in the summary of grades below:

- Normal (5): withstands strong pressure in test position.

- Good plus (4+): withstands moderate to strong pressure.

- Good (4): withstands moderate pressure.

- Good minus (4-): withstands slight to moderate pressure.

- Fair plus (3+): withstands slight pressure.

- Fair (3): holds test position against gravity but tolerates no additional pressure.

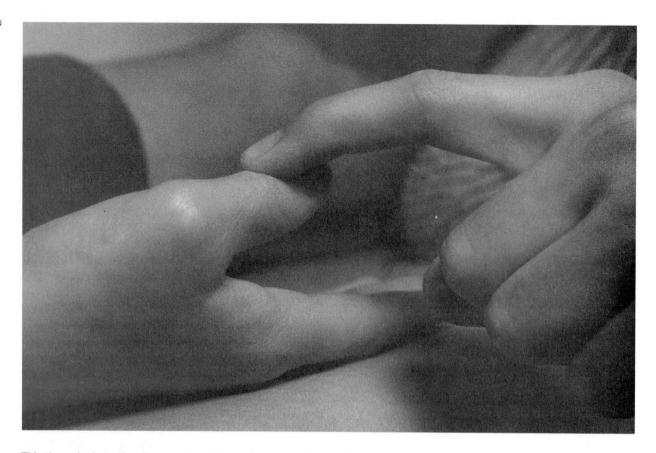

This therapist is testing the muscles of the patient's hand by pressing on the thumb. *(Photograph by John Watney. Science Source/Photo Researchers. Reproduced by permission.)*

- Fair minus (3-): sags from test position or only moves through partial range of motion against gravity (>50% of motion).

- Poor plus (2+): moves through 50% of motion or less in antigravity position, or holds against resistance in gravity-eliminated position (horizontal plane).

- Poor (2): moves through complete range in horizontal plane.

- Poor minus (2-): moves through partial range in horizontal plane.

- Trace (1): slight contraction, but no visible movement of body part detected.

- Zero (0): complete lack of muscle contraction.

It is important to note that manual muscle grades are an ordinal level of measurement, meaning that the categories do not represent equal magnitudes. In other words, the strength required to move from zero to trace is different from the amount of strength required to move from good to normal. Therefore, manual muscle grades are not useful for arithmetical computations.

Manual muscle testing is a relatively quick and inexpensive method of evaluating strength; however, results often do not denote a person's ability to perform functional activities. In addition, a normal muscle grade does not necessarily indicate a patient's ability to return to his or her normal level of activity, especially if it includes sports participation. This ability is better tested with functional tests.

Functional muscle testing

Functional muscle testing allows for the assessment of muscles to perform components of, or entire, tasks related to daily activities. Functional tests look at the ability of muscle groups to decelerate, stabilize or accelerate movement in all three planes of motion in a measurable way. Specific tests can be chosen to look at movements at specific joints or those that are dominant in a certain plane of motion. For example, a single-leg squat provides valuable information about the quadriceps' performance. An anterior jump test provides the same type of information on a more challenging level for the patient.

Categories of functional muscle testing include the following: balance, excursion, lunge, step-up, step-down, jump and hop tests. In performing tests, patient safety is key. Clinical judgment should be used to determine when functional testing is appropriate; for example, a person with a weight-bearing restriction should not perform a balance test on that lower extremity. Testing should be done in a progressive manner; for example, a balance test should be performed before an excursion test, a straight plane lunge test before a rotational lunge test. Tests can be used to document progress by measuring distance of reach, time, degrees of excursion, etc., as appropriate to the specific test.

Dynamometry

Isokinetic dynamometry uses a device that measures the force used in contraction of a muscle group. The device is able to apply maximal resistance at all points in the body part's range of motion at a specified speed. Isokinetic testing can be used to objectively assess strength, power and endurance. Strength is assessed using slow velocity testing to look at peak torques produced. Power testing uses fast velocity settings to look at the amount of work performed during a particular amount of time. **Endurance testing** looks at the patient's ability to maintain sorce output during numerous repetitions at high velocities.

Advantages of isokinetic testing include the ability to maximally load the muscle throughout its range of motion; stabilization of proximal body parts to prevent substitute motions; measurement of concentric and eccentric loading; and objectivity. As in manual muscle testing, however, isokinetic testing does not necessarily provide an accurate picture of how a muscle will function during actual activities of daily living or sports. In addition, unlike manual muscle testing, it requires expensive equipment and space.

Hand-held and grip dynamometers are smaller, less expensive alternatives for measuring muscle strength in an objective manner. Information regarding force produced during a contraction such as knee extension or hand grip is displayed in units (often pounds) on a display or dial. Use of these instruments, however, is limited to the body parts they were designed to measure; i.e., a grip dynamometer is useful only for measuring grip strength.

Results

Results are recorded as described above, by the use of grades or force units. Regardless of the type of muscle testing used, the results can be used to help determine specific sites of impairment, in addition to providing data for assessing progress.

Manual muscle testing—levels of muscle performance	
Level of performance	**Definition**
Normal	Completes full range of motion against gravity, and holds test position against strong pressure.
Good	Completes full range of motion against gravity, and holds test position against moderate to strong pressure.
Fair	Completes full range of motion against gravity, and holds test position with slight or no added pressure. There may a gradual release from test position.
Poor	Completes partial range of motion against gravity, and moves through complete range of motion in horizontal plane.
Poor–	Completes partial range of motion in horizontal plane.
Trace	No visible movement of the part, but examiner may observe or palpate contractile activity in the muscle.
Zero	No contraction detected in the muscle.

SOURCE: Rothstein, J.M., S.H. Roy, and S.L. Wolf. *The Rehabilitation Specialist's Handbook.* 2nd ed. Philadelphia: F.A. Davis Co., 1998.

Health care team roles

Muscle testing is performed by physicians, especially orthopedic doctors and physiatrists, in addition to physical therapists and occupational therapists. Manual muscle testing often is an integral part of a PT or OT evaluation of muscle function. The following knowledge is required for any health care practitioner to perform an accurate test:

• location, origin and insertion of muscle(s) being tested

• direction of muscle fiber orientation

• function of muscle being tested, in addition to functions of its synergists and antagonists

• appropriate positioning for the test

• recognition of substitution or compensation by other muscles

• recognition of the effects of factors such as restricted range of motion and pain

• specific contraindications

• ability to palpate muscle contraction

• ability to modify a test due to inability to attain a certain position

• ability to communicate to the patient regarding purpose, procedures and patient requirements for the test

Resources

BOOKS

American Physical Therapy Association. *Guide to Physical Therapist Practice*. 2nd ed. Fairfax, VA: American Physical Therapy Association, 2001.

Gray, Gary W. *Lower Extremity Functional Profile*. Adrian, MI: Wynn Marketing, Inc., 1995.

Hislop, Helen J. and Jacqueline Montgomery. *Daniels and Worthingham's Muscle Testing: Techniques of Manual Examination*. 6th ed. Philadelphia: W.B. Saunders Company, 1995.

Kendall, Florence Peterson, et. al. *Muscles: Testing and Function*. 4th ed. Baltimore: Williams & Wilkins, 1993.

PERIODICALS

Bohannon, R.W. "Measurement of Hand Grip Strength: Manual Muscle Testing Versus Dynamometry." *Physiotherapy Canada* 51 (Fall 1999): 268-72.

Bohannon, R.W. "Measuring Knee Extensor Strength." *American Journal of Physical Medicine and Rehabilitation* 80 (January 2001): 13-8.

Peggy Campbell Torpey, MPT

Muscular dystrophy

Definition

Muscular dystrophy is the name for a group of inherited disorders in which strength and muscle bulk gradually decline. Nine types of muscular dystrophies are generally recognized.

Description

The muscular dystrophies include:

- Duchenne muscular dystrophy (DMD). DMD affects young boys, causing progressive muscle weakness, usually beginning in the legs. It is a severe form of muscular dystrophy. DMD occurs in about 1 in 3,500 male births, and affects approximately 8,000 boys and young men in the United States. A milder form occurs in a very small number of female carriers.

- Becker muscular dystrophy (BMD). BMD affects older boys and young men, following a milder course than DMD. BMD occurs in about one in 30,000 male births.

- Emery-Dreifuss muscular dystrophy (EDMD). EDMD can appear as an autosomal dominant or recessive form of dystrophy. Thus, both young boys and girls can be affected. It causes contractures and weakness in the calves, weakness in the shoulders and upper arms, and problems in the way electrical impulses travel through the **heart** to make it beat (heart conduction defects). Fewer than 300 cases of EDMD have been identified.

- Limb-girdle muscular dystrophy (LGMD). LGMD begins in late childhood to early adulthood and affects both men and women, causing weakness in the muscles around the hips and shoulders and also the muscles of the arms and legs. It is the most variable of the muscular dystrophies, and there are several different forms of the condition now recognized. Many people with suspected LGMD have probably been misdiagnosed in the past, and therefore the prevalence of the condition is difficult to estimate. The highest prevalence of LGMD is in a small mountainous Basque province in northern Spain, where the condition affects 69 persons per million.

- Facioscapulohumeral muscular dystrophy (FSH). FSH, also known as Landouzy-Dejerine condition, begins in late childhood to early adulthood and affects both men and women, causing weakness in the muscles of the face, shoulders, and upper arms. The hips and legs may also be affected. FSH occurs in about one out of every 20,000 people, and affects approximately 13,000 people in the United States.

- Myotonic dystrophy. This is also known as Steinert's disease and affects both men and women, causing generalized weakness first seen in the face, feet, and hands. Other systems of the body can also be affected. It is accompanied by the inability to relax the affected muscles (myotonia). Symptoms may begin from birth through adulthood. It is the most common form of muscular dystrophy, affecting more than 30,000 people in the United States.

- Oculopharyngeal muscular dystrophy (OPMD). OPMD affects adults of both genders, causing weakness in the eye muscles and throat. It is most common among French Canadian families in Quebec, and in Spanish-American families in the southwestern United States.

- Distal muscular dystrophy (DD). DD is a group of rare muscle diseases that have in common weakness and wasting of the distal (farthest from the center) muscles of the forearms, hands, lower legs, and feet. In general, the DDs are less severe, progress more slowly, and involve fewer muscles than the other dystrophies. DD usually begins in middle age or later, causing weakness in the muscles of the feet and hands. It is most common in Sweden, and rare in other parts of the world.

- Congenital muscular dystrophy (CMD). CMD is a rare group of muscular dystrophies that have in common the presence of muscle weakness at birth (congenital). Biopsies of muscles from persons affected with CMD are abnormal. CMD results in generalized weakness, and usually progresses slowly. A subtype, called Fukuyama CMD, also involves mental retardation and lissencephaly. It is more common in Japan.

The muscular dystrophies are genetic conditions, meaning they are caused by alterations in genes. Genes, which are linked together on chromosomes, have two functions. They code for the production of **proteins** and they are the material of inheritance. Parents pass along genes to their children, providing them with a complete set of instructions for making their own proteins.

Because both parents contribute genetic material to their offspring, each child carries two copies of almost every gene, one from each parent. For some conditions to occur, both copies must be altered. Such conditions are called autosomal recessive conditions. Some forms of LGMD, OPMD and DD exhibit this pattern of inheritance, as does CMD. Persons with only one altered copy, called carriers, will not have the condition, but may pass the altered gene on to their children. When two carriers have children, the chances of having a child with the condition is one in four for each **pregnancy**.

Other conditions occur when only one altered gene copy is present. Such conditions are called autosomal dominant conditions. Other forms of LGMD exhibit this pattern of inheritance, as do DM, FSH, OPMD, and some forms of DD. When a person affected by the condition has a child with someone not affected, the chances of having an affected child are one in two. Autosomal dominant conditions tend to be variable in their symptoms even among members of the same family.

Because of chromosomal differences between the genders, some genes are not present in two copies. The chromosomes that determine whether a person is male or female are called the X and Y chromosomes. A person with two X chromosomes is female, while a person with one X and one Y is male. While the X chromosome carries many genes, the Y chromosome carries almost none. Therefore, a male has only one copy of each gene on the X chromosome, and if it is altered, he will have the condition that alteration causes. Such conditions are said to be X-linked. X-linked conditions include DMD, BMD, and EDMD. Women are not usually affected by X-linked conditions, since they will likely have one unaltered copy between the two chromosomes. Some female carriers of

DMD have a mild form of the condition, probably because their one unaltered gene copy is shut down in some of their cells.

Women carriers of X-linked conditions have a one in two chance of passing the altered gene on to each child born. Daughters who inherit the altered gene will be carriers. A son born without the altered gene will be free of the condition and cannot pass it on to his children. A son born with the altered gene will have the condition. He will pass the altered gene on to each of his daughters, who will then be carriers, but to none of his sons (because they inherit his Y chromosome).

Not all genetic alterations are inherited. As many as one-third of the cases of DMD are due to new mutations that arise during egg formation in the mother. New mutations are less common in other forms of muscular dystrophy.

Causes and symptoms

All of the muscular dystrophies are marked by muscle weakness as the major symptom. The distribution of symptoms, age of onset, and progression are significantly different. **Pain** is sometimes a symptom of each, usually due to the effects of weakness on joint position.

Duchenne muscular dystrophy

A boy with Duchenne muscular dystrophy usually begins to show symptoms before ever entering school, making walking difficult and causing balance problems. Most boys begin to walk three to six months later than expected and have difficulty running. Later on, a boy with DMD will push his hands against his knees to rise to a standing position, to compensate for leg weakness. About the same time, his calves will begin to enlarge with fibrous tissue rather than with muscle, and feel firm and rubbery; this condition gives DMD one of its alternate names, pseudohypertrophic muscular dystrophy. He will widen his stance to maintain balance, and walk with a waddling gait to advance his weakened legs. Contractures (permanent muscle tightening) usually begin by age five or six, most severely in the calf muscles. This pulls the foot down and back, forcing the boy to walk on tip-toes. This is called equinus and further decreases balance. Frequent **falls** are common beginning at this age. Climbing stairs and rising unaided may become impossible by age nine or ten, and most boys use a wheelchair for mobility by the age of 12. Weakening of the trunk muscles around this age often leads to **scoliosis** (a side-to-side spine curvature) and kyphosis (a front-to-back curvature of the spine).

The most serious weakness of DMD is weakness of the diaphragm, the sheet of muscles at the top of the abdomen that perform the main work of breathing and coughing. Diaphragm weakness leads to reduced energy and stamina, and increased lung **infection** because of the inability to cough effectively. Young men with DMD often live into their twenties and beyond, provided they have mechanical **ventilation assistance** and good respiratory hygiene.

Among males with DMD, the incidence of cardiomyopathy (weakness of the heart muscle), increases steadily in teenage years. Almost all affected men have cardiomyopathy after 18 years of age. It has also been shown that carrier females are at increased risk for cardiomyopathy and should also be screened.

About one-third of males with DMD experience specific learning disabilities, including trouble learning by ear rather than by sight and trouble paying attention to long lists of instructions. Individualized educational programs usually compensate well for these disabilities.

Becker muscular dystrophy

The symptoms of BMD usually appear in late childhood to early adulthood. Though the progression of symptoms may parallel that of DMD, the symptoms are usually milder and the course more variable. The same pattern of leg weakness, unsteadiness, and contractures occur later for a young man with BMD, often allowing independent walking into the twenties or early thirties. Scoliosis may occur, but is usually milder and progresses more slowly. Cardiomyopathy occurs more commonly in BMD. Problems may include irregular heartbeats (arrhythmias) and congestive **heart failure**. Symptoms may include fatigue, shortness of breath, chest pain, and dizziness. Respiratory weakness also occurs, and may lead to the need for mechanical ventilation.

Emery-Dreifuss muscular dystrophy

This type of muscular dystrophy usually begins in early childhood, often with contractures preceding muscle weakness. Weakness initially affects the shoulder and upper arm, along with the calf muscles, leading to foot-drop. Most men with EDMD survive into middle age, although a defect in the heart's rhythm (heart block) may be fatal if not treated with a pacemaker.

Limb-girdle muscular dystrophy

While there are several genes that cause the various types of LGMD, two major clinical forms of LGMD are currently recognized. A severe childhood form is similar in appearance to DMD, but is inherited as an autosomal recessive trait. Symptoms of adult-onset LGMD usually appear in a person's teens or twenties, and are marked by progressive weakness and wasting of the muscles closest to the trunk. Contractures may occur, and the ability to walk is usually lost about 20 years after onset. Some people with LGMD develop respiratory weakness that requires use of a ventilator. Life-span may be somewhat shortened. Autosomal dominant forms usually occur later in life and progress in a relatively slow manner.

Facioscapulohumeral muscular dystrophy

FSH varies in its severity and age of onset, even among members of the same family. Symptoms most commonly begin in the teens or early twenties, though infant or childhood onset is possible. Symptoms tend to be more severe in those with earlier onset. The condition is named for the regions of the body most severely affected by the condition: muscles of the face (facio-), shoulders (scapulo-), and upper arms (humeral). Hips and legs may be affected as well. More than half of children with FSH may develop partial or complete sensorineural deafness.

The first symptom noticed is often difficulty lifting objects above the shoulders. The weakness may be greater on one side than the other. Shoulder weakness also causes the shoulder blades to jut backward, called scapular winging. Muscles in the upper arm often lose bulk sooner than those of the forearm, giving a "Popeye" appearance to the arms. Facial weakness may lead to loss of facial expression, difficulty closing the eyes completely, and inability to drink through a straw, blow up a balloon, or whistle. Persons with FSH may not be able to wrinkle their foreheads. Contracture of the calf muscles may cause foot-drop, leading to frequent tripping over curbs or rough spots. People with earlier onset often require a wheelchair for mobility, while those with later onset rarely do.

Myotonic dystrophy

Symptoms of myotonic dystrophy include facial weakness and a slack jaw, drooping eyelids (ptosis), and muscle wasting in the forearms and calves. Persons with myotonic dystrophy have difficulty relaxing their grasp, especially if the object is cold. Myotonic dystrophy affects heart muscle, causing arrhythmias and heart block, and the muscles of the **digestive system**, leading to motility disorders and constipation. Other body systems are affected as well. Myotonic dystrophy may cause **cataracts**, retinal degeneration, mental deficiency, frontal balding, skin disorders, testicular atrophy, sleep apnea, and insulin resistance. An increased need or desire for sleep is common, as is diminished motivation. Severe

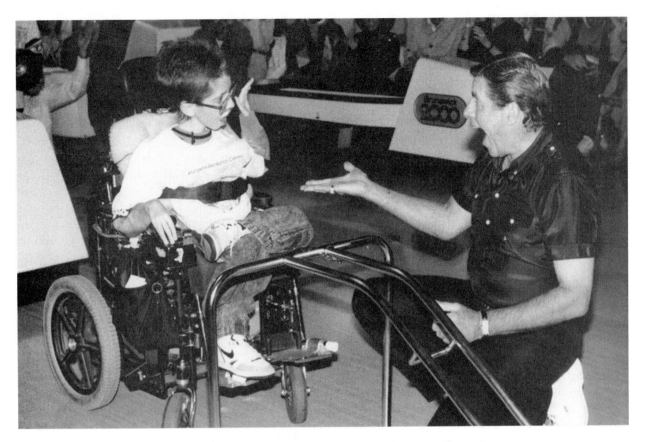

The "Jerry Lewis MDA Labor Day Telethon" raises money for the Muscular Dystrophy Association. *(Muscular Dystrophy Association. Reproduced by permission.)*

disability affects some people with this type of dystrophy within 20 years of onset, although most do not require a wheelchair even late in life. The condition is extremely variable. Some individuals show profound weakness as newborns (congenital myotonic dystrophy), others show mental retardation in childhood, many show characteristic facial features and muscle wasting in adulthood, while the most mildly affected individuals show only cataracts in middle age with no other symptoms.

Oculopharyngeal muscular dystrophy

OPMD usually begins in a person's thirties or forties, with weakness in the muscles controlling the eyes and throat. Symptoms include drooping eyelids, difficulty swallowing (**dysphagia**), and weakness progresses to other muscles of the face, neck, and occasionally the upper limbs. Swallowing difficulty may cause aspiration, or the introduction of food or saliva into the airways. **Pneumonia** may follow.

Distal muscular dystrophy

DD usually begins in the twenties or thirties, with weakness in the hands, forearms, and lower legs.

Difficulty with fine movements such as typing or fastening buttons may be the first symptoms. From that point, symptoms slowly progress and the condition usually does not affect life span.

Congenital muscular dystrophy

CMD is marked by severe muscle weakness from birth, with infants displaying "floppiness" (very poor muscle tone). They often have trouble moving their limbs or head against gravity. Mental function is normal but some are never able to walk. They may live into young adulthood or beyond. In contrast, children with Fukuyama CMD are rarely able to walk, and have severe mental retardation. Most children with this type of CMD die in childhood.

Diagnosis

The diagnosis of muscular dystrophy involves a careful medical history and a thorough physical exam to determine the distribution of symptoms and to rule out other causes. Family history may give important clues, since all the muscular dystrophies are genetic conditions, although no family history will be evident in the event of new mutations. With autosomal recessive inheritance, a family history may also be negative for muscular dystrophy.

Lab tests may include:

- **Blood** level of the muscle enzyme creatine kinase (CK). CK levels rise in the blood due to muscle damage, and may be seen in some conditions even before symptoms appear.

- Muscle biopsy, in which a small piece of muscle tissue is removed for microscopic examination. Changes in the structure of muscle cells and presence of fibrous tissue or other aberrant structures are characteristic of different forms of muscular dystrophy. The muscle tissue can also be stained to detect the presence or absence of particular proteins, including dystrophin.

- Electromyogram (EMG). This electrical test is used to examine the response of the muscles to stimulation. Decreased response is seen in muscular dystrophy. Other characteristic changes are seen in muscular dystrophy.

- Genetic tests. Several of the muscular dystrophies can be positively identified by testing for the presence of the altered gene involved. Accurate genetic tests are available for DMD, BMD, DM, several forms of LGMD, and EDMD. **Genetic testing** for some of these conditions in future pregnancies of an affected individual or parents of an affected individual can be performed before birth through **amniocentesis** or **chorionic villus sampling**. Prenatal testing can only be undertaken after the diagnosis in an affected individual has been genetically confirmed and the couple has been counseled regarding the risks of recurrence.

- Other specific tests as necessary. For EDMD, DMD and BMD, for example, an electrocardiogram may be needed to test heart function, and **hearing** tests are performed for children with FSH.

For most forms of muscular dystrophy, accurate diagnosis is not difficult when performed by someone familiar with the range of conditions. There are exceptions, however. Even with a muscle biopsy, it may be difficult to distinguish between FSH and another muscle condition, polymyositis. Childhood-onset LGMD is often mistaken for the much more common DMD, especially when it occurs in boys. BMD with an early onset appears very similar to DMD, and a genetic test may be needed to accurately distinguish them. The muscular dystrophies may be confused with conditions involving the motor **neurons**, such as spinal muscular atrophy; conditions of the neuromuscular junction, such as myasthenia gravis; and other muscle conditions, as all involve generalized weakness of varying distribution.

Prenatal diagnosis (testing of the baby while in the womb) can be performed for those types of muscular dystrophy where the specific disease-causing gene alteration has been identified in a previously affected family member. Prenatal diagnosis can be accomplished by utilizing DNA extracted from tissue obtained by chorionic villus sampling or amniocentesis.

Treatment

Drugs

There are no cures for any of the muscular dystrophies. Prednisone, a corticosteroid, has been shown to delay the progression of DMD somewhat, for reasons that are still unclear. Some have reported improvement in strength and function in people treated with a single dose. Improvement begins within ten days and plateaus after three months. Long-term benefit has not been demonstrated. Prednisone is also prescribed for BMD, though no controlled studies have tested its benefit. A study is under way in the use of gentamicin, an antibiotic that may slow down the symptoms of DMD in a small number of cases. No other drugs are currently known to have an effect on the course of any other muscular dystrophy.

Treatment of muscular dystrophy is mainly directed at preventing the complications of weakness, including decreased mobility and dexterity, contractures, scoliosis, heart alterations, and respiratory insufficiency.

Physical therapy

Physical therapy, in particular regular stretching, is used to maintain the range of motion of affected muscles and to prevent or delay contractures. Braces are used as well, especially on the ankles and feet to prevent equinus. Full-leg braces may be used in children with DMD to prolong the period of independent walking. Strengthening other muscle groups to compensate for weakness may be possible if the affected muscles are few and isolated, as in the earlier stages of the milder muscular dystrophies. Regular, non-strenuous **exercise** helps maintain general good health. Strenuous exercise is usually not recommended, since it may further damage muscles.

Surgery

When contractures become more pronounced, tenotomy surgery may be performed. In this operation, the tendon of a contracted muscle is cut, and the limb is braced in its normal resting position while the tendon regrows. In FSH, surgical fixation of the scapula can help compensate for shoulder weakness. For a person with OPMD, surgical lifting of the eyelids may help compensate for weakened muscular control. For a person with

DM, sleep apnea may be treated surgically to maintain an open airway. Scoliosis surgery is often needed in boys with DMD, but much less often in other muscular dystrophies. Surgery is recommended at a much lower degree of curvature for DMD than for scoliosis due to other conditions, since the decline in respiratory function in DMD makes surgery at a later time dangerous. In this surgery, the vertebrae are fused together to maintain the spine in an upright position. Steel rods are inserted at the time of operation to keep the spine rigid while the bones grow together.

When any type of surgery is performed in patients with muscular dystrophy, anesthesia must be carefully selected. People with MD are susceptible to a severe reaction, known as malignant hyperthermia, when given halothane anesthetic.

Occupational therapy

An occupational therapist suggests techniques and tools to compensate for the loss of strength and dexterity. Strategies may include modifications in the home, adaptive utensils and dressing aids, compensatory movements and positioning, wheelchair accessories, or communication aids.

Nutrition

Good **nutrition** helps to promote general health in all the muscular dystrophies. No special diet or supplement has been shown to be of particular value in any of the conditions. The weakness in the throat muscles seen especially in OPMD and later DMD may necessitate the use of a gastrostomy tube, inserted directly into the **stomach** to provide nutrition.

Cardiac care

The arrhythmias of EDMD and BMD may be treatable with antiarrhythmic drugs. A pacemaker may be implanted if these do not provide adequate control. Heart transplants are increasingly common for men with BMD. A complete cardiac evaluation is recommended at least once in all carrier females of DMD and EDMD.

Respiratory care

People who develop weakness of the diaphragm or other ventilatory muscles may require a mechanical ventilator to continue breathing deeply enough. Air may be administered through a nasal mask or mouthpiece, or through a tracheostomy tube, which is inserted via a surgical incision through the neck and into the windpipe. Most people with muscular dystrophy do not need a tracheostomy, although some may prefer it to continual use of a mask or mouthpiece. Supplemental oxygen is not needed. Good hygiene of the **lungs** is critical for health and long-term survival of a person with weakened ventilatory muscles. Assisted cough techniques provide the strength needed to clear the airways of secretions; an assisted cough machine is also available and provides excellent results.

Experimental treatments

Two experimental procedures aiming to cure DMD have attracted a great deal of attention in the past decade. In myoblast transfer, millions of immature muscle cells are injected into an affected muscle. The goal of the treatment is to promote the growth of the injected cells, replacing the defective host cells with healthy new ones. Myoblast transfer is under investigation but remains experimental.

Gene therapy introduces good copies of the altered gene into muscle cells. The goal is to allow the existing muscle cells to use the new gene to produce the protein it cannot make with its abnormal gene. Problems with gene therapy research have included immune rejection of the virus used to introduce the gene, loss of gene function after several weeks, and an inability to get the gene to enough cells to make a functional difference in an affected muscle. Researchers are preparing for the first gene therapy trial for LGMD in the United States. The goal will be to replace the missing sarcoglycan gene(s).

Genetic counseling

Individuals with muscular dystrophy and their families may benefit from **genetic counseling** for information on the condition and recurrence risks for future pregnancies.

Prognosis

The expected lifespan for a male with DMD has increased significantly in the past two decades. Most young men will live into their early or mid-twenties. Respiratory infections become an increasing problem as their breathing becomes weaker, and these infections are usually the cause of death.

The course of the other muscular dystrophies is more variable; expected life spans and degrees of disability are hard to predict, but may be related to age of onset and initial symptoms. Prediction is made more difficult because, as new genes are discovered, it is becoming clear that several of the dystrophies are not uniform disorders, but rather symptom groups caused by different genes.

KEY TERMS

Amniocentesis—A procedure in which a needle is inserted through a pregnant woman's abdomen and into her uterus to withdraw a small sample of the fluid that surrounds the fetus (amniotic fluid) for the purposes of analysis.

Autosomal dominant—Conditions that occur when a person inherits only one abnormal copy of a gene.

Autosomal recessive—Conditions that occur when a person inherits two abnormal copies of a gene, one from each parent.

Becker muscular dystrophy (BMD)—A type of muscular dystrophy that affects older boys and men, and usually follows a milder course than DMD.

Chorionic villus sampling—A medical procedure done during weeks 10-12 of a pregnancy. A needle is inserted into the placenta and a small amount of fetal tissue is withdrawn for analysis.

Contractures—A permanent shortening (as of muscle, tendon, or scar tissue) producing deformity or distortion.

Distal muscular dystrophy (DD)—A form of muscular dystrophy that usually begins in middle age or later, causing weakness in the muscles of the feet and hands.

Duchenne muscular dystrophy (DMD)—The most severe form of muscular dystrophy, DMD usually affects young boys and causes progressive muscle weakness, usually beginning in the legs.

Dystrophin—A protein that helps muscle tissue repair itself. Both DMD and BMD are caused by abnormalities in the gene that instructs the body how to make this protein.

Facioscapulohumeral muscular dystrophy (FSH)—This form of muscular dystrophy, also known as Landouzy-Dejerine condition, begins in late childhood to early adulthood and affects both men and women, causing weakness in the muscles of the face, shoulders, and upper arms.

Limb-girdle muscular dystrophy (LGMD)—This form of muscular dystrophy begins in late childhood to early adulthood and affects both men and women, causing weakness in the muscles around the hips and shoulders.

Myotonic dystrophy—This type of muscular dystrophy, also known as Steinert's disease, affects both men and women, causing generalized weakness first seen in the face, feet, and hands. It is accompanied by the inability to relax the affected muscles (myotonia).

Oculopharyngeal muscular dystrophy (OPMD)—This type of muscular dystrophy affects adults of both sexes, causing weakness in the eye muscles and throat.

People with dystrophies having significant heart involvement (BMD, EDMD, myotonic dystrophy) may nonetheless have almost normal life spans, provided that cardiac complications are monitored and aggressively treated. The respiratory involvement of BMD and LGMD similarly requires careful and prompt treatment.

Health care team roles

A pediatrician or family physician often make an initial diagnosis of muscular dystrophy. Pathologists and geneticists evaluate materials collected for testing. Physical therapists may provide supportive services. Braces and other assistive devices may be manufactured by orthotists and others with specialty training. Computer engineers have devised equipment for improving communications. Counselors and nurses provide support to people with muscular dystrophy and their families.

Prevention

There is no way to prevent any of the muscular dystrophies in a person who has the genes responsible for these disorders. Accurate genetic tests, including prenatal tests, are available for some of the muscular dystrophies. Results of these tests may be useful for purposes of family planning.

Resources

BOOKS

Adams, Raymond D., Maurice Victor, and Allan H. Ropper. *Adam's & Victor's Principles of Neurology, 6th ed.* New York, McGraw Hill, 1997.

Barohn, Richard J. "Muscular dystrophies." In *Cecil Textbook of Medicine, 21st ed.*, edited by Goldman, Lee and Bennett, J. Claude. Philadelphia: W.B. Saunders, 2000, 2206-2210.

Fukuyama, Y., Makiko Osawa, and Kayoko Saito. *Congenital Muscular Dystrophies.* New York: Elsevier Science, 1997.

Sarnat, Harvey B. "Muscular dystrophies." In *Nelson Textbook of Pediatrics,* 16th ed. edited by Richard E. Behrman et al. Philadelphia: Saunders, 2000, 1212.

Siegel, Irwin M. *Muscular Dystrophy in Children: A Guide for Families.* Gardena, CA: SCB Distributors, 1999.

PERIODICALS

Cornu, C., F. Goubel, and M. Fardeau. "Muscle and joint elastic properties during elbow flexion in Duchenne muscular dystrophy." *Journal of Physiology* 533, pt. 2 (2001): 605-616.

Kalra, V. "Muscular dystrophies." *Indian Journal of Pediatrics* 67, no. 12 (2000): 923-928.

Kazakov, V. "Why did the heated discussion arise between Erb and Landouzy-Dejerine concerning the priority in describing the facio-scapulo-humeral muscular dystrophy and what is the main reason for this famous discussion?" *Neuromuscular Disorders* 11, no. 4 (2001): 421-434.

Lanza, G. A., A. D. Russo, V. Giglio, L. De Luca, L. Messano, C. Santini, E. Ricci, A. Damiani, G. Fumagalli, G. De Martino, F. Mangiola, and F. Bellocci. "Impairment of cardiac autonomic function in patients with Duchenne muscular dystrophy: relationship to myocardial and respiratory function." *American Heart Journal* 141, no. 5 (2001): 808-812.

Mendell, J. R. "Congenital muscular dystrophy: searching for a definition after 98 years." *Neurology* 56, no. 8 (2001): 993-994.

Vlak, M., E. van der Kooi, and C. Angelini. "Correlation of clinical function and muscle CT scan images in limb-girdle muscular dystrophy." *Neurological Science* 21, 5 Suppl. (2000): S975-S977.

ORGANIZATIONS

American Academy of Neurology, 1080 Montreal Avenue, St. Paul, Minnesota 55116. (651) 695-1940. Fax: (651) 695-2791. <http://www.aan.com/>. info@aan.org.

American Academy of Pediatrics, 141 Northwest Point Boulevard, Elk Grove Village, IL 60007-1098. (847) 434-4000. Fax: (847) 434-8000. <http://www.aap.org/default.htm>. kidsdoc@aap.org.

American Academy of Physical Medicine and Rehabilitation, One IBM Plaza, Suite 2500, Chicago, IL 60611-3604. (312) 464-9700. Fax: (312) 464-0227. <http://www.aapmr.org/consumers/public/amputations.htm>. info@aapmr.org.

Muscular Dystrophy Association - USA, National Headquarters, 3300 E. Sunrise Drive, Tucson, AZ 85718. (800) 572-1717. <http://www.mdausa.org/>. mda@mdausa.org.

OTHER

FacioScapuloHumeral Muscular Dystrophy Society. <http://www.fshsociety.org/>.

Muscular Dystrophy Association of Canada. <http://www.mdac.ca/>.

National Institute of Neurological Disorders and Stroke. <http://www.ninds.nih.gov/health_and_medical/disorders/md.htm>.

National Library of Medicine. <http://www.nlm.nih.gov/medlineplus/musculardystrophy.html>.

Parent Project Muscular Dystrophy. <http://www.parentdmd.org/>.

University of Kansas Medical Center. <http://www.kumc.edu/gec/support/muscular.html>.

West Virginia University. <http://www.wvhealth.wvu.edu/clinical/neurological/muscular.htm>.

L. Fleming Fallon, Jr., MD, DrPH

Muscular system

Definition

The muscular system is the body's network of tissues for both voluntary and involuntary movements. Muscle cells are specialized for contraction.

Description

Body movements are generated through the contraction and **relaxation** of specific muscles. Some muscles, like those in the arms and legs, bring about such voluntary movements as raising a hand or flexing the foot. Other muscles are involuntary and function without conscious effort. Voluntary muscles include the **skeletal muscles**, of which there are about 650 in the human body. Skeletal muscles are controlled by the **somatic nervous system**; whereas the **autonomic nervous system** controls the involuntary muscles. Involuntary muscles include muscles that line the internal organs and the **blood vessels**. These smooth muscles are called visceral and vascular smooth muscles, and they perform tasks not generally associated with voluntary activity. Smooth muscles control several automatic physiological responses such as pupil constriction, which occurs when the muscles of the iris contract in bright light. Another example is the dilation of **blood** vessels, which occurs when the smooth muscles surrounding the vessels relax or lengthen. In addition to the categories of skeletal (voluntary) and smooth (involuntary) muscle, there is a third category, namely cardiac muscle, which is neither voluntary nor involuntary. Cardiac muscle is not under con-

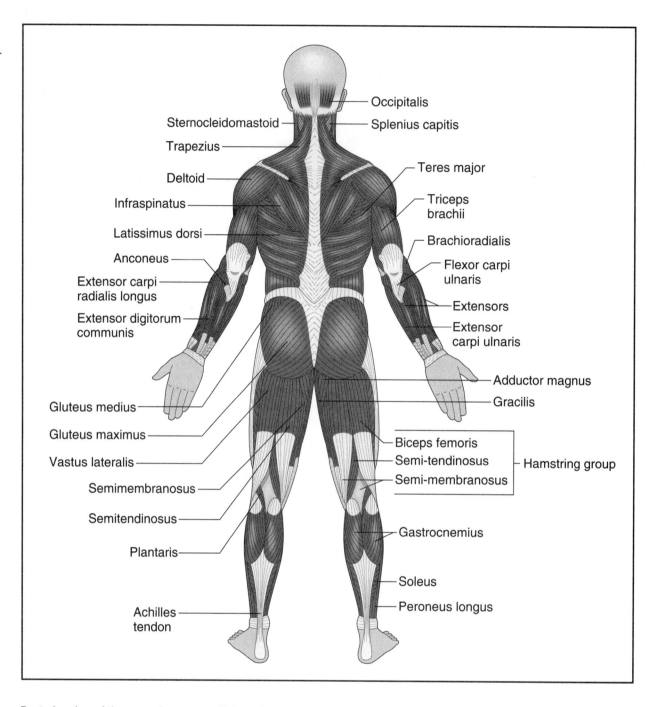

Posterior view of the muscular system. *(Delmar Publishers, Inc. Reproduced by permission.)*

scious control, and it can also function without regulation from the external nervous system.

Smooth muscles derive their name from their appearance under polarized light microscopy. In contrast to cardiac and skeletal muscles, which have striations (appearance of parallel bands or lines), smooth muscle is unstriated. Striations result from the pattern of myofilaments, which are very fine threads of protein. There are two types of myofilaments, actin and myosin, which line the myofibrils within each muscle cell. When many myofilaments align along the length of a muscle cell, light and dark regions create a striated appearance. This microscopic view of muscle reveals that muscles alter their shape to produce movement. Because muscle cells are usually elongated, they are often called muscle fibers. Compared to other cells in the body, striated muscle cells are distinctive in shape, protein composition, and multinucleated structure.

Skeletal muscles

Skeletal muscles are what most people think of as muscle. Skeletal muscles are the ones that ache when someone goes for their first outdoor run in the spring after not running regularly during the winter. Skeletal muscles are also involved when someone carries heavy grocery bags, practices a difficult musical passage, or combs their hair. **Exercise** may increase the size of muscle fibers, but the number of fibers generally remains constant. Skeletal muscles take up about 40% of the body's mass, or weight. They also consume large amounts of oxygen and nutrients from the blood supply. Multiple levels of skeletal muscle tissue receive their own blood supplies.

GROSS ANATOMY OF STRIATED MUSCLE. At the macroscopic level, skeletal muscles usually originate at one point of attachment to a tendon (a band or cord of tough, fibrous connective tissue) and terminate at another tendon at the other end of an adjoining bone. Tendons are rich in the protein collagen, which is arranged in a wavy pattern so that it can stretch out and provide additional length at the junction between bone and muscle.

Skeletal muscles usually act in pairs, such that the flexing (shortening) of one muscle is balanced by a lengthening (relaxation) of its paired muscle or group of muscles. These antagonistic (opposite) muscles can open and close such joints as the elbow or knee. Muscles that cause a joint to bend or close are called flexor muscles, and those that cause a joint to expand or straighten out are called extensors. Skeletal muscles that support the **skull**, backbone, and rib cage are called axial skeletal muscles; whereas the skeletal muscles of the limbs are called distal. Several skeletal muscles work in a highly coordinated manner in such activities as walking.

Skeletal muscles are organized into extrafusal and intrafusal fibers. Extrafusal fibers are the strong, outer layers of muscle. This type of muscle fiber is the most common. Intrafusal fibers, which make up the central region of the muscle, are weaker than extrafusal fibers. Skeletal muscle fibers are additionally characterized as fast or slow according to their activity patterns. Fast or "white" muscle fibers contract rapidly, have poor blood supply, operate anaerobically (without oxygen), and tire easily. Slow or "red" muscle fibers contract more slowly, have a more adequate blood supply, operate aerobically (with oxygen), and do not fatigue as easily. Slow muscle fibers are used in sustained movements, such as holding a **yoga** posture or standing at attention.

The skeletal muscles are enclosed in a dense sheath of connective tissue called the epimysium. Within the epimysium, muscles are sectioned into columns of muscle fiber bundles called primary bundles or fasciculi. Each fasciculus is covered by a layer of connective tissue called the perimysium. An average skeletal muscle may have 20–40 fasciculi which are further subdivided into several muscle fibers. Each muscle fiber (cell) is covered by connective tissue called endomysium. Both the epimysium and the perimysium contain blood and lymph vessels to supply the muscle with nutrients and oxygen, and to remove waste products. The endomysium has an extensive network of capillaries that supply individual muscle fibers. Individual muscle fibers vary in diameter from 10–60 micrometers and in length from a few millimeters in the smaller muscles to about 12 in (30 cm) in the sartorius muscle of the thigh.

MICROANATOMY OF STRIATED MUSCLE. At the microscopic level, a single striated muscle cell has several hundred nuclei and a striped appearance derived from the pattern of myofilaments. Long, cylindrical muscle fibers are formed from several myoblasts in **fetal development**. Multiple nuclei are important in muscle cells because of the tremendous amount of activity. The two types of myofilaments, actin and myosin, overlap one another in a very precise arrangement. Myosin is a thick protein with two globular head regions. Each myosin filament is surrounded by six actin (thin) filaments. These filaments run along the length of the cell in parallel. Multiple hexagonal arrays of actin and myosin exist in each skeletal muscle cell.

Each actin filament slides along adjacent myosin filaments with the help of other **proteins** and ions present in the cell. Tropomyosin and troponin are two proteins attached to the actin filaments that enable the globular heads on myosin to instantaneously attach to the myosin strands. The attachment and rapid release of this bond induces the sliding motion of these filaments that results in **muscle contraction**. In addition, **calcium** ions and ATP (adenosine triphosphate, the source of cellular energy) are required by the muscle cell to process this reaction. Numerous mitochondria (organelles in a cell that produce enzymes necessary for energy **metabolism**) are present in muscle fibers to supply the extensive ATP required by the cell.

The system of myofilaments within muscle fibers are divided into units called sarcomeres. Each skeletal muscle cell has several myofibrils, long cylindrical columns of myofilaments. Each myofibril is composed of myofilaments that interdigitate to form the striated sarcomere units. The thick myosin filaments of the sarcomere provide the dark, striped appearance in striated muscle, and the thin actin filaments provide the lighter sarcomere regions between the dark areas. Muscle contraction creates an enlarged center region called the belly of the muscle. The flexing of a muscle—a bicep for example—makes this region anatomically visible.

Cardiac muscle

Cardiac muscle, as is evident from its name, makes up the muscular portion of the **heart**. While almost all cardiac muscle is confined to the heart, some of these cells extend for a short distance into the cardiac vessels before tapering off completely. Heart muscle is also called myocardium. The myocardium has some properties similar to skeletal muscle tissue, but it also has some unique features. Like skeletal muscle, the myocardium is striated; however, the cardiac muscle fibers are smaller and shorter than skeletal muscle fibers. Cardiac muscle fibers average 5–15 micrometers in diameter and 20–30 micrometers in length. In addition, cardiac muscles align lengthwise more than they do in a side-by-side fashion, compared to skeletal muscle fibers. The microscopic structure of cardiac muscle is also distinctive in that these cells are branched in a way that allows them to communicate simultaneously with multiple cardiac muscle fibers.

Smooth muscle

Smooth muscle falls into three general categories: visceral smooth muscle, vascular smooth muscle, and multi-unit smooth muscle. Visceral smooth muscle fibers line such internal organs as the intestines, **stomach**, and uterus. Vascular smooth muscle forms the middle layer of the walls of blood and lymphatic vessels. Arteries generally have a thicker layer of vascular smooth muscle than veins or lymphatic vessels. Multi-unit smooth muscle is found only in the muscles that govern the size of the iris of the eye. Unlike contractions in visceral smooth muscle, contractions in multi-unit smooth muscle fibers do not readily spread to neighboring muscle cells.

Smooth muscle is innervated by both sympathetic and parasympathetic nerves of the autonomic nervous system. Smooth muscle appears unstriated under a polarized light **microscope**, because the myofilaments inside are less organized. Smooth muscle fibers contain actin and myosin myofilaments that are more haphazardly arranged than their counterparts in skeletal muscles. The sympathetic neurotransmitter, ACh, and parasympathetic neurotransmitter, norepinephrine, activate this type of muscle tissue.

Smooth muscle cells are small in diameter, about 5–15 micrometers, but they are long, typically 15–500 micrometers. They are also wider in the center than at their ends. Gap junctions connect small bundles of cells which are, in turn, arranged in sheets.

Within such hollow organs as the uterus, smooth muscle cells are arranged into two layers. The cells in the outer layer are usually arranged in a longitudinal fashion surrounding the cells in the inner layer, which are arranged in a circular pattern. Many smooth muscles are regulated by hormones in addition to the neurotransmitters of the autonomic nervous system. Moreover, the contraction of some smooth muscles is myogenic or triggered by stretching, as in the uterus and gastrointestinal tract.

Function

Skeletal muscles

Skeletal muscles function as the link between the somatic nervous system and the **skeletal system**. Skeletal muscles carry out instructions from the **brain** related to voluntary movement or action. For instance, when a person decides to eat a piece of cake, the brain tells the forearm muscle to contract, allowing it to flex and position the hand to lift a forkful of cake to the mouth. But the muscle alone cannot support the weight of the fork; the sturdy bones of the forearm assist the muscles in completing the task of moving the bite of cake. Hence, the skeletal and muscular systems work together as a lever system, with the joints acting as a fulcrum to carry out instructions from the nervous system.

The somatic nervous system controls skeletal muscle movement through motor **neurons**. Alpha motor neurons extend from the **spinal cord** and terminate on individual muscle fibers. The axon, or signal-sending end, of the alpha neuron branches to innervate multiple muscle fibers. The nerve terminal forms a synapse, or junction, with the muscle to create a neuromuscular junction. The neurotransmitter acetylcholine (ACh) is released from the axon terminal into the synapse. From the synapse, the ACh binds to receptors on the muscle surface that trigger events leading to muscle contraction. While alpha motor neurons innervate extrafusal fibers, intrafusal fibers are innervated by gamma motor neurons.

Voluntary skeletal muscle movements are initiated by the motor cortex in the brain. Signals travel down the spinal cord to the alpha motor neuron to result in contraction. Not all movement of skeletal muscles is voluntary, however. Certain **reflexes** occur in response to such dangerous stimuli as extreme heat or the edge of a sharp object. Reflexive skeletal muscular movement is controlled at the level of the spinal cord and does not require higher brain initiation. Reflexive movements are

Muscular System

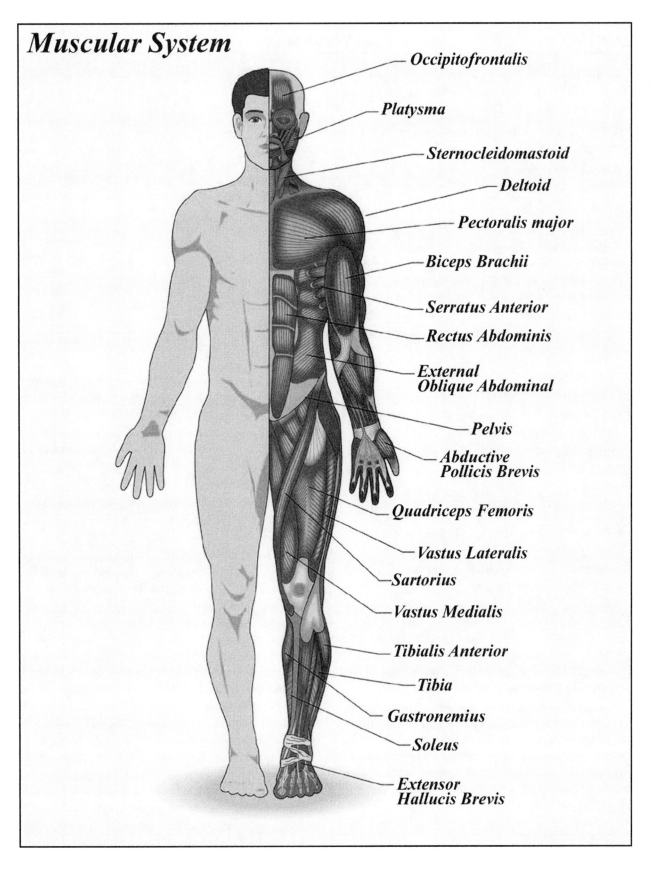

- Occipitofrontalis
- Platysma
- Sternocleidomastoid
- Deltoid
- Pectoralis major
- Biceps Brachii
- Serratus Anterior
- Rectus Abdominis
- External Oblique Abdominal
- Pelvis
- Abductive Pollicis Brevis
- Quadriceps Femoris
- Vastus Lateralis
- Sartorius
- Vastus Medialis
- Tibialis Anterior
- Tibia
- Gastronemius
- Soleus
- Extensor Hallucis Brevis

The muscular system, frontal view. *(Kopp Illustration, Inc. Reproduced by permission.)*

KEY TERMS

Acetylcholine (ACh)—A short-acting neurotransmitter that functions as a stimulant to the nervous system and as a vasodilator.

Actin—A protein that functions in muscular contraction by combining with myosin.

Adenosine triphosphate (ATP)—A nucleotide that is the primary source of energy in living tissue.

Anaerobic—Pertaining to or caused by the absence of oxygen.

Angina pectoris—A sensation of crushing pain or pressure in the chest, usually near the breastbone, but sometimes radiating to the upper arm or back. Angina pectoris is caused by a deficient supply of blood to the heart.

Axial—Pertaining to the axis of the body, i.e., the head and trunk.

Axon—The appendage of a neuron that transmits impulses away from the cell body.

Cardiac muscle—The striated muscle tissue of the heart. It is sometimes called myocardium.

Distal—Situated away from the point of origin or attachment.

Dystrophy—Any of several disorders characterized by weakening or degeneration of muscle tissue

Epimysium—The sheath of connective tissue around a muscle.

Extensor—A muscle that serves to extend or straighten a part of the body.

Fasciculus (plural, fasciculi)—A small bundle of muscle fibers.

Flexor—A muscle that serves to flex or bend a part of the body.

Multinucleated—Having more than one nucleus in each cell. Muscle cells are multinucleated.

Myasthenia gravis—A disease characterized by the impaired transmission of motor nerve impulses, caused by the autoimmune destruction of acetylcholine receptors.

Myosin—The principal contractile protein in muscle tissue.

Parasympathetic—Pertaining to the part of the autonomic nervous system that generally functions in regulatory opposition to the sympathetic system, as by slowing the heartbeat or contracting the pupil of the eye.

Sarcomere—A segment of myofibril in a striated muscle fiber.

Skeletal muscle—Muscle tissue composed of bundles of striated muscle cells that operate in conjunction with the skeletal system as a lever system.

Smooth muscle—Muscle tissue composed of long, unstriated cells that line internal organs and facilitate such involuntary movements as peristalsis.

Sympathetic—Pertaining to the part of the autonomic nervous system that regulates such involuntary reactions to stress as heartbeat, sweating, and breathing rate.

Synapse—A region in which nerve impulses are transmitted across a gap from an axon terminal to another axon or the end plate of a muscle.

Tendon—A cord or band of dense, tough, fibrous tissue that connects muscles and bones.

processed at this level to minimize the amount of time necessary to implement a response.

In addition to motor neuron activity in the skeletal muscles, a number of sensory nerves carry information to the brain to regulate muscle tension and contraction. Muscles function at peak performance when they are not overstretched or overcontracted. Sensory neurons within the muscle send feedback to the brain with regard to muscle length and state of contraction.

Cardiac muscle

The heart muscle is responsible for more than two billion beats in the course of a human lifetime of average

length. Cardiac muscle cells are surrounded by endomysium like the skeletal muscle cells. The autonomic nerves to the heart, however, do not form any special junctions like those found in skeletal muscle. Instead, the branching structure and extensive interconnectedness of cardiac muscle fibers allows for stimulation of the heart to spread into neighboring myocardial cells. This feature does not require the individual fibers to be stimulated. Although external nervous stimuli can enhance or diminish cardiac muscle contraction, heart muscles can also contract spontaneously. Like skeletal muscle cells, cardiac muscle fibers can increase in size with physical conditioning, but they rarely increase in number.

Smooth muscle

The concentric arrangement of some smooth muscle fibers enables them to control dilation and constriction in the blood vessels, intestines, and other organs. While these cells are not innervated on an individual basis, excitation from one cell can spread to adjacent cells through the nexuses that join neighbor cells. Multi-unit smooth muscles function in a highly localized way in such areas as the iris of the eye. Visceral smooth muscle also facilitates the movement of substances through such tubular areas as blood vessels and the **small intestine**. Smooth muscle differs from skeletal and cardiac muscle in its energy utilization as well. Smooth muscles are not as dependent on oxygen availability as cardiac and skeletal muscles are. Smooth muscle uses glycolysis (the breakdown of **carbohydrates**) to generate much of its metabolic energy.

Common diseases and disorders

Mechanical injury

Disorders of the muscular system can result from genetic, hormonal, infectious, autoimmune, poisonous, or neoplastic causes. But the most common problem associated with this system is injury from misuse. Sprains and tears cause excess blood to seep into skeletal muscle tissue. The residual scar tissue leads to a slightly shorter muscle. Muscular impairment and cramping can result from a diminished blood supply. Cramping can be due to overexertion. An inadequate supply of blood to cardiac muscle causes a sensation of pressure or **pain** in the chest called angina pectoris. Inadequate ionic supplies of calcium, sodium, or potassium can also affect most muscle cells adversely.

Immune system disorders

Muscular system disorders related to the **immune system** include myasthenia gravis and tumors. Myasthenia gravis is characterized by weak and easily fatigued skeletal muscles, one of the symptoms of which is droopy eyelids. Myasthenia gravis is caused by antibodies that a person makes against their own ACh receptors; hence, it is an autoimmune disease. The antibodies disturb normal ACh stimulation to contract skeletal muscles. Failure of the immune system to destroy cancerous cells in muscle can result in muscle tumors. Benign muscle tumors are called myomas, while malignant muscle tumors are called myosarcomas.

Disorders caused by toxins

Muscular disorders may also be caused by toxic substances of various types. A bacterium called *Clostridium tetani* produces a neurotoxin that causes tetanus, which is a disease characterized by painful repeated muscular contractions. In addition, some types of **gangrene** are caused by clostridial toxins produced under anaerobic conditions deep within a muscle. A poisonous substance called curare, which is derived from tropical plants of the genus *Strychnos* blocks neuromuscular transmission in skeletal muscle, causing **paralysis**. Prolonged periods of ethanol intoxication can also cause muscle damage.

Genetic disorders

The most common type of muscular genetic disorder is muscular dystrophy, of which there are several kinds. Duchenne's **muscular dystrophy** is characterized by increasing muscular weakness and eventual death. Becker's muscular dystrophy is a less severe disorder than Duchenne's, but both can be classified as X-linked recessive genetic disorders. Other types of muscular dystrophy are caused by a mutation that affects a muscle protein called dystrophin. Dystrophin is absent in Duchenne's and altered in Becker's muscular dystrophies. Other genetic disorders, including glycogen storage diseases, myotonic disorders, and familial periodic paralysis, can affect muscle tissues. In glycogen storage diseases, the skeletal muscles accumulate abnormal amounts of glycogen due to a biochemical defect in carbohydrate metabolism. In myotonic disorders, the voluntary muscles are abnormally slow to relax after contraction. Familial periodic paralysis is characterized by episodes of weakness and paralysis combined with loss of deep tendon reflexes.

Resources

BOOKS

"Muscular Disorders." Chapter 184 in *The Merck Manual of Diagnosis and Therapy*, edited by Mark H. Beers, MD, and Robert Berkow, MD. Whitehouse Station, NJ: Merck Research Laboratories, 1999.

Praemer A, et al., eds. *Musculoskeletal Conditions in the United States*. Rosemont, IL: American Academy of Orthopaedic Surgeons, 1999.

Vesalius, Andreas. *On the Fabric of the Human Body: Book II, The Ligaments and Muscles*. Tr. William Frank Richardson and John Burd Carman. San Francisco, CA: Norman Publishing, 1999.

White, Katherine. *The Muscular System: The Insider's Guide to the Body*. New York: Rosen Publishing Group, 2001.

PERIODICALS

Boskey, Adele L. "Musculoskeletal Disorders and Orthopedic Conditions." *Journal of the American Medical Association* 285, no. 5 (2001): 619-623. Full text available online at <http://jama.ama-assn.org/issues/v285n5/ffull/jsc00335.html>.

ORGANIZATIONS

National Arthritis and Musculoskeletal and Skin Diseases Information Clearinghouse. 1 AMS Circle, Bethesda, MD 20892. (301) 495-4484.

National Center for Complementary and Alternative Medicine (NCCAM), 31 Center Drive, Room #5B-58, Bethesda, MD 20892-2182. (800) NIH-NCAM. Fax: (301) 495-4957. <http://nccam.nih.gov>.

National Institute of Neurological Disorders and Stroke (NINDS). Building 31, Room 8A06, 9000 Rockville Pike, Bethesda, MD 20892. (301) 496-5751. <http://www.ninds.nih.gov>.

Crystal Heather Kaczkowski, MSc.

Mycobacterial culture *see* **Acid-fast culture**

Myelography

Definition

Myelography is a radiographic and fluoroscopic examination of the spinal canal. A contrast agent is injected through a needle into the space around the **spinal cord** (intrathecal sapace) to display the spinal cord, spinal canal, and nerve roots on an x ray.

Purpose

The purpose of a myelogram is to evaluate the spinal cord and/or nerve roots for suspected compression. Pressure on these delicate structures causes **pain** or other symptoms. A myelogram is performed when precise detail about the spinal cord is needed to make a definitive diagnosis. In most cases, myelography is used after other studies, such as **magnetic resonance imaging** (MRI) or a computed tomography scan (CT scan), have not yielded enough information to be sure of the disease process. Sometimes myelography followed by CT scan ("CT myelogram") is an alternative for patients who cannot have an MRI scan, because they have a pacemaker or other implanted metallic device.

A herniated or ruptured intervertebral disc, popularly known as a slipped disc, is one of the most common causes for pressure on the spinal cord or nerve roots. Discs are pads of fiber and cartilage that contain rubbery tissue. They lie between the vertebrae, or individual bones, which make up the spine. Discs act as cushions, accommodating strains, shocks, and position changes. A disc may rupture suddenly, due to injury, or a sudden straining with the spine in an unnatural position. In other cases, the problem may come on gradually as a result of progressive deterioration of the discs with aging. The lower back is the most common area for this problem, but it sometimes occurs in the neck, and rarely in the upper back. A myelogram can help accurately locate the disc or discs involved.

Myelography may be used when a tumor is suspected. Tumors can originate in the spinal cord, or in tissues surrounding the cord. Cancers that have started in other parts of the body may spread or metastasize in the spine. It is important to precisely locate the mass causing pressure, so effective treatment can be undertaken. Patients with known **cancer** who develop back pain may require a myelogram for evaluation.

Other conditions that may be diagnosed using myelography include arthritic bony growths, known as spurs, narrowing of the spinal canal, called spinal stenosis, or malformations of the spine.

Precautions

Patients who are unable to lie still or cooperate with positioning should not have this examination. Severe congenital spinal abnormalities may make the examination technically difficult to carry out. Patients with a history of severe allergic reaction to contrast material (x-ray dye) should report this to their physician. Pretreatment with medications to minimize the risk of severe reaction may be recommended.

Description

The patient lies on the x-ray table on his or her **stomach**. The radiologist first looks at the spine under fluoroscopy, where the images appear on a monitor. This is done to find the best location to position the needle. The procedure starts out like a spinal tap (or lumbar puncture). The skin is cleaned, then numbed with local anesthetic. A needle is placed into the lower back, between two vertebrae, and then inserted into the intrathecal space. A small amount of cerebrospinal fluid, the clear fluid that surrounds the spinal cord and **brain**, is withdrawn through the needle to confirm accurate needle placement and also may be sent for laboratory studies. Then contrast material (a liquid dye that shows up on x rays) is injected.

The x-ray table is tilted slowly. This allows the contrast material to reach different levels in the spinal canal. The flow is observed under fluoroscopy, then x rays are taken with the table tilted at various angles. The patient's head may be below his or her legs (Trendelenburg position). A footrest and shoulder supports keep the patient from sliding while the table is being tilted back and forth.

In many instances, a CT scan of the spine will be performed immediately after a myelogram, while the contrast material is still in the spinal canal. This helps outline internal structures most clearly.

A myelogram takes approximately 30–60 minutes. A CT scan adds about another hour to the examination. If the procedure is done as an outpatient exam, some facilities prefer the patient to stay in a recovery area for up to four hours.

Preparation

Patients should be well hydrated at the time of a myelogram. Increasing fluids the day before the study is usually recommended. All food and fluid intake should be stopped approximately four hours before the myelogram.

Certain medications may need to be stopped for one to two days before myelography is performed. These include some antipsychotics, antidepressants, **blood** thinners, and diabetic medications. Patients should consult with their physician and/or the facility where the study is to be done.

Patients who smoke may be asked to stop the day before the test. This helps decrease the chance of nausea or headaches after the myelogram. Immediately before the examination, patients should empty their bowels and bladder.

Aftercare

After the examination is completed, the patient usually rests for several hours, with the head elevated. Extra fluids are encouraged, to help eliminate the contrast material and prevent headaches. A regular diet and routine medications may be resumed. Strenuous physical activity, especially any that involves bending over, may be discouraged for one or two days. The doctor should be notified if a **fever**, excessive nausea and vomiting, severe headache, or stiff neck develops.

Complications

Headache is a common complication of myelography. It may begin several hours to several days after the examination. The cause is thought to be changes in cerebrospinal fluid pressure, not a reaction to the contrast material. The headache may be mild and easily alleviated with rest and increased fluids. Sometimes, nonprescription medicines are recommended. In some instances, the headache may be more severe and require stronger medication or other measures for relief. Many

---

KEY TERMS

Contrast agent—Also called a contrast medium, this is usually a barium or iodine dye that is injected into the area under investigation. The dye makes the interior body parts more visible on an x-ray film.

---

factors influence whether the patient develops this problem. These include the type of needle used and the age and sex of the patient. Patients with a history of chronic or recurrent headache are more likely to develop a headache after a myelogram.

The chance of reaction to the contrast material is a very small, but a potentially significant risk with myelography. It is estimated that only 5–10% of patients experience any effect from contrast exposure. The vast majority of reactions are mild, such as sneezing, nausea, or **anxiety**. These usually resolve by themselves. A moderate reaction, like wheezing or **hives**, may be treated with medication, but is not considered life threatening. Severe reactions, such as **heart** or **respiratory failure**, happen very infrequently. These require emergency medical treatment.

Rare complications of myelography include injury to the nerve roots from the needle, or from bleeding into the spaces around the roots. Inflammation of the delicate covering of the spinal cord, called arachnoiditis, or infections, can also occur. Seizures are another very uncommon complication reported after myelography.

Results

A normal myelogram shows a spinal canal of normal width, with no areas of constriction or obstruction.

A myelogram may reveal a **herniated disk**, tumor, bone spurs, or narrowing of the spinal canal (spinal stenosis).

Health care team roles

Myelograms can be performed in a hospital x-ray department or in an outpatient radiology facility. The test is performed by a radiologist with the help of a radiologic technologist. The radiologist will interpret the results of the test and recommend any further treatment. A nurse may assist during the procedure, may prepare the patient before the procedure, or may monitor the patient afterwards.

Historical note on contrast media used for myelography

Until the mid- to late 1970s, myelography was performed using an non-aqueous, oil-based, contrast medium. Use of this medium created a significant problem, since it had to be removed from the intrathecal space after the procedure (since it was non-aqueous, it would not be absorbed). More often than not, the removal process caused significant pain for the patient because, after the physician moved the bolus of contrast material to where the needle was, he/she would attach a syringe and attempt to suck the oily fluid out. The negative pressure in the intrathecal space often pulled on the nerve roots in the vicinity of the needle, causing shooting pains and electrical shock-like sensations that extended down to the patients' legs. In many instances, it was not possible to remove all of the contrast material.

In the 1970s, a non-ionic aqueous (water soluble) contrast agent, suitable for injection into the intrathecal space was developed. Its development and adoption for myelography, eliminated the pain and suffering associated with removal because, like contrast agents injected intravenously, it was absorbed and eventually excreted after the procedure.

Resources

BOOKS

Daffner, Richard. *Clinical Radiology, The Essentials.* 2nd ed. Baltimore: Williams and Wilkins, 1999.

Pagana, Kathleen, and Timothy Pagana. *Mosby's Diagnostic and Laboratory Test Reference.* St. Louis, MO: Mosby-Year Book, 1998.

Torres, Lillian. *Basic Medical Techniques and Patient Care in Imaging Technology.* 5th ed. Philadelphia: Lippincott, 1997.

ORGANIZATIONS

The Spine Center. 1911 Arch St., Philadelphia, PA 19103. (215) 665-8300. <http://thespinecenter.org>.

OTHER

CAR Standards and Guidelines for Myelography. Approved: June 1996, Suzanne Fontaine, M.D., Don Lee, M.D., William Maloney, M.D., Harvey Grossman, M.D., and Carla Wallace, M.D. <http://www.car.ca/standards/myelography.htm>.

Patients & Families Center for Diagnostic Imaging. "Diagnostic Injections & Pain Management Procedures & Preparations." <http://www.cdirad.com/p_myelo.htm>.

Stephen John Hage, AAAS, RT-R, FAHRA

Myocardial infarction

Definition

A myocardial infarction, or **heart** attack, is the death or damage of part of the heart muscle because the supply of **blood** to the heart muscle is severely reduced or stopped.

Description

Myocardial infarction (MI) is the leading cause of death in the United States. More than 1.5 million Americans suffer a myocardial infarction every year, and nearly half a million die, according to the American Heart Association. Most myocardial infarctions are the end result of years of silent, undetected, progressive **coronary artery disease**. A myocardial infarction is often the first detected symptom of coronary artery disease. According to the American Heart Association, 63% of women and 48% of men who died suddenly of coronary artery disease had no previous symptoms. Myocardial infarctions are commonly called heart attacks.

A myocardial infarction occurs when one or more of the coronary arteries that supply blood to the heart are completely blocked and blood to the heart muscle is cut off. The blockage is usually caused by atherosclerosis, the build-up of plaque in artery walls, and/or by a blood clot in a coronary artery. Sometimes, a healthy or atherosclerotic coronary artery has a spasm and the blood flow to part of the heart decreases or stops. The result may be a myocardial infarction.

About half of all myocardial infarction patients wait at least two hours before seeking help. This delay dramatically increases the risk of sudden death or disability. The longer the artery remains blocked during a myocardial infarction, the more damage will be done to the heart. If the blood supply is cut off severely, or for longer than 12 hours, muscle cells suffer irreversible injury and die. The patient can die. That is why it is vitally important to teach patients to recognize the signs of a myocardial infarction and seek immediate medical attention at the nearest hospital with 24-hour emergency cardiac care.

About one fifth of all myocardial infarctions are silent, that is, the patient is unaware that the MI has occurred. Although the patient feels no **pain**, silent myocardial infarctions still damage the heart.

The outcome of a myocardial infarction depends on the location of the blockage, whether the heart rhythm is disturbed, and whether there is collateral circulation to the territory supplied by the acutely occluded coronary artery. Blockages in the left coronary artery are usually more serious than those affecting the right coronary artery. Blockages that produce arrhythmia (irregular heartbeat) can cause sudden death.

Causes and symptoms

Myocardial infarctions are generally caused by severe coronary artery disease. Most myocardial infarctions are caused by blood clots that form on atherosclerotic plaque. This impedes the coronary artery from supplying oxygen-rich blood to part of the heart. A number of major and contributing risk factors increase the likelihood of developing coronary artery disease. Some of these risk factors can be modified, but others cannot. Persons with more risk factors are more likely to develop coronary artery disease.

Major risk factors

Major risk factors significantly increase the likelihood of developing coronary artery disease. Risk factors that cannot be changed include:

- Heredity. People whose parents have coronary artery disease, particularly those who develop it at younger ages, are more likely to be diagnosed with it. African Americans are also at increased risk, due to their higher rate of severe **hypertension** than caucasians.

- Gender. Men under the age of 60 years of age are more likely to have myocardial infarctions than women of the same age.

- Age. Men over age 45 and women over age 55 are considered at risk. Older adults (those over 65) are more likely to die of a myocardial infarction. Older women are twice as likely to die within a few weeks of a myocardial infarction as men. This increased mortality may be attributable to other co-existing medical problems.

Major risk factors which can be changed are:

- Smoking. Smoking greatly increases both the risk of developing coronary artery disease and resulting mortality. Smokers have two to four times the risk of non-smokers of sudden cardiac death and are more than twice as likely to have a myocardial infarction. They are also more likely to die within an hour of a myocardial infarction. Second-hand smoke may also increase risk.

- High cholesterol. Cholesterol is produced by the body, and obtained from eating animal products such as meat, eggs, milk, and cheese. Age, gender, heredity, and diet affect cholesterol level. Risk of developing coronary artery disease increases as blood cholesterol levels increase. When combined with other factors, the risk is even greater. Total cholesterol of 240 mg/dL or more poses a high risk, and 200–239 mg/dL a borderline high risk. In LDL (low-density lipoprotein) cholesterol, high risk starts at 130–159 mg/dL, depending on other risk factors. Low levels of HDL (high-density lipoprotein) increases the risk of coronary disease; high HDL protects against it.

- Hypertension (high **blood pressure**). High blood pressure makes the heart work harder, and over time, weakens it. It increases the risk of myocardial infarction, stroke, kidney failure, and congestive **heart failure**. Blood pressure of 140 over 90 or above is considered high. As the numbers increase, high blood pressure progresses from Stage One (mild) to Stage Four (very severe). When hypertension is combined with **obesity**, smoking, high cholesterol, or diabetes, the risk of myocardial infarction or stroke increases several times.

- Sedentary lifestyle and lack of physical activity. Inactivity increases the risk of coronary artery disease. Even modest physical activity is beneficial if done regularly.

Contributing risk factors

Contributing risk factors have been linked to coronary artery disease, but their significance and prevalence are not known yet. Contributing risk factors are:

- Diabetes mellitus. The risk of developing coronary artery disease is seriously increased for diabetics. More than 80% of diabetics die of some type of heart or blood vessel disease.

- Obesity. Excess weight increases the strain on the heart muscle and increases the risk of developing coronary artery disease, even if no other risk factors are present. Obesity increases both blood pressure and blood cholesterol, and can lead to diabetes.

- **Stress** and anger. Stress and anger can produce physiological changes that contribute to the development of coronary artery disease. Stress, the mental and physical reaction to life's irritations and challenges, increases heart rate and blood pressure, and can injure the lining of the arteries. Evidence shows that anger increases the risk of dying from heart disease and more than doubles the risk of having a myocardial infarction right after an episode of anger.

More than 60% of myocardial infarction patients experience symptoms before the myocardial infarction occurs. These symptoms may occur days or weeks before the myocardial infarction. Sometimes, people do not recognize the symptoms of a myocardial infarction or deny

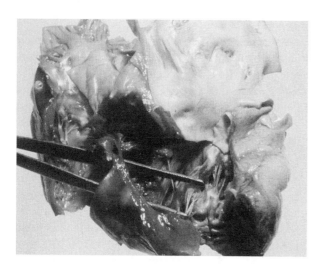

A myocardial infarction, or heart attack, is caused by blockage in a coronary artery, which prevents blood flow to the heart muscle. *(Custom Medical Stock Photo. Reproduced by permission.)*

that they are having symptoms. Common symptoms include:

- Uncomfortable pressure, fullness, heaviness, squeezing, or pain in the center of the chest. The sensation lasts more than a few minutes, or may go away and return.

- Pain that spreads to the shoulders, neck, left arm, or jaw.

- Chest discomfort accompanied by lightheadedness, fainting, sweating, nausea, or shortness of breath.

All of these symptoms do not necessarily occur with every myocardial infarction. Sometimes, symptoms disappear and then reappear. Individuals with any of these symptoms should immediately call an emergency rescue service or be driven to the nearest hospital with a 24-hour cardiac care unit, whichever is quicker.

Diagnosis

Experienced emergency care personnel confirm the diagnosis of MI, by taking a thorough history, checking heart rate and blood pressure, performing an electrocardiogram, and drawing a blood sample. The electrocardiogram shows which of the coronary arteries is blocked. The blood test detects the leak of enzymes or other biochemical markers from damaged cells in the heart muscle. In clinical practice, timely treatment is based on the patient history, **physical examination**, and ECG findings.

Treatment

Treatment is initiated in the emergency department with thrombolytic agents, aspirin, oxygen, and beta-blockers. Oxygen is used to ease the heart's workload or to help patients breathe easier. If oxygen is administered within hours of the myocardial infarction, it also may help limit damage to the heart. Subsequent treatment includes close monitoring, nitrates and morphine if needed, electric shock, drug therapy, re-vascularization procedures, coronary **angioplasty**, and coronary artery bypass surgery.

Patients with complications such as arrhythmias, congestive heart failure, and hypertension or hypotension require additional treatment. A defibrillator may be used to restore a normal rhythm. A temporary pacemaker may be inserted to correct a bradyarrhythmia (slow heart rate). ACE inhibitors may be used to treat congestive heart failure.

Drugs to stabilize the patient and limit damage to the heart include thrombolytics, aspirin, anticoagulants, painkillers, and tranquilizers, beta-blockers, ACE inhibitors, nitrates, anti-arrhthythmics (rhythm-stabilizing) drugs, and diuretics. Thrombolytics, used to limit damage to the heart, work only if given within six to 12 hours of the onset (when the chest pain began) of the myocardial infarction. Thrombolytic drugs act by dissolving the blood clot that is blocking the acutely occluded coronary artery. They increase the likelihood of survival when given as soon as possible after the myocardial infarction. Thrombolytics given within a few hours after a myocardial infarction are the most effective. Injected intravenously, these include acylated plasminogen streptokinase activator complex (APSAC) or anistreplase (Eminase), recombinant tissue-type plasminogen activator (r-tPA, Retevase, or Activase), and streptokinase (Streptase, Kabikinase). Thrombolytics may only be given if they are not contraindicated by disorders such as active bleeding, trauma or surgery within the preceding two weeks, blood pressure greater than 200/120 mm Hg, and **pregnancy**.

To prevent additional myocardial infarctions, aspirin and heparin, an anticoagulant, often follow the thrombolytic drug. These prevent new blood clots from forming and existing blood clots from growing. Anticoagulant drugs help prevent the blood from clotting. The most common anticoagulants are heparin and warfarin. Heparin is given intravenously while the patient is in the hospital. Aspirin helps to prevent the dissolved blood clots from reforming.

To relieve pain, a nitroglycerin tablet taken under the tongue or given intravenously. If the pain continues, morphine sulfate may be prescribed. Tranquilizers such as diazepam (Valium) or alprazolam (Ativan) may be prescribed to lessen the **anxiety** and emotional stress associated with myocardial infarction.

To limit the size of the myocardial infarction and prevent another, beta-blockers are often administered intravenously right after the myocardial infarction. These can also help prevent potentially fatal ventricular fibrillation. Beta-blockers include atenolol (Tenormin), metoprolol (Lopressor), nadolol, pindolol (Visken), propranolol (Inderal), and timolol (Blocadren).

Nitrates, a type of vasodilator, may also be given right after a myocardial infarction to help improve the delivery of blood to the heart and ease chest pain and heart failure symptoms. Nitrates include isosorbide mononitrate (Imdur), isosorbide dinitrate (Isordil, Sorbitrate), and nitroglycerin (Nitrostat).

When a myocardial infarction causes an abnormal heartbeat, arrhythmia drugs may be given to restore the heart's normal rhythm. These include amiodarone (Cordarone), atropine, bretylium, disopyramide (Norpace), lidocaine (Xylocaine), procainamide (Procan), propafenone (Rythmol), propranolol (Inderal), quinidine, and sotalol (Betapace). Angiotensin-converting enzyme (ACE) inhibitors reduce the resistance against which the heart beats and are used to manage and prevent heart failure. They are used to treat myocardial infarction patients whose hearts do not pump well or who have symptoms of heart failure. Taken orally, they include Altace, Capoten, Lotensin, Monopril, Prinivil, Vasotec, and Zestril. Angiotensin receptor blockers, such as losartan (Cozaar) may substitute. Diuretics can help get rid of excess fluids that sometimes accumulate when the heart is not pumping effectively. Usually taken orally, they cause the body to dispose of fluids through urination. Common diuretics include: bumetanide (Bumex), chlorthalidone (Hygroton), chlorothiazide (Diuril), furosemide (Lasix), hydrochlorothiazide (Hydrodiuril, Esidrix), spironolactone (Aldactone), and triamterene (Dyrenium).

Percutaneous transluminal coronary angioplasty, a type of catheter-based intervention, and coronary artery bypass surgery are invasive revascularization procedures that open blocked coronary arteries and improve blood flow. They are usually performed only on patients for whom clot-dissolving drugs do not work, or who have poor **exercise** stress tests, poor left ventricular function, or ischemia. Generally, angioplasty is performed before coronary artery bypass surgery.

Percutaneous transluminal coronary angioplasty, usually called coronary angioplasty, is a non-surgical procedure in which a catheter (a tiny plastic tube) tipped with a balloon is threaded from the femoral or brachial artery (blood vessel in the thigh or arm) into the blocked artery. The balloon is inflated and compresses the plaque to enlarge the blood vessel and open the blocked artery. The balloon is then deflated and the catheter is removed. Coronary angioplasty is performed by a cardiologist in a hospital and generally requires a two-day stay. It is successful about 90% of the time. For one third of patients, the artery restenoses (narrows again) within six months after the procedure. The procedure may be repeated. It is less invasive and less expensive than coronary artery bypass surgery.

In coronary artery bypass surgery, called bypass surgery, a vein taken from the patient's leg, or the internal mammary artery, may be used to reestablish blood flow beyond the coronary artery blockage. The healthy vein or artery then supplies oxygen-rich blood to the heart. Bypass surgery is major surgery appropriate for patients with blockages in two or three major coronary arteries or severely narrowed left main coronary arteries, as well as those who have not responded to other less invasive treatments. It is performed under **general anesthesia** using a heart-lung machine to support the patient while the healthy vein is attached to the coronary artery. About 70% of patients who have bypass surgery experience full relief from angina; about 20% experience partial relief. Long term symptoms recur in only about three or four percent of patients per year. Five years after bypass surgery, survival expectancy is 90%, at 10 years it is about 80%, at 15 years it is about 55%, and at 20 years it is about 40%.

There are three additional catheter-based interventions for unblocking coronary arteries that are currently being performed. During atherectomy, the surgeon shaves off and removes strips of plaque from the blocked artery. Laser angioplasty uses a catheter with a laser tip inserted into the vessel to burn or break down the plaque. Insertion of a metal coil called a stent also may be implanted permanently to keep a blocked artery open.

Prognosis

The sequelae (aftermath) of a myocardial infarction is often severe. Two-thirds of myocardial infarction patients never recover fully. Within one year, 27% of men and 44% of women die. Within six years, 23% of men and 31% of women have another myocardial infarction, 13% of men and 6% of women experience sudden death, and about 20% have heart failure. People who survive a myocardial infarction have a chance of sudden death that is four to six times greater than others and a chance of illness and death that is two to nine times greater. Older women are more likely than men to die within a few weeks of a myocardial infarction.

Health care team roles

Nurses, ECG technicians, laboratory technologists and other allied health professionals have important roles in the diagnosis of acute myocardial infarction as well as institution of timely treatment. Nurses and other practitioners involved in triage or screening in the emergency department must accurately assess patients with chest pain or other indications of myocardial infarction.

ECG technicians and laboratory technologists are responsible for performing the diagnostic tests, ECG and blood chemistries, to confirm the diagnosis of myocardial infarction. In the emergency department and on the hospital floor, nurses and allied health professionals are responsible for closely monitoring patients to prevent complications following myocardial infarction. During the hospitalization, nurses, dieticians, respiratory and physical therapists collaborate to plan a **cardiac rehabilitation** program and provide patient and family education.

Patient education

Nurses, physical therapists, and dieticians work together to educate patients and their families. Patients are taught to recognize and accurately describe symptoms such as pain, pressure, or heaviness in the chest, arm, or jaw. Patients are advised to report any changes in the intensity or quality of their pain to nurses or other health care professionals while in the hospital. When necessary, they are counseled by nursing or pharmacy technicians about the use of sublingual (under the tongue) nitroglycerin to relieve chest pain. They are instructed to seek medical attention immediately should serious symptoms return after they have been discharged.

Along with instruction about medication, follow-up care, and the importance of participating in cardiac rehabilitation, patients are informed about ways to reduce their risk of having another myocardial infarction or other cardiac disorders. This education is tailored to the individual patient's needs. It may include referral to a smoking cessation program; nutritional counseling to reduce dietary fat and sodium and achieve a desirable body weight; and recommendations to increase physical activity. **Patient education** also addresses treatment of any coexisting illnesses such as diabetes, and instruction about ways to more effectively manage stress and anger.

Prevention

Many myocardial infarctions can be prevented through a healthy lifestyle, which can reduce the risk of developing coronary artery disease. For patients who have already had a myocardial infarction, a healthy lifestyle and carefully following doctor's orders can prevent another myocardial infarction. A heart healthy lifestyle includes a low-fat diet, regular exercise, maintaining a healthy weight, no smoking, moderate drinking, no illegal drugs, controlling hypertension, and managing stress.

A healthy diet includes a variety of foods that are low in fat (especially saturated fat), low in cholesterol, and high in fiber; plenty of fruits and vegetables; and limited sodium. Some foods are low in fat but high in cholesterol, and some are low in cholesterol but high in fat. Saturated fat raises cholesterol, and, in excessive amounts, it increases the amount of the **proteins** in blood that form blood clots. Polyunsaturated and monounsaturated **fats** are relatively good for the heart. Fat should comprise no more than 30% of total daily calories.

Cholesterol, a waxy, lipid-like substance, comes from eating foods such as meat, eggs, and other animal products. It is also produced in the **liver**. Soluble fiber can help lower cholesterol. Patients should be advised to limit cholesterol to about 300 mg per day. Many lipid-lowering drugs reduce LDL-cholesterol by an average of 25–30% when combined with a low-fat, low-cholesterol diet. Fruits and vegetables are rich in fiber, **vitamins**, and **minerals**. They are also low calorie and nearly fat free. **Vitamin C** and beta-carotene, found in many fruits and vegetables, keep LDL-cholesterol from turning into a form that damages coronary arteries. Excess sodium can increase the risk of high blood pressure. Many processed foods contain large amounts of sodium. Patients should be advised to limit daily intake to about 2,400 mg—about the amount in a teaspoon of salt.

The "Food Guide Pyramid" developed by the U.S. Departments of Agriculture and Health and Human Services provides easy to follow guidelines for daily heart-healthy eating: six to 11 servings of bread, cereal, rice, and pasta; three to five servings of vegetables; two to four servings of fruit; two to three servings of milk, yogurt, and cheese; and two to three servings of meat, poultry, fish, dry beans, eggs, and nuts. Fats, oils, and sweets should be used sparingly.

Regular aerobic exercise can lower blood pressure, help control weight, and increase HDL ("highly desirable") cholesterol. It may keep the **blood vessels** more flexible. Moderate intensity aerobic exercise lasting about 30 minutes four or more times per week is recommended for maximum heart health, according to the Centers for Disease Control and Prevention and the American College of Sports Medicine. Three 10-minute exercise periods are also beneficial. Aerobic exercise—activities such as walking, jogging, and cycling—uses the large muscle groups and forces the body to use oxygen more efficiently. It can also include everyday activities such as active gardening, climbing stairs, or brisk housework.

Maintaining a desirable body weight is vital for heart health. More than half of American adults are overweight as defined by a body mass index (BMI) greater than 25. The percentage of obese adults (BMI greater than 30) is nearly 25%, a 50% increase over the past 20 years. People who are 20% or more over their ideal body weight have an increased risk of developing coronary artery disease. Losing weight can help reduce total and LDL cholesterol, reduce triglycerides, and boost relative levels of HDL cholesterol. It may also reduce blood pressure.

Smoking has many adverse effects on the heart. It increases the heart rate, constricts major arteries, and can create irregular heartbeats. It also raises blood pressure, contributes to the development of plaque, increases the formation of blood clots, and causes blood platelets to cluster and impede blood flow. Quitting can repair heart damage caused by smoking—even heavy smokers can return to heart health. Several studies have shown that ex-smokers face the same risk of heart disease as non-smokers within five to 10 years of quitting.

Patients should be counseled to drink alcohol in moderation. Modest consumption of alcohol may actually protect against coronary artery disease. This is believed to be because alcohol raises HDL cholesterol levels. The American Heart Association defines moderate consumption as one ounce of alcohol per day—roughly one cocktail, one 8-ounce glass of wine, or two 12-ounce glasses of beer. In some people, however, moderate drinking can increase risk factors for heart disease, such as raising blood pressure. Excessive drinking is always bad for heart health. It usually raises blood pressure, and can poison the heart and cause abnormal heart rhythms or even heart failure. Illegal drugs, like cocaine, can seriously harm the heart and should never be used.

High blood pressure, one of the most common and serious risk factors for coronary artery disease, can be effectively controlled through lifestyle changes and medication. Patients with moderate hypertension may be able to control it through lifestyle changes such as reducing sodium and fat, exercising regularly, managing stress, quitting smoking, and drinking alcohol in moderation. When these changes are ineffective, and for those with severe hypertension, there are eight types of drugs that provide effective treatment.

Stress management means controlling mental and physical reactions to life's irritations and challenges. Techniques for controlling stress include taking life more slowly, spending time with family and friends, thinking

---

KEY TERMS

Angina—Chest pain that occurs when diseased blood vessels restrict the flow of blood to the heart. Angina is often the first symptom of coronary artery disease.

Atherosclerosis—A process in which the walls of the coronary arteries thicken due to the accumulation of plaque in the blood vessels. Atherosclerosis is the cause of coronary artery disease.

Coronary arteries—The two arteries that provide blood to the heart. The coronary arteries surround the heart like a crown, coming out of the aorta, arching down over the top of the heart, and dividing into two branches. These are the arteries where coronary artery disease occurs.

Plaque—A deposit of fatty and other substances that accumulate in the lining of the artery wall.

---

positively, getting enough sleep, exercising, and practicing **relaxation** techniques.

Daily aspirin therapy has been proven to help prevent blood clots associated with atherosclerosis. It can also prevent myocardial infarctions from recurring, prevent myocardial infarctions from being fatal, and reduce the risk of strokes.

Resources

BOOKS

Ahya, Shubhada N, Kellie Flood, and Subramanian Paranjothi. *The Washington Manual of Medical Therapeutics, 30th ed.* Philadelphia: Lippincott Williams & Wilkins, 2001, pp. 105-116.

American Heart Association. *Guide to Myocardial infarction Treatment, Recovery, Prevention.* New York: Time Books, 1996.

DeBakey, Michael E., and Antonio M. Gotto Jr. *The New Living Heart.* Holbrook, MA: Adams Media Corporation, 1997.

PERIODICALS

"Drugs or Angioplasty After a Myocardial Infarction?" In *Harvard Health Letter* 22, no. 10 (August 1997): 8.

Marble, Michelle. "FDA Urged to Expand Uses for Aspirin, Benefits for Women." In *Women's Health Weekly* (February 10, 1997).

"More on Anger and Heart Disease." *Harvard Heart Letter* (May 1997): 6-7.

ORGANIZATIONS

American Heart Association. National Center. 7272 Greenville Avenue, Dallas, TX 75231-4596. (214) 373-6300. <http://www.medsearch.com/pf/profiles/amerh/>.

National Heart, Lung, and Blood Institute Information Center. P.O. Box 30105, Bethesda, MD 20824-0105. <http://www.nhlbi.gov/nhlbi/nhbli.htm>.

Texas Heart Institute Heart Information Service. P.O. Box 20345, Houston, TX 77225-0345. 1-800-292-2221. <http://www.tmc.edu/thi/his.html>.

Barbara Wexler

Myocardial perfusion scan *see* **Thallium heart scan**

Myoclonus *see* **Movement disorders**

Myoglobin test *see* **Cardiac marker tests**

Myopia

Definition

Myopia is the medical term for nearsightedness. People with myopia see objects more clearly when they are close to the eye, while distant objects appear blurred or fuzzy. Reading and close-up work may be clear, but distance **vision** is less sharply defined.

Description

To understand myopia it is necessary to have a basic knowledge of the main parts of the eye's focusing system: the cornea, the lens, and the retina. The cornea is a tough, transparent, dome-shaped tissue that covers the front of the eye (not to be confused with the white, opaque sclera). The cornea lies in front of the iris (the colored part of the eye). The lens is a transparent, double-convex structure located behind the iris. The retina is a thin membrane that lines the rear of the eyeball. Light-sensitive retinal cells convert incoming light rays into electrical signals that are sent along the optic nerve to the **brain**, which then interprets the images.

In people with normal vision, parallel light rays enter the eye and are bent by the cornea and lens (a process called refraction) to focus precisely on the retina, providing a crisp, clear image. In a myopic eye, the focusing power of the cornea (the major refracting structure of the eye) and the lens is too great with respect to the length of the eyeball. Light rays are bent too much, and they converge in front of the retina. This inaccuracy is called a refractive error. In other words, an overfocused fuzzy image is sent to the brain.

There are many varieties of myopia. Some common types include:

- physiologic
- pathologic
- acquired

By far the most common form, physiologic myopia, develops in children sometime between the ages of five and 10 and gradually progresses until the eye is fully grown. Physiologic myopia may include refractive myopia (the cornea and lens-bending properties are too strong) and axial myopia (the eyeball is too long). Pathologic myopia is a far less common abnormality. This condition begins as physiologic myopia, but rather than stabilizing, the eye continues to enlarge at an abnormal rate (progressive myopia). This more advanced type of myopia may lead to degenerative changes in the eye (degenerative myopia). Acquired myopia occurs after infancy. This condition may be seen in association with uncontrolled diabetes and certain types of **cataracts**. **Antihypertensive drugs** and other medications can also affect the refractive power of the lens.

Eyecare professionals have debated the role of genetics in the development of myopia for many years. Most believe that a tendency toward myopia may be inherited, but the actual disorder results from a combination of environmental and genetic factors. Environmental factors include close work, work with computer monitors or other instruments that emit some light (electron microscopes, photographic equipment, lasers, etc.), emotional **stress**, and eye strain.

A variety of genetic patterns for inheriting myopia have been suggested, ranging from a recessive pattern with complete penetrance in people who are homozygotic for myopia to an autosomal dominant pattern; an autosomal recessive pattern; and various mixtures of these patterns. One explanation for this lack of agreement is that the genetic profile of high myopia (defined as a refractive error greater than -6 diopters) may differ from that of low myopia. Some researchers think that high myopia is determined to a greater extent by genetic factors than low myopia.

Another explanation for disagreement regarding the role of heredity in myopia is the sensitivity of the human eye to very small changes in its anatomical structure. Since even small deviations from normal structure cause significant refractive errors, it may be difficult to single out any specific genetic or environmental factor as their cause.

Genetic markers and gene mapping

Since 1992, genetic markers that may be associated with genes for myopia have been located on human chromosomes 1, 2, 12, and 18. There is some genetic information on the short arm of chromosome 2 in highly myopic people. Genetic information for low myopia appears to be located on the short arm of chromosome 1, but it is not known whether this information governs the structure of the eye itself or vulnerability to environmental factors.

In 1998, a team of American researchers presented evidence that a gene for familial high myopia with an autosomal dominant transmission pattern could be mapped to human chromosome 18 in eight North American families. The same group also found a second locus for this form of myopia on human chromosome 12 in a large German/Italian family. In 1999, a group of French researchers found no linkage between chromosome 18 among 32 French families with familial high myopia. These findings have been taken to indicate that more than one gene is involved in the transmission of the disorder.

Family studies

It has been known for some years that a family history of myopia is one of the most important risk factors for developing the condition. Only 6–15% of children with myopia come from families in which neither parent is myopic. In families with one myopic parent, 23–40% of the children develop myopia. If both parents are myopic, the rate rises to 33–60% for their children. One American study found that children with two myopic parents are 6.42 times as likely to develop myopia themselves as children with only one or no myopic parents. As of 2001, the precise interplay of genetic and environmental factors in these family patterns, however, is not yet known.

One multigenerational study of Chinese families indicated that persons in the third generation had a higher risk of developing myopia even if their parents were not myopic. The researchers concluded that, at least in China, the genetic factors in myopia have remained constant over the past three generations while the environmental factors have intensified. The increase in the percentage of people with myopia over the last 50 years in the United States has led American researchers to the same conclusion.

Myopia is the most common eye disorder in humans around the world. It affects between 25 and 35% of the adult population in the United States and the developed countries, but is thought to affect as much as 40% of the population in some parts of Asia. Some researchers have found slightly higher rates of myopia in women than in men.

There is considerable variation in the age distribution of myopia in the United States. The prevalence of myopia rises among children and adolescents in school until it reaches the 25–35% level in the young adult population. It declines slightly in the over-45 age group. Approximately 20% of 65-year-olds have myopia. The figure drops to 14% for Americans over 70.

Other factors that affect the demographic distribution of myopia are income level and education. The prevalence of myopia is higher among people with above-average incomes and educational attainments. Myopia is also more prevalent among people whose work requires a great deal of close focusing, including work with computers.

Causes and symptoms

Myopia is said to be caused by an elongation of the eyeball or a cornea that is steeply curved. This means that the oblong (as opposed to normal spherical) shape of the myopic eye causes the cornea and lens to focus at a point in front of the retina. A more precise explanation is that there is an inadequate correlation between the focusing power of the cornea and lens and the length of the eye.

People are generally born with a small amount of **hyperopia** (farsightedness), but as the eye grows this decreases and myopia does not become evident until later. This change is one reason why some researchers think that myopia is an acquired rather than an inherited trait.

The symptoms of myopia are blurred distance vision, eye discomfort, squinting, and eye strain. Headaches may accompany eye strain.

Diagnosis

The diagnosis of myopia is typically made during the first several years of elementary school when a teacher notices a child having difficulty seeing the chalkboard, reading, or concentrating. The teacher or school nurse often recommends an **eye examination** by an ophthalmologist or optometrist. An ophthalmologist is an MD or DO (Doctor of Osteopathy) who is a medical doctor trained in the diagnosis and treatment of eye problems. Ophthalmologists also perform eye surgery. An optometrist (OD) diagnoses, manages, and treats eye and **visual disorders**. In all states, optometrists are licensed to prescribe diagnostic and therapeutic drugs.

A person's distance vision is tested by reading letters or numbers on a chart posted a set distance away (usually 20 ft [6 m]). The doctor asks the person to view images

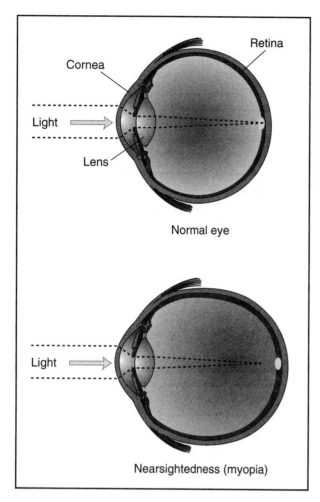

Cornea
Retina
Light
Lens
Normal eye

Light
Nearsightedness (myopia)

Myopia, or nearsightedness, is a condition of the eye in which objects are seen more clearly when close to the eye while distant objects appear blurred or fuzzy. *(Illustration by Electronic Illustrators Group.)*

through a variety of lenses to obtain the best correction. The doctor also examines the inside of the eye and the retina. An instrument called a slit lamp is used to examine the cornea and lens. The eyeglass prescription is written in terms of diopters (D), which measure the degree of refractive error. Mild to moderate myopia usually falls between -1.00D and -6.00D. Normal vision is commonly referred to as 20/20 to describe the eye's focusing ability at a distance of 20 ft (6 m) from an object. For example, 20/50 means that a myopic person must stand 20 ft (6 m) away from an eye chart to see what a normal person can see at 50 ft (15.2 m). The larger the bottom number, the greater the myopia.

Treatment

People with myopia have three main options for treatment: eyeglasses, **contact lenses**, and, for those who meet certain criteria, refractive eye surgery.

Eyeglasses

Eyeglasses are the most common method used to correct myopia. Concave glass or plastic lenses are placed in frames in front of the eyes. The lenses are ground to the thickness and curvature specified in the eyeglass prescription. The lenses cause the light rays to diverge so that they focus further back, directly on the retina, producing clear distance vision.

Contact lenses

Contact lenses are a second option for treatment. Contact lenses are extremely thin, round discs of plastic that are worn on the eye in front of the cornea. Although there may be some initial discomfort, most people quickly grow accustomed to contact lenses. Hard contact lenses, made from a material called PMMA, are virtually obsolete. Rigid gas permeable lenses (RGP) are made of plastic that holds its shape but allows the passage of oxygen into the eye. Some believe that RGP lenses may halt or slow the progression of myopia because they maintain a constant, gentle pressure that flattens the cornea. As of 2001, the National Eye Institute was conducting an ongoing study of RGP lenses called the Contact Lens and Myopia Progression (CLAMP) Study, with results to be released in 2003.

A procedure called orthokeratology acts on this principle of corneal molding. However, when contact lenses are discontinued for a period of time, the cornea will generally go back to its original shape. Rigid gas permeable lenses offer crisp, clear sight. Soft contact lenses are made of flexible plastic and can be up to 80% water. Soft lenses offer increased comfort and have the advantage of extended wear. Some can be worn continuously for up to one week. While oxygen passes freely through soft lenses, bacterial contamination and other problems can occur, requiring replacement of lenses on a regular basis. It is very important to follow the cleaning and disinfecting regimens prescribed because protein and lipid buildup can occur on the lenses, causing discomfort or increasing the risk of **infection**. Contact lenses offer several benefits over glasses, including: better vision, less distortion, clear peripheral vision, and cosmetic appeal. In addition, contacts don't steam up from perspiration or changes in temperature.

Refractive eye surgery

For people who find glasses and contact lenses inconvenient or uncomfortable, and who meet selection criteria regarding age, degree of myopia, general health, etc., refractive eye surgery is a third treatment alternative. As of 2001, four types of corrective surgeries are available:

- **radial keratotomy** (RK)
- photorefractive keratectomy (PRK)
- corneal rings
- laser-assisted in-situ keratomileusis (LASIK), which is still under clinical evaluation by the Food and Drug Administration (FDA)

Refractive eye surgery improves myopic vision by permanently changing the shape of the cornea so that light rays focus properly on the retina. These procedures are performed on an outpatient basis and generally take 10 to 30 minutes.

RADIAL KERATOTOMY. Radial keratotomy (RK), the first of these procedures made available, has a high associated risk of an unfavorable outcome. It was first developed in Japan and the Soviet Union, and introduced into the United States in 1978. The surgeon uses a delicate diamond-tipped blade, a **microscope**, and microscopic instruments to make several spoke-like "radial" incisions in the non-viewing (peripheral) portion of the cornea. As the incisions heal, the slits alter the curve of the cornea, making it more flat, which may improve the focus of images onto the retina. With the advent of laser surgeries, this procedure has become almost obsolete.

PHOTOREFRACTIVE KERATECTOMY. Photorefractive keratectomy (PRK) involves the use of a computer to measure the shape of the cornea. Using these measurements, the surgeon applies a computer-controlled laser to make modifications to the cornea. The PRK procedure flattens the cornea by vaporizing small amounts of tissue from the cornea's surface. As of early 2001, only two excimer lasers are approved by the FDA for PRK, although other lasers have been used. It is important to make sure the laser being used is FDA approved. Photorefractive keratectomy can be used to treat mild to moderate forms of myopia. The cost is approximately $2,000 per eye.

LASER-ASSISTED IN-SITU KERATOMILEUSIS. Laser-assisted in-situ keratomileusis (LASIK) is the newest of these procedures. It is recommended for moderate to severe cases of myopia. A variation on the PRK method, LASIK uses lasers and a cutting tool called a microkeratome to cut a circular flap on the cornea. The flap is flipped back to expose the inner layers of the cornea. The cornea is treated with a laser to change its shape and focusing properties, then the flap is replaced.

Risks

All of these surgical procedures carry risks, the most serious being corneal scarring, corneal rupture, infection, cataracts, and loss of vision. In addition, a study published in March 2001 warned that mountain climbers who have had LASIK surgery should be aware of possible changes in their vision at high altitudes. The lack of oxygen at high altitudes causes temporary changes in the thickness of the cornea.

Since refractive eye surgery doesn't guarantee 20/20 vision, it is important to have realistic expectations before choosing this treatment. In a 10-year study conducted by the National Eye Institute between 1983 and 1993, over 50% of people with radial keratotomy gained 20/20 vision, and 85% passed a driving test (requiring 20/40 vision) after surgery, without glasses or contact lenses. Even if a person gains near-perfect vision, however, there are potentially irritating side effects, such as postoperative **pain**, poor night vision, variation in visual acuity, light sensitivity and glare, and optical distortion. **Refractive eye surgeries** are considered elective procedures and are rarely covered by insurance plans.

Myopia treatments under research include corneal implants and permanent surgically placed contact lenses.

Alternative treatments

Some eye care professionals recommend treatments to help improve circulation, reduce eye strain, and relax the eye muscles. It is possible that by combining exercises with changes in behavior, the progression of myopia may be slowed or prevented. Alternative treatments include: visual therapy (also referred to as vision training or eye exercises), discontinuing close work, reducing eye strain (taking a rest break during periods of prolonged near vision tasks), and wearing bifocals to decrease the need to accommodate when doing close-up work.

Prognosis

Glasses and contact lenses can (but not always) correct a person's vision to 20/20. Refractive surgery can make permanent improvements for the right candidates.

While the genetic factors that influence the transmission and severity of myopia cannot be changed, some environmental factors can be modified. They include reducing close work, reading and working in good light, taking frequent breaks when working at a computer or microscope for long periods of time, maintaining good **nutrition**, and practicing visual therapy (when recommended).

Health care team roles

Ophthalmologists and optometrists diagnose myopia. Both may prescribe corrective lenses (glasses or contact lenses). Ophthalmologists perform surgery to correct myopia. Various individuals can fill prescriptions

KEY TERMS

Accommodation—The ability of the lens to change its focus from distant to near objects. It is achieved through the action of the ciliary muscles that change the shape of the lens.

Cornea—The outer, transparent tissue that covers the front of the eye. The cornea is part of the eye's focusing system.

Diopter (D)—A unit of measure for describing refractive power.

Laser-assisted in-situ keratomileusis (LASIK)—A procedure that uses a cutting tool and a laser to modify the cornea and correct moderate to high levels of myopia.

Lens—The transparent, elastic, curved structure behind the iris (colored part of the eye) that helps focus light on the retina.

Ophthalmologist—A medical doctor (MD or DO) who specializes in the diagnosis and medical and surgical treatment of eye diseases and disorders.

Optic nerve—A bundle of nerve fibers that carries visual messages in the form of electrical signals to the brain.

Optometrist—Doctors of optometry are primary health care professionals who examine, diagnose, treat, and manage diseases and disorders of the visual system, the eye, and associated structures, as well as diagnose related systemic conditions. They prescribe glasses, contact lenses, low vision rehabilitation, vision therapy and medications, as well as perform certain surgical procedures.

Orthokeratology—A method of reshaping the cornea using a contact lens. It is not considered a permanent method to reduce myopia.

Peripheral vision—The ability to see objects and movement to the side, outside of the direct line of vision.

Photorefractive keratectomy (PRK)—A procedure that uses an excimer laser to make modifications to the cornea and permanently correct myopia. As of 2001, two lasers have been approved by the FDA for this purpose.

Radial keratotomy (RK)—A surgical procedure involving the use of a diamond-tipped blade to make several spoke-like slits in the peripheral (non-viewing) portion of the cornea to improve the focus of the eye and correct myopia by flattening the cornea.

Refraction—The bending of light rays as they pass from one medium through another. Used to describe the action of the cornea and lens on light rays as they enter they eye. Also used to describe the determination and measurement of the eye's focusing system by an optometrist or ophthalmologist.

Refractive eye surgery—A general term for surgical procedures that can improve or correct refractive errors by permanently changing the shape of the cornea.

Retina—The light-sensitive membrane that lines the back of the eye. The retinal cells process and send visual signals to the brain through the optic nerve.

Visual acuity—The ability to distinguish details and shapes of objects.

for corrective lenses. This is governed by individual state laws.

Prevention

Eye strain can be prevented by using sufficient light for reading and close work, and by wearing corrective lenses as prescribed. Those with corrective lenses should have regular eye examinations to see if their prescription has changed or if any other problems have developed. This is particularly important for people with high (degenerative) myopia who are at a greater risk of developing retinal detachment, retinal degeneration, **glaucoma**, or other problems.

Resources

BOOKS

Grosvenor, Theodore P., David A. Goss, and Henry W. Hoffstetter. *Clinical Management of Myopia*. Woburn, MA: Butterworth-Heinemann Medical, 1998.

Machat, Jeffrey J., Stephen G. Slade, and Louis E. Probst. *The Art of Lasik*. 2nd ed. Thorofare, NJ: Slack Inc., 1999.

Olitsky, Scott E., and Leonard B. Nelson. "Disorders of Vision." In *Nelson Textbook of Pediatrics*, 16th ed.

Edited by Richard E. Behrman, et al. Philadelphia: Saunders, 2000.

Ong, Editha, and Kenneth J. Ciuffreda. *Accommodation, Nearwork, and Myopia.* Santa Ana, CA: Optometric Extension Program Foundation, 1998.

Rosenfield, Mark, and Bernard Gilmartin. *Myopia and Nearwork.* Woburn, MA: Butterworth-Heinemann Medical, 1998.

PERIODICALS

Chan, C. K., F. C. Lawrence. "Macular Hole After Laser in Situ Keratomileusis and Photorefractive Keratectomy." *American Journal of Ophthalmology* 131, no. 5 (2001): 666-667.

Marr, J. E., et al. "Associations of High Myopia in Childhood." *Eye* 15 (2001): 70-74.

Miller, A. E., et al. "Patient Satisfaction After LASIK for Myopia." *Contact Lens Association of Ophthalmologists Journal* 27, no. 2 (2001): 84-88.

Romano, P. E. "Much Can be Done for Your Child's Myopia." *Optometry and Visual Sciences* 78, no. 4 (2001): 186-187.

Singh, D. "Is Refractive Surgery Justified?" *Journal of the Indian Medical Association* 98, no. 12 (2001): 748-767.

Wu, H. M., et al. "Does Education Explain Ethnic Differences in Myopia Prevalence? A Population-based Study of Young Adult Males in Singapore." *Optometry and Visual Sciences* 78, no. 4 (2001): 234-239.

ORGANIZATIONS

American Academy of Ophthalmology. PO Box 7424, San Francisco, CA 94120. (415) 561-8500. <http://www.eyenet.org>.

American Optometric Association. 243 North Lindbergh Blvd., St. Louis, MO 63141. (314) 991-4100. <http://www.aoanet.org>.

Optometric Extension Program Foundation, Inc. 1921 E. Carnegie Ave., Ste. 3-L, Santa Ana, CA 92705-5510. (949) 250-8070. <http://www.healthy.net/oep>.

OTHER

American Optometric Association. <http://www.aoanet.org/cvc-myopia.html>.

Harvard Medical School. <http://www.med.harvard.edu/publications/On_The_Brain/Volume4/Number3/Myopia.html>.

Internet Ophthalmology. <http://www.ophthal.org>.

Massachusetts Eye and Ear Infirmary. <http://www.meei.harvard.edu/shared/ophtho/ophtho.html>.

Mayo Clinic. <http://www.mayo.edu/ophtha-rst>.

Rush University School of Medicine. <http://www.rush.edu/worldbook/articles/013000a/013000207.html>.

Stanford University School of Medicine. <http://www.med.stanford.edu/school/eye>.

L. Fleming Fallon, Jr., MD, DrPH

Naproxen *see* **Nonsteroidal anti-inflammatory drugs**

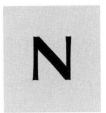

Nasal cannula/face mask application

Definition

A nasal cannula is a narrow, flexible plastic tubing used to deliver oxygen through the nostrils of patients using nasal breathing. It connects to an oxygen outlet, a tank source or compressor, on one end and has a loop at the other end with dual pronged extended openings at the top of the loop. The prongs are slightly curved to fit readily into the front portion of a patient's nostrils. The tubing of the loop is fitted over the patient's ears and is brought together under the chin by a sliding connector that holds the cannula in place.

A simple oxygen face mask is a plastic device that is contoured to fit over a patient's nose and mouth. It is used to deliver oxygen as the patient breathes through either the nose or the mouth. A simple oxygen mask has open side ports that allow room air to enter the mask and dilute the oxygen, as well as allowing exhaled carbon dioxide to leave the containment space. It also has narrow plastic tubing fixed to the bottom of the mask that is used to connect the mask to an oxygen source. An adjustable elastic band is connected to each side of the mask and slides over the head and above the ears to hold the mask securely in place.

A partial rebreather oxygen mask is similar to a simple face mask, however, the side ports are covered with one-way discs to prevent room air from entering the mask. This mask is called a rebreather because it has a soft plastic reservoir bag connected to the mask that conserves the first third of the patient's exhaled air while the rest escapes through the side ports. This is designed to make use of the carbon dioxide as a respiratory stimulant.

A non-rebreather oxygen mask is similar to a simple face mask but has multiple one-way valves in the side ports. These valves prevent room air from entering the mask but allow exhaled air to leave the mask. It has a reservoir bag like a partial rebreather mask but the reservoir bag has a one-way valve that prevents exhaled air from entering the reservoir. This allows larger concentrations of oxygen to collect in the reservoir bag for the patient to inhale.

A Venturi oxygen mask is similar to a simple face mask but the tubing that connects to the oxygen source is larger than that of other masks. The connector has interchangeable adaptors that widen or narrow the diameter of the flow through the tubing to allow settings of specific concentrations of oxygen through the mask.

Purpose

The purpose of nasal cannulas and oxygen face masks is to deliver oxygen in as concentrated a form as required for patients who are hypoxic. There are many conditions that cause hypoxemia and require the administration of supplemental oxygen, including respiratory disease, cardiac disease, **shock**, trauma, severe electrolyte imbalance (hypokalemia), low hemoglobin or severe **blood** loss, and seizures. Prompt treatment of these conditions with non-invasive oxygen administration can prevent the need for more invasive procedures such as intubation and mechanical ventilation.

A nasal cannula is used to deliver low concentrations of oxygen. It can deliver from 24% to 40% oxygen at a flow rate of 0.26-1.58 gal (1-6 L) per minute. A simple mask is used to deliver moderate to high concentrations of oxygen. It can deliver from 40% to 60% oxygen at a flow rate of 2.64-3.17 gal (10-12 L) per minute. A partial rebreather mask is used to deliver high concentrations of oxygen. It can deliver 70% to 90% oxygen at a flow of 1.58-3.96 gal (6-15 L) per minute. A non-rebreather mask is used to deliver high flow oxygen. It can deliver 90% to 100% oxygen at a flow of 3.96 gal (15 L) per minute. A variable flow rate mask has interchangeable adaptors that may be set to deliver oxygen at 24%, 28%, 31%, 35%, 40%, or 50%.

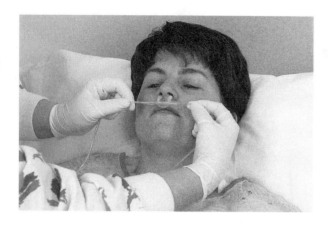

Insertion of nasal cannula. *(Delmar Publishers, Inc. Reproduced by permission.)*

Precautions

Oxygen is flammable. "No Smoking" signs should be posed when a patient is receiving oxygen. Electrical equipment must have special grounding adaptors on plugs to avoid sparks. The patient and family should be warned of the dangers involved in using oxygen at home, such as exercising care when using oxygen near stoves, portable heating units, and ungrounded electrical equipment. Oxygen cylinders must be place in a cart or base to avoid dropping or bumping the tank. Oxygen tanks or compressors should be turned off when not in use and oxygen valves should be checked routinely to be sure that they are secure. Oxygen levels in reserve tanks should be monitored to ensure continuous therapy.

Patients receiving oxygen should be closely monitored. Arterial **blood gas analysis** or the use of a **pulse oximeter** will ensure that the oxygen concentration being delivered is sufficient to meet the patient's needs. Monitor the patient's condition and **vital signs** frequently, according to the policy of the medical setting. The fit of the nasal cannula or mask and all of the oxygen connections should be evaluated, to ensure that no part of the system has been blocked or diverted and the oxygen is being delivered correctly, as ordered.

The use of a face mask can cause a patient to perspire and feel warm, claustrophobic or nauseated. Explain the importance of the oxygen to the patient and encourage him to relax and breathe slowly. A cold cloth on the forehead and moral support can help the patient overcome these anxious feelings. If a patient with an oxygen mask begins to vomit, quickly remove the mask. There is a danger of aspirating vomit into the **lungs** if it collects in the mask over the nose and mouth. Support the patient, assist them in cleaning the mouth after vomiting by rinsing with water or mouthwash, clean off the mask

and the attached tubing, and replace it. The physician should be notified and antiemetics may be ordered.

A nasal cannula is more comfortable for a patient than a mask but can only deliver low concentrations of oxygen. Nasal cannulas should only be used in patients who breathe adequately through their noses. Use of cannulae is not indicated in patients who have severe hypoxia, poor respiratory effort, blocked nasal passages, apnea, or are mouth breathers.

Be cautious about giving oxygen to patients with chronic obstructive pulmonary disease because they may retain carbon dioxide. Oxygen may depress the hypoxic drive in these patients. They should be observed for decreased respirations, an altered mental state or further elevations of their carbon dioxide levels.

Description

Before applying a nasal cannula, the oxygen-flow meter should be turned to the setting in liters per minute that is ordered by the physician. The nurse should use his or her finger tips to ensure that oxygen is flowing through the prongs of the cannula. The nurse should apply a nasal cannula by placing the nasal prongs gently into the patient's nostrils, draping the tubing over the patient's ears, and sliding the fit connector up under the chin to hold the tubing securely in place. Two small pieces of clear plastic tape can be used to hold the cannula against the patient's cheeks to secure the cannula in place if necessary. This is only necessary if the patient is restless, confused, or is a young child who may bat the cannula out of place.

Before applying an oxygen face mask, the nurse should turn on the oxygen flow-meter to the setting in liters per minute that is ordered by the physician. If using a Venturi mask, the adaptor device should be selected and applied to deliver the oxygen concentration that is ordered. Use the finger tips to ensure that oxygen is flowing through the face mask. An oxygen face mask is applied by placing the molded plastic mask onto the patient's face, over the nose and mouth. The nurse should pull the elastic strap over the patient's head to the back of the head and adjust the strap on both sides of the mask to secure the mask in a position that seals it against the face. Some masks have a nose-clip that can be gently squeezed to mold the mask over the bridge of the nose. The mask should fit snugly against the face but must not press so tightly as to leave impressions in the skin. If the mask has a reservoir bag and its purpose is to serve as an oxygen reservoir, the nurse should check that oxygen is filling the bag before applying the mask.

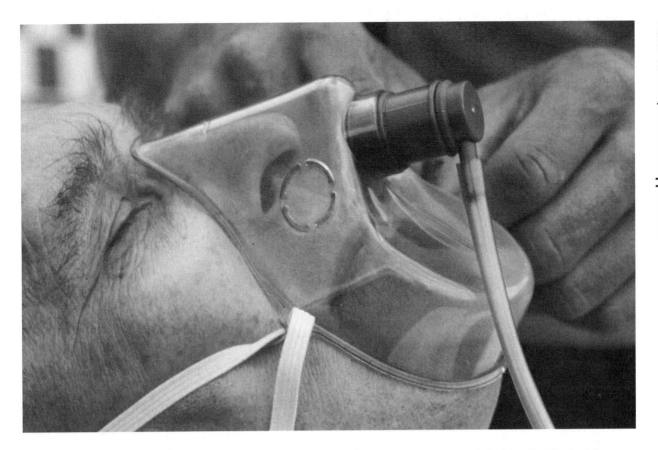

A man is given oxygen via a face mask before being transported to the hospital. *(Photograph by Adam Hart-Davis. Science Source/Photo Researchers. Reproduced by permission.)*

Preparation

The nurse should place the patient in a comfortable position, preferably semi-Fowler's or full Fowler's position (to assist breathing). She or he should take baseline vital signs and note the patient's level of consciousness. A pulse-oximetry reading or draw **blood gases** should be done as ordered for baseline lab values. Oxygen delivery to the patient should be explained, including what equipment is to be used (such as a mask or nasal cannula) and the importance of keeping the apparatus in place. The patient should know of the flammability of oxygen and a "No Smoking" sign should be posted. The nurse should instruct the patient to notify him or her of increasing distress, air hunger, nausea, **anxiety**, dry nasal passages, or "sore throat" (due to drying). The equipment needed should be assembled, including the oxygen-flow meter, humidity bottle if ordered, nasal cannula, or appropriate face mask. The mask or cannula should be connected securely to the oxygen flow-meter. Extension tubing should be used between the mask tubing and the oxygen flow-meter if necessary so that the patient may move about without pulling the mask off or pulling the tubing out of the oxygen source. The nurse should place a pulse-oximeter machine at hand if ordered, to monitor the patient's response to **oxygen therapy**.

Aftercare

After initiating oxygen therapy, the nurse should stay with the patient for a while to reassure the patient and observe his or her reactions to the therapy. The patient's vital signs should be monitored, along with the level of consciousness, comfort with the oxygen apparatus, and oximetry levels, as ordered by the physician or as directed by policy of the medical setting. Oxygen connections and settings should be checked. The nurse should observe the patient, either for improvements in color, respiratory rate and rhythm, and comfort levels, or for increased or decreased respiratory effort, diaphoresis, alteration in mental status, anxiety and restlessness. Facemasks will interfere with communication and eating. Oxygen will dry out the mucous membranes of the nose and mouth. The nurse should briefly remove the mask periodically to allow the patient to drink or eat, for mouth care, or to communicate clearly. When the mask or cannula is off, the skin on the face and above the ears should be checked for signs of skin irritation. If the skin is irritated above the ears, cotton padding can be placed between the ears and the elastic band or the cannula tubing to protect the skin. If the skin of the face is irritated, the face can be massaged gently and a water-based moisturizer applied. The mask can be loosened slightly to decrease irritation. The use of petroleum ointment to the lips or nose should be avoided because it can obstruct the cannula prong openings. If a humidifier is used with the oxygen apparatus, the humidity bottle should be refilled with distilled water according to the medical setting routine or at least once every eight hours. Blood gas analysis should be done as ordered when a patient is receiving oxygen to determine whether levels of oxygen flow should be decreased or need to be increased. When higher levels of oxygen are no longer needed, a patient using a face mask should be changed to a nasal cannula to improve comfort, the ability to communicate, and the ability to eat and drink more easily during therapy.

Complications

The most serious complication of oxygen therapy is the depression of the hypoxic drive to breathe in patients with chronic lung disease. High levels of oxygen may cause elevated levels of trapped carbon dioxide, which may lead to a decrease in respirations, a state of narcosis, and eventually to respiratory stasis or arrest.

Less serious complications include skin breakdown around the mask or cannula, a dry mouth, nose or lips, **sore throat**, and a decrease in appetite.

Results

Oxygen therapy using a nasal cannula or facemask is usually effective in increasing oxygen levels in the body to a normal or near normal state, providing time for treatment of the underlying disease or impediment causing the hypoxemia. Patients who do not respond to non-invasive oxygen therapy will usually be intubated (endotracheal intubation) and placed on mechanical ventilation with oxygen either as an assist device or as a full-capacity respirator.

Health care team roles

Oxygen is considered a drug and in this context is administered by a licensed nurse or respiratory therapist in the medical setting. Once oxygen therapy has been initiated, non-professional staff may assist in caring for the patient using oxygen therapy, including removing and replacing the mask or cannula for skin care, meals or brief ambulation to the bathroom. Nonprofessional staff must be instructed to remember to turn the oxygen flow back on after removal. They may also be trained to check oxygen apparatus such as, checking tubing connections, replacing the oximeter probe, filling the humidity bottles and cleaning or wiping humidity out of the oxygen mask. This should be performed under the direct supervision of the licensed nurse and the nurse or respiratory therapist will continually assess the patient's respiratory status and oxygen levels. When a patient is going home with oxygen, the licensed nurse or respiratory therapist will educate the patient and the patient's caregivers about the safe use of oxygen in the home. Patients using oxygen in the home should have initial and follow-up visits by a **home care** nurse or respiratory technician to check the patient's status and equipment function in the home. Patients receiving oxygen in the home should be scheduled for regular visits to the physician for follow-up assessment, including pulse oximetry and other therapy.

Resources

BOOKS

"Oxygen Delivery Systems." In *The Harriet Lane Handbook*, 15th ed. Ed. by George K. Siberry and Robert Iannone. Mosby, Inc., 2000.

OTHER

"Airway Management." *Respiratory Therapist.* Continuing Education Online. June 2000. <http://www.continuinged-ucation.com/resptherapist/airway/supadmin.html>.

Auerbach, Paul S., M.D. "Oxygen Administration." *Medicine for the Outdoors.* Adam.com Online. The Lyons Press, 1999. <http://www.adam.com/b2b/products/demos/odh/oxygen_admin.html>.

"Inpatient Oxygen Therapy." *Standards for the Diagnosis and Care of Patients with Chronic Obstructive Pulmonary Disease.* American Thoracic Society. Epocnet Online. 2001. <http://www.epocnet.com/area_m/normas/b_4_03f.html#up>.

"Oxygen Administration." *Nursing Interventions and Clinical Skills. 2nd ed.* Harcourt Health Online. Mosby, Inc., 2000. <http://www.harcourthealth.com/MERLIN/Elkin/Skills/31-01.html>.

"Respiratory Function and Therapy," Chapter 10. In *The Lippincott Manual of Nursing Practice.* Books at Ovid Online. 2001. <http://pco.ovid.com/lrppco/>.

Mary Elizabeth Martelli, R.N., B.S.

Nasal culture *see* **Nasopharyngeal culture**

Nasal instillation

Definition

A nasal installation is a medicine solution prepared for administration into the nose. Nasal medicine is given in the form of nose drops or nasal sprays.

Purpose

The purpose of a nasal instillation is to deliver medicine directly into the nose and onto the nasal membranes, where it will be absorbed into the body. The most common nasal medicines are decongestant, antihistamine, and steroid nasal sprays used to relieve nasal congestion secondary to colds or **allergies**. Some nasal installations are unrelated to the nose, but are given by this method because of the ease of administration and the quick uptake through the nasal membranes.

Precautions

Nasal membranes are sensitive and can be traumatized by overuse of medication and by forceful insertion of a nasal spray or dropper tip.

Description

To instill nose drops, have the client sit in an upright position with the head and nose tilted slightly back. Hold the dropper near the entry to the nostril and instruct the client to inhale as you drop the appropriate dose into the nostril. Keep the client's head back for two to three minutes to allow the drops to roll to the back of the nostril. Repeat in the other nostril. To instill nasal spray, have the client sit erect with the head and nose upright or tilted slightly forward. Remove the cap from the nasal spray, shake the bottle, and gently place the tip of the spray bottle well into the nostril. Instruct the client to exhale, and then inhale vigorously as you squeeze the bottle to deliver the spray. Repeat in the other nostril.

Preparation

The nurse should wash his or her hands before instilling nasal medicine. Each time the medicine is administered, the medication label should be checked to avoid medication errors. It should be confirmed that it is the right medicine, the correct dose (i.e., strength), the proper time, the right patient, and the appropriate method. The expiration date on the label should be checked to ensure that the medication is not outdated. Prior to administration of the medicine, the bottle or canister should be shaken. The patient should blow his or her nose before nasal instillations. It is not unusual for nasal instillations to stimulate a sneeze. Tissues should be kept at hand so that residue can be wiped away and for the client to use to cover the mouth and nose when sneezing.

Aftercare

After rinsing the dropper or nasal spray tip with warm water, the cap should be replaced. Soiled tissues should be placed in a bag that can be sealed and discarded. When the procedure has been completed, the nurse should wash his or her hands.

Complications

Nasal medicines can irritate the lining of the nasal membranes and cause inflammation or nosebleeds when used to excess. Additionally, patients can develop a functional dependence for certain nasal sprays if used to excess.

Results

Most nasal instillations work promptly because of the quick uptake of medicine through the nasal membranes. If signs of nasal irritation occur or if the desired effect is not achieved after several days, the physician should be consulted.

Health care team roles

Administering any medicine is the responsibility of a licensed nurse (i.e., R.N. or L.P.N) in most health care settings. The patient or a patient's family member or friend can be instructed on how to administer nasal medicine in the home setting.

Resources

BOOKS

Smith-Temple, Jean, and Joyce Young Johnson. *Nurses' Guide to Clinical Procedures.* 3rd ed. Philadelphia: Lippincott, 1998.

OTHER

"Doctor, Should I Take Antihistamines?" American Association of Otolaryngology—Head and Neck Surgery Online. 2000. <http://www.entnet.org/antihistamines.html>.

"How to Use Nose Drops." National Pharmaceutical Association. PharmWeb Online. 2001. <http://www.pharmweb.net/pwmirror/pwz/patient/pharm webpatinf6.html>.

"Nasal Sprays: How to Use Them Correctly." *Information from Your Family Doctor.* American Academy of Family Physicians Online. 2000. <http://familydoctor.org/hand-outs/104.html>.

"Oxymetazoline (Nasal)." Medline. *National Library of Medicine Online* June 2000. <http://www.nlm.nih.gov/medlineplus/druginfo/oxymeta-zolinenasal202432.html>.

Mary Elizabeth Martelli, R.N., B.S.

▌Nasal packing

Definition

Nasal packing is gauze, foam, or cotton that has been packed into the nasal chambers. The term nasal packing may refer to individual gauze strips or cotton pledgets that are packed as they are inserted into the nose to form a plug or may refer to a pre-shaped pack of foam, gauze, or cotton that is inserted into the nose as a unit. Nasal packing may be coated with petrolatum, **antibiotics** or agents that aid in clot formation. Some types of nasal packing have tails made of sutures or ties, which remain outside the nose to assist in repositioning or removing the nasal packing. Pre-formed nasal packs may include small tubes in the center of the pack to allow some air exchange while the packing is in place.

Purpose

Nasal packing is inserted into the nose by a physician to control severe nosebleeds. The purpose of the packing is to apply direct pressure onto the **blood vessels** located in the nasal membranes. Nasal packing may be used after nasal surgery to provide support to the nasal septum, control bleeding and absorb drainage.

Precautions

Nasal packing prevents air exchange through the nose. If both sides of the nose are packed, the client must breathe through his mouth while the packs are in place. Clients with nasal packing should be placed with the head of the bed elevated 30 degrees and observed for respiratory distress. Continued bleeding may not be apparent on the external end of nasal packing. Check the posterior oropharynx area regularly to see if **blood** is trickling into the back of the throat. Nasal packing can slip back or out with movement or sneezing. Check the positioning of the nasal pack routinely both at the external opening of the nose and by examining the oropharynx.

Description

When assisting the physician with nasal packing insertion, tilt the client back into a semi-reclining position to allow visualization into the nose. Monitor the client's respiratory status and **anxiety** during the procedure. Assist them to keep their hands down out of the way during the procedure if necessary. Assist the physician with positioning of the client, the light, suction and the instruments as instructed.

Local packing is a procedure used when only a small part of the nose must be packed. Typically, this occurs when one blood vessel is prone to bleeding, and there is no need to block breathing through the nose. Local packing is used when the pack can remain in place by itself. This situation can be found at the turbinates. Turbinates are folds of tissue on the insides of the nose. The folds are sufficiently firm to support packing. A small piece of gauze or cotton is wedged in between the turbinates where the blood vessel being treated is located. Local packing is left in place for up to 48 hours and then removed. The main advantage to this type of packing is that it enables the patient to breathe through his or her nose. Local packing is also more comfortable than complete packing, although the patient will still experience a sensation that something is in the nasal cavity.

A postnasal pack is used to treat bleeding in the postnasal area. This is a difficult area to pack. Packs used in this area are pre-formed or made from cotton balls or gauze that have been tied into a tubular shape with heavy gauge suture or umbilical tape. Long lengths of suture or tape are left free. The lengths of suture or tape are used to help position the pack during installation and to remove it. After being tied, the pack is soaked with an antibiotic ointment. Generally, packs are formed larger than needed, so that they completely block the nasal passage. A catheter is passed through the nose and pulled out through the mouth. Strings from one end of the pack are tied to the catheter and the pack is pulled into place by passing through the mouth and up the back of the nasal cavity. The pack is removed in a similar manner. The end of the nose may be taped to keep the packing in place or to prevent the patient from pulling them out. More often a gauze 4x4 is folded and taped across the entrance to the nose to collect excess drainage and remind the client not to interfere with or probe the packing while it is in place.

In patients who are chronic nose pickers, frequent bleeding is common and ulceration of nasal tissue is possible. To promote healing and to prevent nose picking, both sides of the nose are packed with cotton that contains antibiotics. The nose is taped shut with surgical tape to prevent the packing from being removed. The packing is left in the nose for seven to 10 days. If the wound is high up in the nasal cavity, gauze strips treated with petrolatum and antibiotics are used. The strips are placed into the nose one layer at a time, folding one layer on top of the other until the area is completely packed.

Modern pre-formed nasal packs are lubricated with water-soluble lubricant and easily inserted as a unit in a compressed state. They are moistened after insertion by squirting them with saline or nasal medication, which causes them to expand to fill the nose. Newer polymer nasal packs are designed with a non-stick coating and absorbent core to enhance absorption but avoid re-opening the vessels when the pack is removed.

Preparation

When nasal packing is to be inserted in the clinic or emergency room setting, the nurse should wash the hands and put on gloves and a disposable gown. The client should be placed in a sitting position with the nose tilted forward and slightly upward until the physician is ready to insert the packing. The patient should be given 4x4 gauze pads or a washcloth to hold below the nose to catch the blood with one hand, and he or she should apply pressure to the bridge of the nose with the thumb and forefinger of the other hand, while the nurse prepares the equipment. A drape or towel should be placed around the client's neck and shoulders. The nurse should prepare and instrument tray, which includes nasal speculum, hands free light, flash light, nasal packing material, nasal instruments, tongue blades, suction apparatus, sterile saline, lubricant, and medications as requested by the physician. The nurse should explain the procedure to the client, instructing him or her to keep the hands down during the procedure and breathe through the mouth. The patient may feel discomfort while the nose is being packed such as a feeling of congestion or pressure. If he or she has to sneeze, the patient should warn the staff and to sneeze with the mouth open. Medical personnel should wear gowns, gloves, masks and goggles during the insertion of nasal packing because of the potential for blood spraying if the client sneezes.

Aftercare

The patient should be placed in a semi-reclining position with the head elevated at least 30 degrees and should be allowed to rest. Old blood on the face, neck, and hands should be cleaned away with a warm wet wash cloth, and the soiled linens discarded in a contaminated linen bag. Instruments should be handled according to the contaminated instrument policy of the medical setting. Soiled gowns, gloves, gauze 4x4's, and disposable equipment should be placed in a trash bag that can be sealed and discarded. The nurse should wash the hands again.

The staff should check the nasal drip pad and the oropharynx for bleeding every 15-30 minutes, and notify the physician if the patient drains through four drip pads in an hour or if frank bleeding is observed in the oropharynx. Mouth breathing will cause the patient to have a dry mouth. The patient should be offered ice chips or mouthwash to moisten the mouth. The use of a room humidifier will also help keep the mouth moist. The patient should sneeze with their mouth open to avoid increased pressure in the nose. He or she should not "snuff" drainage in their throat, but spit secretions out into a basin or the sink rather than swallow them. The patient should have tissues on hand for secretions and/or sneezing, and be monitored for respiratory distress, especially for the first hour after packing and during sleep. The patient should know that **analgesics** can be given if they experience a headache after the procedure. The nurse should monitor the patient for nausea or vomiting of old or fresh blood and warn the client to avoid spicy food and smoking while the packing is in place. The patient may

KEY TERMS

Asphyxiation—Smothering. A severe decrease in oxygen concentration in the body, leading to death.

Cautery—Intentional destruction of tissue cells to remove abnormal tissue or form a scar to stop bleeding. Cautery is performed with chemical agents, laser instruments or electrical instruments that burn the tissue.

Oropharynx—An area of the throat visible through the open mouth located between the epiglottis and the soft palate.

Pledget—A small compressed cotton pad that is flat and absorbent.

Turbinate—Ridge-shaped cartilage or soft bony tissue inside the nose.

Ulcer—A sore on the skin or mucous tissue that produces pus and in which tissue is destroyed.

smell a foul odor as the nasal pack ages over the next 48 hours. He or she may also develop bruising or swelling of the eyelids secondary to nasal packing. The patient should not pick at the packing or rub the nose while the packing is in place.

Complications

Because of the complications of using nasal packing, physicians will attempt other methods to control nasal bleeding, such as external pressure, cold packs, cautery or **topical medicine application** before the use of nasal packing. The most common complication of nasal packing is that the removal of the packing dislodges healing tissue and causes the nose to bleed again. Nasal packing can cause a lack of oxygen in those who have difficulty breathing through their mouths such as elderly clients or those with chronic obstructive pulmonary disease (COPD). Nasal packing can lead to a drop in the blood oxygen content and an increase in blood carbon dioxide levels (CO_2). This, in turn, can cause respiratory and cardiac complications, including a racing pulse. Airway obstruction and asphyxiation can occur if the nasal packing slips back into the airway, particularly during sleep. Complications may occur if a pack compresses the Eustachian tube, causing ear problems. Infections can develop in the nose, sinus or middle ear after nasal packing insertion. These infections are not common but can lead to **septic shock**.

Results

Nasal packing is usually an effective method to stop nasal bleeding. In cases of nasal surgery, packing is frequently removed within 24-48 hours following surgery. In the case of nosebleeds, packing may be left in for extended periods of time to promote healing and to prevent the patient from removing scar tissue which might reopen the wound.

Health care team roles

Nasal packing is inserted by a physician. A licensed nurse will routinely assess a client with nasal packing for signs of bleeding, respiratory distress or **infection** while they are in the health care setting. Nasal packing is usually removed by the physician but may be removed by a licensed nurse as ordered by the physician. Clients and care providers can be instructed in the care of a client with nasal packing in the home setting but the client must return to the health care setting for removal of the nasal packing.

Resources

BOOKS

Bluestone, C. D., S. E. Stool, and M. A. Kenna. *Pediatric Otolaryngology.* Philadelphia: W.B. Saunders Company, 1996.

Cohen, M., and R.M. Goldwyn. *Mastery of Plastic and Reconstructive Surgery.* Boston: Little, Brown and Company, 1994.

Schuller, D.E., and A.J. Schleuning II. *DeWeese and Saunder's Otolaryngology-Head and Neck Surgery.* St. Louis: Mosby, 1994.

OTHER

Graber, Mark, M.D. and Beaty, Laura, M.D. "Otolaryngology: Nose." *University of Iowa Family Practice Handbook. Virtual Hospital Online,* July 1999. <http://www.vh.org/Providers/ClinRef/FPHandbook/Chapter19/03-19.html>.

Moses, Scott, M.D. "Epistaxsis." *Family Practice Notebook Online,* March 2001. <http://www.fpnotebook.com/ENT109.htm>.

PACU A/P Septoplasty Protocol. Department of Nursing. *UNC Hospitals Online,* May 2000. <http://www.med.unc.edu/nursing/manuals/protocol/SEPTOPLA.pdf>.

Shippert, Ron, M.D. "The History of Nasal Packing." *Shippert Library Online,* November 2000. <http://www.shippertmedical.com/>.

Mary Elizabeth Martelli, R.N., B.S.

Nasogastric intubation and feeding

Definition

Nasogastric intubation refers to the process of placing a soft plastic nasogastric (NG) tube through a patient's nostril, past the pharynx and down the esophagus into a patient's **stomach**.

Purpose

Nasogastric tubes are inserted to deliver substances directly into the stomach, remove substances from the stomach or as a means of testing stomach function or contents.

The most common purpose for inserting a nasogastric tube is to deliver tube feedings to a patient when they are unable to eat. Patients who may need a NG tube for feedings include: premature babies, patients in a **coma**, patients who have had neck or facial surgery or patients on mechanical ventilation. Other substances that are delivered through a NG tube may include ice water to stop bleeding in the stomach or medications to neutralize swallowed poisons.

Another purpose for inserting a nasogastric tube is to remove substances from the stomach. A NG tube is used to empty the stomach when accidental **poisoning** or drug **overdose** has occurred. A NG tube is used to remove air that accumulates in the stomach during **cardiopulmonary resuscitation (CPR)**. It is used to remove stomach contents after major trauma or surgery to prevent aspiration of the stomach contents. Placing a NG helps prevent nausea and vomiting by removing stomach contents and preventing distention of the stomach when a patient has a bleeding ulcer, bowel obstruction or other gastrointestinal diseases.

A NG tube may be inserted to take samples of stomach contents for laboratory studies and to test for pressure or motor activity of the gastrointestinal tract.

Precautions

Do not use force when inserting a NG tube. If resistance occurs, rotate and retract the tube slightly and try again. Forcing the tube can cause traumatic injury to the tissue of the nose, throat or esophagus.

Always check the tube positioning before giving feedings. If the tube is out of place the patient may aspirate the feeding solution into the **lungs**.

Keep the patient in an upright or semi-upright sitting position when delivering a tube feeding to enhance peristalsis and avoid regurgitation of the feeding.

Check patients who are receiving continuous feedings via a pump or gravity hourly or according to the medical settings policy, to assure that the tube is in position, the formula is flowing at the correct rate and the patient is comfortable with no signs of distention or distress.

Cap or clamp off the NG tube when not in use to prevent backflow of stomach contents or accumulation of air in the stomach.

If a patient has severe sinus conditions, nasal obstruction or has had facial surgery, it may be necessary to place a oral-gastric tube to avoid further nasal trauma.

If the amount of gastric aspirate is large prior to a bolus or intermittent feeding, notify the physician and follow the protocol of the medical setting for re-instilling the gastric aspirate. The feeding size may need to be decreased if the patient is not digesting it.

NG tube placement is meant to be a short-term solution for feeding problems. Patients that require long term tube feeding should have surgical placement of a gastrostomy tube or gastrostomy button. Long-term NG tube usage can cause nasal erosion, sinusitis, esophagitis, gastric ulceration, esophageal-tracheal fistula formation, oral infections and respiratory infections.

Description

To insert a nasogastric tube, have the patient tilt his head slightly back and gently ease the lubricated tubing into the nares. As the tube rounds the bend into the throat, have the patient tilt his head forward into a neutral upright position, hold his breath and swallow. Gently rotate the tubing 180 degrees to redirect the curve of the tube. Ease the tubing down the throat past the closed epiglottis. Gravity and swallowing will help move the tube down the esophagus as you gently continue to advance the tube. The patient can assist by swallowing and can even take sips of water to help move the tubing down into the stomach. Advance the tubing until you reach the marker tape that you applied when measuring the distance to the patient's stomach. Secure the tubing with tape and check the tubing for placement. If the patient gags during the procedure, stop advancing the tube and allow the patient to rest. If the tubing comes out of the mouth, retract the tubing and try again. If the patient is unconscious, advance the tube between respirations to avoid placing the tube into the trachea. If the patient becomes cyanotic, coughs or displays any signs of respiratory distress, remove the tubing, allow the patient to rest and begin again.

Once the NG tube is inserted, there are several methods for checking tube placement. Ask the patient to talk. If the patient cannot make sound, the tube has passed through the vocal cords and into the trachea. Remove the tube and start again. If the patient can talk, use a flashlight to look into the patient's mouth to view the tubing. It should appear straight in the back of the throat with no coiling into the mouth. Next, connect a 30 or 60cc catheter tip syringe to the end of the NG tube and aspirate to see if stomach contents return into the tubing. Stomach aspirate is often clear or yellow appearing but this depends upon what is in the patient's stomach. Stomach aspirate has a pH of 1-4 and an effective way to establish that the tube is in the stomach is to check the pH of the aspirate. Methods for checking tube placement, however, vary according to the medical setting. Follow the medical setting policy for checking tube placement. Another, more traditional method for checking tube placement is to draw 10-20 cc of air into the syringe, place the **stethoscope** over the patient's stomach and quickly inject the bolus of air into the stomach. A whooshing sound should be audible through the stethoscope over the stomach if the tube is in the stomach. If the tube is in the esophagus or trachea, the air sounds will be absent or muffled. The most accurate way to check for tube placement is an x ray of the abdomen. The NG tube is radiographic and will show up clearly on the x ray. A **chest x ray** is rarely done for NG tube placement because of the cost, but if performed for other purposes the radiologist will usually note the positioning of the NG tube on the report.

Preparation

Position the patient in bed with the head of the bed elevated 45-90 degrees and place a towel across the chest up to the patient's neck. Explain the nasal intubation procedure to the patient. Let them know that by holding their breath as the tube is passed through the pharynx, they will close off the airway and that if they swallow when instructed, it will help move the tubing down the esophagus into the stomach. Have the patient blow their nose to clear out the nasal passages and remove dentures if they have them. Question the patient about whether they have had sinus problems, nasal problems such as nosebleeds or nasal surgery in the past. Consult with the physician if the patient has a history of nasal problems. Select a nostril to use for intubation. Assemble the equipment needed, including a nasogastric tube, flash light, emesis basin, tissues, 30cc-60cc catheter tip syringe and irrigation set, a glass of water, water-soluble lubricant, clear plastic tape, a transparent dressing, stethoscope and gloves. Obtain a suction apparatus and connection tubing if the NG tube is to be used for suctioning the stomach.

Prepare a piece of 1-inch tape that is cut horizontally half way through the piece of tape to make two tails. The uncut end will be placed along the patient's nose and the tails wrapped around the tube in opposite directions to secure the tube to the nose after insertion. Develop a hand signal with the patient so that they can ask to stop the procedure to let them rest if they are in distress during the procedure.

NG tubes are available in a variety of types, lengths and sizes. Large-bore tubes (some with a second lumen) are used for suctioning stomach contents. Small-bore tubing is used for feedings. Select the tube appropriate to the patient's size and the purpose for which the tube is being inserted. Wash the hands and put on gloves. Remove the tube from the packaging and uncoil it. Examine the tubing for flaws. Run some water through the tubing to check for leaks. To find the distance to the patient's stomach, use the tube to measure from the tip of the patient's nose back to the ear and then down to the tip of the sternum. Mark this place on the tube using a small piece of tape. Moisten the tip and first few inches of the tubing with water-soluble lubricant and lay it back into the packaging.

Aftercare

After correct positioning of the NG tube has been established, secure the NG tube to the nose with a second piece of plastic tape or use a transparent dressing to hold the tubing to the nose. The intent is to secure the tube so that it will not slip in or out, the method of securing the tube may vary according to the size of the patient, their type of skin and the amount of perspiration on the nose. Securing the other end of the NG tube to the patient's gown with a looped rubber band and safety pin can prevent accidental pulling on the NG tube as the patient moves around. The end of the NG tube should be plugged or clamped when not connected to suction or in use for feedings. Ongoing care of the patient with a NG tube includes encouraging good mouth care and cleansing the nares routinely. Change the tape position daily and examine the tissue around the nose and under the tape for signs of irritation or breakdown. Keep the head of the bed elevated 30 degrees at all times to decrease gastric reflux. Place the head of the bed 30-45 degrees during tube feedings and for 30-60 minutes after intermittent tube feedings if the patient can tolerate this position.

When a NG tube is used to administer tube feedings, they may be given by gravity or by pump. Tube feedings may also be given either intermittently or continuously. The physician will calculate the patient's nutritional needs within a 24-hour period and order the solution, frequency and rate of flow. Tube feedings are supplemented liquid **nutrition** and may be prepared by the dietary department in a medical setting or provided in prepared cans of formula (such as Ensure) that are manufactured for this purpose. There are a large number of formulas to select from according to the patient's nutritional needs. Be certain that the formula used for tube feeding exactly matches the physician's orders.

Intermittent tube feedings may be given using a large catheter tip syringe or a feeding bag. Check the position of the NG tube according to the policy of the medical center. Aspirate the stomach contents for residual formula from the last feeding. If the residual exceeds 100 cc for an adult, hold the feeding and notify the physician. Re-instill the gastric aspirate according to the policy of the medical center or the physician's order. Review the physician's order and select the appropriate type and amount of feeding. Be sure that the patient remains in an upright position during the feeding. Shake prepared formulas before administering them. Formulas that have been refrigerated should be allowed to warm up to room temperature before administering them. To give the feeding using a syringe, remove the barrel from the syringe. Open the end of the NG tube and connect it to the end of the syringe. Pour the feeding into the wide end of the syringe and hold or secure the syringe to the bed or an IV pole just above the patient's head so that it will flow in slowly by gravity over 15-30 minutes. If more feeding is needed than can be held in the syringe, watch the syringe and refill the syringe until the feeding is complete. When the feeding is complete, rinse the tube with 30 cc of water. Disconnect and recap the end of the NG tube and rinse the syringe according to the medical setting's policy. To give an intermittent feeding using a feeding bag, pour the correct feeding amount into the bag and through the tubing connected to the bag down to the tip of the tubing. Clamp the tubing using the roller clamp apparatus. Hang the bag on an IV pole just above the patient's head. Open the NG tube and connect it to the feeding bag tubing. Open the feeding bag roller clamp apparatus and adjust the flow rate to run the feeding in over the prescribed amount of time (usually 15-30 minutes). When the feeding is complete, purge the line by putting 30 cc of water into the bag and allowing it to flow in wide open. Clamp and disconnect the feeding bag tubing. Recap the NG tube. Rinse and reuse the feeding bag according to the medical center's policy. Feeding bags and syringes are usually replaced every 24 hours to prevent bacterial contamination.

Continuous tube feedings are given using a feeding bag with connected tubing and an automatic food pump to deliver the feeding at a specific rate of flow. Patients receiving continuous tube feedings should be kept in an upright position of 30-45 degrees to prevent reflux of for-

mula. The feeding bag is filled with formula solution for no more than four hours and the pump is set at the flow rate that the physician has ordered. Check the NG tube for correct placement every four hours and aspirate the NG tube to check for formula residual. If the residual is 1.5 times greater than the amount administered each hour, notify the physician. Re-instill the residual by gravity using a syringe and flush the line with 30-60 cc of water. Refill the formula bag for the next four hours. Observe the patient hourly to be sure that the patient is in no distress, the patient's abdomen is not distended, the formula is flowing at the correct rate and that the tubing connections are secure. Refill the bag as necessary or every four hours. The feeding bag and tubing should be changed according to the medical setting's policy, usually every 24 hours to prevent bacterial contamination.

Complications

The complications of nasogastric intubation may include:

- aspiration of the stomach contents leading to asphyxia, **abscess** formation or aspiration pneumonia;

- trauma injury including perforation of the nasal, pharyngeal, esophageal or gastric tissue

- pulmonary hemorrhage, empyema, pneumothorax, pleural effusion or pneumonitis from a malpositioned tube

- nosebleeds

- secondary **infection** in the sinus, throat, esophagus or stomach

- development of a tracheal-esophageal fistula

- erosion and/or necrosis of nasal, pharyngeal, esophageal or gastric tissue

The complications of nasogastric tube feedings may include:

- obstruction of the tube

- perforation of the tube

- tube migration out of correct position

- regurgitation and aspiration of the feeding

- diarrhea

- nausea and vomiting

- abdominal distention, cramping and discomfort from too much feeding or a rate of feeding that is too rapid

- any of the complications listed above in the complications of nasogastric intubation

KEY TERMS

Empyema—A collection of pus in the lung cavity.

Fistula—A passageway or connecting duct that is abnormal and connects body cavities or tissues that should not be connected. Fistulas develop as the result of injury, disease or congenital deformity.

Gastrostomy button—A soft plastic apparatus with a button closure that is surgically inserted and sutured onto the surface of the abdomen. The gastrostomy button is placed in a surgical opening that leads from the stomach to the surface of the abdomen and is used for long term tube feedings in patients who cannot eat to prevent malnutrition.

Gastrostomy tube—A soft plastic tube that is inserted and sutured into a surgical opening that leads from the stomach to the surface of the abdomen. A gastrostomy tube is used for long term tube feedings in patients who cannot eat to prevent malnutrition.

Peristalsis—Muscular contractions of the gastrointestinal tract that move food, fluids and refuse in a wave-like motion through the system.

Reflux—A backward flow of food or fluid from the stomach into the esophagus.

Regurgitation—A vigorous reversed flow of the stomach contents up the esophagus and out of the mouth.

Results

The use of a nasogastric tube for feedings can effectively prevent malnutrition in the patient who is unable to eat. A nasogastric tube is also an effective temporary measure for decompression and removal of stomach contents and free air in a variety of gastrointestinal illnesses, major trauma, or surgery.

Health care team roles

Nasogastric intubation is usually performed by a licensed nurse or physician in the medical setting. Paramedics or other emergency personnel may receive special training to insert NG tubes as appropriate in the field. Patients' families may be trained to insert or change nasogastric tubes in the home setting if a patient is discharged with a NG tube in place. It is unusual, however, to continue NG tube feedings in the home setting. Most patients who require long-term tube feedings will have a gastrostomy tube or gastrostomy button placed for feedings.

Tube feedings are usually administered by a licensed nurse in the medical setting. Non-licensed personnel may receive special training to start, stop or check tube feedings under the direction of a licensed nurse in some medical settings. Patients and patients' families may be taught by a licensed nurse to administer tube feedings in the home. Patients receiving tube feedings in the home should be monitored by visiting nurses or undergo frequent medical check-ups to assess the their responses to the feedings and the their ongoing nutritional needs.

Resources

OTHER

Elliott, Noel R.N., B.S.N., C.R.N.A. "Care of the Patient Requiring a Nasogastric Tube." *Nursewise Online*, 1998. <http://www.nursewise.com/courses/ng_hour.htm>.

"Enteral Feeding." Chapter 20. Nutritional Problems. In *Lippincott Manual of Nursing Practice*. Books at Ovid Online. 2001. <http://pco.ovid.com/lrppco/>.

"Enteral Nutrition." *Adult Guidelines for Parenteral and Enteral Nutrition*. University of California Davis Online. February 1998. <http://wellness.ucdavis.edu/diet_exercise/nutrition/parenteral_and_enteral_nut/>.

Hendrickson, Gail R.N., B.S. "Stomach Tube Insertion." *Health Answers.com*, May 2000. <http://www.healthanswers.com>.

Knies, Robert C. R.N., M.S.N., C.E.N. "Confirming Safe Placement of Nasogastric Tubes." *Emergency Nursing World Online*, 2001. <http://www.enw.org/Research-NGT.htm>.

"Nasal Gastric Bolus Feeding." *Patient Education Program*. Children's Hospital Medical Center Cincinnati Online. August 1998. <http://www.cincinnatichildrens.org/family/pep/homecare/2110/>.

"Nasogastric Feeding Tube Insertion." *Patient Education Program*. Children's Hospital Medical Center Cincinnati Online. August 1998. <http://www.cincinnatichildrens.org/family/pep/homecare/2010/>.

"Tube Feeding with Gravity Feeding Set." *Patient Education Program*. Children's Hospital Medical Center Cincinnati Online. September 1998. <http://www.cincinnatichildrens.org/family/pep/homecare/2006>.

Mary Elizabeth Martelli, R.N., B.S.

Nasopharyngeal culture

Definition

A nasopharyngeal culture is a microbiology test used to identify pathogenic organisms present in the nasal cavity that may be the cause of an upper respiratory tract illness or may be transmitted by carriers to persons susceptible to **infection**.

Purpose

Some of the organisms responsible for upper respiratory infections are carried primarily in the nasopharynx. Nasopharyngeal cultures are performed to isolate these organisms. These include **viruses** such as **influenza**, parainfluenza, and respiratory syncytial virus, which are the most common causes of respiratory infection in young children, and pathogenic **bacteria** such as *Bordetella pertusis* and *Corynebacterium diphtheriae,* which are infrequent causes of infections in the United States. In addition, nasopharyngeal cultures are used to identify carriers of *Staphylococcus aureus, Streptococcus pneumoniae,* and *Neisseria meningitidis.* These organisms usually do not cause disease in the nasopharynx or throat. However, asymptomatic carriers may transmit these organisms via nasal secretions to others that will develop serious infections. *Staphylococcus aureus* and *Streptococcus pneumoniae* can cause **pneumonia** and septicemia and *N. meningitidis* can cause outbreaks of **meningitis**.

Bacteria that cause pharyngeal infection (**sore throat**) such as *Haemophilus influenzae, Streptococcus pyogenes* (group A streptococcus), *Candida albicans,* and *Mycoplasma pneumoniae* may also be isolated from the nasopharynx. The procedure can also be used as a substitute for a **throat culture** in infants, the elderly patient, the debilitated patient, or in cases where a throat culture is difficult to obtain.

Precautions

For best results, the specimen should be obtained prior to initiating any therapy. The health care worker obtaining the specimen should wear gloves to prevent spreading infectious organisms.

Description

Collection and transport

A sample is obtained from the nasopharynx by means of a swab, aspirate, or wash. Swabbing is most commonly used for collection. A **calcium** algenate (wool) or polyester swab on a flexible wire is most commonly used. The nose is cleared of mucus and the swab is inserted into the nasal cavity and moved forward along the septum until it reaches the rear of the pharynx. The swab is rotated several times and then removed. For viral culture, the swab should be transported in a small amount of veal infusion or sucrose-phosphate broth. For bacterial culture, the swab should be placed in Stuart's or Amie's transport medium. If pertussis is suspected, the swab should be placed directly onto Regan-Lowe media before transporting to the lab. Aspirates are collected by placing a thin flexible catheter or plastic tube onto the end of a 10 mL syringe and applying suction. Washings are collected by irrigating the nasal cavity with 7-10 mL of sterile phosphate buffered saline using a suction bulb and then aspirating the fluid.

VIRUSES. Nasopharyngeal swabs are most often used to collect samples from neonates or young children who have an upper respiratory infection. Most respiratory infections in young children are caused by viruses. Cultures are not routinely ordered for influenza, parainfluenza, or respiratory syncytial virus. Influenza and parainfluenza are cultured in primary monkey kidney cells or chick egg embryos. RSV is most often cultured in HEp2 cells (malignant human epithelioma cells). Since viral cultures can take up to seven to 12 days, tests for viral antigens using fluorescent or enzyme immunoassay are performed frequently.

BACTERIA. Bacterial culture and **Gram stain** are performed routinely for nasopharyngeal specimens. Gram stain is helpful in suggesting the presence of *Candida albicans* (gram-positive budding yeast), *Corynebacterium diphtheriae* (small gram-positive rods arranged like Chinese letters), and *Neisseria meningitidis* (small gram-negative diplococci).

The Gram stain is performed by:

- Transferring a small portion of the specimen to the center of a glass slide, which is then heat-fixed and cooled before staining.

- Placing a few drops of crystal violet on the slide and allowing it to set for 30-60 seconds.

- Rinsing off the crystal violet, gently, with water.

- Applying a few drops of Gram's iodine on the slide and allowing it to set for 60 seconds.

- Rinsing off the iodine, gently, with water.

- Decolorizing by rinsing with 95% ethanol, drop by drop, until the alcohol rinses clear.

- Placing a few drops of safranin on the slide and allowing it to set for 30 seconds.

- Rinsing off the safranin, gently, with water.

Antibiotic—A drug given to stop the growth of bacteria. Antibiotics are ineffective against viruses.

Bacilli—Rod-shaped bacterium.

Cocci—Spherical shape bacterium.

Nasopharynx—The back wall of the nasal cavity where it meets the throat.

- Blotting excess water with bibulous paper.
- Allowing the slide to air dry.
- Observing the slide under oil immersion.

Gram-positive cells retain the crystal violet and appear dark purple, while gram-negative cells do not retain the crystal violet. They are stained with the safranin and appear red.

Specimens should be plated on sheep blood agar, which supports the growth of most of the pathogenic bacteria encountered in nasopharyngeal specimens except *Chlamydia, Haemophilus*, and *Mycoplasma*; chocolate (heated blood) agar for *Haemophilus*; and a selective medium for gram-positive cocci such as colistin-nalidixic acid (CNA). If *Corynebacterium diphtheriae* is suspected, the specimen should be plated on Loeffler or Tinsdale agar, which permit faster growth than blood agar. If *Bordetella pertussis* is suspected the specimen should be plated on Regan-Lowe (charcoal-horse blood agar) or Bordet-Gengou agar. Cultures should be incubated at 35°C in air at high humidity. Plates should be examined for growth each day and suspect colonies Gram stained and subcultured (that is, transferred to an appropriate medium). If *C. diphtheriae* or *B. pertussis* is suspected, plates should be held for six to seven days. Otherwise, plates showing no growth of suspected pathogens may be discarded after 48 hours. Preliminary identification of the organism can be made from catalase, coagulase, urease, nitrate reduction, sucrose fermentation, and characteristic colonial morphology.

Antibiotic susceptibility testing is performed by the Kirby-Bauer or broth microdilution method for *Haemophilus, Neisseria, Streptococcus pneumoniae,* or *Staphylococcus aureus*. **Antibiotics** usually included are ampicillin, chloramphenicol, cephalosporins, meropenem, oxacillin, vancomycin, and trimethoprim-sulfamethoxazole. Antibiotic susceptiblity is not performed for *C. diphtheriae, B. pertussis,* or *M. pneumoniae* because they are susceptible to erythromycin, and are difficult to grow in

MIC broth for susceptibility testing. *Streptococcus* is susceptible to penicillin.

Alternative procedures

In most cases of upper respiratory tract infections, a throat culture is more appropriate than a nasopharyngeal culture. However, the nasopharyngeal culture should be used in cases where throat cultures are difficult to obtain or to detect the carrier states especially meningococcal disease.

Preparation

The patient should clear their nose of excess secretions prior to sample procurement. To prevent contamination, the swab should not touch the patient's tongue or side of the nostrils.

Aftercare

None.

Complications

There is little to no risk of complications involved in a nasopharyngeal culture.

Results

Preliminary results may be reported in one or two days followed by confirmation which usually takes additional time depending upon the organisms isolated. Bacteria that normally grow in the nasal cavity will be identified by a nasopharyngeal culture. These include nonhemolytic streptococci, alpha-hemolytic streptococci, some *Neisseria* species, diphtheroids, and some types of staphylococci.

Pathogenic organisms that might be identified by this culture include:

- group A beta-hemolytic streptococci
- *Bordetella pertussis*, the causative agent of whooping cough
- *Corynebacterium diptheriae*, the causative agent of diptheria
- *Neisseria gonorrhoeae*, the causative agent of gonorrhea which may be isolated from persons who have engaged in oral sex
- *Chlamydia trachomatis*, the causative agent of pelvic inflammatory disease and urethritis which may cause a nasopharyngeal infection in the neonate from transmission in the womb

In addition, some bacteria normally present in the nasal cavity may be the cause of infection or disease when they are present in large amounts. These include:

- *Haemophilus influenzae*, a causative agent of bronchitis, inner ear infection, and meningitis

- *Streptococci pneumoniae*, a causative agent of pneumonia

- *Candida albicans*, the causative agent of thrush

Asymptomatic carriers may contain the following organisms in the nasopharynx:

- *Neisseria meningitidis*, a causative agent of meningitis

- *Streptococci pneumoniae*, a causative agent of pneumonia

- *Staphylococcus aureus*, the causative agent of many Staph infections

Health care team roles

A physician orders a nasopharyngeal culture. A physician, physician assistant, or nurse collects the specimen. A clinical laboratory scientist/medical technologist who specializes in microbiology performs the culture and antibiotic sensitivity test when required. The physician determines the appropriate antimicrobial treatment.

Resources

BOOKS

Byrne, J., Saxton, D. F., Pelikan, P. K., and Nugent, P. M. *Laboratory Tests, Implication for Nursing Care.* 2nd ed. Menlo Park, CA: Addison-Wesley Publishing Company.

Chernecky, Cynthia C, and Berger, Barbara J. *Laboratory Tests and Diagnostic Procedures.* 3rd ed. Philadelphia, PA: W. B. Saunders Company, 2001.

Loeb, S., ed. *Illustrated Guide to Diagnostic Tests.* Springhouse, PA: Springhouse Corporation, 1994.

ORGANIZATIONS

The American Medical Association, Kids Health. <http:www.ama-assn.org/KidsHealth>.

National Center for Infectious Disease, Centers for Disease Control and Prevention. 1600 Clifton Rd., NE, Atlanta GA 30333. <http://www.cdc.gov> and <http://www.cdc.gov/ncidod/diseases>.

Victoria E. DeMoranville

NCV *see* **Electromyography**
Nearsightedness *see* **Myopia**

Near-drowning

Definition

Near-drowning is the term used for survival after suffocation caused by submersion in water or other fluid or liquid.

Description

An estimated 15,000–70,000 near-drownings occur in the United States each year; insufficient reporting prevents a more precise estimate. A typical person experiencing near-drowning is young and male. Nearly half of all drownings and near-drownings involve children less than four years old. Because home swimming pools are the sites for 60–90% of drownings in the 0–4 age group, they pose the greatest risk for children. Teenage boys are also at heightened risk for drowning and near-drowning; drugs and alcohol are implicated in 40–50% of teenage drownings. Overall, roughly four out of five drowning victims are males.

Causes and symptoms

On many occasions, near-drownings are secondary to an event such as a heart attack that causes unconsciousness or a head or spinal injury that prevents a diver from resurfacing. Near-drownings, moreover, can occur in shallow as well as deep water. Small children have drowned or almost drowned in bathtubs, toilets, industrial-size cleaning buckets, and washing machines. Bathtubs are especially dangerous for infants between six months and one year of age, who can sit up straight in a bathtub but may lack the ability to pull themselves out of the water if they slip under the surface.

A reduced concentration of oxygen in the **blood** (hypoxemia) is common to all near-drownings. When drowning begins, the larynx (air passage) closes involuntarily, preventing both air and water from entering the **lungs**. In 10–15% of cases, hypoxemia results because the larynx stays closed; this is called dry drowning. Hypoxemia also occurs in wet drownings, the 85–90% of cases where the larynx relaxes and water enters the lungs. Only a small amount of either freshwater or saltwater is needed to damage the lungs and interfere with the body's oxygen intake. Within three minutes of submersion, most people are unconscious. Within five minutes, the **brain** begins to suffer from lack of oxygen. Abnormal **heart** rhythms (cardiac dysrhythmias) often occur in near-drowning cases, and the heart may stop pumping (cardiac arrest). An increase in blood acidity (acidosis) is another consequence of near-drowning and, under some circum-

KEY TERMS

Acidosis—An increase in acid content of the blood manifested by a decrease in blood pH below 7.40.

Cardiac arrest—Cessation of heartbeats.

Cardiac dysrhythmias—Abnormal heart rhythms.

Cyanosis—A blue color of the skin caused by inadequate oxygen in the blood.

Dry drowning—Hypoxemia due to closure of the larynx.

Endotracheal intubation—Inserting a tube in the trachea to maintain an open airway.

Hypothermia—A decrease in the internal temperature of the body to a core temperature below 96°F (35.6°C).

Hypoxemia—A reduced concentration of oxygen in the blood.

Tachycardia—Rapid heart rate.

Tachypnea—Rapid breathing.

Trachea—Windpipe.

Wet drowning—Water entering the lungs due to relaxation of the larynx.

stances, near-drowning can cause a substantial increase or decrease in the volume of circulating blood. Many individuals experience a severe drop in body temperature (hypothermia).

The signs and symptoms of near-drowning can differ widely from person to person. Some people are alert but agitated, while others are comatose. Breathing may have stopped in one person, while another may be gasping for breath. Bluish skin (**cyanosis**), coughing, and frothy pink sputum (material expelled from the respiratory tract by coughing) are often observed. Rapid breathing (tachypnea), a rapid heart rate (tachycardia), and a low-grade **fever** are common during the first few hours after rescue. People who have experienced near-drowning but remain conscious may appear confused, lethargic, or irritable.

Diagnosis

Diagnosis relies on a **physical examination** and on a wide range of tests and other procedures. Blood is taken to measure oxygen levels. Pulseoximetry is another way of assessing oxygen levels. An electrocardiograph is used to monitor heart activity. X rays, computed tomography (CT) scans, or **magnetic resonance imaging** (MRI) scans can detect head and neck injuries and excess tissue fluid (**edema**) in the lungs.

Treatment

Treatment begins with removing the victim from the water and performing **cardiopulmonary resuscitation** (**CPR**). One purpose of CPR is to bring oxygen to the lungs, heart, brain, and other organs by breathing into a person's mouth. When someone's heart has stopped, CPR also attempts to get the heart pumping again by pressing down on the chest. After CPR has been performed and emergency medical help has arrived on the scene, oxygen is administered. If the person's breathing has stopped or is otherwise impaired, a tube is inserted into the windpipe (trachea) to maintain the airway (endotracheal intubation). The person is also checked for head, neck, and other injuries, and intravenous fluids are given. Hypothermia cases require careful handling to protect the heart.

In the emergency department, victims who have experienced near-drowning continue receiving oxygen until blood tests show a return to normal. About one-third of the patients are intubated and initially need mechanical support to breathe. Re-warming is undertaken when hypothermia is present. People may arrive requiring treatment for cardiac arrest or cardiac dysrhythmias. Comatose patients present a special problem. Although various treatment approaches have been tried, none have proved beneficial. Many of these patients die.

People can be discharged from the emergency department after four to six hours if their blood oxygen level is normal, and no signs or symptoms of near-drowning are present. Because lung problems can arise 12 or more hours after submersion, the medical staff must emphasize that the individuals must seek further medical help, if necessary. Admission to a hospital for at least 24 hours for further observation and treatment is a must for people who do not appear to recover fully in the emergency department.

Prognosis

Neurological damage is the major long-term concern in the treatment of people experiencing near-drowning. Those who arrive at an emergency department awake and alert usually survive with brain function intact, as do about 90% of those who arrive mentally impaired (lethargic or confused) but not comatose. Death or permanent neurological damage is very likely when individuals arrive in a comatose condition. Early rescue of people experiencing near-drowning (within five minutes of submersion) and prompt application of CPR (within less than 10 minutes of submersion) seem to be the best predictors of a complete recovery.

Health care team roles

First aid can be administered by anyone with proper training. This may include CPR. Paramedics may provide support during transport to a hospital. Physicians commonly evaluate and provide treatment in an emergency department. Nurses provide emergency and supportive care. Therapists may be called upon to provide follow-up counseling.

Prevention

Prevention depends on educating parents, other adults, and teenagers about water safety.

Parents must realize that young children who are left in or near water without adult supervision, even for a short time, can easily get into trouble. Experts consider putting up a fence around a home swimming pool an essential precaution, and estimate that 50–90% of child drownings and near-drownings could be prevented if fences were widely adopted. The fence should be at least five feet (1.5 m) high, have a self-closing and self-locking gate, and completely surround the pool.

Pool owners and all other adults should consider learning CPR. Everyone should follow the rules for safe swimming and boating. Those who have a medical condition that can cause a seizure or otherwise threaten safety in the water are advised always to swim with a partner. People need to be aware that alcohol and drug use substantially increase the chances of an accident.

Resources

BOOKS

Dix, Jay. *Asphyxia and Drowning: An Atlas*. Boca Raton, FL: CRC Press, 2000.

Fletemeyer, John A., and Samuel J. Freas. *Drowning: New Perspectives on Intervention and Prevention*. Boca Raton, FL: CRC Press, 1999.

Kallas, Harry J. "Drowning and Near Drowning." In *Nelson Textbook of Pediatrics, 16th ed.*, edited by Richard E. Behrman et al. Philadelphia: W. B. Saunders, 2000, 279-87.

Modell, Jerome H. "Drowning and Near Drowning." In *Harrison's Principles of Internal Medicine, 14th ed.*, edited by Anthony S. Fauci et al. New York: McGraw-Hill, 1998, 2555-56.

Piantadosi, Claude A. "Physical, Chemical, and Aspiration Injuries of the Lung." In *Cecil Textbook of Medicine, 21st ed.*, edited by Lee Goldman and J. Claude Bennett. Philadelphia: W. B. Saunders, 2000, 425-33.

PERIODICALS

Blum, C., and J. Shield. "Toddler Drowning in Domestic Swimming Pools." *Injury Prevention* 6 no. 4 (2000): 288-90.

Frison, Y. M. "Pediatric Near-Drownings." *Nursing Spectrum* 8 no. 16 (1998): 11, 24, 1998.

Gheen, K. M. "Near-Drowning and Cold Water Submersion." *Seminars in Pediatric Surgery* 10 no. 1 (2001): 26-7.

Giesbrecht, G. G. "Cold Stress, Near Drowning and Accidental Hypothermia: A Review." *Aviation, Space and Environmental Medicine* 71 no. 7 (2000): 733-52.

Zuckerman, G. B, and E. E. Conway. "Drowning and Near Drowning: A Pediatric Epidemic." *Pediatric Annuals* 29 no. 6 (2000): 360-66.

ORGANIZATIONS

American College of Emergency Physicians. P.O. Box 619911, Dallas, TX 75261-9911. (800) 798-1822. (972) 550-0911. (972) 580-2816. <http://www.acep.org/>. info@acep.org.

American College of Osteopathic Emergency Physicians. 142 E. Ontario Street, Suite 550, Chicago, IL 60611. (312) 587-3709. (800) 521-3709. (312) 587-9951. <http://www.acoep.org>.

National Safe Kids Campaign. 1301 Pennsylvania Avenue, Suite 1000, Washington, D.C. 20004-1707. <http://pedsccm.wustl.edu/AllNet/english/neurpage/protect/drown.htm>.

Search and Rescue Society of British Columbia. P.O. Box 1146, Victoria, BC Canada V8W 2T6. (250) 384-6696. <http://www.sarbc.org/homepage.html>. sarbc@sarbc.org.

OTHER

Columbia Presbyterian Medical Center. <http://cpmcnet.columbia.edu/texts/guide/hmg13_0005.html>.

Consumer Products Safety Commission. <http://www.life-saver.com/stats.htm>.

Diving Medicine Online. <http://www.gulftel.com/~scubadoc/hypoth.htm>.

Merck Manual. <http://www.merck.com/pubs/mmanual_home/sec24/283.htm>.

National Library of Medicine. <http://medlineplus.adam.com/ency/article/000046.htm>.

L. Fleming Fallon, Jr., M.D., Dr.P.H.

Neck pain, physical therapy for *see* **Back and neck pain, physical therapy for**

Needles *see* **Syringe and needle**

Neonatal care

Definition

Neonatal care refers to that care given to the newborn infant from the time of delivery through about the first month of life. The term "neonate" is used for the newborn infant during this 28-30 day period.

Purpose

The purpose of neonatal care in the delivery room and newborn nursery is to:

- Assess and evaluate the newborn as s/he transitions from intrauterine life to extrauterine life.

- Evaluate and monitor the newborn system-by-system for normal versus abnormal functioning, providing maintenance of normal and potential treatment of abnormal findings.

- Foster bonding between infant and parent/s.

- Provide a safe environment at all times.

Description

Neonatal care begins as soon as the baby is born. In fact, suctioning of the nose and mouth may take place as the baby is in the process of being delivered—with the head out, and while the mother is taking a pause before the next push. *In utero* the infant is swimming in amniotic fluid. As he or she comes down the birth canal, the contractions exert pressure on the body and push some of the amniotic fluid out of the **lungs**. It is this fluid that is suctioned out during those first few moments. Shortly after delivery, the umbilical cord is clamped and then cut. Shortly after clamping, the cord will be checked for the presence of two arteries and one vein. Once the cord is clamped, the baby must breathe and function independently from the mother. The first few breaths cause several internal changes to occur. These will be discussed in the Results section below.

Because of the internal environment, the baby is very wet when born. Drying the baby off right away is critical, as the baby can lose considerable body heat through evaporation, convection, radiation, and conduction. This is especially true of the head, which has a large surface area in relation to the rest of the body. Also, head hair retains considerable moisture if not well dried. A cap placed on the head once it has been dried helps to maintain body temperature. The nurse may place the newborn on the mother's skin while drying the skin, both to begin the bonding process as well as to allow the mother's body heat to warm the infant. The rubbing that takes place to dry the infant provides tactile and sensory stimulation. The neonate may cry, bringing more oxygen into the lungs. A certain amount of pressure is needed in the **heart** and lungs in order to convert from fetal circulation to neonatal circulation. A color change is noticeable as the infant's skin changes from a bluish hue to pink. In some circumstances, oxygen from a mask may be placed near the mouth while the infant is being dried off to increase the initial intake of oxygen. Once dry, the infant is wrapped in several warm receiving blankets and may be placed at the mother's breast for an initial breastfeeding. If the mother will not be breastfeeding, she may choose to hold the newborn at this point.

The first breastfeeding helps to trigger the involution process of the uterus, as it stimulates the production of natural oxytocin, which helps the uterus contract. Also, in the first hour or so after birth, the neonate is usually quite alert, unless the mother was given **pain** medications late in labor.

While the infant is being dried off, the mother is delivering the placenta. The amniotic fluid is clear, perhaps tinged with **blood**. If it appears murky in any way, the baby most likely had a bowel movement during the stressful labor and delivery process. This first bowel movement is called meconium. If present in the amniotic fluid, it is possible that the infant inhaled some into its lungs. This is called meconium aspiration. The neonate with meconium in the amniotic fluid may be intubated to avoid aspiration. Meconium aspiration can lead to tachypnea (rapid respirations) and also **pneumonia**, and may require the neonate to spend some time under observation in the neonatal intensive care unit (NICU), instead of being kept with its mother. As the infant is being suctioned, assessed and dried, it may be placed in a slight Trendelenburg position, depending on the hospital. This downward slant of about 10 degrees allows gravity to assist in draining mucous.

At one and five minutes after birth the neonate is assessed for Apgar scores. The infant's heart rate, respiratory effort, muscle tone, reflex, irritability, and color are each given a score of 0, 1, or 2. Each score is then added together for a highest possible score of 10. The normal range is 7-10. It is rare to receive a 10, as some **cyanosis** in the hands and feet (called acrocyanosis) is quite normal.

In the birthing room a rapid **physical examination** is performed to assess any gross abnormalities as well as any heart-related problems, and to determine the need for any immediate intervention. The spine will be assessed, and should be free of any openings or dimpling. It will be flat, as the lumbar and sacral curves develop later when the child learns to sit and walk. A more detailed examination will take place about 24 hours later. The umbilical cord and placenta will also be examined for any abnormalities. Any medications given to the mother during labor and delivery are recorded in the neonate's chart, as the medication could affect the infant's respirations and its own ability for tissue oxygenation. The physician or nurse-midwife will also make sure the entire placenta has been expelled to avoid the risk of **infection** for the mother due to any retained tissue.

Because the neonate has difficulty maintaining its temperature, any examination that is immediately needed usually takes place under a source of radiant heat. During the first 24 hours the neonate is adjusting to extrauterine life and some normal fluctuations are expected. It is for this reason that the more thorough examination will take place a bit later on, once the initial fluctuations stabilize. The expected findings of the head-to-toe neonatal assessment will be discussed in the Results section below.

Before leaving the delivery room the nurse will:

• Place an identification band on the neonate's hands and feet.

• Place an ID band with the same number as the baby's on the mother's (and in some hospitals) on the father's wrist.

• Take a foot print of the infant (in some hospitals).

• Give an intramuscular (IM) injection of **vitamin K** to the neonate.

• Administer an antibacterial eye ointment into both eyes.

To assist the neonate's blood's ability to clot in its early life, infants receive an IM injection of vitamin K in the delivery room. The injection is usually given in the thigh muscle, as this is the largest and safest muscle in which to give an infant an injection. The antibacterial eye ointment used prevents contracting an infection from one present in the birth canal, such as gonorrhea or chlamydia.

Hospitals differ in which identification system they use, but the premise is the same: before the infant leaves the delivery room, he or she should receive an ID band with a number on it. The same ID number is on a band for the mother, as well as possibly for the father. Before leaving the baby with the parents, the bands should be checked by the nurse or nursing student to avoid any mix-up. Some hospital ID bands contain a microchip in it that causes an alarm bell to ring if the infant is taken out of a certain area. Also, some hospitals require that if the mother is going to take a nap or a shower, the infant must be returned to the nursery so that the infant is not unattended in the mother's room. Some hospitals use a band on each of the baby's hands and feet, so that if one or two fall off, proper ID still remains on the neonate. In addition to the ID band, a print of the infant's foot is made along with the mother's fingerprint. Both are recorded on the same sheet of paper.

If the neonate appears physiologically unstable, she will be taken either to the nursery or to the NICU for further evaluation or treatment. Once the mother's condition is stable, she may be wheeled to the infant's location if she desires.

Weight and length are measured, either in the birthing room or in the newborn nursery, **vital signs** are closely monitored and skin color is assessed for signs of **jaundice**. Jaundice that appears in the first 24 hours is of a different nature than that which sets in after 24 hours. If undressed, the infant is kept under radiant heat to assist in maintaining proper body temperature. Temperature may be regulated for several hours with a monitor attached to the chest skin. A rectal temperature may be taken to check for a patent anus. After any examinations, the infant will be swaddled in several layers of receiving blankets, a cap will be placed on the head to further reduce loss of body heat, and the newborn is placed in a bassinette either on its side, with a rolled blanket behind the back to prevent tipping, or on its back. To prevent sudden infant death syndrome (SIDS), infants should not be placed on their **stomach**.

Most insurance plans allow hospital stays of only 48 hours after an uncomplicated vaginal delivery, so much takes place within that time. Twenty-four to seventy-two hours after the neonate's first intake of protein her blood is checked via a heel-stick for the presence of phenylketonuria (PKU), a protein **metabolism** disorder that requires strict nutritional guidelines for treatment to avoid **central nervous system** (CNS) damage. Neonates whose mothers had **gestational diabetes** will have their blood sugar monitored in the nursery. During the second day of life the infant will have a detailed physical assessment done cephalocaudal (head-to-toe). The normal ranges for this will be discussed in the Results section. Parents who wish to have their male infants circumcised in the hospital will make those arrangements. The nursery nurses will monitor the circumcised infant for any signs of infection or abnormal bleeding.

Hospitals may differ in terms of how much time the infant spends with the mother in her room. The aim is for a balance between the mother's need for rest to ensure more rapid healing, the need for the parents and baby to form a strong bond, and the safety of the infant if unattended. Most hospitals bring the breast-feeding infant to the mother on demand. Formula-fed babies may spend more time in the nursery with staff feeding the baby, if the mother needs more rest time after a difficult delivery.

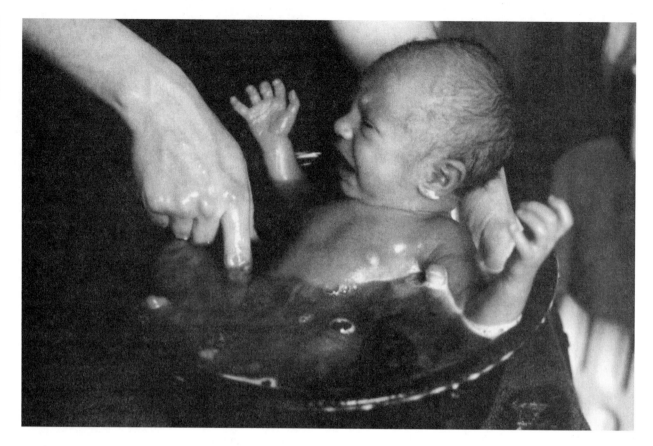

A newborn girl receives a bath. *(Photograph by James Stevenson. Science Source/Photo Researchers. Reproduced by permission.)*

In July 1999 the Centers for Disease Control (CDC) determined that hepatitis B immunizations, which had been routinely given to newborns, should no longer be administered to neonates until the preservative thimerosal is removed from vaccines. Since thimerosal is derived from ethylmercury, and even though there is no evidence that exposure to low levels of thimerosal is harmful, concerns about the exposure to mercury compounds led to the decision as a precautionary measure.

Results

The clamping of the umbilical cord signals the neonate's abrupt transition from intrauterine to extrauterine life. *In utero* the fetus's blood was oxygenated through the placenta and the mother's circulation. Now the neonate's lungs must take over. With the first breath, the lungs expand and create a pressure difference in the chest, pulmonary artery and heart. This leads to the closing of the *ductus arteriosus* and the *foramen ovale*. The blood flow through the cord stops and any blood within the cord will clot, causing the vessels to dry out, allowing the cord to fall off within about 10 days. Assessment of the cord area can be done with each diaper change.

The cord site should remain dry, with no evidence of redness, bleeding or discharge.

Infants born by cesarian section do not have the force of the birth canal pushing amniotic fluid out of the lungs. Because of this, some infants may have some initial difficulty with respirations, due to the excess of fluid still remaining in their lungs.

During the first hour after birth, the neonate is very alert. He or she may be interested in nursing, or may spend time just gazing at the mother or parents. The initial breastfeeding establishes the neonate's ability to coordinate breathing, sucking and swallowing.

Variability is normal in the newborn, so pulse and respirations should be monitored for an entire minute. If abnormal values are noted, yet the infant does not appear in distress, wait a minute or two and then recheck. Normal values for the neonate include:

- Apical pulse (recorded over the heart) between 120 and 160. The sleeping newborn may have a pulse of 100, the crying infant may have a pulse of 180. Rates below 100 and above 180 should be investigated.

- Respirations range from 30 to 60 breaths per minute. Infants are nose-breathers, so a clear nasal passage is critical. Poor breastfeeding position can block the nose and requires repositioning. Respirations can be counted by watching the abdomen move up and down. While short periods of crying can be beneficial in bringing more oxygen into the lungs, long periods of crying exhausts the neonate's **cardiovascular system** and should be avoided.

- The average weight of a newborn is 7.5 pounds (3.4 kg), with a normal range of 5.5 to 8.5 (2.5-3.8 kg). A weight above 10 pounds (4.5 kg) may indicate that the mother had gestational diabetes. The average length of the newborn is 20-21 inches (50-53 cm) long.

- Initially, the newborn is very sensitive to temperature changes, as her ability to regulate her temperature is not yet well developed. A normal rectal temperature ranges from 97.8-99°F (36.5-37.2°C). A newborn experiencing heat loss will increase his or her respirations.

- Within the first 24 hours, the newborn should void and pass meconium, a sticky, tar-like first stool. The neonate does not take in a great deal within the first few days, but intake and output should increase after the first few days. Bowel sounds are present.

A head-to-toe assessment is usually done without the parents present, but can be very helpful if done in front of the first-time parent for reassurance. The head will appear large in relation to the body. Average head circumference is about 13.5–14 inches (34–35 cm) in diameter. A circumference of less than 33 cm or greater than 37 cm may indicate a neurological abnormality and warrants further evaluation. The head of a baby born vaginally may look misshapen at first. This is called molding. The baby's **skull** allows for movement so that it can pass through the birth canal. Within a few days it takes on its normal shape. Infants delivered with the help of forceps or vacuum aspiration may have bruising on the head, or even a cephalhematoma. Cephalhematoma is a collection of blood under the scalp, such as can result from **blood vessels** that have ruptured during birth. It does not cross the midline of the skull. Caput succedaneum is an area of **edema** under the scalp. It may cross the midline. These will resolve over time, although the increased amount of blood being processed from the cephalhematoma may result in jaundice. Infants born by cesarian delivery have normally shaped heads right at birth if it is a scheduled caesarian delivery. If the mother has been in prolonged labor and a caesarian delivery is deemed necessary, the newborn's head may still be molded. Newborns may have a full head of hair, although most often falls out during the first month. The two soft spots on top of the head are called fontanels. The anterior fontanel should close after

12 to 18 months; the smaller, posterior fontanel should close by the third month. A bulging fontanel in a quiet infant indicates increased intracranial pressure. A depressed fontanel indicates **dehydration**. It is normal to be able to feel the pulsing of each heart contraction at the anterior fontanel. The eyes and ears should be in good proportion. Low-set ears indicate a chromosomal abnormality, such as trisomy 13 or 18. The nose, which is large at this age for the face, may have little white dots called milia. These are blocked sebaceous glands, and will disappear in a few weeks. These should not be squeezed or scratched, to avoid creating a portal for infection. The mouth should have an intact palate. Small round dots may be present and are called *Epstein pearls*. They are a form of **calcium** deposit and will disappear. Parents may confuse them with white patches of thrush, which is a Candida infection.

Newborn skin may be somewhat mottled, and early acrocyanosis in the hands and feet is common. Central cyanosis in the trunk should be investigated, as it indicates decreased oxygenation. Jaundice that sets in after the first 24 hours is common, but the bilirubin level should be closely monitored if the jaundice travels below the nipple line. Birthmarks, or hemangiomas, are common. Some are flat and reddish-purple in color. They may fade or disappear over time, but some larger ones may remain. Laser treatment in later life is becoming more common to remove those marks that are large or prominent enough to interfere with an individual's self-esteem. Raised, cavernous hemangiomas may indicate similar lesions on internal organs which can rupture and bleed with a blow to the child's abdomen. Mongolian spots are gray-purple-blue patches seen on children of Asian, Mediterranean, or African descent. They can resemble bruises, and are usually found on the buttocks and sacrum.

Newborns may be covered in *vernix caseosa*, a waxy substance that acts as a skin lubricant. It is especially noticeable in skin folds. Babies born post-dates (over 40 weeks) have very dry skin and may have cracks in the skin folds. The color of the vernix is an indicator of intrauterine life. It may be green-tinged, indicating the presence of meconium in the amniotic fluid. Yellow vernix indicates bilirubin. Lanugo is a fine, downy hair that may cover the shoulders, back, and upper arms. **Premature infants** have more lanugo; post-dates infants usually have none at all. The neonate's skin is sensitive and may respond to washing products with a rash.

The hormones circulating in the mother are passed into the fetus. Newborns may have enlarged genitalia in response to the circulating maternal hormones. Female neonates may have some white or blood-tinged discharge from the vagina for a week or so after birth. There should be no evidence of trauma, however.

The neonate is able to move her arms and legs symmetrically. Lack of movement or limpness indicates an injury and needs careful evaluation. A broken clavicle may be the result of a difficult birth, but should heal to full movement. The examiner will check for extra digits, or fused/webbed digits. The legs are normally bowed at this time, and will straighten with growth. Feet may appear twisted, due to a long-held intrauterine position. If they can be easily brought into alignment, this will usually revert to normal with growth and weight bearing. A foot that does not come into alignment may indicate talipes, or clubfoot. Early treatment brings the best success. The hips are checked for symmetrical abduction. Clicking heard during examination may indicate subluxation, and treatment is usually begun right away.

Neonatal **reflexes** are checked to assess for any neuromuscular abnormalities. Intact reflexes provide a safety/survival mechanism for the newborn. These reflexes include:

- Rooting; present from birth until about six weeks of age. To elicit the reflex, stroke the corner of the mouth. The neonate should turn his head in that direction. This reflex assists the infant in finding the breast.

- Sucking; from birth until about six months of age. Touching the lips begins the sucking reflex. When the lips are touched by the breast or bottle nipple, the infant begins to suck, taking in nourishment.

- Swallowing; as food reaches the back of the tongue, the swallowing reflex is elicited and the food is swallowed.

- Palmar grasp; disappears by three months of age. Placing an object, such as a finger, into the neonate's palm elicits this reflex. The infant will grasp tightly onto whatever has been placed into her hand.

- Stepping; present from birth until about three months of age. Hold the infant upright with his feet just touching a flat surface. The infant will take small weight-bearing "steps." These are not true steps, and the infant must be fully supported.

- Babinski; present until about three months of age. To elicit the response, stroke the sole of the neonate's foot, starting at the heel. The newborn will curl and fan his toes upward and outward. Once the reflex disappears, the same motion should cause the toes to flex, as in the neurologically intact adult.

- Moro; strongest from birth through two months of age, then fades until it disappears around the fifth month. This is a startle reflex, so evaluation is done somewhat gently. One method is for the examiner to clap her hands near the newborn, but out of eyesight. Another method is to hold the infant above a padded mat, then either let the head fall backwards by an inch or so, or quickly lower the infant's body towards the mat. This gives the infant a sense of falling. The reflex action is for the neonate to first extend both arms and legs, then to pull his legs up towards his abdomen while making the shape of a "C" with his fingers. For some very sensitive infants, walking quickly down the stairs may elicit this response. Such infants may feel more comforted being swaddled.

A neonate's **hearing** and **vision** will be assessed. The fetus is able to hear inside the uterus, and after birth it will clearly respond to the voices of the mother and father but may ignore unfamiliar voices. The neonate focuses best on an object 9-12 inches (23-30 cm) away. This is approximately the distance between its face and the face of the mother when held in a breastfeeding position. There should be no redness or drainage from the eye on inspection. The blink reflex should be intact, elicited by briefly shining a bright light at the eye. Depending on the birthing position, there may be edema around the eye, although this fluid should reabsorb in a few days after birth.

Health care team roles

At birth, the physician or nurse-midwife is in attendance, along with the labor and delivery nurse. If the fetus has been in distress, a neonatalogist may also be present. After birth the newborn is handed to the nurse who begins the drying off of the newborn, and addresses the other issues mentioned above. Nurses perform the neonatal care tasks discussed above in the nursery. Blood drawn drom the neonate's heel is usually done by the nursery nurse, and then sent to the laboratory for processing by the laboratory technicians. In some hospitals nurses may care for both the newborn and the mother as a unit. Nurses provide all the necessary teaching provided to the new mother.

Neonatal care continues through about the fourth week after birth. During this time the infant and mother may receive a home nursing visit to ensure that breastfeeding is well established, that no jaundice is present in the neonate, and that the mother is healing well from the delivery. At the follow-up office visit, the nurse or medical assistant will weigh and measure the length of the infant.

Patient education

Parent education, especially for the first-time parent is extremely important. Nurses or nurse-midwives will provide breastfeeding and postpartum teaching for the mother, as well as explaining the care needed for the newborn. This may include cord care, normal number of daily feedings and diapers, how to determine the presence of jaundice, how and when to bathe the infant, as well as answer any questions the new parents may have. A follow-up appointment is usually established before the infant leaves the hospital. The nurse will often be the one to ensure that a car seat is present and properly installed in the car before allowing the mother and baby to leave the hospital, as mandated by state law. Nurses also provide information when parents call with questions to the doctor's office.

Resources

BOOKS

Curtis, Glade B. and Judith Schuler. *Your Baby's First Year Week by Week.* Tucson, AZ: Fisher Books, 2000.

Doenges, Marilynn E. and Mary Frances Moorhouse. *Maternal/Newborn Plans of Care; Guidelines for Individualizing Care.* Philadelphia: F. A. Davis Company, 1999.

Klaus, Marshall H. and Phyllis H. Klaus. *Your Amazing Newborn.* Reading, MA: Perseus Books, 1998.

The Parents' Answer Book from Birth Through Age Five. New York: St. Martin's Griffin, 1998.

Pasquariello, Patrick S. *The Children's Hospital of Philadelphia: Book of Pregnancy and Child Care.* New York: John Wiley & Sons, Inc., 1999.

Pillitteri, Adele. *Maternal & Child Health Nursing 3rd Edition.* Philadelphia: Lippincott, 1999.

Swanson, Jennifer, ed. *Infant and Toddler Sourcebook 1st Edition.* Detroit: Omnigraphics, 2000.

ORGANIZATIONS

The American Academy of Pediatrics. 141 Northwest Point Boulevard, Elk Grove Village, IL 60007-1098. (847) 434-4000. <http://www.aap.org>.

Medscape, Inc. 20500 NW Evergreen Parkway, Hillsboro, OR 97124. (503) 531-7000. <http://www.medscape.com>.

OTHER

The American Academy of Family Physicians, The American Academy of Pediatrics, The Advisory Committee on Immunization Practices, and The United States Public Health Service. *"Joint Statement Concerning Removal of Thimerosal From Vaccines."* Centers for Disease Control website. June 22, 2000. <http://www.cdc.gov/nip/vacsafe/concerns/thimerosal/joint_statement_00.htm>.

Esther Csapo Rastegari, R.N., B.S.N., Ed.M

Neonatal jaundice

Definition

Neonatal **jaundice** and hyperbilirubinemia are terms used when a newborn has a higher-than-normal level of bilirubin in the **blood**. Bilirubin is an end-product of the breakdown of the hemoglobin present in the red blood cells at the end of their life cycle. Hemoglobin carries oxygen to tissues and cells. Before birth the placenta is not as efficient in providing oxygen as the baby's **lungs** will be after birth. Because of this, infants *in utero* have more red blood cells than they will need after birth to provide enough oxygen. Therefore, newborns have an excess of red blood cells that they need to process, and an immature **liver** with which to complete the job. Jaundice refers to the yellow discoloration of the skin and sclera (whites) of the eyes, which results as the breakdown of bilirubin goes faster than the rate at which it can leave the body, causing its level to rise in the blood.

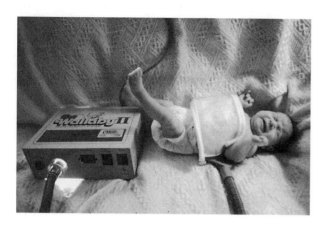

A newborn receives home health care to treat jaundice with bilirubin lights. *(Photograph by Cindy Roesinger, Photo Researchers, Inc. Reproduced by permission.)*

Description

When the fetus is *in utero*, bilirubin is processed through the placenta and the maternal-fetal circulation. After birth, the infant's often-immature liver must take over this task. Clinical jaundice (serum bilirubin levels of 5-7 mg/dL and above) occurs in about 60-70% of term newborns, and about 80% of **premature infants**. Ever since hospital stays after delivery decreased to 24-48 hours postpartum, hyperbilirubinemia has become the leading cause of hospital readmissions in the first two weeks of life. The greatest concern with hyperbilirubinemia is that the unexcreted bilirubin will begin to deposit in the **brain** of the neonate, resulting in a serious, potentially life-threatening condition called kernicterus. Another term used for kernicterus is brain encephalopathy.

Causes and symptoms

An elevated bilirubin level may be due to its increased production, a decreased rate of conjugation, or abnormalities of the liver. In order for the bilirubin to be excreted in the urine and stool, it must be converted, or conjugated from a fat- or lipid-soluble form to a water-soluble form. Bilirubin that has not been excreted can be reabsorbed and contributes to increased blood levels.

Initial symptoms of a rising bilirubin level can be subtle, and usually include increased drowsiness, which leads to poor feeding, and the subsequent decreased urine and stool output. The diaper may contain orange spots, an indication of the presence of uric acid crystals, a sign of **dehydration**. A change in the infant's cry to a high-pitched tone may indicate early neurological damage.

There are several types of jaundice. The most common form of neonatal jaundice appears between the first 24-72 hours after birth and is usually considered a benign form. It is often referred to as early-onset breast milk jaundice, and is related to insufficient breastfeeding, which results in decreased nutritional intake and decreased stooling. With decreased stooling the bilirubin in the stool is not being excreted, and is also available for reabsorption. Increasing the feedings from six to 12 times a day, and checking for latching-on and a good suck and swallow pattern, can lead to a decreasing bilirubin level to within normal limits. To encourage adequate maternal milk production, supplementation with water or glucose is discouraged.

Late-onset breast milk jaundice may occur in 10-30% of breast-fed infants and appears in the second to sixth weeks of life. This form of jaundice is believed to be related to a substance present in the mother's milk that affects the infant's absorption of bilirubin.

Jaundice that sets in within the first 24 hours after birth is usually due to an **Rh factor** or ABO blood incompatibility between the mother and infant.

Risk factors for the development of hyperbilirubinemia include:

- premature birth
- Asian and Native American descent—including more rapid rise and higher peak levels of bilirubin
- maternal diabetes
- hemolytic disease in the neonate
- sepsis
- family history of jaundice
- presence of excessive bruising due to traumatic birth, and cephalhematoma
- oxytocin-induced delivery
- mother's use of sulfa medications during **pregnancy**
- history of familial liver disease
- delayed cord clamping
- thyroid gland abnormalities
- G6PD (glucose-6-phosphate dehydrogenase) deficiency

Diagnosis

Diagnosis of hyperbilirubinemia usually begins with the observation of jaundice at the time of **physical examination**. However, a delay in recognition of jaundice may occur since many infants have already gone home prior to its onset. Pediatric practices vary as to times of follow-up after hospital discharge. Parents may call their pediatric care provider's office because of jaundice, or because of a decreased ability of the infant to feed. Examination of the infant is best done next to a window so that the jaundice can be assessed in natural light. Blood tests to check the bilirubin level, blood type, and for signs of dehydration will usually be ordered.

Treatment

Treatment is primarily focused on decreasing the bilirubin level to prevent the progression of the condition to kernicterus. In kernicterus, the bilirubin deposits in the brain. This leads to **central nervous system** damage, and can progress to **hearing loss**, seizures, and death.

Phototherapy

For many infants, increasing breastfeeding will be sufficient to bring about adequate hydration and an increase in gastric motility and stooling, so that the bilirubin is effectively excreted from the body. Some infants may need the additional assistance of **phototherapy**. The light source most effective in treating hyperbilirubinemia occurs in the blue-green spectrum. Phototherapy may be provided in the hospital. In the hospital the infant is usually placed in a special bassinet, with an overhead light source. The skin is uncovered, exposing as much surface area to the light. The infant's eyes and genitals are usually shielded from direct light and heat, depending on the intensity of the light. If the bilirubin level is under about 15–20 mg/dL, phototherapy may be administered via a fiberoptic source referred to as a blanket or belt in the home. The home unit is designed to encourage parent-infant bonding. The blanket/belt wraps around the infant's bare middle so that the cool light source is next to the skin. There is no need to shield the eyes from the light, and parents can hold, feed and interact with the infant as usual. Most insurance companies cover the cost of the home rental for the phototherapy equipment and the accompanying daily home nursing visits.

In 1994 the American Academy of Pediatrics (AAP) developed guidelines for care and management of neonatal jaundice. As of March 2001 these guidelines were being reviewed, but the 1994 guidelines remain in effect. In studies where experienced pediatric practitioners evaluated the same infants for jaundice, considerable discrepancies existed. Despite all the research done in this area, there are no consistent predictors of which infants will continue from benign jaundice to kernicterus. Research studies express concern over finding a balance between treating those that need treatment, without treating well infants unnecessarily.

KEY TERMS

Bilirubin—A yellowish-brown substance in the blood that forms as old red blood cells are broken down.

Jaundice—The yellow discoloration of the skin and sclera of the eyes as a result of poor liver function.

Kernicterus—A serious condition in which bilirubin deposits in the brain leading to permanent neurological damage and potentially death.

Prognosis

Jaundice addressed in its early stages rarely progresses to kernicterus, and therefore the prognosis for complete resolution of the problem is excellent. Phototherapy is extremely effective in bringing down the bilirubin levels. Some extreme cases may require a blood transfusion, but those situations are relatively rare. Infants who do develop kernicterus may continue to have long-term neurological effects present if the kernicterus was well established at the time of initiation of treatment.

Health care team roles

The nurse may participate in the care of the infant in the hospital nursery, where he or she may be the first to notice the jaundice. The nurse may also be the one to take the parent's call about the jaundice in the pediatric care provider's office. In the home setting, the nurse's role involves daily visits to the home for infant assessment and blood draws via a heel stick for bilirubin evaluation, parent teaching on bottle or breastfeeding and neonatal and postpartum issues. The nurse should inform the parents that phototherapy increases the baby's **metabolism**, resulting in increased output to clear the bilirubin. This means that the infant will require more feedings to compensate for the fluids lost. The nurse should also inform the parents that the stool containing bilirubin may be more loose than usual and of a greenish color. Some pediatric practices may have the parents bring the infant into the laboratory where the technician would be the one to draw the infant's blood for bilirubin evaluation. Heel sticks on an infant can be difficult when the infant is dehydrated. Ways to facilitate a more successful blood draw include:

• Use of a heel warmer to increase circulation to the foot.

• Having a parent hold the infant in a seated position so that the foot is below the level of the heart.

• Having the parent feed the infant prior to the lab visit.

Prevention

Primary prevention begins with addressing the risk factors mentioned above. Prevention of kernicterus requires early detection, monitoring and potential treatment of jaundice with rising bilirubin levels. Frequent feedings of ten or more per day help to ensure adequate hydration, **nutrition**, gastric motility, and stool and urine output.

Resources

BOOKS

Behrman, Richard E., Robert M. Kliegman, and Hal B. Jenson. *Nelson Textbook of Pediatrics, 16th Edition.* Philadelphia: W. B. Saunders Company, 2000.

Burns, Catherine E., Margaret A. Brady, Ardys M. Dunn and Nancy Barber Starr. *Pediatric Primary Care A Handbook for Nurse Practitioners, 2nd Edition.* Philadelphia: W. B. Saunders Company, 2000.

Pasquariello, Patrick S. *The Children's Hospital of Philadelphia: Book of Pregnancy and Child Care.* New York: John Wiley & Sons, 1999.

Taeusch, H. William, and Roberta A. Ballard. *Avery's Diseases of the Newborn, 7th Edition.* Philadelphia: W. B. Saunders Company, 1998.

PERIODICALS

Moyer, Virginia A., Chul Ahn, and Stephanie Sneed. "Accuracy of Clinical Judgement in Neonatal Jaundice." *Archives of Pediatric and Adolescent Medicine* 154 (2000): 391-394.

Newman, Thomas B. and M. Jeffrey Maisels. "Less Aggressive Treatment of Neonatal Jaundice and Reports of Kernicterus: Lessons About Practice Guidelines." *Pediatrics* 105, no. 1 Pt 3 (2000): 242-245.

Wiley, Catherine C., Naline Lai, Christopher Hill, and Georgine Burke. "Nursery Practices and Detection of Jaundice After Newborn Discharge." *Archives of Pediatric and Adolescent Medicine* 152 (1998): 972-975.

ORGANIZATIONS

Archives of Pediatric and Adolescent Medicine; Journal of the American Medical Association. <http://www.archpedi.ama-assn.org>.

Esther Csapo Rastegari, R.N., B.S.N., Ed.M.

Neonatal respiratory care

Definition

Respiratory care of the newborn is the systematic process by which health care providers ensure consistent and appropriate oxygenation levels through assessment and therapeutic intervention.

Purpose

Adequate respiratory function is of utmost importance in newborn care and must be assessed frequently.

Precautions

Health care providers should practice **universal precautions** when caring for newborns.

Description

Respiratory care is guided by the Apgar score which is obtained at one minute and five minutes after birth through observation of the newborn. The caregiver assesses the newborn for **heart** rate, respiratory effort, muscle tone, reflex irritability, and color. The newborn receives scores of 0, 1, or 2 for each category and all five scores are added together. An infant scoring less than 4 is in grave danger and requires immediate resuscitation. A score of 4 to 6 indicates that the newborn's condition is serious and that the baby may require clearing of the airway and **oxygen therapy**. A score of 7 to 10 indicates that the infant is doing well. The highest score a newborn can receive is 10.

Respiratory care of the newborn can be separated into two general categories: care of the healthy, term newborn and care of the high-risk newborn.

Respiratory care of the healthy, term newborn

RESPIRATORY EFFORT. A healthy, term newborn generally releases a lusty, spontaneous cry within 30 seconds after delivery. By one minute, the newborn normally maintains regular, but often rapid respirations. If the mother received large amounts of narcotic analgesia or a general anesthetic in labor or birth the baby's respirations might be depressed. The administration of a medication to counter this effect, such as naloxone (Narcan) may be indicated.

The newborn should be able to maintain a clear airway with little assistance and should have a respiratory rate of 30 to 60 breaths per minute. Physical signs of respiratory distress are retractions (the skin is pulling against the ribs), nasal flaring, and grunting. The **lungs** should sound clear when listened to with a **stethoscope** (auscultated).

Care of the normal newborn's respiratory status includes the following actions:

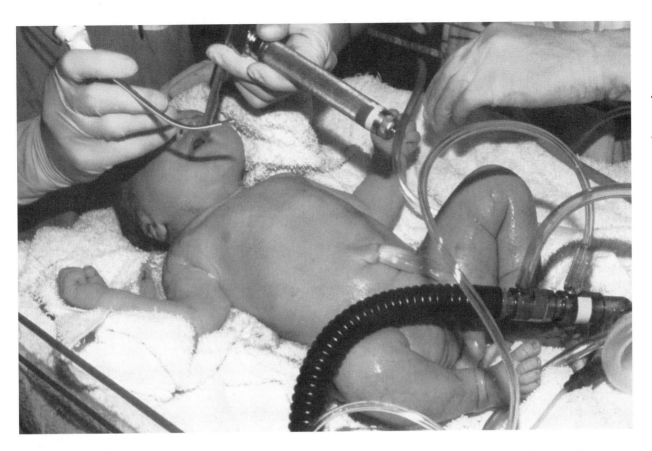

Newborns commonly have some amniotic fluid in their lungs, and it may need to be removed with suction through an endotracheal tube. *(Photograph by David Nunuk. Science Source/Photo Researchers. Reproduced by permission.)*

- Assess the baby's respiratory rate every 15 minutes for 1 hour. Observe for an increase in respiratory rate, the development of retractions, nasal flaring, or grunting.

- Position the newborn with the head down and on one side to aid in the drainage of secretions from the respiratory tract.

- Suction the baby's mouth first with a bulb syringe and then the nose. Suctioning the nose before the mouth can induce the aspiration of secretions through the mouth.

- Frequently change the baby's position to encourage the drainage of secretions thereby helping the lungs to aerate and expand.

- Keep the baby warm either by wrapping loosely with a blanket and placing a hat on the baby's head or by placing the baby under a radiant warmer. Check the baby's temperature frequently at first. A cold baby experiences an increase in metabolic rate that raises oxygen requirements resulting in a more rapid respiratory rate.

Respiratory care of a high-risk newborn

The high-risk newborn may be premature, may have a congenital condition, or may have experienced some degree of asphyxia in utero from compression of the umbilical cord, maternal anesthesia or analgesia, **placenta previa**, or a partial separation of the placenta. The manner in which the first few moments of life are managed will determine the eventual outcome for the high-risk newborn. It is imperative that respirations are established within two minutes of birth or severe respiratory acidosis may develop that is difficult to reverse. Any baby that does not take a first breath or has difficulty breathing adequately requires resuscitative intervention.

Resuscitation of the newborn consists of three sequential steps:

ESTABLISHING AN AIRWAY. If the baby does not initiate spontaneous respirations, suction the mouth and nose with a bulb syringe. Stimulating the skin by rubbing the baby's back may initiate breathing. If the baby's skin color is not pink, hold an oxygen tube with warmed oxygen by the baby's nose or provide oxygen by face mask. If these interventions are ineffective, administer oxygen by a positive pressure bag and mask.

EXPANDING THE LUNGS. A baby who cannot sustain effective breathing may need oxygen via bag and mask. The mask should cover the mouth and the nose but should not cover the eyes. The bag and mask deliver 100% oxygen and are compressed at a rate of 40 to 60 compressions per minute until the baby breathes spontaneously.

If the baby's Apgar score remains low, deeper suctioning with a suction catheter may be required. Position the infant on his or her back and place a folded towel beneath the baby's shoulders. Pass a catheter above the infant's tongue to the rear of the throat and suction for no longer than 10 seconds. A baby who initiates no respiratory effort is likely to require immediate placement of an endotracheal tube into the airway through a technique called intubation. The instrument used to open the airway so that the endotracheal tube can be placed in the airway is called a laryngoscope. After placement of the endotracheal tube, deeper suctioning of the trachea through the endotracheal tube is possible. A pressure bag can then be attached to the endotracheal tube and deliver 100% oxygen. The bag is compressed 40 to 60 times a minute.

If the amniotic fluid was meconium-stained, stimulation of the baby's breathing by rubbing the back or the administration of oxygen under pressure could cause the infant to aspirate meconium into the lungs. Instead, only provide oxygen therapy by mask without pressure. Passing a laryngoscope and suctioning the trachea should remove the meconium. Then tactile stimulation and oxygen therapy under pressure can be initiated.

MAINTAINING EFFECTIVE VENTILATION. All newborns, particularly those who encountered respiratory problems at birth, should be carefully assessed for several hours after birth. It is also of utmost importance to keep the baby warm. If the baby continues to produce copious secretions from the respiratory tract he or she should be suctioned out with a catheter or bulb syringe. If the baby is intubated, preventilating with a bag means suctioning can be performed through the endotracheal tube. If the baby's respiratory status remains critical, administration of pressure and oxygen via a ventilator or by continuous positive airway pressure (CPAP) may be necessary.

Preparation

It is essential that a well stocked area for infant resuscitation be maintained and frequently checked. Necessary equipment includes oxygen; various sized laryngoscopes and endotracheal tubes for preterm to large infants; suction catheters of different sizes; bulb syringes; and blankets. Supplies are usually placed alongside a radiant warmer.

Health care team roles

Nurses, respiratory therapists, and physicians should become certified in neonatal resuscitation. Health care practitioners who are trained to intubate with a laryngoscope include: obstetricians, midwives, pediatricians, neonatologists, anesthesiologists, and neonatal nurse practitioners. At least one person who can intubate an infant should be present at every delivery of a high-risk infant.

Resources

BOOKS

Maternal & Child Health Nursing. 3rd ed. Philadelphia: Lippincott, 1999.

ORGANIZATIONS

American Heart Association (AHA). 7272 Greenville Avenue, Dallas, TX 75231. 1-877-AHA-4-CPR. <http://www.americanheart.org/>.

Nadine M. Jacobson, R.N.

Nephrostomy tube care

Definition

A percutaneous nephrostomy tube (PNT) is a urinary diversion system comprised of a collection bag, a nephrostomy tube at an exit site (usually in the skin over the flank area), and a nephrostomy tube that enters and ends in the renal pelvis of the kidney. This allows for direct drainage of urine from the kidney when normal urinary flow is impeded. The PNT is most often used for a urinary obstruction such as a calculus.

Purpose

The purpose of PNT care is to prevent complications when a PNT is in use.

Precautions

Aspiration of fluid from the nephrostomy tube is prohibited as such action will damage the renal pelvis. Gravity drainage is used to collect specimens, and the nurse should never use force when irrigating the tube. A tube should never be irrigated with more than 5 ml of solution, since the capacity of the renal pelvis is between 4 and 8 ml. The nurse must avoid dislodging the tube while removing the dressing.

Preparation

The nurse should wash hands prior to beginning the procedure, then assemble all of the following equipment:

- disposable underpad
- clean gloves
- measuring tape
- sterile gloves
- sterile cotton tip applicators (4)
- sterile 0.9% NaCl or povidone-iodine solution or sponges
- sterile 4x4 pad or transparent dressing
- sterile 2x2 pads
- tape
- pouch belt

Description

The nurse should provide privacy for the patient in preparation for the procedure. He or she should position the patient on the side opposite the tube site with the nephrostomy site up. This provides better viewing of the tube and allows an easier dressing change.

The nurse should put on clean gloves and place a disposable underpad beneath to the patient to absorb any drainage. To minimize tension at the site and to prevent dislodging, the nephrostomy tube should be anchored with a small piece of tape. The collection bag must be emptied. The old dressing can be removed by carefully loosening the edges, and then moving to the center of dressing. Care should be taken to avoid dislodging the tube while removing the dressing. A sterile cotton-tip applicator placed on the catheter will help stabilize the catheter while removing the dressing. The site is then assessed for signs of **infection**, any moisture, or other drainage. The PNT is then measured from exit site to tip. If the PNT length is longer than the measurement at time of insertion, the catheter may have migrated out, and the physician should be notified at that point. The nurse should remove the soiled gloves at this time and replace with sterile ones. The exit site should be cleansed with the agent of choice (0.9% saline or povidone-iodine solution), using sterile 2x2 pads. Each pad can only be used once. Cleansing should start at the exit site and work outward in a circular motion; this action should be repeated twice. If there is any crusted matter at the site, this must be loosened and removed by using a cotton-tip applicator moistened with 0.9% saline. Then, sterile dressing should be applied. After removing the old tape, the tube must be secured with new tape to the skin below the dressing, approximately 2.5 inches (6.5 cm) from the exit site. The patient will need to be assisted in the application of the pouch belt. Anchoring the PNT with tape reduces trauma and minimizes the possibility of dislodging or kinking the tubing; adding the belt further secures the PNT. The nurse may remove gloves at this point and wash hands. The patient's dressing needs to be dated and initialed, and will need to be changed daily, or more often if necessary.

Aftercare

The used equipment needs to be disposed of properly. Upon completion of the procedure, the nurse should again wash hands. Then the nurse will need to document observations and the techniques used, including the assessment of the site, the external catheter length, the type of dressing applied, and the devices used to secure the PNT.

Complications

There is an increased risk of infection because the PNT provides a direct pathway to the kidney. There is also a risk for dislodging the PNT during this procedure.

Patient education

The patient may shower 48 hours post-insertion. The patient should be given all of the following instructions:

- Cover the dressing and exit site with a waterproof covering before showering.
- Empty the collection bag prior to showering.

- Securely tape the PNT at the exit site and use a belt for the collection bag in the shower to prevent tube migration.

- Generally, after 14 days, if there are no complications, the site may be left uncovered when showering.

The patient should notify the doctor if any problems arise such as:

- signs of infection at the exit site of the PNT, including warmth, redness, swelling, tenderness, and discharge

- drainage from the PNT

- decreased urine output

- inability to flush the PNT

- presence of any bleeding, clots, stones, sediment, and odor

- incontinence or inadequate bladder emptying

- inadequate **pain** control, nausea, or vomiting

- fever

- accidental dislodgement of the PNT, or suspected migration of the PNT

Results

The site should not display any signs of infection. PNT measurement should be consistent with the baseline value. Abnormal findings are signs of infection, suspected migration, or a dislodged PNT. In the collection bag, any bleeding, clots, stones, sediment, and odor are all abnormal findings.

Health care team roles

Registered nurses (RNs) and licensed practical nurses (LPNs) may perform this procedure. After returning home, the patient may simply cleanse the insertion site with soap and water, and change the dressing daily. In an inpatient setting, an **aseptic technique** must be maintained.

Nurses are responsible for:

- dressing changes

- proper disposal of equipment

- documentation of the procedure

- **patient education**

Resources

BOOKS

Modic, Mary Beth, and Dorothy Calabrese. "Renal and Urologic Care" In *Nursing Procedures, Third Edition* Springhouse, PA: Springhouse Corporation, pp. 595-597.

ORGANIZATIONS

American Nephrology Nurses Association. ANNA National Office, East Holly Avenue, Box 56, Pitman, NJ 08071-0056. (888) 600-2662. <http://anna.inurse.com/>.

Society of Urologic Nurses and Associates. National Headquarters, East Holly Avenue, Box 56, Pitman, NJ 08071-0056. (888) TAP-SUNA. <http://www.suna.org/>.

OTHER

"What Do I Need to Know about My Child's Nephrostomy Tube?" Patient Education Program Children's Hospital, Cincinnati. <http://www.cincinnatichildrens.org/family/pep/home-care/2106/>.

Maggie Boleyn, R.N., B.S.N.

Nerve conduction velocity testing *see* **Electromyography**

Nervous system, autonomic

Definition

The autonomic nervous system is a network of nerves that regulate involuntary control of cardiac muscle, organ smooth muscle, and glands such that basic biological processes such as digestion and breathing can occur without conscious thought.

Description

The peripheral nervous system consists of nerves that must travel outside of the **brain** and **spinal cord** in order to contact organs, glands, and muscles. Under the umbrella of the peripheral nervous system are the somatic and autonomic nervous systems. The **somatic nervous system** is responsible for controlling voluntary movements during activities such as walking while the autonomic nervous system regulates involuntary tasks such as food digestion. More specifically, the somatic division mediates voluntary or reflexive control of **skele-**

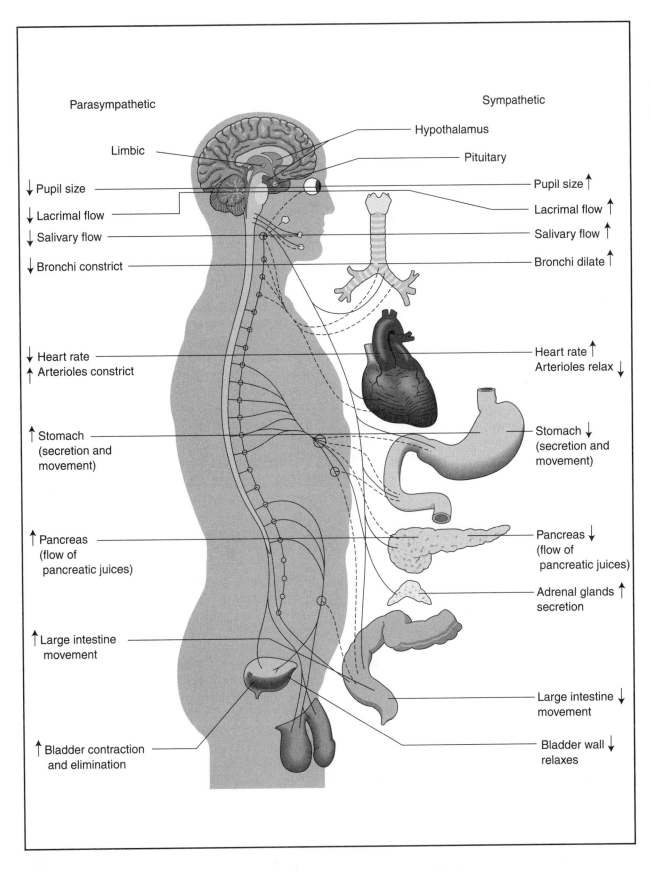

Parasympathetic

Sympathetic

Limbic

Hypothalamus

Pituitary

↓ Pupil size

↓ Lacrimal flow

↓ Salivary flow

↓ Bronchi constrict

Pupil size ↑

Lacrimal flow ↑

Salivary flow ↑

Bronchi dilate ↑

↓ Heart rate
↑ Arterioles constrict

Heart rate ↑
Arterioles relax ↓

↑ Stomach
(secretion and
movement)

Stomach ↓
(secretion and
movement)

↑ Pancreas
(flow of
pancreatic juices)

Pancreas ↓
(flow of
pancreatic juices)

Adrenal glands ↑
secretion

↑ Large intestine
movement

Large intestine ↓
movement

↑ Bladder contraction
and elimination

Bladder wall ↓
relaxes

The autonomic nervous system (ANS). *(Delmar Publishers, Inc. Reproduced by permission.)*

tal muscles while the autonomic nervous system is responsible for the involuntary and reflexive control of glands, organ smooth muscle, and cardiac muscle.

The autonomic nervous system has three components:

- sympathetic nervous system
- parasympathetic nervous system
- enteric nervous system

The enteric nervous system is the less common of the three and is responsible for coordinating the digestive functions of the gastrointestinal tract, **pancreas**, and gall bladder. The two other subdivisions of the autonomic nervous system, parasympathetic and sympathetic, work in concert to subconsciously control other bodily functions, such as **heart rate**, **blood pressure**, digestion, **metabolism**, reproduction, breathing, excretion, sweating, and temperature.

The parasympathetic and sympathetic divisions have similar organizations but are distinguishable at the anatomical, biochemical, and functional levels. Both systems are organized into a two-neuron chain. The first neuron in this chain is referred to as a preganglionic neuron and the second as a postganglionic neuron. The nucleus containing cell bodies of preganglionic **neurons** are found in the brain and spinal cord of the **central nervous system**. The preganglionic neuron extends a fiber process, known as an axon, outside of the central nervous system to make contact with the cell body of the postganglionic neuron. The place where the axon of the preganglionic neuron meets the cell body of the postganglionic neuron is called a synapse. The synapses of the autonomic nervous system are outside of the brain and spinal cord of the central nervous system in specialized structures known as autonomic ganglia.

The preganglionic neurons of the parasympathetic nervous system originate in the brainstem and sacral spinal cord. These preganglionic neurons communicate with postganglionic neurons by extending very long axons that release the neurotransmitter, acetylcholine. The synapses of the parasympathetic ganglia are usually in or near the targeted organ. The postganglionic neuron expresses protein receptors on the surface that are capable of responding to acetylcholine. The postganglionic neurons have very short axons that release acetylcholine onto the targeted organ to modulate the intrinsic activity of that particular organ. These organs include the eye, lacrimal gland, salivary gland, heart, bronchi and **lungs**, **small intestine**, **stomach**, **gallbladder**, **liver**, pancreas, **large intestine**, rectum, genitalia, **blood vessels**, and bladder. Each of these targeted organs expresses acetyl-

choline receptors to respond to the parasympathetic nervous system.

The preganglionic neurons of the sympathetic nervous system originate in the thoracic and upper lumbar regions of the spinal cord. These preganglionic neurons send very short axons to synapse in the paravertebral or in the prevertebral ganglia. The paravertebral ganglia lie in close proximity to the spinal cord. The postganglionic neurons of the paravertebral ganglia send axons to the head, trunk, and limb regions. The other organs in the body receive inputs from the prevertebral ganglia which is further away from the spinal cord and closer to the target organ. An exception to organization is the adrenal gland which is directly contacted by preganglionic neurons of sympathetic nervous system. Identical to the parasympathetic nervous system, the preganglionic neurons of the sympathetic nervous system communicate by releasing the neurotransmitter acetylcholine. However, the postganglionic neurons of the sympathetic nervous system differ in that they release norepinephrine onto the targeted organ. An exception to this is in the sweat glands where sympathetic postganglionic neurons release acetylcholine instead of norepinephrine. The target organs of the sympathetic nervous system include many of the same ones as the parasympathetic nervous system.

Function

The autonomic nervous system maintains internal balance (homeostasis) but also enables humans to respond to changes in the environment. This is achieved because the parasympathetic and sympathetic divisions of the systems are antagonistic. The parasympathetic and sympathetic nervous system usually have opposing effects on target organs. The predominate resting tone of an organ is established by either the sympathetic or parasympathetic system. For example, the predominate resting tone of the eye pupil is constriction, maintained by the parasympathetic nervous system. However, a fearful situation may induce pupil dilation, mediated by the sympathetic nervous system. In other words, the autonomic nervous system enables humans to deviate from normal functions to respond to changes in the environment. The parasympathetic nervous system is often referred to as "rest and digest" and the sympathetic nervous system as "fight or flight."

Each organ has a predominate resting tone that is influenced in a distinct way by the sympathetic and parasympathetic nervous systems. The sympathetic nervous system increases heart rate, while the parasympathetic slows it down. Likewise, the sympathetic system constricts **blood** vessels while the parasympathetic dilates them and therefore both systems influence blood pressure. The sympathetic nervous system reduces motility of the stomach and intestines while the parasympathetic increases motility. Most of the organs and glands controlled by the autonomic nervous system have this dual but opposing mechanism of regulation.

In some situations it is beneficial to override the autonomic nervous system. The postganglionic neurons and the targeted organs express protein receptors that sense and respond to the neurotransmitters acetylcholine and norepinephrine. The practice of autonomic **pharmacology** uses drugs to modify these receptors to override the existing setting. In this manner, dysfunctions such as high blood pressure can be treated and maintained.

Role in human health

The autonomic nervous system has a crucial role in human health because it maintains the internal balance as well as allows the individual to respond to environmental stimuli. Problems can arise when this system is over- or underactive. The role of **stress** on the autonomic nervous system is of serious consequence. The autonomic nervous system is designed to respond to stress but too much stress can lead to abnormal resting organ tones. This is exemplified by heart disease and high blood pressure which can be treated by drugs that block the autonomic nervous system.

Common diseases and disorders

Holmes-Adie's syndrome

This is believed to be a disorder of the autonomic nervous system characterized by loss of the ability to constrict the eye pupil. This syndrome is also referred to as tonic pupil. The presenting patient maintains a dilated pupil and has decreased **reflexes**. The ciliary ganglion, where the parasympathetic pre- and postganglion fibers meet, has been observed to degenerate. This loss of the parasympathetic tone renders the patient unable to constrict the pupil in response to light and nearby objects. The underlying cause is unknown but possibilities include viral infections that induce inflammation of the ciliary ganglion.

Familial dysautonomia

Familial dysautonomia is also referred to as Riley-Day syndrome and is an inherited disorder of the autonomic nervous system. The inheritance is autosomal recessive with widespread prevalence in patients of Ashkenazi Jewish decent. It is characterized by an increase in **pain** sensation, decreased lacrimation, an inability to regulate temperature, excessive sweating, and

---

hypertension. It is usually diagnosed early in life and impairs development. There is evidence that there are a decreased number of sensory and autonomic nervous system neurons. Recently, the gene has been mapped to chromosome 9 and codes for a protein called IKAP. The function of IKAP is unknown, but it is hypothesized to be involved in gene activation mechanisms.

Horner's syndrome

Horner's syndrome is characterized by a lack of sympathetic tone to one side of the face. Therefore, symptoms that present are dropping eyelids, pupil constriction, and dryness to the face. The underlying cause of this is not clear but may originate within the spinal cord due to injury or tumor formation.

Shy-Drager syndrome

Patients with Shy-Drager syndrome have general autonomic nervous system dysfunction as well as parkinsonian like symptoms. The autonomic symptoms included a decrease in blood pressure, orthostatic hypotension, constipation, urinary incontinence, and abnormal sweating. Some patients may also develop irregular heartbeats and have difficulty breathing. The parkinsonian like symptoms included, tremor, slowness of movement, and problems maintaining balance. A key feature of the syndrome is dizziness or fainting due to the inability to maintain blood pressure. The underlying cause of the disease is unknown but neurons in the spinal cord have been observed to degenerate.

Resources

BOOKS

Guyton A.C. and J.E. Hall. *Medical Physiology.* Philadelphia, PA: W.B. Saunders Company, 2000.

Powley, Terry L. "Central Control of Autonomic Functions." *Fundamental Neuroscience*, edited by M.J. Zigmond, F. E. Bloom, S. C. Landis, J. L. Roberts, and L. R. Squire. San Diego, CA: Academic Press, 1999, pp.1027–1036.

PERIODICALS

Slaugenhaupt, Susan A., et. al. "Tissue-Specific Expression of a Splicing Mutation in the IKBKAP Gene Causes Familial Dysautonomia." *American Journal of Human Genetics* 68 (March 2001): 6803-6806.

OTHER

Atkins, David L. *The Autonomic Nervous System.* <http://gwis2.circ.gwu.edu/~atkins/Neuroweb/autonomic.html>.

Susan M. Mockus, Ph.D.

Nervous system, somatic

Definition

The somatic nervous system (SNS) is a division of the peripheral nervous system (PNS). The SNS controls voluntary activities, such as movement of **skeletal muscles**. It includes both sensory and motor nerves. Sensory nerves convey nerve impulses from the sense organs to the **central nervous system** (CNS), while motor nerves convey nerve impulses from the CNS to skeletal muscle effectors.

Description

Nervous tissue

All nervous tissue—including that of the SNS—consists of two main cell types: neurons and glial cells. **Neurons** transmit nerve signals and are surrounded by glial cells, that provide mechanical and physical support as well as electrical insulation between neurons.

Neurons

A neuron consists of a cell body, the soma, which contains the nucleus and surrounding cytoplasm, several short thread-like projections, called dendrites, and of one long filament, called the axon. The dendrites receive information from other nearby cells and transmit the signals to the soma and the axon carries signals away from the neuron. Both axons and dendrites are surrounded by a white protective coating called the myelin sheath. The average adult **brain** contains about 100 billion neurons. Neurons are also the longest cells of the body, a single axon can be several feet long. There are two types of neu-

rons found in the SNS: sensory neurons, which typically have long dendrites and short axons, and carry messages from sensory receptors to the CNS, and motor neurons, which have a long axon and short dendrites and transmit signals from the CNS to muscles or glands.

The nervous system

The nervous system of the human body is divided into the central nervous system (CNS), consisting of the **spinal cord** and brain, and the peripheral nervous system (PNS), consisting of all the nerves that connect the CNS with organs, muscles, **blood vessels** and glands. The PNS is subdivided into the somatic nervous system (SNS) and the **autonomic nervous system** (ANS). The ANS is further divided by function into sympathetic and parasympathetic systems.

The somatic nervous system (SNS)

The somatic nervous system (SNS) consists of sensory and motor nerve divisions. The sensory division, also called the afferent division, contains neurons that receive signals from the tendons, joints, skin, skeletal muscles, eyes, nose, ears and tongue, and many other tissues and organs. These signals are conveyed to the cranial and spinal nerves. The motor division, also called the efferent division, contains pathways that go from the brain stem and spinal cord to the lower motor neurons of the cranial and spinal nerves. When these nerves are stimulated, they cause the skeletal muscles to contract. This is called voluntary contraction of the skeletal muscles.

The nerves of the sensory-somatic system are:

THE CRANIAL NERVES (12 PAIRS).

• olfactory nerve, a sensory nerve for the sense of **smell**

• optic nerve, a sensory nerve for **vision**

• oculomotor nerve, a motor nerve for eyelid and eyeball muscle control

• trochlear nerve, a motor nerve for eyeball muscle control

• trigeminal nerve, a mixed nerve, the sensory part for facial and mouth sensation and the motor part for chewing

• abducens nerve, a motor nerve for eyeball movement control

• facial nerve, a mixed nerve, the sensory part for **taste** and the motor part for the control of facial muscles and salivary glands

• auditory nerve, a sensory nerve for **hearing** and balance control

Axon—Long filament of a neuron that carries outgoing electrical signals from the cell body towards target cells. Each neuron has one axon, which can be longer than a foot. Neurons communicate with each other by transmitting signals from branches located at the end of their axons. At the end of the axons, nerve impulses are transmitted to other nerve cells or to effector organs.

Brachial plexus—A group of lower neck and upper back spinal nerves supplying the arm, forearm and hand.

Brain stem—Lowest part of the brain that connects with the spinal cord. It is a complicated neural center with several neuronal pathways between the cerebrum, spinal cord, cerebellum, and motor and sensory functions of the head and neck. It consists of the medulla oblongata, the part responsible for cardiac and respiratory control, the midbrain, which is involved in basic, involuntary body functions, and the pons, where some cranial nerves originate.

Central nervous system (CNS)—One of two major divisions of the nervous system. The CNS consists of the brain, the cranial nerves and the spinal cord.

Cranial nerve—In humans, there are 12 cranial nerves. They are connected to the brain stem and basically 'run' the head as well as help regulate the organs of the thoracic and abdominal cavities.

Dendrites—Threadlike extensions of the cytoplasm of a neuron.

Effector—Any molecule, chemical, organ, structure or agent that regulates a pathway by changing the pathway's reaction rate.

Ganglia—A mass of nerve tissue or a group of neurons.

Mechanoreceptors—Receptors specialized to detect mechanical signals and relay that information centrally in the nervous system. Mechanoreceptors include hair cells involved in hearing and balance.

Myelin—The substance making up the protective sheath of nerve axons.

Nervous system—The entire system of nerve tissue in the body. It includes the brain, the brain stem, the spinal cord, the nerves and the ganglia, and is divided into the peripheral nervous system (PNS) and the central nervous system (CNS).

Neurons—Cells of the nervous system. Usually consist of a cell body, the soma, that contains the nucleus and the surrounding cytoplasm; several short thread-like projections (dendrites); and one long filament (the axon)

Neuropathy—A general term describing functional disorders and/or abnormal changes in the peripheral nervous system. If the involvement is in one nerve it is called mononeuropathy, and if in several nerves, mononeuropathy multiplex.

Oculomotor nerve—Cranial nerve responsible for motor enervation of the upper eyelid muscle, the extraocular muscle and the eye pupil muscle.

Parasympathetic nervous system—One of the two divisions of the autonomic nervous system. Parasympathetic nerves emerge from the skull as fibres from the oculomotor, facial, glossopharyngeal and vagus nerves and from the sacral region of the spinal cord.

Peripheral nerves—The nerves outside of the brain and spinal cord, including the autonomic, cranial, and spinal nerves. These nerves contain cells other than neurons and connective tissue as well as axons.

Peripheral nervous system (PNS)—One of the two major divisions of the nervous system. The PNS consists of the somatic nervous system (SNS), which controls voluntary activities, and of the autonomic nervous system (ANS), which controls regulatory activities. The ANS is further divided into sympathetic and parasympathetic systems.

Plexus—A network or group of nerves.

Sensory cells—Cells that contain receptors on their surface.

Sensory nerve—A nerve that receives input from sensory cells, such as the skin mechanoreceptors or the muscle receptors.

Spinal cord—Elongated part of the central nervous system that lies in the vertebral column and from which the spinal nerves emerge.

Sympathetic nervous system—One of the two divisions of the autonomic nervous system. The sympathetic neurons have their cell bodies in the thoracic and lumbar regions of the spinal cord and connect to the paravertebral chain of sympathetic ganglia. They innervate heart and blood vessels, sweat glands, organs and the adrenal medulla.

- glossopharyngeal, a mixed nerve, the sensory part for taste and the motor part for the control of swallowing

- vagus, a mixed nerve, main PNS nerve that controls the gut, **heart** and larynx

- accessory, a motor nerve for swallowing and moving the head and shoulders

- hypoglossal, a motor nerve for the control of tongue muscles

THE SPINAL NERVES (31 PAIRS). All of the spinal nerves are mixed nerves containing both sensory and motor neurons. They consist of eight cervical, 12 thoracic, five lumbar, five sacral, and one coccygeal. In spinal nerves, some nerves fibers are ascending, meaning that they carry messages to the brain, while others are descending, meaning that they carry messages from the brain.

Sensory input to the nervous system occurs through the senses, which are: vision, taste, smell, touch and hearing, also called the *special senses*. Additional input is provided by the *somatic senses*, which are **pain**, temperature, and pressure. This sensory input uses sensors, also called sensory receptors. The major sensory receptors are:

- mechanoreceptors that respond to hearing and stretching

- photoreceptors that are sensitive to light

- chemoreceptors that respond mostly to smell and taste

- thermoreceptors that are sensitive to changes in temperature

- electroreceptors that detect electrical currents in the environment

Function

The major function of the SNS is the voluntary control of the muscle system of the body and the processing of sensory information to the CNS. All conscious knowledge of the external world and all the motor activity performed by the body to respond to it operates through the SNS.

Role in human health

The overall role of the nervous system is to act as an internal communications system that allows the body to react to environmental changes and to perform all activities required to maintain life. The PNS is the message carrier between the CNS and the rest of the body and it can not function with an impaired SNS. Thus, the role of the SNS in human health is crucial.

Common diseases and disorders

Somatic nervous system diseases are diseases of the peripheral nerves that are external to the brain and spinal cord. Thus, they include diseases of the nerve roots, ganglia, sensory and motor nerves. A functional disorder and/or abnormal change that occurs in any region of the peripheral nervous system is called a *neuropathy*. If the involvement is in one nerve only, it is called a mononeuropathy, and if in several nerves, mononeuropathy multiplex or polyneuropathy. The most common disorders are the following:

- Brachial plexus neuropathies: Diseases of the peripheral nerve components of the brachial plexus, a group of lower neck and upper back spinal nerves supplying the arm, forearm and hand. Symptoms include local pain, muscle weakness, and decreased sensation (hypesthesia) in the upper extremity.

- Cranial nerve diseases: Disorders and diseases of the cranial nerves.

- Cranial nerve neoplasms: Benign or cancerous growth in cranial nerve tissues. Examples are: acoustic neuroma, optic nerve glioma, optic nerve meningioma.

- Diabetic neuropathies: Peripheral and cranial nerve disorders that are associated with diabetes. A common condition associated with diabetic neuropathy includes third nerve palsy, which affects the oculomotor nerve.

- Guillain-Barre syndrome: An acute inflammatory autoimmune neuritis caused by the body attacking the myelin coating of its own peripheral nerves. The syndrome often occurs as a result of viral or bacterial **infection**, surgery, immunization, lymphoma, or exposure to toxins.

- Mononeuropathies: Disease or trauma involving a single peripheral nerve. Mononeuropathies result from a wide variety of causes such as traumatic injury; nerve compression, and connective tissue diseases.

- Myasthenia gravis (MG): MG (and also the less common Lambert-Eaton syndrome) are neuromuscular junction diseases, that is, diseases affecting how nerve impulses are transmitted to muscle at the neuromuscular junction. They are autoimmune diseases, meaning that the body generates an **immune system** attack against its own skeletal muscles.

- Nerve compression syndromes: These syndromes are due to the compression of nerves or nerve roots from internal or external causes and result in the blocking of nerve impulses due to myelin sheath or axon damage.

- Neuralgia: Neuralgias are disorders of the cranial nerves that result in intense or aching pain occuring along a peripheral or cranial nerve. Neuralgias are associated with all of the cranial nerves: trigeminal neuralgia in the facial area, glossopharyngeal neuralgia in the throat, occipital neuralgia in the rear and side of the head, geniculate neuralgia in the ear, and vegal neuralgia in the jaw.

- Neuritis: Inflammation of a peripheral or cranial nerve.

- Peripheral nervous system neoplasms: Benign or cancerous growths that arise from peripheral nerve tissue. They include neurofibromas, granular cell tumors and malignant peripheral nerve sheath tumors.

- Trigeminal neuralgia (TN): Most common neuralgia. It affects the fifth cranial (trigeminal) nerve and causes episodes of intense, stabbing, electric shock-like pain in the areas of the face where the branches of the nerve are distributed, that is lips, eyes, nose, scalp, forehead, upper jaw, and lower jaw.

Resources

BOOKS

Afifi, A. K. and R. A. Bergman. *Functional Neuroanatomy: Text and Atlas.* New York: McGraw Hill, 1999.

Rowland, L. P., ed. *Textbook of Neurology,* 9th ed. Media: Williams and Wilkins, 1995.

Senneff, John A. *Numb Toes and Aching Soles: Coping with Peripheral Neuropathy.* San Antonio: Medpress, 1999.

PERIODICALS

Vaillancourt, P. D., and Langevin, H. M. "Painful peripheral neuropathies." *The Medical Clinics of North America* 83 (1999): 627-642.

ORGANIZATIONS

Guillain-Barre Syndrome Foundation International, P.O. Box 262, Wynnewood, PA 19096. (610) 667-0131. Fax: (610) 667-7036.

National Institute of Neurological Disorders and Stroke. NIH Neurological Institute, P.O. Box 5801, Bethesda, MD 20824. (800) 352-9424.

Neuropathy Association. 60 East 42nd Street, Suite 942, New York, NY 10165-0999. (212) 692-0662; (800)-247-6968. info@neuropathy.org. <http://www.neuropathy.org>.

OTHER

Kimball's Biology Pages. "The Sensory-Somatic Nervous System." <http://www.ultranet.com/~jkimball/BiologyPages/P/PNS.html#sensory-somatic>.

NINDS Peripheral Neuropathy Information Page. <http://www.ninds.nih.gov/health_and_medical/disorders/peripheralneuropathy_doc.htm>.

Monique Laberge, Ph.D.

Neural tube defect

Definition

Neural tube defects, or NTDs, are a group of severe birth defects in which the **brain** and **spinal cord** are malformed and lack the protective encasement of soft tissue and bone. They are called neural tube defects because they develop out of a tube formed in the early embryo by the closure of the outer germ layer of tissue. This tube later develops into the brain and spinal cord.

Description

Incomplete formation and protection of the brain or spinal cord with bony and soft tissue coverings that occur during the fourth week of embryo formation are known collectively as neural tube defects. These lesions may occur anywhere in the midline of the head or spine. Neural tube defects are among the most common serious birth defects, but they vary considerably in their severity. In some cases, the brain or spinal cord is completely exposed; in some cases it is protected by a tough membrane (meninges); and in other cases it is covered by skin.

Spina bifida is a congenital defect that accounts for about two-thirds of all neural tube defects. Its name comes from two Latin words that mean "cloven backbone." The spinal defect may appear anywhere from the neck to the buttocks. In its most severe form, termed "spinal rachischisis," the entire spinal canal is open, exposing the spinal cord and nerves. More commonly, the defect appears as a localized mass on the back that is covered by skin or by the meninges.

Anencephaly, the second most common neural tube defect, accounts for about one-third of cases. Two major subtypes occur. In the most severe form, all of the **skull** bones are missing and the brain is exposed in its entirety. The second form, in which only a part of the skull is missing and a portion of the brain exposed, is termed "meroacrania."

Encephaloceles are the least common form of neural tube defects, comprising less than 10% of the total. With encephaloceles, a portion of the skull bones is missing, leaving a bony hole through which the brain and brain coverings herniate, or protrude abnormally. Encephaloceles occur in the midline from the base of the nose to the junction of the skull and neck. As with spina bifida, the severity of encephaloceles varies greatly. At the mildest end of the spectrum, an encephalocele may appear as only a small area of faulty skin development with or without any underlying skull defect. At the severe end of the spectrum, most

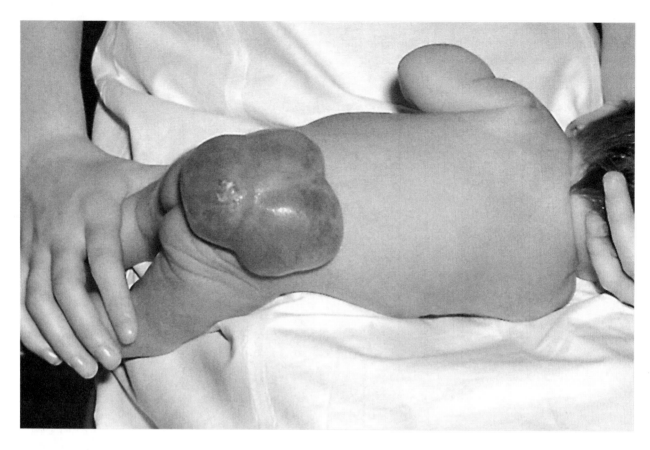

An infant with spina bifida. *(Photograph by Biophoto Associates, Photo Researchers, Inc. Reproduced by permission.)*

of the brain may be herniated outside of the skull into a skin-covered sac.

Genetic profile

Most neural tube defects (80–90%) occur as isolated events. In the United States and Canada, NTDs occur in the Caucasian population in about 1.5 of every 1,000 live births. Neural tube defects of this variety are believed to arise through the combined influence of genetic and environmental forces. This multifactorial causation presumes that one or more predisposing genes collaborate with one or more environmental influences to result in the birth defect. Poor **nutrition** is believed to be an environmental risk factor; hereditary defects in the absorption and utilization of **folic acid** are presumptive genetic predisposing factors. After a couple has one infant with a neural tube defect, the risk of recurrence is 3–5%. After the birth of two infants affected with neural tube defects, the risk increases to 8–10%. A parent with a multifactorial NTD has a 3–4% chance of having a child with an NTD.

When neural tube defects occur concurrently with other malformations, there is a greater likelihood of an underlying specific genetic or environmental cause.

Genetic causes include chromosome aberrations and single gene mutations. Environmental causes include maternal **diabetes mellitus**, exposure to prolonged hyperthermia, and taking seizure medications during the early months of **pregnancy**.

Demographics

Neural tube defects occur worldwide. It appears that the highest prevalence (about one in 100 pregnancies) exists in certain northern provinces in China; an intermediate prevalence (about one in 300–500 pregnancies) has been found in Ireland and in Central and South America; the lowest prevalence (fewer than one in 2,000 pregnancies) has been found in the Scandinavian countries. In the United States, the highest prevalence tends to occur in the Southeast. Worldwide there has been a steady downward trend in prevalence rates over the past 50–70 years.

Causes and symptoms

Because of the incorrect development of the spinal cord and nerves, a number of consequences are commonly seen in spina bifida. As a rule, the nerves below the level of the defect develop in an abnormal manner and fail to function, resulting in **paralysis** and loss of sensation below the level of the spinal lesion. Since most defects occur in the lumbar region, the lower limbs are paralyzed and lack normal sensation. Furthermore, the bowel and bladder have inadequate nerve connections, leading to the inability to control bladder and bowel function. Sexual function is likewise impaired. Hydrocephaly, which is an abnormal accumulation of fluid within the ventricles or cavities of the brain, develops in most of these infants either before or after surgical repair of the spine defect.

In anencephaly, the brain is destroyed by its exposure during intrauterine life. Most infants with anencephaly are stillborn or die within the first few days or weeks after birth.

Infants with encephaloceles have variable neurologic impairments depending on the extent of brain involvement. When only the brain covering is involved, the individual may escape any adverse effect. When the brain is involved in the defect, however, impairments of the special senses such as sight and **hearing**, as well as cognitive impairments, commonly result.

Diagnosis

At birth, the diagnosis of a neural tube defect is usually obvious based on external findings. Prenatal diagnosis may be made with ultrasound examination after 12–14 weeks of pregnancy. Screening of pregnancies can be carried out at 16 weeks by testing the mother's **blood** for the level of alpha-fetoprotein. Open neural tube defects leak this fetal chemical into the surrounding amniotic fluid, a small portion of which is absorbed into the mother's blood.

Treatment

No treatment is available for anencephaly. Aggressive surgical and medical management has improved survival and function of infants with spina bifida. Surgery closes the defect, providing protection against injury and **infection**. Walking may be achieved with orthopedic devices. A common complication that may occur before or after surgical correction is the accumulation of excessive cerebral spinal fluid (hydrocephaly) in the major cavities within the brain. Hydrocephaly is usually treated with the placement of a mechanical shunt, which allows cerebral spinal fluid from the ventricles to drain into the circulation or into another body cavity. A number of medical and surgical procedures have been used to protect the **urinary system**. Encephaloceles are usually repaired by surgery

---

KEY TERMS

Anencephaly—Absence of all or a portion of the bones of the skull.

Embryo—An organism during an early development period when organs and other specialized structures are being formed. In humans, the embryonic period is considered to be the first eight weeks after conception.

Encephalocele—A hole in the bony covering of the spinal cord through which portions of the brain, spinal cord or meninges may herniate.

Folic acid—A water-soluble vitamin that is essential to the formation of purine and thymine in the body. A deficiency of folic acid causes a form of anemia.

Herniate—To protrude abnormally through an opening in bone or surrounding tissues.

Hydrocephaly—An abnormal accumulation of cerebrospinal fluid in the cavities of the brain.

Meninges—The three-layered membrane that covers the brain and spinal cord.

Neural tube—A tube that forms in the early embryo when the outer germ layer of tissue (ectoderm) closes. The neural tube develops into the spinal cord and the brain.

Spina bifida—A congenital defect in the covering of the spine.

Spinal rachischisis—A lack of covering over the entire spinal canal, exposing the spinal cord and nerves.

---

soon after birth. The success of surgery often depends on the amount of brain tissue involved in the encephalocele.

It has been found that 400 mcg of folic acid taken for two to three months prior to conception and two to three months following conception protects the fetus against most neural tube defects. While there are a number of foods (green leafy vegetables, legumes, liver, orange juice) that are good sources of natural folic acid, synthetic folic acid is available in over-the-counter multivitamins and a number of fully fortified breakfast cereals.

In addition, a population-wide increase in folic acid intake has been achieved through the fortification of enriched cereal grain flours since January 1998, a measure authorized by the U.S. Food and Drug Administration. The increased blood levels of folic acid in the general population achieved in recent years has likely resulted from the synergy of dietary, supplementation, and fortification sources.

Prognosis

The prognosis for infants with anencephaly is grim; they are usually stillborn or die within the first days of life. In contrast, 80–90% of infants with spina bifida survive with surgery. Paralysis below the level of the defect, including an inability to control bowel and bladder function, and hydrocephaly are complications experienced by most infants who survive. Intellectual function, however, is normal in most cases.

The prognosis for infants with encephaloceles varies considerably. Small encephaloceles may cause no disability whether surgical correction is performed or not. Infants with larger encephaloceles may have residual impairment of **vision**, hearing, nerve function, and intellectual capacity.

Health care team roles

Pediatricians, family physicians, obstetricians, or nurse midwives usually diagnose previously unknown neural tube defects at birth. Testing maternal blood for alpha-fetoproteins can often diagnose neural tube defects. Surgeons often repair neural tube defects. Physical therapists, social workers, and counselors may provide ongoing care to children with neural tube defects and their families. Support groups are often helpful to these families.

Prevention

Taking folic acid supplements (400 mcg per day) from two to three months prior to conception and the first trimester of pregnancy offers some protection against many neural tube defects. Pregnant women should be advised to avoid certain medications and recreational drugs, especially some anticonvulsants and hallucinogens.

Resources

BOOKS

Adams, Raymond D, Maurice Victor, and Allan Ropper. *Adams' and Victor's Principles of Neurology*, 6th ed. New York: McGraw-Hill, 1997.

Cunningham, F. Gary, et al. *Williams Obstetrics*, 21st ed. New York: McGraw-Hill, 2001.

Elias, Sherman, Joe Leigh Simpson, and Allan T. Bombard. "Amniocentesis and Fetal Blood Sampling." In *Genetic Disorders in the Fetus: Diagnosis, Prevention, and Treatment*, 5th ed., edited by Aubrey Milunsky. Baltimore, MD: Johns Hopkins University Press, 1998.

Haslam, Robert H. A. "Neural tube defects." In *Nelson Textbook of Pediatrics*, 16th ed., edited by Richard E. Behrman et al. Philadelphia: Saunders, 2000.

"Multifactorial Inheritance." Chapter 286 in *The Merck Manual of Diagnosis and Therapy*, edited by Mark H. Beers, MD, and Robert Berkow, MD. Whitehouse Station, NJ: Merck Research Laboratories, 1999.

Rapp, Rayna. *Testing Women, Testing the Fetus: The Social Impact of Amniocentesis in America.* New York: Routledge, 2000.

Shannon, Joyce B. "Amniocentesis and chorionic villus sampling (CVS)." In *Health Reference Series, Medical Tests Sourcebook.*, ed. Joyce B. Shannon. Detroit, MI, Omnigraphics, Inc., 1999.

PERIODICALS

Gelabert-Gonzalez M, Cutrin-Prieto JM, Garcia-Allut A. "Spinal arachnoid cyst without neural tube defect." *Children's Nervous System* 17, no. 3 (2001): 179-181.

Gross SM, Caufield LA, Kinsman SL, Ireys HT. "Inadequate folic acid intakes are prevalent among young women with neural tube defects." *Journal of American Dietetic Association* 101, no. 3 (2001): 342-345.

Hernandez-Diaz S, Werler MM, Walker AM, Mitchell AA. "Neural tube defects in relation to use of folic acid antagonists during pregnancy." *American Journal of Epidemiology* 153, no. 10 (2001): 961-968.

Richter B, Stegmann K, Roper B, Boddeker I, Ngo ET, Koch MC. "Interaction of folate and homocysteine pathway genotypes evaluated in susceptibility to neural tube defects (NTD) in a German population." *Journal of Human Genetics* 46, no. 3 (2001): 105-109.

van der Put NM, van Straaten HW, Trijbels FJ, Blom HJ. "Folate, homocysteine and neural tube defects: An overview." *Experimental Biology and Medicine (Maywood)* 226, no. 4 (2001): 243-270.

Viner-Brown SI, Cain R, Simon PR. "Open neural tube defects among newborns in Rhode Island." *Medicine and Health in Rhode Island* 84, no. 4 (2001): 138-139.

ORGANIZATIONS

American Academy of Neurology. 1080 Montreal Avenue, St. Paul, MN 55116. (651) 695-1940. Fax: (651) 695-2791. <http://www.aan.com>. info@aan.org.

American Academy of Pediatrics. 141 Northwest Point Boulevard, Elk Grove Village, IL 60007-1098. (847) 434-4000. Fax: (847) 434-8000. <http://www.aap.org/default.htm>. kidsdoc@aap.org.

American Association for Clinical Chemistry. 2101 L Street, NW - Suite 202, Washington, DC 20037-1558. (800) 892-1400 or (202) 857-0717. Fax: (202) 887-5093. <http://www.aacc.org>. info@aacc.org.

American Board of Obstetrics and Gynecology. 2915 Vine Street Suite 300, Dallas, TX 75204. (214) 871-1619. Fax: (214) 871-1943. <http://www.abog.org>. info@abog.org.

American College of Obstetricians and Gynecologists. 409 12th St., S.W., PO Box 96920, Washington, DC 20090-6920. <http://www.acog.org>.

American Society for Reproductive Medicine. 1209 Montgomery Highway, Birmingham, AL 35216-2809. (205) 978-5000. <http://www.asrm.com>.

OTHER

Arc. <http://www.thearc.org/faqs/folicqa.html>.

Association for Spina Bifida and Hydrocephalus. <http://www.asbah.org/folicacid.html>.

Centers for Disease Control and Prevention. <http://www.cdc.gov/ncbddd/folicacid>.

Columbia Presbyterian Medical Center. <http://cpmcnet.columbia.edu/texts/gcps/gcps0052.html>.

National Library of Medicine. <http://www.nlm.nih.gov/medlineplus/neuraltubedefects.html>.

Surgical Tutor. <http://www.surgical-tutor.org.uk/default-home.htm>.

L. Fleming Fallon, Jr., MD, DrPH

Neuroleptics *see* **Antipsychotic drugs**

Neuromuscular physical therapy

Definition

Neuromuscular **physical therapy** involves the examination, treatment, and instruction of persons in order to detect, assess, prevent, correct, alleviate, and limit physical disability and bodily malfunction.

Purpose

The purpose of neuromuscular physical therapy is to help individuals experiencing structural distortion, biomechanical dysfunction, and the accompanying **pain** that is often symptomatic of the underlying problem. It is used to locate and release tissue spasms and hypercontraction; eliminate trigger points that cause referred pain; restore postural alignment, proper biomechanics and flexibility to the tissues; rebuild the strength of injured tissues and assist venous and lymphatic flow.

Precautions

A physician's referral is recommended.

Description

The practice of neuromuscular physical therapy includes the administration, interpretation, and evaluation of tests; measurements of bodily functions and structures; and the planning, administration, evaluation, and modification of treatment and instruction, including the use of physical measures, activities, and devices, for preventive and therapeutic purposes. Neuromuscular physical therapy may also be referred to as neuromuscular reeducation, physical therapy, or physiotherapy.

Neuromuscular physical therapy is employed to treat patients with a variety of health conditions and diseases including accident victims, and individuals with disabling conditions such as low back pain, arthritis, **heart** disease, **fractures**, head injuries, and **cerebral palsy**.

In an effort to restore, maintain, and promote overall fitness and health, neuromuscular physical therapists examine patients' medical histories, test and measure patients' strength, range of motion, balance, coordination, posture, muscle performance, respiration, and motor function. Neuromuscular physical therapists determine patients' ability to be independent and reintegrate into the community or workplace. Based on a patient's medical history and test results, therapists develop treatment plans that describe treatment strategy, purpose, and anticipated outcome.

Neuromuscular physical therapy treatment often includes **exercise** for patients who have been immobilized or who lack flexibility, strength, or endurance. As part of the treatment, patients are encouraged to improve flexibility, range of motion, strength, balance, coordination, and endurance. The goal is to improve an individual's function at work and home.

Neuromuscular physical therapy may involve the use of electrical stimulation, hot packs, cold compresses, or ultrasound to relieve pain and reduce swelling. Traction or deep-tissue massage may be employed to relieve pain. Patients are instructed in the use of assistive and adaptive devices including crutches, prostheses, and wheelchairs. Patients are often shown how to perform exercises to do at home.

During treatment, neuromuscular physical therapists document the patient's progress, conduct periodic examinations, and modify treatments when necessary. Therapists rely on this documentation to track the patient's progress, and identify areas requiring more or less attention.

Neuromuscular physical therapy may be used to treat a wide range of patients with conditions presenting in areas such as pediatrics, geriatrics, orthopedics, sports medicine, neurology, and cardiopulmonary physical therapy.

Length of treatment varies depending upon several factors, including the severity of the condition being treated. Treatment costs also vary depending upon a number of factors including geographic location and the diagnostic tests conducted. Many insurance policies cover neuromuscular physical therapy treatments provided that a physician's referral is obtained prior to treatment.

There are a number of alternative neuromuscular therapies. Among the most popular are the following:

Alexander technique

The goal of this discipline is to bring the body's muscles into natural harmony. Hence it can aid in the treatment of a wide variety of neurological and musculoskeletal conditions, including disorders of the neck, back and hip; traumatic and repetitive strain injuries; chronic pain; arthritis; breathing and coordination disorders; **stress** related disorders; and even migraine.

People with **sciatica**, **scoliosis**, **osteoporosis**, **osteoarthritis**, rheumatoid arthritis, and neck and low back syndrome may find the Alexander technique useful in improving overall strength and mobility. Others with Lyme disease, chronic fatigue syndrome, lupus, or **fibromyalgia** may use it for **pain management**. It is also used to improve functioning in people with **multiple sclerosis**, stroke, or **Parkinson's disease**. Because the technique requires active participation by the patient, it is impossible to test its effectiveness with conventional scientific procedures.

Aston patterning

This specialized program of physical training and massage is designed to relieve muscle tension and pain, speed recovery from injuries, and aid in general **relaxation** and stress reduction. It is particularly appropriate for such problems as back and neck pain, headache, and repetitive stress injuries like tennis elbow.

Like most forms of bodywork and movement training, Aston patterning does not lend itself to controlled clinical trials, and its effectiveness has therefore not been scientifically verified. Furthermore, it requires a significant patient commitment; it involves much more than a program of passive massage.

Feldenkrais

The Feldenkrais method is a supportive therapy that may help in situations where improved movement patterns (and awareness of those patterns) can help with recovery from illness or injury. Practitioners consider it useful for many types of chronic pain, including headache, temporomandibular joint disorder, other joint disorders, and neck, shoulder, and back pain. It is sometimes used as supportive therapy for people with neuromuscular disorders, such as multiple sclerosis, cerebral palsy and stroke. It is also helpful for improving balance, coordination, and mobility. Many athletes, dancers, and other performers use the Feldenkrais method as part of their overall conditioning.

Hellerwork

Hellerwork is a combination of deep tissue massage and movement reeducation. It is advocated by its practitioners for a variety of problems related to muscle tension and stress. Hellerwork is said to relieve respiratory problems, **sports injuries**, and pain in the back, neck, and shoulders. Like most forms of bodywork, it has undergone little in the way of scientific testing.

Trager

This light, gentle form of massage seeks to release deeply ingrained tensions, promoting a sense of relaxation and freedom. It may be helpful for those with chronic neuromuscular pain, including back problems and sciatica, and it has also been advocated for stress-related conditions, high **blood pressure**, strokes, migraine, and **asthma**. Proponents say that it can benefit patients with polio, multiple sclerosis, and **muscular dystrophy** as well.

Preparation

There are no typical pre-treatment preparations. However, a physician's referral is recommended.

Aftercare

Patients are often shown how to perform exercises to do at home.

Results

There are a number of beneficial results realized through neuromuscular therapy, including decreased body toxicity, greater flexibility, greater freedom of movement, increased circulation, increased energy and vitality, increased sense of well-being, and improved postural patterns.

Health care team roles

Neuromuscular physical therapists often consult and practice with physicians, dentists, nurses, educators, social workers, occupational therapists, speech-language pathologists, rehabilitation counselors, vocational counselors, and audiologists.

Neuromuscular physical therapists practice in hospitals, clinics, and private offices. They may also treat patients in the patient's home or at school.

Over two-thirds of neuromuscular physical therapists are employed in either hospitals or physical therapists' offices. Other work settings include home health agencies, outpatient rehabilitation centers, physicians' offices and clinics, and **nursing homes**. Some neuromuscular physical therapists maintain a private practice and provide services to individual patients or contract to provide services in hospitals, rehabilitation centers, nursing homes, home health agencies, adult daycare programs, or schools. They may be engaged in individual practice or be part of a consulting group. Some therapists teach in academic institutions and conduct research.

Neuromuscular physical therapists are required to pass a licensure exam after graduating from an accredited educational program before they can practice.

According to the American Physical Therapy Association, in 1999 there were 189 accredited programs. Of the accredited programs, 24 offered bachelor's degrees, 157 offered master's degrees, and eight offered doctoral degrees. By 2002 the Commission on Accreditation in Physical Therapy Education will require all physical therapist programs seeking accreditation to offer degrees at the master's degree level.

Resources

BOOKS

American Physical Therapy Association. *Guide to Physical Therapist Practice, 2nd Edition.* American Physical Therapy Association., 2001.

Carr, Janet and Shepherd, Roberta. *Movement Science: Foundations for Physical Therapy in Rehabilitation, 2nd Edition.* Aspen Publishers, Inc. 2000.

ORGANIZATIONS

American Center for the Alexander Technique (ACAT). 129 West 67th Street New York, NY 10023. 212-799-0468.

American Physical Therapy Association, 1111 North Fairfax Street, Alexandria, VA 22314-1488. <http://www.apta.org>.

Aston Training Center. P.O. Box 3568 Inclined Village, NV 89450. 702-831-8228.

Feldenkrais Guild. P.O. Box 489 Albany, OR 97321. 503-926-0981 or 800-775-2118.

Hellerwork. 406 Berry St. Mount Shasta, CA 96067. 916-926-2500.

Trager Institute. 33 Millwood Mill Valley, CA 94941. 415-388-2688.

Bill Asenjo, PhD, CRC

Neuromuscular electrical stimulation *see* **Electrotherapy**

Neurons

Definition

A neuron is a specialized cell of the nervous system designed to rapidly communicate with other neurons and organs by sending chemical and electrical signals.

Description

The nervous system contains two major types of cells, neurons and glia. Neurons are specialized cells of the central and peripheral nervous systems that play key roles in transmitting and propagating information from one neuron to another. The role of glial cells is less clear, but they are involved in supporting the functions of the neuron. There are many different types of neurons, such as motor neurons, sensory neurons, and interneurons. Each class of neuron is specially designed to perform certain functions, and therefore neuronal populations differ in structure and chemical composition. Most neurons are polarized, which means that fibers extend from the cell in a certain direction or orientation. Polarization is determined by the direction and length of structures unique to neurons, which are axons, dendrites, and the cell body.

Neurons are similar to other types of cells in that they contain all the basic cell organelles such as a nucleus, mitochondria, ribosomes, lysosomes, endoplasmic reticulum, and Golgi apparatus. However, neurons differentiate into polarized cells that contain three basic structural components: cell body (soma), axon, and dendrites. The cell body contains the nucleus and other cellular organelles and is the major place where protein synthesis occurs.

Dendrites are branched fibers extending from the cell body. The number and organization of dendrites is unique to each neural population and most neurons extend multiple dendrites that are relatively short processes. Dendrites contain small protrusions called spines. These spines express protein receptors on the sur-

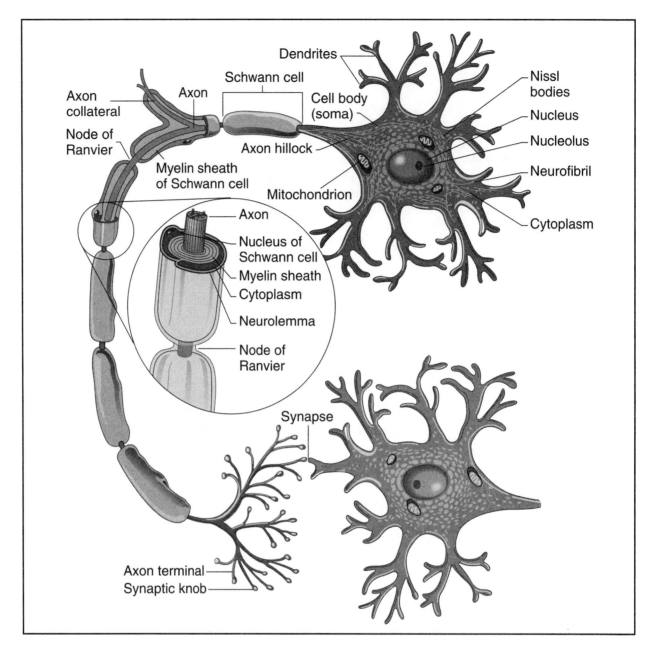

Neuron. *(Diagram by Hans & Cassidy. Courtesy of Gale Group.)*

face that are capable of responding to chemical neurotransmitters such as acetylcholine. The dendritic spines contact axon terminals of other neurons at a connection point called a synapse. The dendrites send this chemical information to the cell body. The cell body integrates the chemical signal from all the dendrites and generates an electrical signal called an axon potential that is sent down the length of the axon to signal the next neuron.

The axon is a fiber neurite process that extends from the cell body and can be up to a meter in length. The axon protrudes from a bulge at the base of the cell body at a region called the axon hillock. Most neurons have only one axon but may have hundreds of dendrites. The axon is specially designed to send electrical signals known as action potentials down the length of the axon to the axon terminals. The axon terminal releases chemical neurotransmitters in response to the action potential onto the dendrite of another neuron. The place where the axon terminal of one neuron meets the dendrite of another neuron is called a synapse. The axon contains a cytoskeletal structure designed to transport **proteins** and other molecules down the length of the axon to the axon terminal and from the axon terminal back up to the cell

Zigmond M.J., F.E. Bloom, S.C. Landis, J.L. Roberts, and L.R. Squire. *Fundamental Neuroscience.* San Diego, CA: Academic Press, 1999.

Susan M. Mockus, Ph.D.

KEY TERMS

Axon—A fiber process extended from the neuronal cell body that carries action potentials.

Dendrite—A branch-like projection from the cell body of a neuron.

Synapse—Meeting place between the axon terminal of one neuron and the dendrite of another neuron.

body. This cytoskeletal structure is composed of actin filaments, neurofilaments, and microtubules.

Function

Neurons are specially designed to communicate with other neurons by converting chemical signals into electrical ones. This is accomplished by the axon. A covering called myelin insulates the outside of the axon. Myelin is a sheath of stacked membranes and is very high in lipid. Axon myleination is conduction by the glia, oligodenrocytes, and Schwann cells. There are periodic interruptions in the myelin at the nodes of Ranvier. Electrical signals referred to as action potentials are rapidly transmitted down the axon by jumping from one node of Ranvier to the next. The action potential induces the release of chemical neurotransmitters from the axon terminal. The axon terminal contains vesicles containing packaged neurotransmitters. The action potential triggers the release of neurotransmitters onto the next neuron that then generates an axon potential to propagate the signal for cell-cell communication. This process allows signaling to occur over very long distances within milliseconds.

Common diseases and disorders

Neurons are implicated in numerous nervous system diseases from **Alzheimer's disease** to Huntington's disease to certain types of **brain cancer**. In many neural diseases, neurons degenerate due to abnormalities in basic cellular function. Populations of neurons can also become cancerous, such as in neuroblastomas.

Resources

BOOKS

Behbehani, Michael M. "Biology of Neurons." In *Cell Physiology.* Edited by Nicholas Sperelakis. San Diego, CA: Academic Press, 1998, pp. 429-434.

Neurophysiology

Definition

Neurophysiology is the study of the functions of the nervous system. Clinical neurophysiology is the study of the functions of the nervous system in the clinical setting, for diagnostics, treatment, and intensive care purposes.

Description

Neurophysiology is a broad field of study because many different levels are involved in the overall functioning of the nervous system and its components. For example, the transmission of a nervous impulse across the synapses, or the cleft that connects nerve cells, involves chemical reactions at the cellular level of organization. Understanding how messages are relayed from the **brain** to the hand is best explained at the system level. This involves studying the relationship and pathways between the brain and the organs of the body and the nerves that connect them, both sensory, meaning nerves that receive input from sensors, and motor, meaning the nerves that activate muscle. Thus, neurophysiology studies nervous function ranging from individual nerve cells to the complex behaviors of the **central nervous system**. Additionally, the nervous system not only functions at the cell and system levels of organization, but also at a mechanistic level, that involves the study of the control or regulatory processes that occur.

The neurophysiology of systems

A branch of neurophysiology describes the function of the major system components of the nervous system of the human body at the system level. The overall nervous system of the body consists of the central nervous system (CNS), and the peripheral nervous system (PNS). The neurophysiology of the CNS studies the function of the brain and **spinal cord** while that of the PNS studies the function of all the nerves that connect the CNS with organs, muscles, **blood vessels** and glands. The neurophysiology of the PNS further subdivides into the **somatic nervous system** (SNS) and the **autonomic nervous system** (ANS), with the ANS being further divided by function into the sympathetic and parasympathetic sys-

KEY TERMS

Axon—The part of the nerve cell used to carry impulses away from the cell body.

Electroencephalography (EEG)—Recording of electrical impulses that reflect brain function, used to diagnose extensive variety of nervous system disorders.

Electromyography (EMG)—Electrical testing of nerves and muscles, used to diagnose nervous disorders.

Evoked potentials (EP)—Electrical signals of the nerves, spinal cord and brain in response to light stimulation of the eyes, or sound stimulation of the ears or mild electrical stimulation of the nerves in the arms or legs, used to diagnose nervous system disorders, such as multiple sclerosis, hearing loss, and various spinal cord disorders.

Microneurography—Technique used primarily for research purposes that enable recording of electrical activity of a single axon from the peripheral nerves of awake human subjects.

Nerve condition velocity (NCV)—Technique for studying nerve or muscle disorders, measuring the speed at which nerves transmit signals.

Neurophysiology—The study of the functions of the nervous system.

Polysomnography reduction—Technique used to monitor brain patterns, eye movements, muscle tension, air flow and respiratory effort, oxygen levels and heart beat during sleep to study sleep disorders.

tems. PNS nerves are of two types: the sensory—or afferent—nerves that transmit information from the sensory organs, muscles, joints, internal organs and all other parts of the body to the CNS, and the motor—or efferent—nerves that transmit signals from the CNS to the body, for example, to the muscles or to internal organs.

The neurophysiology of nerve cells

Neurophysiology is also the study of the physiology, structure and function of nerve cells, or **neurons**, meaning how individual neurons receive and transmit information using chemical and electrical signals. The most important feature of neurons as compared to other cell types in the body is their high degree of electrical excitability. The transmission of nervous signals is based

on changes in this electrical excitability, and neurophysiology studies these effects at the cellular level as well as the electrical properties of neurons. It also seeks to understand the differences between the excitability of muscle and nervous tissue. Examples are: the release of neurotransmitters, substances that are activated by the excitation of neurons; the specific chemical features of the various neurotransmitters; the study of the redistribution of charged ions inside and outside nervous cells, including the pumps used to transport them across **cell membranes**; and the properties of the various special channels used for this transport.

The neurophysiology of control mechanisms

The control activities of the nervous system are performed through very complex mechanisms and pathways. In the brain and the spinal cord there are complex regulatory pathways for functions like food and water intake, sleep, **pain**, and muscle control, to name a few. Investigations of such control systems are of central interest in neurophysiology. This includes, for example, the mechanisms involved in the regulation of sleep, pain, breathing, and the **cardiac cycle**. The understanding of these mechanisms provides a basis for understanding changes in the functions that may result in diseases. Also the treatment of diseases, for instance the use of drugs to correct dysfunctions, requires that the underlying mechanisms of the disorder be understood. One of the most important topics of neurophysiology is the study of **feedback systems** that constantly monitor and regulate numerous aspects of body function, such as the levels of oxygen and carbon dioxide, nutrients, hormones, and other chemical substances in the **blood**. Other higher functions, such as language, learning and **memory**, and emotions, while being mostly studied by neuropsychology, are also affected by neurophysiological mechanisms and these aspects are also included in neurophysiology.

Measurement techniques in neurophysiology

The electrical signals of the nervous system propagate throughout the body to control movement, breathing, **heart** rate, and the capacity to think and remember. Neurophysiology also includes all the electrical measuring techniques used to provide information on the function of the brain and nerves. These include:

• Electroencephalography (EEG): EEG is a recording of electrical impulses that reflect brain function. It is used to test for a wide variety of disorders of the nervous system, such as tumor growth and infections as well as the development of the brain in babies and children. EEG is also used in the diagnosis of epilepsy and strokes. EEG is often performed during surgery on the arteries of the neck to ensure that the blood flow to the brain is adequate.

• Evoked potentials (EP): This technique evaluates the condition of nerve pathways. EPs are electrical signals of the nerves, spinal cord, and brain in response to light stimulation of the eyes, sound stimulation of the ears, or mild electrical stimulation of the nerves in the arms or legs. EPs are used to diagnose disorders of the nervous system such as **multiple sclerosis**, **hearing loss**, and various spinal cord disorders. EPs are also used during neurosurgery to locate brain structures or check on the patient's response to surgery.

• Polysomnography (PSG): This technique monitors brain wave patterns, eye movements, muscle tension, air flow, respiratory effort, oxygen levels, and heart beat during sleep. It is mostly used to diagnose and treat various sleep disorders.

• Electromyography (EMG): EMG refers to electrical testing of nerves and muscles. The technique is used to diagnose nervous disorders such as muscle spasticity and pinched nerves in the back or neck as well as other nerve or muscle disorders.

• Nerve conduction velocity (NCV): NCV is another technique used to study nerve or muscle disorders, it measures the speed at which nerves transmit signals.

• Microneurography (MN): Microneurography is mostly used for research purposes, it is a technique that makes it possible to record the electrical activity of a single axon from the peripheral nerves of awake human subjects.

The spectacular advances in knowledge of the nervous system during the past decades and the promising developments in the treatment of nervous disorders have made neurophysiology one of the most active branches of modern biology and medicine. The understanding that neurophysiology provides about nervous system functions from the level of the cell to the level of the systems also makes it the foundation stone of other clinical fields like neurology and psychiatry. The development of drugs to control and cure disease also requires an understanding of how drugs affect the nervous system, which is only possible if the detailed neurophysiology of the systems they target is well understood. Neurophysiology research fulfills that role, thus creating a strong link to neuropharmacology and general health care practice.

Resources

BOOKS

Baddeley, R., Hancock, P. J. B. and P. Foldiak, eds. *Information Theory and the Brain.* New York: Bantam Doubleday Dell, 1999.

Johnston, D. and Samuel Miao-Sin Wu. *Foundations of Cellular Neurophysiology.* Cambridge: MIT Press, 1995.

Levin, K. H. and H. O. Luders. *Comprehensive Clinical Neurophysiology.* Philadelphia: W. B. Saunders Co., 2000.

Nicholls, John G., A. Robert Martin, Bruce G. Wallace, and Paul A. Fuchs. *From Neuron to Brain.* 4th ed. Sunderland: Sinauer and Associates, 1999.

Sanes, D. H., Reh, T. A. and W. A. Harris, eds. *Development of the Nervous System.* New York: Academic Press, 2000.

OTHER

EMG and Nerve Conduction Homepage. <http://www.teleemg.com/>.

Clinical Neurophysiology on the Web. <http://www.neuro-phys.com/>.

Monique Laberge, Ph.D.

Newborn hearing screening

Definition

A newborn **hearing** screening assesses infants for adequate hearing levels.

Purpose

Three out of 1,000 babies are born with permanent **hearing loss**, making congenital hearing impairment the most common birth defect. Without screening, children with dysfunctions in hearing are usually not identified until two and a half to three years of age and many are not diagnosed properly until five to six years of age. A postponement in diagnosis results in considerable delays in the attainment of essential speech, language, social, cognitive, and emotional development skills that are central to later success in school and life. Even children with a hearing impairment in one ear suffer significant detrimental effects and are more likely to be held back at least one grade when compared with a group of children without hearing impairments.

Because simple, cost-effective technology now exists to detect hearing loss in newborns, many hospitals have implemented universal screening programs. When diagnosed shortly after birth, infants can start to wear amplification devices as early as one month of age. Children who were identified prior to six months of age and received early intervention and amplification devices were found to be one to two years ahead in language, cognitive, and social skills as compared to children who were not identified early.

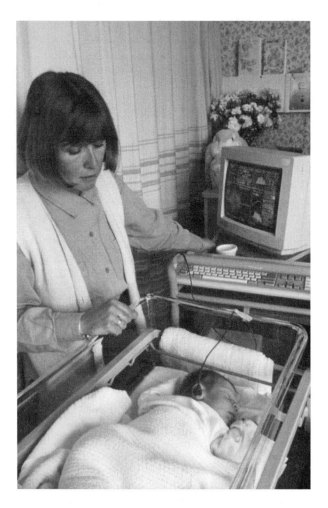

The otoacoustic emission (OAE) test detects the response of the newborn's inner ear to sounds and registers them on the computer. The test can be administered while the baby sleeps. *(Photograph by James King-Holmes. Science Source/Photo Researchers. Reproduced by permission.)*

Description

In 1993, the National Institutes of Health concluded that all newborns should receive screening for hearing impairment. Screening was determined to be most appropriate prior to discharge from the hospital.

Some hospitals screen only newborns who are at risk of hearing loss—about 10% of the population. Risk factors include a history of childhood hearing impairment in the family, **infection** (cytomegalovirus, rubella, herpes, toxoplasmosis, or **syphilis**), congenital malformations of the head or neck, weight at birth less than 3.3 pounds (1,500 grams), severe **jaundice** (hyperbilirubinemia), **antibiotics**, bacterial **meningitis**, and severe asphyxia at birth. Because research has indicated that only about half of children identified as having congenital hearing loss had any risk factors, and because of the availability of

new screening techniques, many hospitals have adopted the universal hearing screening of newborns.

The majority of newborn hearing screening programs use one of three types of equipment: automated auditory brainstem response (AABR), distortion product otoacoustic emissions (DPOAE), or transient evoked otoacoustic emissions (TEOAE).

The general technique for the exam is to place an earphone or probe on the baby's ear and to attach an electrode to the scalp. A sound or click is then transmitted to the baby. A microcomputer or miniature microphone interprets the electrical potential created by the brainstem responding to the sound or the echo from the cochlea (located in the inner ear).

The cost of the equipment ranges from $4,000 to $25,000 for each individual unit. Training of personnel takes approximately two to four hours, and time involved to perform each test varies from 15 minutes to 40 minutes for each baby.

Preparation

If the environment is quiet and the baby is restful, testing results will be the easiest to obtain.

Aftercare

Infants who do not appear to have adequate hearing at the screening should obtain a follow-up hearing evaluation before six months of age.

Results

Results should be the detection of infant hearing loss. It is possible that mild hearing loss will not be detected.

Health care team roles

Any member of the health care team can be trained in administering the test. Generally, most hospitals have nurses involved in the screening process.

Resources

BOOKS

Pilliterri, Adele. *Maternal & Child Health Nursing.* 3rd ed. Philadelphia: Lippincott, 1999.

ORGANIZATIONS

American Speech-Language-Hearing Association (ASHA). 10801 Rockville Pike, Rockville, MD 20852. (888) 321-ASHA. <http://professional.asha.org/index7.htm>.

National Center for Hearing Assessment and Management (NCHAM). Utah State University, 2880 Old Main Hill,

KEY TERMS

Asphyxia—A deficiency of oxygen or state of carbon dioxide over-saturation within the body.

Cochlea—A component of the bony labyrinth of the inner ear that is involved in hearing.

Logan, UT 84322. (435) 797-3584. <http://www.infant-hearing.org/>.

OTHER

Issue Brief: Early Hearing Loss Detection, Diagnosis and Intervention. ASHA, 1999. <http://professional.asha.org/governmental_affairs/issue_walsh.htm>.

Selecting Equipment for a Newborn Hearing Screening Program. NCHAM, 2001. <http://www.infanthearing.org/resources/equipment.html>.

Universal Newborn Hearing Screening: Fact Sheet. NCHAM, 2000. <http://www.infanthearing.org/ehdi/screening.html>.

Nadine M. Jacobson, R.N.

Newborn life support *see* **Ventilation assistance**

Niacin

Description

Niacin, also known as Vitamin B$_3$, is important for the normal function of many bodily processes. Like other B **vitamins**, it is water-soluble and plays a role in turning food into energy, as well as in the **metabolism** of **fats** and **carbohydrates**. Niacin can also act as an antioxidant within cells, which means it can destroy cell-damaging free radicals. In conjunction with **riboflavin** and pyridoxine, it helps to keep the skin, intestinal tract and nervous system functioning smoothly.

General use

The recommended daily allowance (RDA) of niacin for infants under six months is 5 mg. Babies from six months to one year of age require 6 mg. Children need 9 mg at one to three years of age, 12 mg at four to six years, and 13 mg at seven to 10 years. Women need 15 mg at 11–50 years, and 13 mg thereafter. Somewhat more is required for **pregnancy** (17 mg) and **lactation** (20 mg). Men require 17 mg from 11 to 14 years of age, 20 mg from 15 to 18 years, 19 mg from 19 to 50 years, and 15 mg at 51 years and older.

Niacin, in the form of nicotinic acid, can be taken in very large doses to decrease cholesterol and reduce the risk of **heart** attack. The amount required is between 2 and 3 g. This is not a therapy that should be undertaken without professional medical advice and supervision. Certain conditions preclude the use of high doses of niacin. These include **gout**, diabetes, peptic ulcer, **liver** or kidney disease, and high **blood pressure** requiring medication. Even in the absence of these conditions, a patient on high doses of niacin should be closely monitored to be sure the therapy is both effective and without complications. A frequent side effect of this therapy is extreme flushing of the face and neck. It is harmless, but can be unpleasant. An alternative form of nicotinic acid that does not cause flushing is inositol hexaniacinate. "Slow release" niacin also causes less flushing, but should not be taken as there is higher risk of liver inflammation.

There is some evidence that niacinamide used on a long-term basis can prevent the onset of juvenile diabetes in many susceptible children. Those who have been newly diagnosed with juvenile diabetes may also benefit by extending the time that the **pancreas** continues to produce a small amount of insulin. The advice of a health care provider should be sought for these uses.

Inositol hexaniacinate can be helpful for people suffering from intermittent claudication. This condition causes leg **pain** with **exercise** due to poor **blood** flow to the legs. Dilation of the **blood vessels** caused by the inositol hexaniacinate relieves this condition to some extent, allowing the patient to walk farther with less pain.

Other conditions that may be benefited by supplemental niacinamide include vertigo, tinnitus, premenstrual syndrome (PMS) headaches, and **osteoarthritis**. Raynaud's phenomenon reportedly may be improved by large doses of inositol hexaniacinate. A health care provider should be consulted for these uses. Niacin is not effective for the treatment of **schizophrenia**.

Preparations

Natural sources

Tuna is one of the best sources of niacin, but many foods contain it. Most processed grain products are fortified with niacin, as well as other B vitamins. Although niacin is not destroyed by cooking, it does leach into water, so cooking with minimal liquid best preserves it. The amino acid tryptophan is widely found in foods high

KEY TERMS

Antioxidant—Any one of a group of substances which function to destroy cell-damaging free radicals in the body.

Gout—A painful condition of joints, especially the feet and hands, caused by the presence of uric acid crystals.

Myopathy—A disease of muscle tissue.

Sprue—A chronic disease of malabsorption characterized by diarrhea.

in protein, and about half of the tryptophan consumed is used to make niacin. Cottage cheese, milk, fowl, and tuna are some of the foods that are highest in tryptophan.

Supplemental sources

Niacin can be purchased as an oral single vitamin product. A balanced B complex supplement is preferred over high doses of an individual vitamin unless there is a specific indication. Supplements should be stored in a cool, dry place, away from light, and out of the reach of children.

Deficiency

A serious deficiency of niacin causes a condition called pellagra. Once quite common, it has become rare outside of areas where poor **nutrition** is still the norm. The symptoms include dermatitis, **dementia**, and **diarrhea**.

Milder deficiencies of niacin can cause similar, but less severe symptoms. Dermatitis, especially around the mouth, and other rashes may occur, along with fatigue, irritability, poor appetite, indigestion, diarrhea, headache, and possibly delirium.

Risk factors for deficiency

Severe niacin deficiency is uncommon in most parts of the world, but some people may need more than the RDA in order to maintain good health. Vegans, and others who do not eat animal protein, should consider taking a balanced B vitamin supplement. Others that may need extra niacin and other B vitamins may include people under high **stress**, including those experiencing chronic illnesses, liver disease, sprue, or poor nutritional status. People over 55 years old are more likely to have a poor dietary intake. Certain metabolic diseases also increase the requirement for niacin. Those who abuse nicotine,

alcohol or other drugs are very frequently deficient in B vitamins, but use of niacin with alcohol can cause seriously low blood pressure. A health care professional can determine if supplementation is appropriate.

Precautions

Niacin should not be taken by anyone with a B vitamin allergy, kidney or liver impairment, severe hypotension, unstable angina, arterial hemorrhage, or **coronary artery disease**. Supplemental niacin can exacerbate peptic ulcers. Diabetics should use caution as supplements of either niacin or niacinamide can alter medication requirements to control blood glucose. Supplements can raise uric acid levels, and aggravate gout in people with this condition. Pregnant women should not take high doses of niacin, or any supplement, except on the advice of a health care provider.

Health care should be sought immediately if certain symptoms occur following niacin supplementation. These include abdominal pain, diarrhea, nausea, vomiting, yellowing of the skin, faintness, or headache. Such symptoms may indicate excessively low blood pressure or liver problems. Heart palpitations and elevated blood sugar are also potential effects.

Side effects

High doses of niacin can cause a harmless, but unpleasant, flushing sensation and darkening of the urine. The "no-flush" form can lessen this complication.

Interactions

Niacin supplements should not be taken by anyone on medication for high blood pressure, due to the potential for hypotension. Isoniazid, a drug used to treat **tuberculosis**, inhibits the body's ability to make niacin from tryptophan. Extra niacin may be required. Supplements may also be needed by women taking oral contraceptives. Concomitant use of niacin with statin class drugs to lower cholesterol can cause myopathy. Cholestyramine and cholestipol, older medications to lower cholesterol, should be taken at a different time than niacin or they will reduce its absorption. Transdermal nicotine used with niacin is likely to cause flushing and dizziness. Carbamazepine, an antiseizure medication, is more likely to cause toxicity in combination with niacin.

Resources

BOOKS

Bratman, Steven, and David Kroll. *Natural Health Bible.* Prima Publishing, 1999.

Griffith, H. Winter. *Vitamins, Herbs, Minerals & supplements: the complete guide.* Arizona: Fisher Books, 1998.

Jellin, Jeff, Forrest Batz, and Kathy Hitchens. *Pharmacist's letter/Prescriber's Letter Natural Medicines Comprehensive Database.* California: Therapeutic Research Faculty, 1999.

Pressman, Alan H., and Sheila Buff. *The Complete Idiot's Guide to Vitamins and Minerals.* New York: alpha books, 1997.

Judith Turner

Nightmares *see* **Sleep disorders**

Nitrite test *see* **Urinalysis**

Nitrous oxide

Definition

Nitrous oxide is a colorless, sweet-smelling gas used as an anesthetic, most commonly during dental procedures.

Purpose

Nitrous oxide, also called laughing gas, is the weakest form of sedation to aid in the **relaxation** of the anxious dental patient. When inhaled, nitrous is absorbed by the body and has a quick-acting calming effect on the patient.

Description

The nitrous gas used in dental offices is actually a blend of two gases: oxygen and nitrous oxide. Mixed together it has a sweet-smelling aroma that gives a sense of well-being and aids in relaxation of the entire body. It causes light, conscious sedation, while the patient still retains the ability to respond to verbal commands.

Nitrous oxide has three kinds of sedative characteristics, including:

• Conscious sedation: Being awake and able to interact vocally with the dental staff, but feeling completely relaxed.

• Inhalation sedation: Becoming sedated through inhalation with the nose or mouth with a sedative agent such as nitrous oxide.

• Psychosedation: Nitrous oxide acts on the psyche or the **central nervous system** in such a way that **pain**

KEY TERMS

Anesthesia—A complete or partial loss of sensation.

Conscious sedation—Being awake during a procedure, able to respond to questioning, but completely relaxed.

General sedation—Being completely asleep during the procedure.

Inhaled sedation—Reaching a sedated state through inhalation of the nose or mouth with a sedating agent, such as nitrous oxide.

Sedative—An agent having a calming, relaxing effect.

---

impulses are not relayed to the cerebral cortex or their interpretation is altered.

According to the American Academy of Pediatric Dentistry, nitrous oxide/oxygen is the safest sedative in dentistry. It is non-addictive, mild, and easily administered to the patient. It is a safe, effective technique for calming patient fears of the dental office and procedures to be performed.

Operation

The concentration of nitrous oxide in the oxygen mixture varies, allowing for a range from light to deep sedation, depending on the apprehension, **anxiety**, fear, and pain the patient is experiencing. Consideration of the patient risks due to health issues or age may determine the amount of gas used during the dental procedure. Commonly used first in the dental office as a calming agent before an injection of a local anesthetic, nitrous oxide is inhaled through a nosepiece attached to the patient's face. From two separate tanks, two tubes carry the oxygen and the nitrous oxide gases to the nosepiece, where they are combined into one gas. Each tank has separate controls that indicate how much oxygen and nitrous are being used at any given time. The minimum number of people involved in the administration of the gas should be two, the dentist or other licensed professional and an assistant trained to monitor the patient during the procedure to make certain the amount of gas flowing through both tubes is correct. The effectiveness of all procedures using nitrous oxide is greatly enhanced by a quiet environment. Near the end of the dental procedure the flow of nitrous oxide is shut off and the patient is allowed to inhale 100% oxygen. The body quickly dissipates the nitrous oxide, and the patient begins to come out of the conscious sedated state.

Pregnant women should not use or handle nitrous oxide, because studies of pregnant mice and rats exposed to nitrous oxide have linked the use of the gas with birth defects.

Maintenance

Monitoring the control panels from each tank of oxygen and nitrous oxide at the beginning of each day is essential for safe practice. Daily checking of the tubes and nosepiece is vital to make certain they are free of blockages and small tears.

The tanks of oxygen and nitrous oxide should have an oxygen fail-safe system that is calibrated weekly. All emergency equipment should be functional and within reach.

Health care team roles

The dental office staff, including the dentist, dental hygienist, and dental assistant working as team, help create a calm environment. To ensure an adequate supply, the supervising dental assistant should monitor the amount of gas in each tank of oxygen and nitrous oxide, and schedule tank replacements as necessary. At least one back-up tank of each gas should be on hand, in addition to the ones being actively used with patients.

The front office staff maintains a current **health history** on each patient seen in the office. This health history has all known **allergies** or medical problems kept up to date for the dentist to refer to when deciding if nitrous oxide is safe for a particular patient.

The dental assistant in charge of the patient during the conscious sedation needs to document the **heart** rate, **blood pressure**, respiratory rate, and responsiveness of the patient periodically during the procedure, including the few minutes of recovery period when the patient is inhaling 100% oxygen.

Training

Many state laws require dental offices to have a license for housing a nitrous oxide unit and administering the gas. Dentists and dental hygienists receive training for using the gas in their degree courses. Continuing education courses on how to administer nitrous oxide are offered for the dental assistant. However, the dental assistant can only monitor the patient under the guidance of a licensed general dentist or licensed dental hygienist. A separate test is required to become fully licensed for use without supervision.

Resources

PERIODICALS

Nitrous Oxide. Brochure. American Academy of Pediatric Dentistry (AAPD) Brochure. 2001. <http://aapd.org/publications/brochures/nitrous.html>.

ORGANIZATIONS

Academy of General Dentistry (AGD). 211 East Chicago Ave., Chicago, IL 60611. (312) 440-4300. <http://www.agd.org>.
American Academy of Pediatric Dentistry. 211 East Chicago Avenue, Suite 700. Chicago, IL 60611-2663. <http://aapd.org>.

OTHER

Anesthesia. Academy of General Dentistry. <http://www.agd.org/consumer/factsheets/anesthesia.html>.

Cindy F. Ovard, RDA

Nonsteroidal anti-inflammatory drugs

Definition

Nonsteroidal anti-inflammatory drugs are medications other than **corticosteroids** that relieve **pain**, swelling, stiffness, and inflammation.

Purpose

Nonsteroidal anti-inflammatory drugs (NSAIDs) are prescribed for a variety of painful conditions, including arthritis, **bursitis**, tendinitis, **gout**, menstrual cramps, sprains, strains, and other injuries.

Description

The nonsteroidal anti-inflammatory drugs are a group of agents inhibiting prostaglandin synthetase, thereby reducing the process of inflammation. As a group, they are all effective **analgesics**. Some, including the salicylates, ibuprofen, and naproxene, are also useful antipyretics (fever-reducers).

Although the NSAIDs fall into discrete chemical classes, they are usually divided into the nonselective NSAIDs and the COX-2 specific agents. Among the non-specific NSAIDs are diclofenac (Voltaren), etodolac (Lodine), flurbiprofen (Ansaid), ibuprofen (Motrin, Advil, Rufen), ketorolac (Toradol), nabumetone (Relafen), naproxen (Naprosyn), naproxen sodium (Aleve, Anaprox, Naprelan), and oxaprozin (Daypro). The COX-2 specific drugs are celecoxib (Celebrex) and rofecoxib (Vioxx).

Nonselective NSAIDS inhibit both cyclooxygenase 1 and cyclooxygenase 2 (COX-2). Cyclooxygenase 1 is important for homeostatic maintenance, such as platelet aggregation, the regulation of **blood** flow in the kidney and **stomach**, and the regulation of gastric acid secretion. The inhibition of cyclooxygenase 1 is considered the primary cause of NSAID toxicity, including gastric ulceration and **bleeding disorders**. COX-2 is the primary cause of pain and inflammation. Note that both celecoxib and rofecoxib are relatively selective, and may cause the same adverse effects as the nonselective drugs, although with somewhat reduced frequency.

The analgesic activity of NSAIDs has not been fully elucidated. Antipyretic activity may be caused by the inhibition of prostaglandin E2 (PGE2) synthesis.

Although not all NSAIDs have approved indications for all uses, as a class, they are used for:

• ankylosing spondylitis

• bursitis

• fever

• gout

• headache

• juvenile arthritis

• mild to moderate pain

• osteoarthritis

• PMS

• primary dysmennorhea

• rheumatoid arthritis

• tendinitis

Recommended dosage

Recommended doses vary, depending on the patient, the type of nonsteroidal anti-inflammatory drug prescribed, the condition for which the drug is prescribed, and the form in which it is used. Consult specific sources for detailed information.

Common nonsteroidal anti-inflammatory drugs (NSAIDs)

Generic name (trade name)	Comparison to other NSAIDs
Aspirin (many trade names)	Most widely used NSAID for analgesic and anti-inflammatory effects; also used frequently for antipyretic and anticoagulant effects.
Diclofenac (Voltaren)	Substanially more potent than naproxen and several other NSAIDs; adverse side effects occur in 20% of patients.
Diflunisal (Dolobid)	Has potency 3–4 times greater than aspirin in terms of analgesic and anti-inflammatory effects but lacks antipyretic activity.
Etodolac (Lodine)	Effective as analgesic/anti-inflammatory agent with fewer side effects than most NSAIDs; may have gastric-sparing activity.
Fenoprofen (Ansaid)	Similar to aspirin's benefits and side effects; also available as topical ophthalmic preparation (Ocufen).
Ibuprofen (Motrin, Rufen, others)	First nonaspirin NSAID also available in nonprescription form; fewer GI side effects than aspirin but GI effects still occur in 5–15% of patients.
Indomethacin (Indameth, Indocin)	Relative high incidence of dose-related side effects; problems occur in 25–50% of patients.
Ketoprofen (Orudis)	Similar to aspirin's benefits and side effects but has relatively short half-life (1–2 h).
Ketorolac (Toradol)	Can be administered orally or by intramuscular injection; parenteral doses provide postoperative analgesia equivalent to opioids.
Nabumetone (Relafen)	Effective as analgesic/anti-inflamatory agent with fewer side effects than most NSAIDs.
Naproxen (Anaprox, Naprosyn)	Similar to ibuprofen in terms of benefits and adverse effects.

SOURCE: Rothstein, J.M., S.H. Roy, and S.L. Wolf. *The Rehabilitation Specialist's Handbook.* 2nd ed. Philadelphia: F.A. Davis Co., 1998.

Precautions

The most common hazard associated with NSAID use is gastrointestinal intolerance and ulceration. This may occur without warning, and is a greater risk among patients over the age of 65. The risk appears to rise with increasing length of treatment and increasing dose. Patients should be aware of the warning signs of gastrointestinal (GI) bleeding.

Allergic reactions are rare, but may be severe. Patients who have allergic reactions to aspirin should not be treated with NSAIDs.

Because NSAID metabolites are eliminated by the kidney, renal toxicity should be considered. Clinicians should monitor kidney function before and during NSAID use.

Among the NSAIDs that are classed as **pregnancy** category B are ketoprofen, naproxen, naproxen sodium, flurbiprofen, and diclofenac. Etodolac, ketorolac, mefenamic acid, meloxicam, nabumetone, oxaprozin, tolmetin, piroxicam, rofecoxib, and celecoxib are category C. Breastfeeding is not advised while taking NSAIDs.

Many other rare but potentially serious adverse effects have been reported with NSAIDs. Consult specific references.

Drug interactions

Many **drug interactions** have been reported with NSAID therapy. The most serious are those that may affect the bleeding hazards associated with NSAIDs. A partial list of interacting drugs follows. Consult specific references for further information.

- blood thinning drugs, such as warfarin (Coumadin)
- other nonsteroidal anti-inflammatory drugs
- heparin
- tetracyclines
- cyclosprorine
- digitalis drugs
- lithium
- phenytoin (Dilantin)
- zidovudine (AZT, Retrovir)

Samuel D. Uretsky, Pharm.D.

Nonsurgical periodontal therapy

Definition

Nonsurgical treatment of periodontal disease is the management of gum disease with cleanings and **antibiotics**. Both of these modalities can be implemented by a general dentist or a periodontist (a dentist specially trained in the periodontal field), who also prescribe any necessary antibiotics.

Purpose

The primary goals of periodontal treatment are the eradication of the disease process from the gums, ligaments, and bones that surround the teeth, and restoration of health that can be maintained on a daily basis. This nonsurgical approach is the conservative method of treating periodontal disease; it is for the patient who is fearful of surgery or wants the most conservative, noninvasive treatment. This approach is also used for the patient who presents a case of mild-to-medium severity of periodontal disease.

Precautions

The patient medical history is vital information that should be known by the entire dental staff. For example, it is crucial for them to know if the patient has **allergies** to certain medications—especially antibiotics—which cannot be tolerated, or will not mix well with prescriptions the patient is already taking. A nonsurgical treatment will be chosen by some patients, even after surgery has been recommended by the dentist or periodontist because it is the optimal treatment.

Description

Periodontal disease is the number one chronic infectious disease in the world. Surveys and studies show that over 50% of the American adult population have **gingivitis** and that 36% have periodontal disease. Periodontal disease increases with age. Most children and teenagers show some forms of gingivitis, but the harmful **bacteria** linked to gum disease is not present in young children. **Periodontitis** affects 1% of American teenagers and 3.6% of young adults aged 18–34. Among people aged 70 years or older, the rate of periodontitis increases to 86% due to the bacteria linked to this disease. It is the leading cause of tooth loss, and begins as a painless **infection** in the gums that is caused by buildup of bacteria. The bacteria buildup becomes dental plaque. If left untreated, pockets of plaque form around the gum tissue and plaque continues to accumulate below the gum line. Inflammation results, destroying the soft tissue and bone that support the teeth. Dr. Robert Schoor, the former president of the American Academy of Periodontology (AAP), has concluded that this bacteria can travel into the bloodstream and other parts of the body, putting a person's health at risk.

Treatment for periodontal disease differs depending on the severity of the case the patient presents to the office. Nonsurgical therapy for periodontal disease needs to be taken in steps and cannot be treated in a one visit trip to the dentist. The periodontist will divide the mouth into four quadrants—upper left; lower left; upper right; and lower right. Each quadrant is treated during a single visit. Different nonsurgical approaches to treating this disease are:

- **oral hygiene** instruction
- scaling and tooth planing
- systemic antibiotic therapy (medication taken by mouth)
- topical and local antibiotic therapy

Oral hygiene instruction is a procedure designed to educate the patient on its importance, and to train the patient, via a hands-on approach, how to properly clean and brush the teeth.

Scaling and root planing, also known as deep cleaning, is the conservative approach to the removal of plaque from and the prevention of infection beneath the gum line. During the scaling, a vibrating ultrasonic unit is used to clean tartar and visible particles from the teeth. Scaling removes deposits of bacterial plaque, food debris, and any pus that has accumulated in the infected pocket as a result of periodontitis. For areas that are more difficult to reach, a curet is used. This probes and cleans the pockets that the receding gums form around the teeth. Root planing smooths and cleans the root of the tooth so that the gum tissue may heal next to the tooth. The curette is used to plane the tooth root to make the surface smooth.

This procedure also removes the source of bacteria from the pockets around the tooth. It is helpful in reducing the opportunity for more bacteria to invade as a result of an inherent characteristic of plaque: it does not adhere well to smooth surfaces.

Scaling and root planing are done one quadrant at a time, and thus require several visits to the dental office to have the other quadrants treated. A local anesthetic can be used if there is any discomfort or **pain**. Scaling and root planing treatment are often effective in allowing the healing of early stages of periodontitis, and can help to reduce time spent in subsequent surgical treatment.

Systemic antibiotics (antibiotics taken by mouth) may be used in conjunction with other treatments to help rid the mouth of the bacteria causing periodontitis. Systemic antibiotics, however, are used conservatively because of the danger of a patient developing antimicrobial resistance. In fact, topical antibiotics are used more frequently than systemic antibiotics. Studies by the AAP reveal that taking antibiotics after undergoing scaling and root planing reduce the need for surgery by stopping the progression of the disease.

Systemic antibiotic administration may include the use of:

- Augmentin 500 mg: taken twice daily for at least eight days.
- Metronidazole (Flagyl), 500 mg: taken twice daily for at least eight days.
- Clindamycin (for penicillin-allergic patients), 300 mg: twice daily for at least eight days.
- Tetracycline 500 mg: taken for at least 14 days.
- Doxycycline 100 mg: taken twice daily for at least 14 days.

As mentioned previously, topical, or local antibiotic therapy, is another method of delivering antibiotics to the infected space in the gum tissue of the affected teeth. Here, the medication is applied directly to the affected area(s). This nonsurgical treatment approach is used mainly when scaling and root planing are considered insufficient to treat the infected tissue. The drugs that may be used include:

- Atridox (block drug)
- PerioChip (chlorhexidine)
- Periostat

Atridox was approved by the U.S. Food and Drug Administration (FDA) in late 1998 as the first and only locally delivered antibiotic treatment for periodontal disease. It contains the antibiotic "doxycycline," a proven antibiotic that kills bacteria associated with periodontal disease. The American Dental Association (ADA) awarded Atridox their Seal of Approval in 2000. Atridox gives dental professionals a practical, highly effective, and pain-free therapeutic option for treating moderate-to-severe periodontal disease before costly and invasive treatments become necessary. This type of treatment is used in conjunction with scaling and root planing. Anesthetics are not needed.

PerioChip treatment releases chlorhexidine as the antibiotic to fight against the disease. The entire chip must be used to insure adequate concentration of chlorhexidine for the seven to ten day treatment period. The PerioChip has three considerations during usage.

KEY TERMS

Adjunct—One connected to the other in a dependent or subordinate nature.

Calculus—Calcium deposits on teeth from the buildup of plaque that has not been removed.

Conjunction—In combination or association with.

Local or topical antibiotics—Method of therapy that delivers medications to local area of the body.

Periodontal—Tissue and structures that surround and support the teeth.

Periodontist—A dentist with specialized training for periodontal treatment and care.

RDA—Registered dental assistant. Individual trained to assist the dentist in dental procedures.

RDH—Registered dental hygienist. An individual trained for the specific purpose of oral hygiene, which includes the performance of teeth cleanings and home care instruction.

Root planing—Making the tooth smooth by removing built up calculus and tartar from below the gum tissue.

Scaling—The removal of food and debris from the portion of the tooth above the gum line.

Systemic antibiotics—Antibiotic medications that affect the whole body.

First, it is designed to be placed in a periodontal pocket of 5 mm or more. It is 5 mm long and 4 mm wide, with a curved end. This end is inserted into the pocket, into which it completely disappears. A patient who might be a candidate for this treatment approach might be one who is medically compromised in some way; someone in for whom surgery is contraindicated. Lastly, the PerioChip can be used where probing produces bleeding—where other forms of care have been unsuccessful, but root planing has been achieved. Initially, the area to be treated should be scaled and root planed; any subgingival plaque must be removed.

Published studies by the AAP have indicated the subgingival administration of this drug in a controlled release device reduces the bacteria and improves gingival health. Controlled clinical trials compared the benefits of scaling and root planing (SRP) alone to that of scaling, root planing and the use of the PerioChip, and revealed statistically significant benefits of adjunctive chip use

with regard to reducing probing pocket depths (0.65 mm versus 0.95 mm) and a gain of clinical attachment (0.58 mm versus 0.78 mm). The changes were small, but change did occur. Currently in studies performed by the AAP, two-chip applications have produced a result if any result is going to be seen. If no clinical result is seen after the two-chip application, additional chip therapy may be limited, but not produce any results at all. No data to date have been found by the AAP regarding further need of surgical or non-surgical treatment of sites after PerioChip treatment.

Periostat therapy, available in a 20 mg capsule as doxycycline hyclate (tetracycline) for oral administration, is indicated as an adjunct to scaling and root planing. It has been available in pharmacies since November 1998. It is listed under local and topical antibiotic treatment rather than systemic antibiotic treatment because its use is only for the treatment of periodontal disease and no other. Periostat works by attacking the enzymes that are produced by the cells within the pockets and inside the gum tissue itself. These enzymes are produced in response to a bacterial invasion of the gum and pockets with adult periodontitis. Periostat is the only treatment that suppresses the pathologically elevated levels of tissue-destroying enzymes that may lead to tooth loss in adult periodontitis. Periostat treats all periodontal pockets throughout the mouth simultaneously and therefore may be called a systemic type of therapy. Periostat administered for nine months revealed statistically significant benefits of adjunctive Periostat use with regard to reducing probing pocket depths from 1.48 mm to a gain of 1.17 mm pocket attachment and depth of 1.36 mm to a gain of 0.86 mm pocket depth. The magnitude of these changes is quite small (0.17 mm to 0.48 mm) and patients were required to use Periostat for the duration of the study. Periostat can be taken for a period of three to nine months. The length of duration depends upon the treating periodontist and the severity of the periodontal disease being treated. The AAP found no data regarding further need of surgical or non-surgical treatment of sites after using Periostat.

Preparation

Preparation for nonsurgical treatment of periodontal disease is limited to reading the medical history of the patient if any allergies to antibiotics exist and if the patient has any sensitivity to the medication prescribed. It is vital to know all existing medical conditions of the patient and what other medications being taken, especially in older patients with advanced periodontal disease. A need to know what type of medications might interact with ones prescribed is also vital knowledge in preparing for nonsurgical treatment.

Aftercare

Since periodontal treatment is done in quadrants, root planing and scaling can leave the gums and teeth tender to the touch. Chewing soft foods and rinsing with salt-water rinses will help heal the tissue. If treatment is accomplished using systemic antibiotics, aftercare is limited to following the prescription directions prescribed by the periodontist. If topical or local antibiotic treatment has been performed in quadrants, eating soft foods and light use of the quadrants will be advised. Brushing is recommended, but using a soft bristle toothbrush will be advised. If Atridox or the PerioChip have been used during treatment, flossing will not be advised until the treatment is completed.

Maintenance of periodontal disease is ongoing to prevent recurrence of the disease. Visits to the dental office for evaluations and checkups should occur on a regular basis. The examination should include observation of the gums, checking the bite, and removing any new plaque and tartar. How often the appointments are made depends upon the patients' willingness to control the disease. Most maintenance is practicing good daily hygiene habits at home. All patients should go back to the basics with regard to toothbrushing, flossing, and rinsing.

Complications

There are some concerns by the ADA that use of systemic therapy should be reserved for patients with continuing periodontal breakdown. The concern stems from the frequent use of antibiotics, because bacteria are increasing developing strains that are resistant to systemic therapy. This will make treating the disease harder, and is a growing health concern around the world. Incorporating this type of therapy into a routine management for adult periodontitis is not justified at this time. Periostat offers some solution because the antibiotic dosage level is very low, but it still poses some concern.

Results

Periodontal disease can be eradicated with the help and cooperation of the patient.

Health care team roles

A recent poll done by the AAP of 165 periodontists found that half of the patients seen in the offices reported feeling fearful of pain before they were treated, but only 10% reported feeling extreme discomfort or pain during treatment. Most patients making appointments with a periodontist are being referred by their general dentist and are aware of the periodontal disease they present. It is vital that periodontal office have a good rapport with local general dental offices to keep a specialty office running.

As a health care team, all areas of the office are helpful to the treating and healing of a patient. A registered dental hygienist (RDH) is most often seen by patients for root planing and scaling. Pocket depth charting is accomplished by the RDH and then relayed to the periodontist, who then plans the treatment with the patient. The registered dental assistant (RDA) assists the periodontist in organizing and sterilizing the instruments. The RDA keeps the patient flow running smoothly. A patient is greeted by the receptionist, who is also the last to see the patient. A warm and courteous front office staff is vital to the operation of any dental office at which the patient's disease is managed and his or her healing is accomplished.

Resources

Hodges, Kathleen. *Nonsurgical Periodontal Therapy.* Albany: Delmar Publishers, 1998.

PERIODICALS

American Association of Periodontology, Committee on Research, Science, and Therapy. Informational Paper. "The pathogenesis of periodontal disease." *Journal of Periodontology* 70 (1999): 457–70. <http://www.healthatoz.com>.

"Atridox Periodontal Disease Treatment." *Doctor's Guide to Medical and Other News.* <http://www.docguide.com>. January 4, 2000.

"Two Step Non-surgical Procedure." *Journal of Periodontology* 72, no. 3 (March 2001).

OTHER

About Gums.com. *Maryland's Top Periodontists.* <http://www.aboutgums.com>. (January 2001).

American Academy of Periodontology, 4157 Mountain Road, PBN 249 Pasadena, MD 21122. (410) 437-3749. <http://www.perio.org>.

American Dental Association, 211 East Chicago Avenue, Chicago, IL 60611. (312) 440-2500. <http://www.ada.org>.

Health A to Z. "How Serious Is Periodontal Disease?" <http://www.healthatoz.com>. 1999.

Packman, Harold D.M.D. PA. "Periodontal Specialists." <http://www.packmanperio.com>. (January 2000).

Rosen, David D.M.D. "Warning Signs of Periodontal Disease." *Periodontal News.com* 2001. <http://www.periodont.com>. (February 2001).

"Statement on Periostat." <http://www.perio.org/rsources-products/periostate.htm>. January 2000.

Cindy F. Ovard, R.D.A.

Nose packing *see* **Nasal packing**

Nosocomial infections *see* **Cross infection**

NSAIDs *see* **Nonsteroidal anti-inflammatory drugs**

Nuclear magnetic resonance *see* **Magnetic resonance imaging**

Nuclear medicine technology

Definition

Nuclear medicine technology is the medical specialty concerned with the use of safe and small amounts of radioactive material for diagnostic, therapeutic, and research purposes. Nuclear medicine involves using radioactive materials to perform body function studies and organ imaging, analyze biologic specimens and to treat, manage, and prevent serious disease. Nuclear medicine allows for early detection that can result in more effective treatments and better prognosis.

Description

Nuclear medicine imaging techniques combine the use of radioactive substances, detectors, and computers to provide physicians with a way to see inside the human body. Specific techniques include **positron emission tomography** (**PET**) and single photon emission computed tomography (SPECT). Nuclear medicine imaging is useful for detecting tumors, irregular or inadequate **blood** flow to various tissues, blood cell disorders, and inadequate functioning of organs. During diagnostic procedures, the patient experiences little or no discomfort, and the radiation dose is small.

Nuclear medicine technologists are highly skilled individuals who work closely with nuclear medicine physicians. Responsibilities include in vivo procedures, performing radiation safety and quality control procedures, operating the cameras that create images, and patient positioning and education. The technologist also collects, prepares, and analyzes biologic specimens, and prepares data for the physician's interpretation.

In nuclear medicine, radioactive materials, or radiopharmaceuticals, are used to diagnose and treat disease. Radiopharmaceuticals are attracted to specific organs, bones, or tissues and emit gamma rays that can be detected externally by scintillation cameras. Images are created by computers and provide data and information about the area of the body being imaged. The amount of radiation from a nuclear medicine procedure is comparable to that received during a diagnostic x ray.

Before the procedure, the nuclear medicine technologist explains the test procedure to the patient. The technologist then prepares a dosage of the radiopharmaceutical, which can be administered intravenously, orally, or by inhalation. When preparing radiopharmaceuticals, technologists adhere to safety standards that keep the radiation dose as low as possible. After positioning the patient for imaging, the technologist starts a gamma scintillation camera that scans the radioactive material and creates images of its distribution as it localizes in and emits signals from the patient's body.

Nuclear medicine technologists also perform radioimmunoassay studies. These studies assess the behavior of a radioactive substance inside the body. For example, technologists may add radioactive substances to blood or serum to determine levels of hormones or therapeutic drug content.

Work settings

Nuclear medicine technologists work in a variety of clinical settings including community hospitals, university-affiliated teaching hospitals, research institutions, imaging centers, **public health** institutions, and physicians' offices. Some technologists find work outside the medical profession as sales or training representatives for medical equipment and radiopharmaceutical manufacturing firms, or as radiation safety officers in regulatory agencies or hospitals.

Risks for radiation exposure do exist in the workplace, but it is kept to a minimum by adherence to strict safety guidelines in the field. These include the use of shielded syringes, gloves, and other protective devices. Technologists also wear badges that measure radiation levels.

Education and training

Individuals seeking to go into nuclear medicine need a strong background in anatomy, physiology, mathematics, chemistry, physics, radiation safety, clinical nuclear instrumentation, and laboratory technique.

Nuclear medicine technology programs vary in length from one to four years. Depending on the program, an individual can earn a certificate, associate's degree or bachelor's degree. Generally, healthcare professionals like radiologic technologists will enter a one-year certificate program when they want to specialize in nuclear medicine. Certificate programs are offered in hospitals and community colleges, as well as in bachelor's programs at four-year colleges and universities. A curriculum usually includes physical sciences, the biological effects of radiation exposure, radiation protection and procedures, the use of radiopharmaceuticals, imaging techniques, and computer applications. The Joint Review Committee on Education Programs in Nuclear Medicine Technology accredits most formal training programs in nuclear medicine technology.

Program graduates take two national certification exams: the American Registry of Radiologic Technologists (ARRT) and the Nuclear Medicine Technologist Certification Board (NMTCB). Upon successful completion of the exams, the individual will be a certified nuclear medicine technologist (CNMT).

All nuclear medicine technologists must meet the minimum federal standards on the administration of radioactive drugs and the operation of radiation detection equipment. Licensure is required in about half of the 50 U.S. states.

Advanced education and training

Certified nuclear medicine technologists can continue their education to earn an associate in science degree or enter a baccalaureate degree program at an area university. Some technologists seek to specialize in a clinical area such as nuclear cardiology or computer analysis. Technologists seeking to advance their careers or to become instructors or directors for nuclear medicine technology programs will pursue a bachelor's degree or a master's in nuclear medicine technology. Continuing education allows individuals to advance into positions such as supervisor, chief technologist, department administrator, or department director.

Future outlook

The number of job openings each year in nuclear medicine technology is relatively low because the field is not large. However, technological innovations in the field may spur an increased demand for nuclear medicine technologists. Also, more opportunities may arise with the development of new radiopharmaceuticals and with the wider application of nuclear medical imaging in areas like neurology, cardiology, and oncology. Still, there will be more competition for jobs as many hospitals are combining their nuclear medicine and radiologic departments. Therefore, technologists who can perform both

---

KEY TERMS

Gamma camera—The basic instrument used to produce a nuclear medicine image.

In vivo—In vivo procedures involve trace amounts of radiopharmaceuticals given directly to a patient. The majority of nuclear medicine procedures are in vivo.

Positron emission tomography (PET)—A technique that produces three-dimensional computer-reconstructed images that measure and determine the biochemistry or physiology in a specific organ or site.

Radiopharmaceutical—Also called a tracer, it is the radioactive compound necessary to produce a nuclear medicine image.

Scan—The images produced as the result of a nuclear medicine procedure, often referred to as the actual procedure, examination, or test.

Single photon emission computed tomography (SPECT)—A technique that provides three-dimensional computer-reconstructed images of multiple views and function of the organ being imaged.

---

nuclear medicine and radiologic procedures will have the best prospects.

Resources

BOOKS

Kuni, Christopher C., and Rene P. duCret. *Manual of Nuclear Medicine Imaging*. New York: Thieme, 1997.

PERIODICALS

Chidley, Elise. "Radiopharmaceuticals: Understanding an Underdog." *Radiology Today* (April 23, 2001): 22–25.

Malley, Mary T. "Quality Assurance in Nuclear Medicine." *Radiology Today* (February 12, 2001): 8–11.

"Nuclear Medicine Technologists." *Occupational Outlook Handbook*. 2001. <http://stats.bls.gov/oco/ocos104.htm> (January 5, 2001).

OTHER

Society of Nuclear Medicine. "About Nuclear Medicine." 2001. <http://www.snm.org/nuclear/index.html> (June 16, 2001).

Daniel J. Harvey

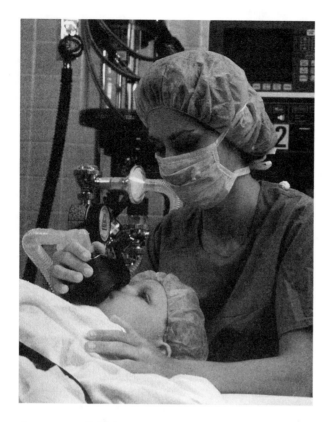

A nurse anesthetist prepares a child for surgery in the operating room. *(Science Source/Photo Researchers. Reproduced by permission.)*

Nurse anesthetist

Definition

Nurse anesthetists, or certified **registered nurse anesthetists** (CRNAs), are advanced practice registered nurses with specialized graduate level education, training, and certification in anesthesiology.

Description

CRNAs provide services similar to those provided by anesthesiologists. CRNAs have administered anesthesia for over 100 years in the United States, and they administer the majority of anesthetics in the United States.

The majority of CRNAs work in conjunction with anesthesiologists (MDs). Their responsibilities, whether in collaboration or functioning independently, are largely related to operative procedures. As the scope of practice for anesthesiologists broadens, so does that of CRNAs. **Pain management** teams established in most hospitals now have CRNA members. The newest Joint Commission on Accreditation of Health Organizations

(JCAHO) accreditation regulations mandate that acute care institutions have a **pain** management (assessment and intervention, with outcomes evaluation) system in place. The CRNA is part of that team. Laws regarding the level of collaboration required between physicians and CRNAs vary from state to state.

The first step in a CRNA's role in the operative setting is evaluation of the patient prior to anesthesia. This includes reviewing the patient's history, ordering diagnostic tests and consultations, interviewing the patient, discussing the anesthesia with the patient, obtaining **informed consent** for anesthesia or assuring that informed consent has been obtained, and ordering preoperative medications and fluids.

The CRNA is responsible for the formulation and implementation of an anesthesia care plan, which should detail the needs, treatment, and expected outcomes for the patient. The CRNA must choose the appropriate mode of anesthesia for the needs of the patient. **Local anesthesia** is numbing of a small, specific area so that a patient can have a procedure free of pain. Sedation alters the patient's level of consciousness so that the patient is more relaxed and less aware of uncomfortable sensations. Regional anesthesia (i.e., spinal blockade, axillary blockade, etc.) causes a loss of sensation to a specific region of the body. **General anesthesia** results in a loss of consciousness and lack of sensation throughout the body and as such carries the greatest risk of all anesthesias for the patient. The CRNA must assess the risks and benefits of each type of anesthesia in the context of the individual patient.

During the course of the operative procedure, the CRNA administers anesthetics and any adjunctive medications or fluids needed to induce and maintain anesthesia and patient homeostasis. Managing the patient's pulmonary status and oxygen saturation is one of the chief responsibilities of the CRNA, as **respiratory failure** or compromise is a key risk associated with anesthesia or sedation. The CRNA must confirm that the airway remains patent and that ventilation and oxygen equipment is working correctly. Techniques such as endotracheal intubation and extubation, mechanical ventilation, pharmacologic treatment, and **respiratory therapy** help to maintain a patent and functioning pulmonary system. The CRNA is also responsible for carefully checking equipment such as the anesthesia machine, mechanical ventilator, and oxygen equipment for safety and functionality prior to any procedures.

The patient's physiologic status, especially hemodynamics, must be monitored at all times during anesthesia. **Vital signs**, pulse oximetry, **heart** monitors, and monitors on oxygen and ventilation systems are examples of methods for monitoring the patient's response and status of equipment. Neuromuscular function and status must also be monitored when neuromuscular-blocking drugs are administered. The patient's position may need to be shifted during lengthy procedures in order to prevent injuries related to anesthesia-induced immobility, but prevention of anticipated pressure points is the first step. The CRNA is responsible for prevention or correction of any abnormal response to anesthesia. For example, an episode of respiratory compromise may lead to an acid-base imbalance. Symptoms of respiratory compromise or acid-base imbalance can be detected through physiologic changes such as **cyanosis** or hyperventilation and tests such as arterial **blood gases** and oxygen saturation. The CRNA is trained to quickly detect and correct this problem. There are two key abnormal responses that could prove fatal to the patient without early recognition and appropriate intervention by the CRNA: malignant hyperthermia and **anaphylaxis** (systemic allergic response). Both have cardinal signs and prescribed intervention procedures.

Even after the procedure is complete, the CRNA remains involved in extubation, assessing emergence, and initial recovery from anesthesia. The CRNA will follow up postoperatively to evaluate and treat any anesthesia side effects, determine when the patient is safely recovered from anesthesia, and discharge the patient from the postanesthesia care unit (PACU) or recovery room when appropriate.

In addition to the more traditional roles related to surgery, CRNAs are prepared to administer emergency care in any setting, including **airway management**, fluid and medication administration, and other interventions requiring advanced cardiac life support (ACLS) skills.

CRNAs also practice in the area of acute and chronic pain management through specialized techniques using drugs, regional anesthetics, or devices (such as a patient controlled anesthesia pump). They may also be asked to consult in the areas of respiratory care and are required to respond to cardiac arrest codes, especially when they occur with patients in the emergency department.

CRNAs may also choose to specialize in specific patient populations such as pediatrics, geriatrics, cardiovascular, neurology, or obstetrics.

It is important that the CRNA document in the chart descriptions of any of the above roles, providing details about the procedure, techniques, equipment, clinical situation, and patient outcomes.

Work settings

Practice settings for CRNAs include independent or group practice in hospitals (i.e., surgical suites or obstet-

---

KEY TERMS

Arterial blood gases—Measurement of oxygen, carbon dioxide, pH, bicarbonate, and their chemical relationships in the arterial blood in order to determine oxygenation and acid-base balance.

Cyanosis—Blue coloring of the skin around the eyes, lips, or fingers that signals low blood oxygen levels.

Extubation—Removal of an endotrachael tube.

Homeostasis—A state of physiologic balance.

Intubation—Insertion of an endotrachael tube to protect or restore the airway.

Mechanical ventilation—The use of a respirator or manual method to assure that the patient receives adequate oxygenation.

Patent—Open or unobstructed.

Pulse oximetry—Measurement of oxygen levels and heart rate through a device worn on the finger or ear lobe.

---

rical delivery rooms), outpatient surgery facilities, and dental, ophthalmology, podiatry, or plastic surgery offices. Military treatment facilities often use CRNAs as the chief anesthesia providers in facilities such as mobile care units or veterans hospitals. CRNAs may also work in the areas of research, quality assurance, critical care management or oversight, and administrative roles. Currently there are some states where CRNAs are granted the right to independent practice without physician supervision.

Education and training

There are over 80 university-affiliated educational programs for nurse anesthetists in the United States. In order to qualify for CRNA education, the nurse must have a bachelor of science in nursing degree or another science or health care-related baccalaureate-level degree, a current registered nurse license, and a minimum of one year acute care experience. Some CRNA programs require two years experience in either the operating room or critical care. Accredited CRNA programs require a 24- to 36-month program that includes a graduate degree and clinical training. After this training is complete, the nurse anesthetist must pass a national certification exam in order to become a CRNA. CRNAs must be recertified every two years and that requires continuing education credits specific to the specialty as well as proof of a designated number of hours spent giving anesthesia to patients.

Future outlook

It has been projected that more CRNAs will be required and utilized in the future. According to the American Association of Nurse Anesthetists (AANA), 50% of hospitals and 65% of rural hospitals currently use nurse anesthetists as their sole anesthesia providers. Furthermore, the AANA has summarized reports by organizations including the National Academy of Sciences, the Centers for Disease Control, and the US House of Representatives and concluded that CRNAs are a cost-effective and equally safe alternative to anesthesiologists. There is an ongoing controversy between the American Society of Anesthesiologists and the AANA, in the face of requests of managed care companies to cut costs, that contests the independent practice option for CRNAs. The contention by the physician's group is that CRNA independent practice is not as safe for patients as MD supervision would be, but, to date, that has not been proved to the satisfaction of regulatory agencies. The needs for available, safe, and effective care ensure the ongoing need for CRNAs in the health care environment especially in areas where there is a scarcity of anesthesiologists, such as remote centers and rural populations.

Resources

BOOKS

McIntosh, L. *Essentials of Nurse Anesthesia*. New Jersey: McGraw Hill, 1995.

Nagelhout, J. and K. Zaglaniczny. *Nurse Anesthesia*. 2nd ed. Pasadena: Kaiser Permanente, 2001.

ORGANIZATIONS

American Association of Nurse Anesthetists. 222 South Prospect Avenue, Park Ridge, IL 60068-4001. (847) 692-7050. <http://www.aana.com/>.

Joint Commission on Accreditation of Healthcare Organizations. 1 Renaissance Blvd, Oakbrook Terrace, IL 60181. (800) 994-6610. <http://www.jcaho.org/>.

Katherine L. Hauswirth, APRN

Nurse midwifery

Definition

Nurse midwifery is a profession that independently functions within the health care system. Nurse midwives manage the different stages of women's health from pregnancy, to childbirth, through the postpartum period, as well as meeting women's gynecological needs during the menopausal and post-menopausal periods. Nurse midwives additionally may provide newborn care and will occasionally provide prenatal education, all as a part of their philosophy of family-centered care. A nurse midwife is a person trained in the two professions of nursing and midwifery as compared to a certified midwife (CM) who is trained in midwifery but not through the profession of nursing.

The certified nurse midwife (CNM) is an individual who has successfully completed an approved course of study in nurse midwifery and practices in compliance with the *Standards for the Practice of Nurse Midwifery* as defined by the American College of Nurse Midwives (ACNM). Midwives have attended births in America since colonial times, but the actual profession of nurse midwifery was not officially recognized in the United States until the early 1920s.

Description

The nurse midwife provides women during pregnancy with appropriate supervision, care, and advice. During labor and the postpartum period, the nurse midwife performs vaginal deliveries and may care for the newborn while facilitating family involvement, particularly of fathers and siblings. Nurse midwives foster an environment that facilitates minimal intervention while continuously assessing for abnormal conditions in the mother and child that would necessitate medical assistance or emergency procedures.

Nurse midwives promote family-centered maternity care that incorporates counseling and education for the woman and the family. The occupation stresses the importance of antenatal education and preparation for parenthood. The nurse midwife acts as a kind of primary-care provider by providing the woman with family planning and a range of gynecological care.

Many of the clients that a nurse midwife cares for can be classified as "vulnerable" by one or more of the subsequent criteria: less than 16 years of age; level of education less than eight years; race and ethnicity other than white; and source of payment through public programs such as Medicaid, Medicare, and the Indian Health Service or free/self-pay. Women and infants seen by nurse midwives live disproportionately in areas where a higher than average number of people live below the poverty level.

The ACNM is the main professional organization in the Unites States representing CNMs and CMs. The group is the oldest women's health organization in the Unites States with roots back to the 1920s. ACNM con-

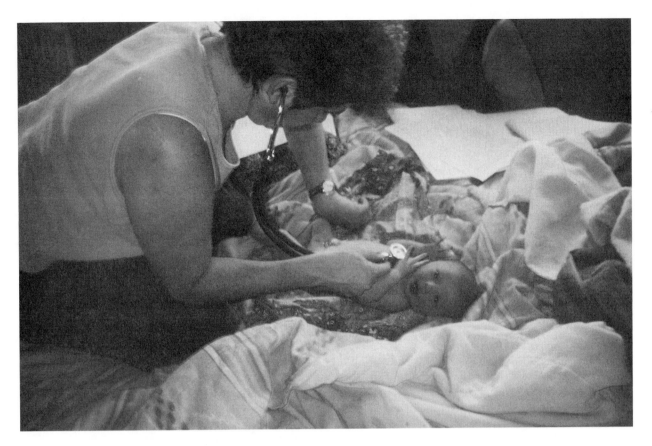

A nurse midwife examines a newborn after a home birth. *(Photograph by Michelle del Guercio. Science Source/Photo Researchers. Reproduced by permission.)*

ducts research in midwifery practice; accredits midwifery schools; coordinates and administers continuing education programs; develops clinical practice standards of care; and works with state and federal agencies and members of Congress in promoting midwifery.

Work settings

The practice of nurse midwifery is legal in all 50 states and the District of Columbia. Most nurse midwives function in a hospital or physician practice and attend deliveries in hospital settings. In 1997, 96% of nurse midwives delivered in hospitals, 2.4% delivered in separate birth centers and 1% delivered in a home setting.

Hospitals

Nurse midwives have various roles in the care facility, from providing solely intrapartal care to antepartal care to well-woman care to all of these combined. One of the more recent developments in hospital labor and delivery is the creation of birthing rooms that provide a more comfortable, home-like ambiance. Comfort features include showers or Jacuzzis, and beds that convert to birthing beds in which a woman can labor, deliver, and recover. Nurse midwives have been strong proponents of such advances and find them very useful in their practice.

Health maintenance organizations (HMOs) and managed care

Nurse midwives fit well into the model of managed care, which emphasizes cost-effective care focusing on prevention. They provide OB/GYN care as well as family planning. In 1992, Kaiser Permanente, a California-based HMO, reported that nurse midwives handled 70% of the low-risk obstetrical patients and had contributed to lowering the cesarean section rate to 12%. The national average for cesarean sections is 23.5%.

Private practices

A great number of nurse midwives work in private practices of different sorts. Some practice in private OB/GYN practices with physicians, others in private nurse midwife only practices with physician consultation available, some in freestanding birth centers and a few perform home births. Private practices give nurse midwives greater autonomy, allowing them to utilize the fullest extent of their training.

Birth centers

Freestanding birth centers offer the patient and her family a place to give birth that is a compromise between the hospital and home. In birthing centers, the nurse midwife tries to foster a home-like atmosphere as much as possible but still has the advantages of specialized equipment and proximity of emergency transportation.

Clinics

Nurse midwives make a major contribution to caring for indigent and under-served populations in **public health** clinics—both independent clinics and those affiliated with a hospital. In these settings, nurse midwives attend to women that are susceptible to poorer than average outcomes of childbirth due to age, socioeconomic status, refugee status, and ethnic background.

Home births

Nurse midwives who assist in home births ensure the patient's and baby's safety while delivering personalized care and emotional support. A woman delivering in her own home experiences a familiar environment that is conducive to the woman retaining control of her birthing experience.

International health

Before nurse midwifery was generally accepted in the United States, a large number of nurse midwives focused on the improvement of maternal-child health on a global level. A large number of international health organizations fund projects for nurse midwives in an effort to improve the health status of women and children throughout the world.

Education and training

The education of nurse midwives consists of a thorough foundation in the health sciences and extensive clinical preparation. Clinical training concentrates on the acquisition of knowledge, decision-making ability, and skills required to provide primary care and independent management of women and newborns. Students learn to function within a health care system where they can obtain medical consultation if necessary, where they can manage patients collaboratively and where they can refer when needed. The ACNM defines the scope of practice of a nurse midwife to include antepartum, intrapartum, postpartum, newborn, family planning, gynecology, and primary care.

The numbers of patient visits and experiences below represent suggested guidelines for nurse midwifery educational programs from the ACNM:

- 10 preconception care visits
- 15 new antepartum visits
- 70 return antepartum visits
- 20 labor management experiences
- 20 births
- 20 newborn assessments
- 10 breastfeeding support visits
- 20 postpartum visits (0-5 days)
- 15 postpartum visits (4-8 weeks)
- Primary care visits:
- 40 common health problems
- 20 family planning visits
- 20 gynecologic visits
- 20 perimenopausal/postmenopausal visits

Nurse midwifery students matriculate in a variety of academic programs and have various options including: diploma or associate degree (AD) **registered nurse** (RN) to certified nurse midwife (CNM) programs; BA/BS to RN/CNM-graduate programs; post-secondary programs; distance education; master's completion programs; and post-master's certificate programs.

Advanced education and training

The ACNM defines continuing education as an educational experience that goes beyond basic midwifery education. Nurse midwives may complete a variety of educational activities, including taking a national certification exam, attending workshops, and completing home study units of study.

Future outlook

The popularity and acceptance of nurse midwifery increased dramatically in the 1970s and 1980s. The number of nurse midwife attended births has steadily increased from year to year. Many more obstetricians and other healthcare providers have concluded that nurse midwifery is a safe, cost-effective way of managing normal pregnancies and deliveries. They are also coming to be accepted as primary care providers in managing women's health.

Resources

BOOKS

Varney, Helen. *Varney's Midwifery,* 3rd ed. Boston: Jones & Bartlett, 1997.

ORGANIZATIONS

American College of Nurse Midwives (ACNM). 818 Connecticut Ave, Suite 900 Washington, DC 20006. (202) 728-9860. <www.acnm.org>.

OTHER

ACNM. "About ACNM." 2000. <www.acnm.org/about/index.htm>.
ACNM. "Midwifery Education." 1999. <www.acnm.org/educ/index.htm>.
ACNM. "Professional Information." 2000. <www.acnm.org/prof/Index.htm>.

Nadine M. Jacobson, R.N.

Nursing assessment *see* **Nursing diagnosis**

Nursing diagnosis

Definition

In 1990, the North American Nursing Diagnosis Association (NANDA) defined nursing diagnosis as "a clinical judgement about individual, family, or community responses to actual or potential health problems/life processes. Nursing diagnoses provide the basis for selection of nursing interventions to achieve outcomes for which the nurse is accountable."

Purpose

The first conference on nursing diagnosis was held in 1973 to identify nursing knowledge and establish a classification system to be used for computerization. At this conference, the National Group for Classification of Nursing Diagnosis was founded; this group was later renamed the North American Nursing Diagnosis Association (NANDA). In 1984, NANDA established a Diagnosis Review Committee (DRC) to develop a process for reviewing and approving proposed changes to the list of nursing diagnoses. The American Nurses Association (ANA) officially sanctioned NANDA as the organization to govern the development of a classification system for nursing diagnosis in 1987. However, the ANA also recognizes the Omaha system and the Home Health Classification system as two additional nursing diagnosis systems currently in use.

The purpose of the NANDA diagnosis list is three fold. First, it provides nurses with a common frame of reference and standardizes language that improves communication among nurses, helps organize research, and is useful in educating new practitioners. Second, nursing diagnoses provide a classification system to describe the scientific foundation of nursing practices—a major criterion necessary for nursing to be recognized as a separate profession, differentiated from medicine and other health care professions. Third, the NANDA diagnosis system has the potential for computer use and may, in the future, provide nomenclature for the reimbursement of nursing activities, not unlike DRGs and ICDs do for medicine.

Precautions

It is important to distinguish nursing diagnoses from medical diagnoses. The two are similar because they are both designed to plan care for a patient. However, nursing diagnoses focus on human response to stimuli, while medical diagnoses focus on the disease process. An example of this difference is the different diagnoses given by a nurse and a doctor to a patient who exhibits difficulty breathing, a productive cough, and crackles throughout lung fields. This patient might be medically diagnosed as having **pneumonia**. Some nursing diagnoses that might be made for this particular patient, however, include activity intolerance, impaired **gas exchange**, and fatigue.

Another feature that is unique to nursing diagnoses is the identification of potential problems. The diagnosis of "at risk for aspiration" is an example of a diagnosis that recognizes the potential for a given problem to occur. In order for a risk diagnosis to be made, risk factors must be present and identified upon assessment. In the above example, the absence of the gag reflex, and the presence of facial droop or **paralysis** may be among the risk factors for impaired swallowing that would lead a nurse to make the diagnosis of "at risk for aspiration." These diagnoses are important because they allow nursing to take a preventive approach to patient care.

KEY TERMS

Expected outcome—A measurable individual, family, or community state, behavior, or perception that is measured along a continuum and is responsive to nursing interventions.

Medical diagnosis—A medical determination of disease or syndrome performed by a physician. The focus is on the disease process and the physical, genetic, or environmental cause of that process.

NANDA, North American Nursing Diagnosis Association—Formed in 1973, this group is responsible for developing a classification system of nursing diagnoses.

NIC, Nursing Interventions Classification—Developed by the Iowa Intervention Project, this is a collection of nursing interventions linked to the NANDA diagnoses. The 2000 publication includes approximately 500 interventions.

NOC, Nursing Outcomes Classification—Developed by the Iowa Outcome Project, this is a comprehensive, standardized classification of patient outcomes developed to evaluate the effects of nursing interventions. The outcomes may be linked to the NANDA diagnoses and other diagnoses systems. The 2000 publication includes 260 outcomes.

Nursing assessment—The way in which a nurse gathers and evaluates data about a client (individual, family, or community). The assessment includes a physical examination, interviewing, and observations. Assessment is also the first step in the nursing process.

Nursing diagnostic statement—The formal, written documentation of a nursing diagnosis. It includes the label or diagnosis, the etiology, and the indicators. In the statement, the etiology is preceeded by the phrase "related to." The indicators are the assessment data that led to the diagnosis. They are preceeded by the phrase, "as evidenced by."

Nursing intervention—Any treatment that a nurse performs on a patient in response to a nursing diagnosis to reach a projected outcome.

Risk diagnosis—A nursing diagnosis that recognizes a potential problem not an existing problem. The indicators for risk diagnoses are risk factors that are identified through assessment.

Description

The term "nursing diagnosis" refers to items on the NANDA list of approved diagnoses, such as **anxiety**. The term "nursing diagnostic statement" refers to the approved or accepted way in which a nursing diagnosis is written in practice. Gordon identifies three structural components of a nursing diagnostic statement: the problem, the etiology (cause), and the signs and symptoms. An example of a nursing diagnostic statement would read, "Anxiety related to hospitalization as evidenced by verbal comments, and increased **heart** rate." When writing an "at-risk" nursing diagnostic statement, the signs and symptoms are replaced by the list of risk factors present for a particular response.

Nursing diagnoses may be made for an individual, a family, or a community. An example of a family nursing diagnosis is "risk for altered parent-infant attachment." The nursing diagnostic statement in this case might read, "risk for altered parent-infant attachment related to maternal distancing as evidenced by lack of eye contact between mother and infant." "Management of therapeutic regimen, ineffective: community," is an example of a nursing diagnosis for a community. The nursing diagnostic statement in this case may read, "Management of therapeutic regimen related to prevention of teen **pregnancy**, ineffective in the community, as evidenced by higher rate of teen pregnancy than surrounding communities."

Preparation

In order to make an appropriate nursing diagnosis, the practitioner must conduct an in-depth interview, physical assessment, and critical observation of the individual, family, or community for which the diagnosis is being made. A complete nursing assessment includes: the patient's current health status, signs and symptoms, strengths, and problem areas. The patient (who can be an individual, a family, or a group) should be the primary source of assessment data.

After compiling data through assessment, the data are grouped or organized into categories that will assist the nurse in identifying appropriate diagnoses. A variety of organizing frameworks exist to assist the nurse in organizing the data, including **Maslow's hierarchy of needs**, NANDA's human response patterns, and Gordon's functional health patterns.

Aftercare

Diagnosis is the second step in the nursing process, following assessment. Once an in-depth assessment has been completed and the appropriate nursing diagnoses are made, the steps of planning and implementing nursing interventions and subsequently evaluating the outcomes based on treatment goals must be undertaken. In planning nursing intervention, priorities must be set and expected measurable outcomes or objectives must be specifically stated.

In 1987, a program begun at the University of Iowa for treatment goals became known as the Iowa Intervention Project. This was a large research project from which the Nursing Interventions Classification system (NIC) was produced. In 2000, the third edition of NIC was published. It included almost 500 nursing interventions. NIC provides a link to the NANDA diagnoses. Using NIC, nurses may look up a NANDA diagnosis and be directed to appropriate nursing interventions for that diagnosis.

Research for the development of the Nursing Outcomes Classification (NOC) began in 1991. The second edition of NOC was completed by the Iowa Outcomes Project in 2000 and contains 260 outcomes. Each outcome has a definition, list of indicators, and a five-point Likert scale to assess patient status. NOC has been linked to the NANDA diagnoses, the NIC interventions, Gordon's functional patterns, the Omaha system of problems, resident admission protocols (RAPs) used in **nursing homes**, and to the OASIS system used in **home care**.

Results

Nursing diagnoses are made to identify current and potential problems for individuals, families, and communities, and to communicate these problems to other practitioners in a standard form. Once a nursing diagnosis is made, it is anticipated that the appropriate nursing interventions will be implemented to either correct or prevent the problem.

Health care team roles

Although nursing diagnoses are almost exclusively generated and used by nurses, members of the nursing profession hope these diagnoses will become more widely recognized and adopted by other health care professions. Using the standardized language that NANDA provides facilitates communication between health care professionals.

Resources

BOOKS

Carpenito, L.J. *Nursing Diagnosis Application to Clinical Practice.* 7th ed. Philadelphia: Lippincott, 1997.

Cox, H.C., et al. *Clinical Applications of Nursing Diagnosis: Adult, Child, Women's, Psychiatric, Gerontic, and Home Health Considerations.* 3rd ed. Philadelphia: F.A. Davis Company, 1997.

PERIODICALS

Laduke, Sharon. "Spotlight What You Really Do With This Powerful Documentation Tool." *Nursing* (June 2000).

ORGANIZATIONS

American Nurses Association, 600 Maryland Avenue, SW, Suite 100 West, Washington, DC 20024. (800) 274-4ANA. <http://www.nursingworld.org>.

Joint Commission on Accreditation of Healthcare Organizations (JCAHO), One Renaissance Boulevard, Oakbrook Terrace, IL 60181. 630-792-5000. Fax: 630-792-5005. <http://www.jcaho.org>.

North American Nursing Diagnosis Association (NANDA), 1211 Locust St., Philadelphia, PA 19107. (215) 545-8105. Fax: (215) 545-8107. <http://www.nanda.org>. info@nanda.org.

The University of Iowa College of Nursing, 101 Nursing Building, Iowa City, IA 52242. (319) 335-8960. <http//coninfo.nursing.uiowa.edu/index.htm>.

Jennifer Lee Losey, R.N.

Nursing education

Definition

Nursing education refers to formal learning and training in the science of nursing. This includes the functions and duties in the physical care of patients, and a combination of different disciplines that both accelerates the patient's return to health and helps maintain it.

Description

Nursing and nursing education have undergone striking changes over the centuries. This history reveals a constant struggle for autonomy and professionalism. There have been many influences on nursing practice in the past, including women's struggle for professional acceptance and status, religion, war, technology, and societal attitudes. These factors still influence nursing today. During the past decades, the profession worked to improve its image.

Nursing education in the United States had its beginnings in Europe. In 1836, in Kaiserwerth, Germany, Theodor Fliedner opened a small hospital and training school called the Order of Deaconesses. Florence Nightingale, the founder of modern nursing, received her formal training at this school. In 1859, she published *Notes on Nursing: What It Is and What It Is Not* in

London. This was not intended as a text for nurses but for the ordinary woman who was the nurse for her family. In 1869, voting rights for women were promoted with the organization of the National Women's Suffrage Association and Lavinia Dock, a nurse, used the organization to promote and expand nurses' rights.

The first training schools in the United States were opened in 1872 in Philadelphia at the Women's Hospital, and in Boston at the New England Hospital for Women and Children in Boston. Linda Richards, American's first trained nurse, graduated from the latter in 1873. The American National Red Cross was organized by Clara Barton in 1882, and in 1885 Clara Weeks Shaw published the first textbook written by an American nurse: *Textbook of Nursing for the Use of Training Schools, Families, and Private Students*. The first home visiting nursing organization in the United States, the Henry Street Settlement in New York, was founded by Lillian Wald and Mary Brewster in 1893. In that same year, the American Society of Superintendents of Training Schools for Nurses (renamed the National League of Nursing Education in 1912), was established.

The Nurses' Associated Alumnae of United States and Canada was established in 1897 and renamed the American Nurses Association in 1911. North Carolina, New Jersey, Virginia, and New York established the first Nurse Practice Acts in 1903. In a study funded by the Rockefeller Foundation in 1920, the Goldmark Report recommended that nursing schools become independent of hospitals, and that students should not be a source of cheap labor. It also advocated financial support of university-based nursing schools.

During the Great Depression, many nurses were unemployed and the number of schools declined, but the outbreak of World War II brought a huge increase in nursing demand. During the war years, new students were still taught by experienced nurses in hospital-based programs called diploma schools of nursing.

In 1948 the Brown Report recommended that education for nursing take place in colleges and universities, not hospitals. In the same year, the National League of Nursing Education established the National Nursing Accrediting Service for nursing educational programs. In 1951, Dr. Mildred Montag suggested that one way to increase the number of nurses was to shorten their education period. She also recommended that they be trained in colleges and universities instead of diploma schools. In her dissertation "The Education of Nursing Technicians," she proposed a two-tiered system in which "technical" nurses, who would be trained for two years, largely in community colleges, would assist "professional" nurses, who would receive four-year degrees.

Although the model was not adopted at that time, Dr. Montag's paper is credited with creating the associate degree in nursing.

In 1965, the American Nurses' Association (ANA) published a position paper urged that all nursing education should take place in institutions of higher learning. As a result, many diploma schools closed and nursing education began its move to collegiate programs. At this time, the ANA also echoed Dr. Montag's proposal that nursing practice consist of two levels: a professional nurse, who would hold a baccalaureate or higher degree, and a technical nurse, who would have an associate degree and would work under the direct supervision of the professional nurse. Since then, as medical knowledge advanced, nurses have had to keep up with new medications, technology, and a rapidly changing health care system as well as appropriate nursing care.

Degree programs

Associate degree programs were originally introduced in the United States in 1952 and are primarily offered by community colleges. This is a two-year program emphasizing technical skills with a foundation in behavioral and biological science. Associate degree graduates take a state licensing examination and are entitled to practice using the initials RN. Since the 1950s, the National League for Nursing (NLN) has been the accrediting body for two and four-year nursing colleges. In recent years, though, four-year colleges have turned to the American Association of Colleges of Nursing (AACN) for their accreditation, an association that does not allow two-year colleges to join.

The baccalaureate program, found in universities and colleges across the United States, takes four years to complete. It provides an education in the arts, sciences, and humanities. Although the program teaches bedside care, the emphasis is placed on leadership and management, community health nursing, and research. These graduates also take the licensing examination and receive the designation of RN.

Advanced practice nurses are RNs who specialize in one of several fields, which include nurse practitioner (NP), certified nurse midwife (CNM), certified **registered nurse** anesthetist (CRNA), and **clinical nurse specialist** (CNS). These nurses have four-year degrees with at least some postgraduate study; most hold master's degrees. Like RNs, advanced practice nurses are licensed and certified.

To obtain a master's or doctoral degree, a student is required to hold a baccalaureate degree from an accredited college or university. Graduate programs emphasize advanced clinical practice, research, and prepare students for roles as educators and administrators.

Nurses can also serve without a college degree. Becoming a practical nurse takes about one year and is comprised of training in a hospital along with classroom work. After graduating from a practical nursing program, students must pass a licensing examination, after which they can use the initials LPN (**licensed practical nurse**) or LVN (licensed vocational nurse) and practice under the supervision of a registered nurse. Compared to RNs, however, LPNs make less money, have less responsibility, and usually are not promoted to supervisory roles.

Of the 2.6 million registered nurses in the United States, 32% have an associate's degree, 27% have a diploma, and 31% have a baccalaureate degree as their highest degree. In 1995, 61% of all new nursing graduates were from associate degree programs, slightly more than 9% had master's degrees and less than 1% held doctorates. In 1998, the Veteran's Administration, one of the nation's largest employers of nurses, stated that they preferred to hire nurses with baccalaureate degrees, but would not require one for entry-level positions. In that year, the VA set aside $10 million for each of the following five years to help associate degree nurses on staff go back to school to obtain a baccalaureate degree. Although many nurses consider their associate degree a valuable first step, higher degrees are necessary to enhance their prospects for advancement.

The nursing shortage

Health care has become a complex business; nurses are becoming managers who are expected to have the education and skill to provide leadership in administrative settings. At the same time, their workloads have increased and the patients for whom they care are more ill. In addition, many other professions are now open to women, diluting the pool of available candidates. The profession is also facing a shortage of nursing faculty. As a result, the number of nurses in the field is dropping, creating a significant shortage.

The average age of all RNs in 1996 was 44.3 years; for practicing nurses, 42.3 years. Worse still, the average age continues to increase at the same time that enrollment in baccalaureate programs is decreasing. Federal figures project that if current trends continue, rising demand will outstrip the supply of RNs in or about the year 2010. According to a U.S. Department of Health and Human Services Division Of Nursing projection, 114,000 jobs for full-time RNs will go unfulfilled in the year 2015.

To meet these future needs, hospitals and other employers have stepped up recruitment. The nursing practice has also been moving away from the acute care setting. Nurses have more opportunities in the community, advanced practice settings, health maintenance organizations, insurance companies and home health, and administrators are now requiring new employees to be bachelor's prepared.

Viewpoints

Changing curriculum

The capacity to develop critical thinkers and proactive professional nurses is driving all aspects of the education process. The scope is broad and highly technical, while requiring knowledge of social change and community development and all specialties in between. Theory and practice are also changing at rates that require nurses to continue their education throughout their careers along with retaining basic nursing values. Nursing practice should foster these attributes in a health care system of challenge and change.

Leading nursing organizations view a bachelor of science degree in nursing as the first step towards a career in professional nursing, and as a requirement for anyone seeking a position as nurse manager or supervisor. Nurses with a baccalaureate degree are prepared to practice in all health care settings, giving graduates a broader employment choice. This level of education includes health care policy, economics, research, outcome measures, quality indicators, fiscal management, legislative advocacy, and managing information systems.

LONG-DISTANCE LEARNING. Nursing students can now obtain an education from anywhere in the world, increasing competition and pressure for quality teaching. The Internet offers a wide range of information, available faster than ever before, along with a choice of curricula, with clinical practice based in the student's community. In addition, today's more diverse and demanding student body expects choices and educational methods that fit in with all aspects of their lives. As institutes of higher learning become increasingly more responsive to education consumers, students will expect flexible learning opportunities in settings that fit their multiple roles as employees, homemakers, and members of communities. Needless to say, all nursing education programs, whatever their format, should foster collaboration, nourish racial and ethnic diversity, and encourage men to enter nursing programs. Mentoring programs starting at the high school level would also encourage more nurses to join the profession.

Professional implications

Nurses at all levels are required to deliver high-quality service while containing costs. To this end, nursing education must foster innovation and prepare students to be critical thinkers and problem solvers. Nursing professionals must be able to search for new solutions, be proactive, and entrepreneurial. Continuous learning for the professional nurse is no longer just a task needed for license renewal, but is critical to staying current in today's nursing workforce.

Legislation is constantly changing the scope of nursing practice, and educators should reflect this in their curriculum. Nursing education shapes practice—it doesn't simply react to changes in government and care environments. Collaboration between nursing educators and practicing nurses to shape nursing curriculum should reflect nursing core values and ethics. Nurses who possess analytical, communicative, and negotiating skills can help improve the health care system by educating both the public and government policymakers.

Teachers must prepare nurses to work in highly technical settings, to be computer literate, and to be highly organized and self-directed. Knowledge of today's advanced medical science is communicated in complex and sophisticated ways, requiring all nursing professionals to have the ability to manage, retrieve, and interpret data, and to be autonomous and flexible. Educators will be obliged to teach technology solutions as well as enhanced personal services. Both students and teachers must be flexible in the ways they teach and learn.

There is also greater demand for nurses in specialty areas: critical care, operating room, radiology special procedures, neonatal, and emergency. Therefore, delivering a more complex level of care is extremely important. Nurses with advanced clinical skills will have greater opportunity in their choice of clinical environments, though they may have to pursue employment in a region other than their own community. Advanced practice nurses are in increasing demand across the United States and in other countries.

Educating future generations of nursing professionals will be a unique challenge in the next decade. While the nursing shortage is just beginning to be felt, nursing faculty may face a decrease as profound as the general nursing shortage. If and when a new generation of students can be persuaded to join the profession, an associate's degree would be the fastest and most economical way into the profession. If only a limited number of faculty are available, this will perpetuate the general shortage. Nursing roles in leadership and legislation will also be severely curtailed.

Many strategies have been suggested to counter the nursing and faculty shortage. Recruiting and retention committees are the focus of many educational institutions and health care facilities in the United States and internationally. Both shortages must addressed because one can not be maintained without the other. The challenge will be a unique and challenging endeavor for the future of nursing education and will doubtless have a major global impact on health care.

Resources

PERIODICALS

Arnovitz, F. "Competition for the Education of Nurses." *Community College Week* (October 2000): 13–16.

Happell, B. "Nurse Education: Is It Responding to the Forces of Supply and Demand?" *Nursing Economics* 17, no. 5 (September/October 1999): 252–256.

Lindeman, C. "A Vision for Nursing Education." *Creative Nursing* (January/February 1996): 2–5.

Lordes, E. *"Two Years or Four? The Question Splits Nursing Education."* Chronicles of Higher Education (September 1999): 46–55.

Richards, J. "Nursing in a Digital Age." *Nursing Informatics* 19, no.1 (January/February 2001): 6 ff.

OTHER

Hinshaw, A. "A Continuing Challenge: The Shortage of Educationally Prepared Nursing Faculty." *Online Journal of Issues in Nursing*. <http://www.nursingworld.org/ojin/topic14/tpc14_3.htm>.

ORGANIZATIONS

American Association of Colleges of Nursing. 1 Dupont Circle, NW, Suite 530, Washington, DC 20036. (202) 463-6930.

René Jackson, R.N.

Nursing ethics *see* **Code of ethics for nurses**

Nursing homes

Definition

A nursing home is a long-term care facility that offers room and board and health care services, including basic and skilled nursing care, rehabilitation, and a full range of other therapies, treatments, and programs. People who live in nursing homes are referred to as residents.

Description

Nursing homes are often the only alternative for patients who require nursing care over an extended period of time. They are too ill to remain at home, with families, or in less structured long-term facilities. These individuals are unable to live independently and need assistance with activities of daily living (ADL). Nursing homes are largely populated by the elderly. Some nursing homes offer specialized care for certain medical conditions such as **Alzheimer's disease**.

Commonly, nursing home residents are no longer able to participate in the activities they once enjoyed. However, it is required by law that these facilities help residents achieve their highest possible quality of life. It is important for residents to have as much control as possible over their everyday lives. Laws and regulations exist to raise nursing home quality of life and care standards.

By law, nursing homes cannot use chemical or physical restraints unless they are essential for treating a medical problem. There are many dangers associated with the use of restraints, including the chance of a fall if a resident tries to walk while restrained. The devices may also lead to depression and decreased self-esteem. A doctor's order is necessary before restraints can be used in a nursing home.

Licensing

The Joint Commission on the Accreditation of Health Care Organizations (JCAHO) offers accreditation to nursing homes through the Long Term Care Accreditation Program established in 1966. This group helps nursing homes improve their quality of care. The JCAHO periodically surveys nursing homes to check on quality issues.

A nursing home may be certified by **Medicare** or **Medicaid** if it meets the criteria of these organizations. Families should be informed of the certifications a nursing home holds. Medicare and Medicaid are the main sources of financial income for nursing homes in the United States.

The state where a nursing home is located conducts inspections every nine to 15 months. Fines and other penalties may be enforced if the inspection reveals areas where the nursing home does not meet requirements set by that state and the federal government. Problem areas are noted in terms of scope and severity. The scope of a problem is how widespread it is, and the severity is the seriousness of its impact on the residents. When a nursing home receives an inspection report, it must post it in a place where it can be easily seen by residents and their guests.

Contract

When a resident checks into a nursing home, a contract is drawn up between him or her and the facility. This document includes information regarding the rights of the residents. It also provides details regarding services provided and discharge policies.

Resident decision-making

Decisions are made by each nursing home resident unless he or she has signed an Advanced Directive giving this authority to someone else. In order for health care decisions to be made by another person, the resident must have signed a document called a Durable Power of Attorney for Health Care.

Costs

Nursing home care is costly. The rate normally includes room and board, housekeeping, bedding, nursing care, activities, and some personal items. Additional fees may be charged for haircuts, telephones, and other personal items.

Medicare covers the cost of some nursing home services, such as skilled nursing or rehabilitative care. This payment may be activated when the nursing home care is provided after a Medicare qualifying stay in the hospital for at least three days. It is common for nursing homes to have only a few beds available for Medicare or Medicaid residents. Residents relying solely on these types of coverage must wait for a Medicare or Medicaid bed to become available.

Medicare supplemental insurance, such as Medigap, assists with the payment of nursing home expenses that are not covered by Medicare.

Medicaid qualifications vary in each state. Families of potential residents should check with their state government to determine coverage options. According to a federal law, a nursing home that drops out of the Medicaid program cannot evict current residents whose care is supported by Medicaid.

Private insurance, such as **long-term insurance**, may cover costs associated with a nursing home. People may enroll in these plans through their employers or other group insurance policies.

In many cases, nursing homes are paid for by the residents' personal funds. When these funds are exhausted, the residents sometimes become eligible for Medicaid assistance.

KEY TERMS

Long-term care—Residential care over a period of time. A nursing home is a type of long-term care facility that offers nursing care and assistance with daily living tasks.

Restraint—A physical device or a medication designed to restrict a person's movement.

Viewpoints

The quality of care in nursing homes is an important issue. Quality issues include:

• Ratios of staff to patients. Advocacy groups are pushing for increased staff-to-patient ratios in nursing homes. The National Citizens' Coalition for Nursing Home Reform recommends one direct care staff (R.N., L.V.N., or C.N.A.) per five residents during the day shift, 10 residents during the evening shift, and 15 residents during the night shift.

• Elder abuse. It is important for nursing home personnel to look for signs of abuse or neglect when a resident checks in and during a resident's stay. Signs of abuse include bodily injuries that appear suspicious, visible harm to the wrist or ankles that may indicate the use of restraints, skin ulcers that seem neglected, poor hygiene, inadequate **nutrition**, unexplained **dehydration**, untreated medical problems, or **personality disorders** such as excessive nervousness or withdrawal. The nurse or allied health professional is to report any signs of abuse to the supervisor or physician.

• Nurses' salaries. Salaries may be lower in long-term facilities than in acute care hospitals.

• Reimbursement. Nursing home administrators report that reimbursements do not cover the expenses, while nursing home advocates would like a higher portion of revenues to be allocated for direct patient care.

Professional implications

Long-term care is a growing trend, making nursing homes a viable career alternative for nurses and allied health professionals. Approximately one out of twenty Americans over age 65 live in nursing homes, although younger adults may require the special services a nursing home offers. There are about 17,000 nursing homes in the United States caring for over 1.5 million people. Nursing homes have an average occupancy rate of 80 percent.

Nursing homes must meet the physical, emotional, and social needs of its residents. The leadership staff may include an administrator, medical director, director of nursing, and directors for other allied health services. It is important for nursing home staff to understand the policies regarding care in these types of facilities.

These professionals provide care and treatments in nursing homes:

• physicians

• nurses

• nursing assistants

• dietitians

• physical, occupational, and speech therapists

• pharmacists

• social activities staff

• dentists

• social workers or psychological counselors

• other staff, such as custodians and office personnel

Required care plans

There are federal laws regarding the care given in a nursing home, and it is essential that staff members become aware of these regulations. It is required that staff conduct a thorough assessment of each new resident during the first two weeks following admission. The assessment includes the resident's ability to move and his or her rehabilitation needs, the status of the skin, any medical conditions that are present, nutritional state, and abilities regarding activities of daily living.

In some cases, the nursing home residents are unable to communicate their needs to the staff. Therefore, it is particularly important for nurses and other professionals to look for problems during their assessments. Signs of malnutrition and dehydration are especially important when assessing nursing home residents.

It is not normal for an elderly person to lose weight. However, some people lose their ability to **taste** and **smell** as they age and may lose interest in food. This can result in malnutrition, which can lead to confusion and impaired ability to fight off disease.

Older people are also more susceptible to dehydration. Their medications may lead to dehydration as a side effect, or they may limit fluids because they are too afraid of uncontrolled urination. It is very dangerous to be without adequate fluid, so the nurse and other staff must be able to recognize early signs of dehydration.

When the assessment is complete, a care plan is developed. This plan is subject to change as changes in the resident's condition occur.

Patients' rights

It is important for the professionals working in nursing homes to be aware of the residents' rights. Residents are informed of their rights when they are admitted. Residents have the right to:

- Manage their finances.
- Have privacy (for themselves and their belongings).
- Make decisions (unless Advanced Directives or Durable Power of Attorney exist).
- See visitors in private.
- Receive information regarding their medical care and treatments.
- Have social services.
- Leave the nursing home after giving the required amount of notice. A stay in a nursing home is normally considered voluntary; however, the facility will consider a variety of factors before discharging a resident. These factors include the resident's health, safety and potential danger to self or others, as well as the resident's payment for services. The contract will state how much notice is required before a resident may transfer to another facility, return home, or move in with a family member.

Family involvement

In some cases, a nursing home is chosen after the family has only a short time to prepare for the change. For example, when a patient is unable to care for himself or herself due to a sudden illness or injury, the family must turn to nursing home care without having the luxury of researching this option over time. The nursing home's costs must be explained to the resident or family prior to admission. It is important for the nursing home staff to be willing to answer the family's questions and reassure them about the care their loved one will receive.

Nursing home professionals have an opportunity to continue to work closely with the resident's family and loved ones over the course of a resident's stay. In these facilities, concerned family members and friends of the resident are involved in his or her care, and may have guardianship or other decision-making responsibility. These individuals may voice their concerns through meetings between staff and family members. Those with legal guardianship are entitled to see a resident's **medical records**, care plans, and other related material.

Communication

As in other health care settings, communication among nursing home staff is very important. In nursing homes, the care is based on a team approach. Physicians, nurses, and allied health professionals work together to make sure the resident is able to experience the highest quality of life possible.

In many cases, physicians who have had a long-term relationship with a patient continue treatment after the patient has been admitted to a nursing home. It is important for the nursing home staff to leave blocks of time open in the schedule for physician visits. It is also the staff's duty to keep the personal physicians apprised of a resident's medical condition.

The resident, physician, and resident's legal guardian and family must be told immediately if any of the following situations arise: an accident involving the resident, the need for a major treatment change, and a decision regarding discharge or transfer. Unless an emergency arises, the nursing home must give 30 days written notice of discharge or transfer. The family may appeal the decision.

Resources

BOOKS

Hosley, Julie B. "Geriatric Patients." In *Lippincott's Textbook for Medical Assistants*, edited by Julie B. Hosley, Shirley A. Jones, and Elizabeth A. Molle-Matthews. Philadelphia: Lippincott, 1997, pp.1021–22.

ORGANIZATIONS

Health Care Financing Administration. 7500 Security Boulevard, Baltimore, MD 21244. (410) 786-3000. <http://www.hcfa.gov>.

Joint Commission on the Accreditation of Health Care Organizations, 601 13th Street NW, Suite 1150N, Washington D.C. 20005. (202) 783-6655. <http://www.jcaho.org>.

OTHER

Federwisch, Anne. "A Good Home?" *NurseWeek* (September 6, 1999): <http://www.nurseweek.com/features/99-9/goodhome.html>.

"New law bars nursing homes from dumping patients." *NurseWeek* (March 29, 1999): <http://www.nurseweek.com/news/99-3/29f.html>.

"Your Guide to Choosing a Nursing Home." *U.S. Department of Health and Human Services, Health Care Financing Administration.* (August 2000): <http://www.medicare.gov/Publications/Pubs/pdf/nhguide.pdf>.

Rhonda Cloos, R.N.

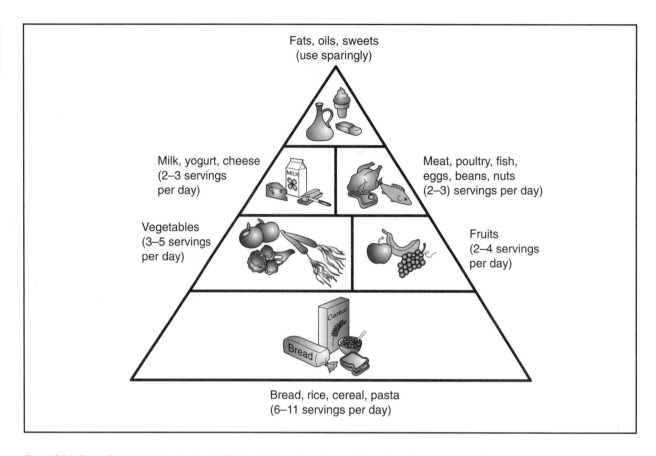

Fats, oils, sweets
(use sparingly)

Milk, yogurt, cheese
(2–3 servings
per day)

Meat, poultry, fish,
eggs, beans, nuts
(2–3) servings per day)

Vegetables
(3–5 servings
per day)

Fruits
(2–4 servings
per day)

MILK

Cereal

Bread

Bread, rice, cereal, pasta
(6–11 servings per day)

The USDA Food Pyramid. *(Illustration by Electronic Illustrators Group. Reproduced by permission.)*

Nutrition

Definition

Good nutrition can help prevent disease and promote health. There are six categories of nutrients that the body needs to acquire from food: protein, **carbohydrates**, fat, fibers, **vitamins** and **minerals**, and water.

Proteins

Protein supplies amino acids to build and maintain healthy body tissue. There are 20 amino acids considered essential because the body must have all of them in the right amounts to function properly. Twelve of these are manufactured in the body but the other eight amino acids must be provided by the diet. Foods from an animal source such as milk or eggs often contain all these essential amino acids while a variety of plant products must be taken together to provide all these necessary protein components.

Fat

Fat supplies energy and transports nutrients. There are two families of fatty acids considered essential for the body: the omega-3 and omega-6 fatty acids. Essential fatty acids are required by the body to function normally. They can be obtained from canola oil, flaxseed oil, cold-water fish, or fish oil, all of which contain omega-3 fatty acids, and primrose or black currant seed oil, which contains omega-6 fatty acids. The U.S. diet often contains an excess of omega-6 fatty acids and insufficient amount of omega-3 **fats**. Increased consumption of omega-3 oils are recommended to help reduce risk of cardiovascular diseases and **cancer** and alleviate symptoms of rheumatoid arthritis, premenstrual syndrome, dermatitis, and inflammatory bowel disease.

Carbohydrates

Carbohydrates are the body's main source of energy and should be the major part of total daily intake. There are two types of carbohydrates: simple carbohydrates (such as sugar or honey) and complex carbohydrates (such as grains, beans, peas, or potatoes). Complex carbohydrates are preferred because these foods are more nutritious yet have fewer calories per gram compared to fat and cause fewer problems with overeating than fat or sugar. Complex carbohydrates are also preferred over simple carbohydrates by diabetics because they allow better **blood** glucose control.

Fiber

Fiber is the material that gives a plant texture and support. Although it is primarily made up of carbohydrates, it does not have a lot of calories and usually is not broken down by the body for energy. Dietary fiber is found in plant foods such as fruits, vegetables, legumes, nuts, and whole grains.

There are two types of fiber: soluble and insoluble. Insoluble fiber, as the name implies, does not dissolve in water because it contains high amount of cellulose. Insoluble fiber can be found in the bran of grains, the pulp of fruit and the skin of vegetables. Soluble fiber is the type of fiber that dissolves in water. It can be found in a variety of fruits and vegetables such as apples, oatmeal and oat bran, rye flour, and dried beans.

Although they share some common characteristics such as being partially digested in the **stomach** and intestines and have few calories, each type of fiber has its own specific health benefits. Insoluble fiber speeds up the transit of foods through the **digestive system** and adds bulk to the stools, therefore, it is the type of fiber that helps treat constipation or **diarrhea** and prevents colon cancer. On the other hand, only soluble fiber can lower blood cholesterol levels. This type of fiber works by attaching itself to the cholesterol so that it can be eliminated from the body. This prevents cholesterol from recirculating and being reabsorbed into the bloodstream.

Vitamins and minerals

Vitamins are organic substances present in food and required by the body in a minute amount for regulation of **metabolism** and maintenance of normal growth and functioning. The most commonly known vitamins are A, B_1 (**thiamine**), B_2 (**riboflavin**), B_3 (**niacin**), B_5 (pantothenic acid), B_6 (pyridoxine), B_7 (**biotin**), B_9 (**folic acid**), B_{12} (cobalamin), C (ascorbic acid), D, E, and K. The B and C vitamins are water-soluble, excess amounts of which are excreted in the urine. The A, D, E, and K vitamins are fat-soluble and will be stored in the body fat.

Minerals are vital to our existence because they are the building blocks that make up muscles, tissues, and bones. They also are important components of many life-supporting systems, such as hormones, oxygen transport, and enzyme systems.

There are two kinds of minerals: the major (or macro) minerals and the trace minerals. Major minerals are the minerals that the body needs in large amounts. The following minerals are classified as major: **calcium**, **phosphorus**, magnesium, sodium, potassium, sulfur, and chloride. They are needed to build muscles, blood, nerve cells, teeth, and bones. They are also essential electrolytes that the body requires to regulate blood volume and **acid-base balance**.

Unlike the major minerals, trace minerals are needed only in tiny amounts. Even though they can be found in the body in exceedingly small amounts, they are also very important to the human body. These minerals participate in most chemical reactions in the body. They are also needed to manufacture important hormones. The following are classified as trace minerals: **iron**, **zinc**, iodine, **copper**, manganese, fluoride, chromium, selenium, molybdenum, and boron.

Many vitamins (such as vitamins A, C, and E) and minerals (such as zinc, copper, selenium, or manganese) act as antioxidants. They protect the body against the damaging effects of free radicals. They scavenge or "mop up" these highly reactive radicals and change them into inactive, less harmful compounds. In so doing, these essential nutrients help prevent cancer and many other degenerative diseases, such as premature aging, **heart** disease, autoimmune diseases, arthritis, **cataracts**, **Alzheimer's disease**, and **diabetes mellitus**.

Water

Water helps to regulate body temperature, transports nutrients to cells, and rids the body of waste materials.

Origins

Unlike plants, human beings cannot manufacture most of the nutrients that they need to function. They must eat plants and/or other animals. Although nutritional therapy came to the forefront of the public's awareness in the late twentieth century, the notion that food affects health is not new. John Harvey Kellogg was an early health-food pioneer and an advocate of a high-fiber diet. An avowed vegetarian, he believed that meat products were particularly detrimental to the colon. In the 1870s, Kellogg founded the Battle Creek Sanitarium, where he developed a diet based on nut and vegetable products.

Benefits

Good nutrition helps individuals achieve general health and well-being. In addition, dietary modifications might be prescribed for a variety of complaints including **allergies**, anemia, arthritis, colds, depressions, fatigue, gastrointestinal disorder, high or low **blood pressure**, insomnia, headaches, **obesity**, **pregnancy**, premenstrual syndrome (PMS), respiratory conditions, and **stress**.

Nutritional therapy may also be involved as a complement to the allopathic treatments of cancer, diabetes, and **Parkinson's disease**. Other specific dietary measures include the elimination of food additives for attention deficit hyperactivity disorder (ADHD), gluten-free diets for **schizophrenia**, and dairy-free for chronic respiratory diseases.

A high-fiber diet helps prevent or treat the following health conditions:

• High cholesterol levels. Fiber effectively lowers blood cholesterol levels. It appears that soluble fiber binds to cholesterol and moves it down the digestive tract so that it can be excreted from the body. This prevents the cholesterol from being reabsorbed into the bloodstream.

• Constipation. A high-fiber diet is the preferred non-drug treatment for constipation. Fiber in the diet adds more bulk to the stools, making them softer and shortens the time foods stay in the digestive tract.

• Hemorrhoids. Fiber in the diet adds more bulk and softens the stool, thus reducing painful hemorrhoidal symptoms.

• Diabetes. Soluble fiber in the diet slows down the rise of blood sugar levels following a meal and helps control diabetes.

• Obesity. Dietary fiber makes a person feel full faster.

• Cancer. Insoluble fiber in the diet speeds up the movement of the stools through the gastro-intestinal tract. The faster food travels through the digestive tract, the less time there is for potential cancer-causing substances to work. Therefore, diets high in insoluble fiber help prevent the accumulation of toxic substances that cause cancer of the colon. Because fiber reduces fat absorption in the digestive tract, it may also prevent **breast cancer**.

A diet low in fat also promotes good health and prevents many diseases. Low-fat diet can help treat or control the following conditions:

• Obesity. High fat consumption often leads to excess caloric and fat intake, which increases body fat.

• Coronary artery disease. High consumption of saturated fats is associated with coronary artery disease.

• Diabetes. People who are overweight tend to develop or worsen existing diabetic condition due to decreased insulin sensitivity.

• Breast cancer. A high dietary consumption of fat is associated with an increased risk of breast cancer.

Description

The four basic food groups, as outlined by the United States Department of Agriculture (USDA) are:

• dairy products (such as milk and cheese)

• meat and eggs (such as fish, poultry, pork, beef, and eggs)

• grains (such as bread cereals, rice, and pasta)

• fruits and vegetables

The USDA recommendation for adults is that consumption of meat, eggs, and dairy products should not exceed 20% of total daily caloric intake. The rest (80%) should be devoted to vegetables, fruits, and grains. For children age two or older, 55% of their caloric intake should be in the form of carbohydrates, 30% from fat, and 15% from **proteins**. In addition, saturated fat intake should not exceed 10% of total caloric intake. This low-fat, high-fiber diet is believed to promote health and help prevent many diseases, including heart disease, obesity, and cancer.

Allergenic and highly processed foods should be avoided. Highly processed foods do not contain significant amounts of essential trace minerals. Furthermore, they contain lots of fat and sugar as well as preservatives, artificial sweeteners and other additives. High consumption of these foods causes build up of these unwanted chemicals in the body and should be avoided. Food allergy causes a variety of symptoms including food cravings, weight gain, bloating, water retention. It may also worsen chronic inflammatory conditions such as arthritis.

Preparations

An enormous body of research exists in the field of nutrition. Mainstream Western medical practitioners point to studies that show that a balanced diet, based on the USDA Food Guide Pyramid, provides all of the necessary nutrients.

The Food Guide Pyramid recommends the following daily servings in six categories:

• Grains: Six or more servings.

• Vegetables: Five servings.

• Fruits: Two to four servings.

• Meat: Two to three servings.

• Dairy: Two to three servings.

• Fats and oils: Use sparingly.

Precautions

Individuals should not change their diets without the advice of nutritional experts or health care professionals. Certain individuals especially children, pregnant and lactating women, and chronically ill patients should only change their diets under professional supervision.

Side effects

It is best to obtain vitamins and minerals through food sources. Excessive intake of vitamins and mineral supplements can cause serious physiological problems.

The following is a list of possible side effects resulting from excessive doses of vitamins and minerals

- vitamin A: birth defects, irreversible bone and **liver** damage
- vitamin B_1: deficiencies in B_2 and B_6
- vitamin B_6: damage to the nervous system
- vitamin C: affects the absorption of copper; diarrhea
- vitamin D: hypercalcemia (abnormally high concentration of calcium in the blood)
- phosphorus: affects the absorption of calcium
- zinc: affects absorption of copper and iron; suppresses the immune system

Research and general acceptance

Due to the large volume of scientific evidence demonstrating the benefits of the low-fat, high-fiber diet in disease prevention and treatment, this diet has been accepted and advocated by most health care practitioners.

Resources

BOOKS

Bruce, Debra Fulghum, and Harris H. McIlwain. *The Unofficial Guide to Alternative Medicine.* New York: Macmillan, 1998.

Cassileth, Barrie R. *The Alternative Medicine Handbook.* New York: W.W. Norton, 1998.

Credit, Larry P., Sharon G. Hartunian, and Margaret J. Nowak. *Your Guide to Complementary Medicine.* Garden City Park, NY: Avery Publishing Group, 1998.

U.S. Preventive Services Task Force Guidelines. "Counseling to Promote a Healthy Diet." *Guide to Clinical Preventive Services.* 2nd edition. <http://cpmcnet.columbia.edu/texts/gcps/gcps0066.html>.

Winick, Myron. *The Fiber Prescription.* New York: Random House, Inc., 1992.

PERIODICALS

Halbert, Steven C. "Diet and Nutrtion in Primary Care: From Antioxidants to Zinc." *Primary Care: Clinics in Office Practice* (December 1997): 825–843.

Turner, Lisa. "Good 'n Plenty." *Vegetarian Times* (February 1999):48

Vickers, Andrew, and Catherine Zollman. "Unconventional approaches to nutritional medicine." *British Medical Journal* (November 27, 1999): 1419.

ORGANIZATIONS

American Association of Nutritional Consultants. 810 S. Buffalo Street, Warsaw, IN 46580. (888) 828-2262.

American Dietetic Association. 216 W. Jackson Boulevard, Suite 800, Chicago, IL 60606-6995. (800) 366-1655. <http://www.eatright.org/>.

Mai Tran

Nutrition assessment *see* **Dietary assessment**

Nutrition counseling *see* **Dietary counseling**

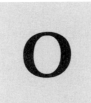

Obesity

Definition

Obesity is an abnormal accumulation of body fat, usually 20% or more over an individual's ideal body weight. Obesity is associated with increased risk of illness, disability, and death.

Description

Obesity is defined by both the U.S. Department of Agriculture and the U.S. Department of Health and Human Services as the presence of a Body Mass Index (BMI) greater than or equal to 30. BMI is a measure of body weight relative to height and is computed as weight/height^2, where weight is measured in kilograms and height in meters. Obesity is considered a subset of overweight, which is indicated by a BMI of 25 or higher.

Approximately 55% of the U.S. population is overweight, and almost one in five is obese. Excessive weight can result in many serious, and potentially deadly, health problems, including **hypertension**, Type II **diabetes mellitus** (non-insulin dependent diabetes), increased risk for coronary disease, increased unexplained **heart** attack, hyperlipidemia, **infertility**, and a higher prevalence of colon, prostate, endometrial, and, possibly, **breast cancer**. Approximately 300,000 deaths a year are attributed to obesity, prompting leaders in **public health**, such as former Surgeon General C. Everett Koop, M.D., to label obesity "the second leading cause of preventable deaths in the United States."

Causes and symptoms

The mechanism for excessive weight gain is clear—more calories are consumed than the body burns, and the excess calories are stored as fat (adipose) tissue. However, the exact cause is not as clear and likely arises from a complex combination of factors.

Genetic factors significantly influence how the body regulates the appetite and the rate at which it turns food into energy (metabolic rate). Studies of adoptees confirm this relationship—the majority of adoptees followed a pattern of weight gain that more closely resembled that of their birth parents than their adoptive parents. Yet genetic factors do not explain the rapid increase in the prevalence of obesity in the U.S. and other industrialized countries in the past 10–15 years.

A genetic predisposition to weight gain, however, does not automatically mean that a person will be obese. Eating habits and patterns of physical activity also play a significant role in the amount of weight a person gains.

Recent studies have indicated that the amount of fat in a person's diet may have a greater impact on weight than the number of calories it contains. **Carbohydrates** (cereals, breads, fruits, and vegetables) and protein (fish, lean meat, turkey breast, skim milk) are converted to fuel almost as soon as they are consumed. Most fat calories are immediately stored in fat cells, which add to the body's weight and girth as they expand and multiply.

A sedentary life-style, particularly prevalent in affluent societies, such as in the United States, can contribute to weight gain. Psychological factors, such as depression and low self-esteem may, in some cases, also play a role in weight gain.

At what stage of life a person becomes obese can effect his or her ability to lose weight. Some studies suggest that during two critical periods of a person's life—in early childhood and **puberty**, excess calories are converted into new fat cells (hyperplastic obesity), while excess calories consumed in adulthood only serve to expand existing fat cells (hypertrophic obesity). Since dieting and **exercise** can only reduce the size of fat cells, not eliminate them, persons who were obese as children can have great difficulty losing weight, since they may have up to five times as many fat cells as someone who became overweight as an adult. An estimated 13% of

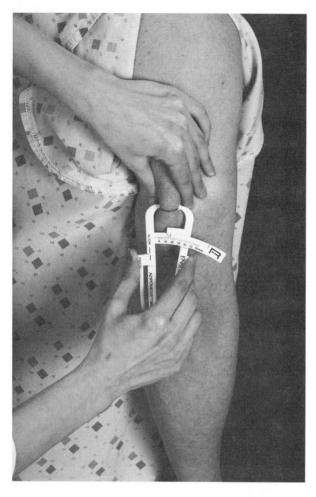

Measurement of triceps skinfold, which is an indicator of total body fat. *(Delmar Publishers, Inc. Reproduced by permission.)*

children ages 6–11 years and 14% of adolescents ages 12–19 years are currently overweight.

Obesity can also be a side-effect of certain disorders and conditions, including Cushing's syndrome, a disorder involving the excessive release of the hormone cortisol; hypothyroidism, a condition caused by an underactive **thyroid gland**; neurologic disturbances, such as damage to the hypothalamus, a structure located deep within the **brain** that helps regulate appetite; and consumption of certain drugs, such as steroids or antidepressants.

The major symptoms of obesity are excessive weight gain and the presence of large amounts of fatty tissue. Obesity can also give rise to several secondary conditions, including arthritis and other orthopedic problems, such as lower back **pain**; heartburn; high cholesterol levels; high **blood pressure**; menstrual irregularities or cessation of menstruation (amenorrhea); shortness of breath that can be incapacitating; and skin disorders, arising from the bacterial breakdown of sweat and cellular mate-

rial in thick folds of skin or from increased friction between folds.

Diagnosis

Diagnosis of obesity is made by observation and by comparing the patient's weight to ideal weight charts. Many doctors and obesity researchers refer to the body mass index (BMI), which uses a height-weight relationship to calculate an individual's ideal weight and personal risk of developing obesity-related health problems.

Since this method can be misleading, due to its failure to account for body composition and muscle mass, physicians may also obtain direct measurements of an individual's body fat content by using calipers to measure skin-fold thickness at the back of the upper arm and other sites. The most accurate means of measuring body fat content involves hydrostatic weighing, or having a person let as much air as possible out of his **lungs**, immersing him in water and measuring relative displacement; however, this method is very unpleasant and impractical, and is usually only used in scientific studies requiring very specific assessments. Women whose body fat exceeds 32% and men whose body fat exceeds 27% are generally considered obese.

Doctors may also note how a person carries excess weight on his or her body. Studies have shown that this factor may indicate whether or not an individual has a predisposition to develop certain diseases or conditions that may accompany obesity. "Apple-shaped" individuals who store most of their weight around the waist and abdomen are at greater risk for **cancer**, heart disease, stroke, and diabetes than "pear-shaped" people whose extra pounds settle primarily in their hips and thighs.

Treatment

Treatment of obesity depends primarily on how overweight a person is and his or her overall health. However, to be successful, any treatment must affect life-long behavioral changes rather than short-term weight loss. A report issued by the National Institutes of Health-sponsored group, the National Heart, Lung, and Blood Institute, *The Practical Guide to Identification, Evaluation, and Treatment of Overweight and Obesity in Adults,* recommends a combination of diet modification, increased physical activity, and behavior therapy as the means most likely to prove effective.

"Yo-yo" dieting, in which weight is repeatedly lost and regained, has been shown to increase a person's likelihood of developing fatal health problems more than if the weight had been lost gradually or not lost at all. Behavior-focused treatment should concentrate on:

HEIGHT AND WEIGHT GOALS

	Men		
Height	**Small Frame**	**Medium Frame**	**Large Frame**
5'2"	128-134 lbs.	131-141 lbs.	138-150 lbs.
5'3"	130-136	133-143	140-153
5'4"	132-138	135-145	142-153
5'5"	134-140	137-148	144-160
5'6"	136-142	139-151	146-164
5'7"	138-145	142-154	149-168
5'8"	140-148	145-157	152-172
5'9"	142-151	148-160	155-176
5'10"	144-154	151-163	158-180
5'11"	146-157	154-166	161-184
6'0"	169-160	157-170	164-188
6'1"	152-164	160-174	168-192
6'2"	155-168	164-178	172-197
6'3"	158-172	167-182	176-202
6'4"	162-176	171-187	181-207

	Women		
Height	**Small Frame**	**Medium Frame**	**Large Frame**
4'10"	102-111 lbs.	109-121 lbs.	118-131 lbs.
4'11"	103-113	111-123	120-134
5'0"	104-115	113-126	112-137
5'1"	106-118	115-129	125-140
5'2"	108-121	118-132	128-143
5'3"	111-124	121-135	131-147
5'4"	114-127	124-141	137-151
5'5"	117-130	127-141	137-155
5'6"	120-133	130-144	140-159
5'7"	123-136	133-147	143-163
5'8"	126-139	136-150	146-167
5'9"	129-142	139-153	149-170
5'10"	132-145	142-156	152-176
5'11"	135-148	145-159	155-176
6'0"	138-151	148-162	158-179

Source: Doctors On-Line, Inc. "Height and Weight Goals as Determined by the Metropolitan Life Insurance Company." http://www.doli.com/weight.htm. (Standley Publishing. Reproduced by permission.)

• What and how much a person eats. This aspect may involve keeping a food diary and developing a better understanding of the nutritional value and fat content of foods. It may also involve changing grocery-shopping habits (e.g. buying only what is on a prepared list and only going on a certain day), timing of meals (to prevent feelings of hunger, a person may plan frequent, small meals), and actually slowing down the rate at which a person eats.

• How a person responds to food. This may involve understanding what psychological issues underlie a person's eating habits. For example, one person may binge eat when under **stress**, while another may always use food as a reward. In recognizing these psychological triggers, an individual can develop alternative coping mechanisms that do not focus on food.

• How they spend their time. Making activity and exercise an integrated part of everyday life is a key to

Obesity

achieving and maintaining weight loss. Starting slowly and building endurance keeps individuals from becoming discouraged. Varying routines and trying new activities also keeps interest high.

For most individuals who are mildly obese, these behavior modifications entail life-style changes they can make independently while being supervised by a family physician. Other mildly obese persons may seek the help of a commercial weight-loss program (e.g. Weight Watchers). The effectiveness of these programs is difficult to assess, since programs vary widely, drop-out rates are high, and few employ members of the medical community. However, programs that emphasize realistic goals, gradual progress, sensible eating, and exercise can be very helpful and are recommended by many doctors. Programs that promise instant weight loss or feature severely restricted diets are not effective and, in some cases, can be dangerous.

For individuals who are moderately obese, medically supervised behavior modification and weight loss are required. While doctors will put most moderately obese patients on a balanced, low-calorie diet (1200–1500 calories a day), they may recommend that certain individuals follow a very-low-calorie liquid protein diet (400–700 calories) for as long as three months. This therapy, however, should not be confused with commercial liquid protein diets or commercial weight-loss shakes and drinks. Doctors tailor these diets to specific patients, monitor patients carefully, and use them for only a short period of time.

In addition to reducing the amount and type of calories consumed by the patient, doctors will recommend professional therapists or psychiatrists who can help the individual effectively change his or her behavior in regard to eating. For individuals who are severely obese, dietary changes and behavior modification may be accompanied by surgery to reduce or bypass portions of the **stomach** or **small intestine**. Such obesity surgery, however, can be risky, and it is only performed on patients for whom other strategies have failed and whose obesity seriously threatens their health. Other surgical procedures are not recommended, including liposuction, a purely cosmetic procedure in which a suction device is used to remove fat from beneath the skin, and jaw wiring, which can damage gums and teeth and cause painful muscle spasms.

Appetite-suppressant drugs are sometimes prescribed to aid in weight loss. These drugs work by increasing levels of serotonin or catecholamine, which are brain chemicals that control feelings of fullness. Appetite suppressants, though, are not considered truly effective, since most of the weight lost while taking them is usually regained after stopping them. Also, suppressants containing amphetamines can be potentially abused by patients.

While most of the immediate side-effects of these drugs are harmless, the long-term effects of these drugs, in many cases, is unknown. Two drugs, dexfenfluramine hydrochloride (Redux) and fenfluramine (Pondimin) as well as a combination fenfluramine-phentermine (Fen/Phen) drug, were taken off the market when they were shown to cause potentially fatal heart defects.

Other weight-loss medications available with a doctor's prescription include: sibutramine (Meridia), diethylpropion (Tenuate, Tenuate dospan) mazindol (Mazanor, Sanorex) phendimetrazine (Bontril, Plegine, Prelu-2, X-Trozine) and phentermine (Adipex-P, Fastin, Ionamin, Oby-trim).

Phenylpropanolamine (Acutrim, Dextarim) is the only nonprescription weight-loss drug approved by the FDA, but in November, 2000, the FDA announced that it was considering withdrawing its approval. These over-the-counter diet aids have been found to increase the risk of hemorrhagic stroke (bleeding into the brain or into tissue surrounding the brain) in women, and men may also be at risk.

Combined with diet and exercise and used only with a doctor's approval, prescription anti-obesity medications enable some patients to lose 10% more weight than they otherwise would. Most patients regain lost weight after discontinuing use of either prescription medications or nonprescription weight-loss products. Prescription medications or over-the-counter weight-loss products can cause: constipation, dry mouth, headache, irritability, nausea, nervousness, and sweating. None of them should be used by patients taking monoamine oxidase inhibitors (MAO inhibitors).

Doctors sometimes prescribe fluoxetine (Prozac), an antidepressant that can increase weight loss by about 10%. Weight loss may be temporary and side effects of this medication include **diarrhea**, fatigue, insomnia, nausea, and thirst.

Weight-loss drugs currently being developed or tested include ones that can prevent fat absorption or digestion; reduce the desire for food and prompt the body to burn calories more quickly; and regulate the activity of substances that control eating habits and stimulate overeating.

In April, 1999, the U.S. Food and Drug Administration (FDA) approved Xenical (orlistat), which works in the intestines, where it blocks some fat from being absorbed. This undigested fat is then eliminated in the patient's bowel movements. Available only with a doctor's prescription, many gastrointestinal side-effects can occur with Xenical. This medication should not be used by patients who have problems absorbing food or have **gallbladder** problems.

The Chinese herb ephedra (*Ephedra sinica*), combined with **caffeine**, exercise, and a low-fat diet in physician-supervised weight-loss programs, can cause at least temporary weight loss. However, the large doses of ephedra required to achieve the desired result can also produce serious side effects including chest pain, **myocardial infarction**, hepatitis, stroke, seizures, psychosis, and death. Mixing this with caffeine (a diuretic) also promotes **dehydration**, which can cause a number of other health problems. Ephedra should not be used by anyone with a history of diabetes, heart disease, or thyroid problems.

Getting the correct ratios of protein, carbohydrates, and good-quality **fats** can help in weight loss via enhancement of the **metabolism**. Support groups that are informed about healthy, nutritious, and balanced diets can offer an individual the support he or she needs to maintain this type of eating regimen.

Prognosis

As many as 85% of dieters who do not exercise on a regular basis regain their lost weight within two years. In five years, the figure rises to 90%. Repeatedly losing and regaining weight (yo-yo dieting) encourages the body to store fat and may increase a patient's risk of developing heart disease. The primary factor in achieving and maintaining weight loss is a life-long commitment to regular exercise and sensible eating habits.

Health care team roles

Physicians diagnose obesity and prescribe drugs to control it, but others can also play a role in treatment. Nutritionists and dietitians design effective and safe meal plans while taking into account the person's individual needs. Registered nurses also make nutritional recommendations and monitor the person's daily dietary intake.

Many obese people with back or knee problems cannot exercise, exacerbating the weight problem. Physical therapists design exercise programs for these individuals to improve the body's physical functionality, so more exercise can be done at higher levels of intensity. Personal trainers and fitness instructors help with weight training and cardiovascular exercise, to increase the amount of lean muscle mass and decrease body fat.

KEY TERMS

Body Mass Index (BMI)—A way of computing an individual's relative weight to height ratio, used in determining the degree to which an individual may be overweight.

Obesity—An abnormal accumulation of body fat, usually 20% or more over an individual's ideal body weight.

Since obesity often causes self-esteem problems, psychiatrists and psychologists use therapies including hypnotism and imagery to help improve a person's emotional well being or body image. Psychologists prescribe drugs to treat depression and **anxiety** disorders resulting from obesity. Treatments such as sound therapy, **relaxation**, and **yoga**, monitored by holistic health professionals, also may be helpful.

Prevention

Obesity experts suggest that a key to preventing excess weight gain is monitoring fat consumption rather than counting calories, and the National Cholesterol Education Program maintains that only 30% of calories should be derived from fat. Only one-third of those calories should be contained in saturated fats (the kind of fat found in high concentrations in meat, poultry, and dairy products).

Because most people eat more than they think they do, keeping a detailed food diary is a useful way to assess eating habits. Eating three balanced, moderate-portion meals a day—with the main meal at mid-day—is a more effective way to prevent obesity than fasting or crash diets.

Exercise increases the metabolic rate by creating muscle, which burns more calories than fat. When regular exercise is combined with regular, healthful meals, calories continue to burn at an accelerated rate for several hours.

Finally, encouraging healthful habits in children is a key to preventing childhood obesity and the health problems that follow in adulthood.

Resources

ORGANIZATIONS

HCF Nutrition Research Foundation, Inc. P.O. Box 22124, Lexington, KY 40522. (606) 276-3119.

National Institute of Diabetes and Digestive and Kidney Diseases. 31 Center Drive, USC2560, Building 31, Room 9A-04, Bethesda, MD 20892-2560. Phone: (301) 496-3583. Website: <http://www. niddk.nih/gov>.

National Obesity Research Foundation. Temple University, Weiss Hall 867, Philadelphia, PA 19122.

The Weight-Control Information Network. 1 Win Way, Bethesda, MD 20896–3665. Phone: (301) 951–1120. Website: <http://www.navigator.tufts.edu/special/win.html>.

OTHER

U.S. Department of Health and Human Services. Centers for Disease Control and Prevention and National Center for Health Statistics. *Prevalence of Overweight and Obesity Among Adults in the United States; Prevalence of Overweight Among Children and Adolescents: United States, 1999.* Hyattsville, MD: Division of Data Services, pp. 20782–2003.

U.S. Food and Drug Administration. Center for Drug Evaluation and Research. <http://www.fda.gov/cder/index.html>.

U.S. Food and Drug Administration. "Dietary Supplements Containing Ephedrine Alkaloids." 21 CFR Part 111, Docket No. 95N-0304, RIN 0901-AA59.

Maia Appleby

Obstetric sonogram *see* **Pelvic ultrasound**

Occlusion *see* **Malocclusion**

Occult blood test *see* **Fecal occult blood test**

Occupational Safety and Health Act

Definition

The United States Congress passed the Occupational Safety and Health Act of 1970 to ensure that work environments are safe and free of dangerous hazards for both employees and their employers.

Description

When the Act was signed into law by President Richard M. Nixon on December 29, 1970, it called for the creation of the Occupational Safety and Health Administration (OSHA), the regulating governmental body that inspects workplaces for unsafe and unhealthy conditions. The first standards were adopted by OSHA in 1971. The Act also created the National Institute for Occupational Safety and Health (NIOSH), a federal agency under the Centers for Disease Control (CDC) that researches work-related injuries and workplace hazards. NIOSH also is charged with making recommendations on how to prevent accidents in the workplace and, at the request of business owners or its employees, investigates businesses where hazards may exist. The agency is the clearinghouse for dissemination of workplace safety information and trains occupational safety and health professionals. NIOSH follows the National Occupational Research Agenda (NORA), a research agenda developed by 500 organizations that outlines the top 21 research priorities among workplace safety issues.

The law applies to all employers and employees in the United States, District of Columbia, Puerto Rico, and any other jurisdiction of the U.S. federal government. The law is not enforceable among federal or state employees, or farms where only immediate family members are employed. Those who are self-employed or whose workplaces are covered under other federal regulations, such as nuclear energy, mining, or nuclear weapons manufacturing, also are exempt from the Act.

Employers covered by the law are required to implement proper policies and procedures within their businesses that comply with the regulations. Regulations cover, but are not limited to, hazardous waste handling, fall protection at construction sites, asbestos, ergonomics, and respiratory protection. States have the option of enforcing the federal regulations or adopting their own job safety programs that are at least as strict as the OSHA regulations. In 1972, South Carolina, Montana, and Oregon were the first states to approve their own programs.

Employees who work in environments covered by the Act have certain rights under the law. Employees are permitted to file complaints with OSHA regarding the safety conditions of their workplaces. Complaints are kept confidential from employers. In order to enforce the Act, OSHA employs compliance safety and health officers (CSHOs) that are authorized to perform inspections of workplaces that are covered under the law. OSHA conducts two kinds of inspections, programmed and unprogrammed. Unprogrammed inspections are triggered when a fatality or catastrophe occurs, or if a complaint is filed.

Violations

A violation of an OSHA standard covered under the Act carry several penalties depending on the severity of the violation. Violations are classified as other than serious, serious, willful, or repeated.

Other-than-serious violation. An other-than-serious violation directly affects job safety, but likely would not cause serious injury or death. It is within the CSHO's discretion to impose up to a $7,000 penalty for each violation. However, if the business owner shows a good-faith effort to make the appropriate corrections to comply with the law, the $7,000 penalty can be reduced by up to 95%. The size of the business and whether there have been previous violations also are taken into consideration when reducing a penalty.

Serious violation. A serious violation occurs when it is likely that serious injury or death could occur because of a violation of an OSHA standard that the employer knew or should have known was harmful or hazardous. In cases of serious violations, up to a $7,000 penalty can be imposed. But, again, the penalty can be decreased on the basis of previous violations, how serious the violation, good-faith effort to correct the problem, and the size of the business.

Willful violation. An employer willfully commits a violation when he or she is aware the violation exists. Either the employer knows a violation is being committed or does not try to eliminate a dangerous condition that exists. An employer who commits a willful violation faces a penalty of at least $5,000 and not more than $70,000. The only considerations taken into account when decreasing the penalty for a willful violation is the number of previous violations and the size of the business. If a death has occurred as a result of a willful violation, an employer could face up to six months of prison and/or a fine imposed by the courts. If criminal charges are levied and a conviction results, the employer's corporation could face a $500,000 fine and the individual a $250,000 fine, enforceable under the Comprehensive Crime Control Act of 1984.

Repeated violation. If upon reinspection by OSHA officers a similar violation is found, a $70,000 penalty may be imposed.

Other violations. Once a violation is found, and a deadline imposed as to when the violation must be corrected, employers could face a $7,000 penalty for every day the problem goes uncorrected. Additionally, employers found doctoring records or applications could face a fine of up to $10,000 and/or six months in prison. Any kind of interference with an OSHA compliance officer who is attempting to perform an inspection, whether it be by resisting or intimidating the officer, is considered a crime and could carry up to a $250,000 penalty for an individual and $500,000 for a corporation.

KEY TERMS

Ergonomics—The study of the relationship between people and their working environment.

Musculoskeletal disorder—Injuries that affect the muscles and skeleton, such as repetitive stress injuries to the hand and wrist.

Viewpoints

One of the most controversial OSHA standards debated in Congress was the Ergonomics Rule issued by the agency in November 2000. The measure, which would have applied to 1.6 million employers in the United States, aimed to prevent nearly a half million musculoskeletal disorders (MSDs) in more than 102 million workers in the country's workplaces. The proposed standard would have affected manual handling, manufacturing, and occupational job sites where MSDs are reported. Employers would have been required to implement ergonomics programs that would decrease the risk of MSDs. However, many employers, particularly owners of small businesses, claimed the measure would be far too costly. OSHA reported that compliance with the regulation would cost businesses $4 billion a year, but would be offset by eliminating the estimated $20 billion a year spent on lost wages and medical costs of those absent from work because of MSDs and other workplace injuries. The National Coalition on Ergonomics (NCE), one of OSHA's staunchest opponents, estimated costs at $26 billion a year for businesses.

After the 2000 election in which George W. Bush was elected President, the U.S. House of Representatives and the Senate voted to overturn the rule. Those voting to overturn the rule were most concerned about the cost of implementation, and the lack of sound scientific grounding for the standard. The U.S. Department of Labor began drafting a new ergonomics rule in early 2001.

Professional implications

When OSHA first proposed a new ergonomics rule, officials turned to occupational therapists because the discipline is the most appropriate in dealing with the application of workplace safety regulations. The American **Occupational Therapy** Association identified ergonomics and workplace safety consulting as a major emerging job market at the turn of the new millennium. Occupational therapists have a strong background in basic health education, physiology, and anatomy. Applying those skills in the workplace setting makes occupational therapists the experts to turn to for consulting needs.

Resources

BOOKS

Dell Orto, Arthur E. and Robert P. Marinelli, eds. *Encyclopedia of Disability and Rehabilitation.* New York: Simon & Schuster Macmillan, 1995.

PERIODICALS

Gourley, Meghan. "Refining OT's Edge in Ergonomics." *OT Practice*(11 September 2000): 14–17.

ORGANIZATIONS

The American Occupational Therapy Association. 4720 Montgomery Lane, Bethesda, MD 20824-1220. (301) 652-2682. <http://www.aota.org>.

The Centers for Disease Control, National Institute for Occupational Safety and Health, 200 Independence Avenue, SW, Washington, DC 20201. (800) 356-4674. <http://www.cdc.gov/niosh>.

The Environmental Protection Agency. Ariel Building, 1200 Pennsylvania, NW, Washington, DC 20210. (202) 260-2090. <http://www.epa.gov>.

National Coalition on Ergonomics. 1615 H Street, NW, Washington, DC 20062. (202) 293-3384. <http://www.ncergo.org>.

The U.S. Department of Labor, Occupational Safety and Health Administration. 200 Constitution Avenue, NW, Washington, DC 20210. (202) 693-4650. <http://www.osha.gov>.

Meghan M. Gourley

Occupational therapy

Definition

Occupational therapy is a holistic, patient-centered, occupation-based approach to life skill development. This health profession helps people whose lives have been altered by physical or mental disease, injury, or other health problems. People of any age can benefit from occupational therapy to prevent injury and improve skills needed to perform everyday tasks or "occupations" at home, work, or school. Examples include activities of daily living such as dialing a phone, using a computer, writing a check, and driving a car.

Description

Occupational therapists first came onto the scene during World War I, when practitioners worked with sol-diers suffering from shell shock, amputations, and other injuries. Also in the early 20th century, occupational therapists treated persons with **tuberculosis** and polio.

Today, the role of occupational therapists is varied and broad. For the last several decades, occupational therapists have treated patients suffering from physical and developmental disabilities such as **brain** injury, **spinal cord injury**, repetitive **stress** injury, stroke, Alzheimer's, diabetes, attention deficit disorder, mental retardation, and Parkinson's, among others. At the turn of the new millennium, however, practitioners began to prove their worth in areas such as **vision** treatment, mental health, ergonomics consulting, and home modification.

Through activities of daily living (ADL) evaluations, it is determined by the practitioner how independent a client is in performing his or her daily tasks at home, at work, and within his or her social environment. After evaluation, an occupational therapist may implement an intervention to facilitate a more independent lifestyle. The goal of occupational therapy practitioners is to facilitate the patients physical independence. One way that they do this is by implementing exercises that aid in mobility. When a patient has impaired vision, a therapist might analyze lighting and contrast needs in the home, and equip the patient with tools to make the home and work environment more functional. Such tools might include a magnifying glass, or auxiliary lighting. In ergonomics consulting, a therapist might advise businesses and industries about functional and comfortable work stations that minimize repetitive stress injuries caused by repetitive movements, such as typing or assembly line work. Interventions that help patients—such as those with developmental disabilities, or those in mental health settings—to function on a daily basis, such as stress management and communication skills, might also be facilitated by occupational therapists.

Work settings

Occupational therapy practitioners may work in a variety of settings; the scope of their practice may be vast. Traditional work settings are long-term-care (LTC) and skilled nursing facilities (SNFs), outpatient clinics, and other **nursing homes**, in which practitioners provide direct care to patients with physical and developmental problems (e.g., arthritis, hand injuries, and **dementia**). Occupational therapists and occupational therapy assistants have found their place in mental health facilities, home health agencies, and, more recently, community-based settings and private practice. No matter what the setting in which a practitioner practices, the approach is patient-centered; the patient's needs and the environment

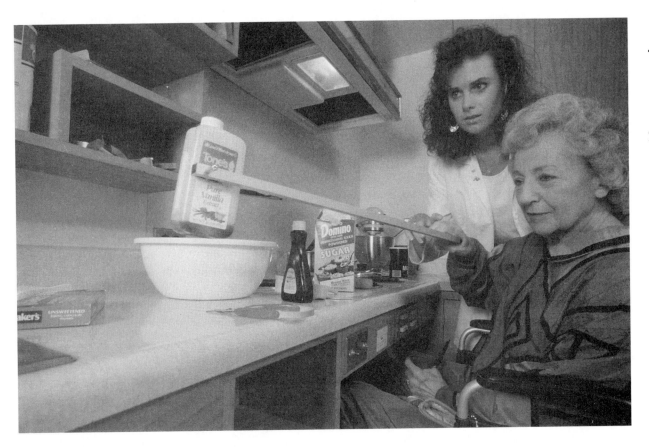

A therapist works with a patient recovering from a stroke. *(Photograph by Will & Deni McIntyre. Science Source/Photo Researchers. Reproduced by permission.)*

in which the patient lives are considered when developing a treatment plan.

Many occupational therapy practitioners work with children in the school systems. The focus of a therapist in an educational environment may be to implement a handwriting intervention program, with the goal of improving finger dexterity in young children. According to a compensation survey of its members that the American Occupational Therapy Association (AOTA) conducted in 2000, nearly a quarter of members who responded are employed by school systems. Practitioners reported that they are also finding more opportunities in community-based settings, such as workplace ergonomics consulting and work rehabilitation programs.

Education and training

Current practitioners are credentialed as either occupational therapists, considered professionals after completing an accredited bachelor's degree program, or as occupational therapy assistants, who are considered at the technical level after completing a two-year associate program.

Prior to graduation, students must complete a supervised fieldwork program through their college or university program, and pass a national certification exam administered by the National Board of Certification in Occupational Therapy (NBCOT). The NBCOT is currently developing a recertification program.

The Accreditation Council for Occupational Therapy Education (ACOTE), following a resolution by the AOTA's Representative Assembly, moved to require a master's degree upon entry into the field of occupational therapy. By the year 2007, all educational institutions offering occupational therapy programs must do so under the standards of ACOTE's post-baccalaureate requirements. However, there are many practitioners in the field who have already earned master's and doctorate degrees. As of 2001, the number of practitioners with advanced degrees had nearly doubled (since 1990).

Licensure

The profession of occupational therapy is regulated in every state; in 43 states, as well as the District of Columbia, Puerto Rico, and Guam, occupational therapists are required to be licensed. Licensure is important because

KEY TERMS

Activities of daily living (ADL)—Activities of daily living are an individual's skills and practices that determine how well he or she can function in daily life and how well he or she relates to and participates in his or her environment.

Alzheimer's Disease—A progressive, neurodegenerative disease characterized by loss of function and death of nerve cells in several areas of the brain, leading to loss of mental functions, such as memory and learning. Alzheimer's disease is the most common cause of dementia.

Arthritis—Inflammation of one or more joints.

Attention deficit disorder (ADD)—A condition characterized by an attention span that is less than expected for the age of the person. There is often age-inappropriate hyperactivity and impulsive behavior, as well.

Ergonomics—The study of the relationship between people and their working environment.

Home modification—Altering the physical environment of the home so as to remove hazards and provide an environment that is more functional for the patient. Examples of home modification include the installation of grab bars and no-slip foot maps in the bathroom, to prevent falls.

Parkinson's disease—A disorder of the brain characterized by shaking and difficulty with walking, movement, and coordination. The disease is associated with damage to a part of the brain that controls muscle movement.

Stroke—A group of brain disorders involving loss of brain functions that occur when the blood supply to any part of the brain is interrupted.

it defines the scope of practice for therapists and provides guidance to facilities and health care providers on the appropriate application of occupational therapy services.

The field of occupational therapy has been playing catch-up with its allied health counterparts, such as **physical therapy** and speech–language pathology. More sophisticated and specialized education was necessary for occupational therapists to remain competitive and prove their worth when interacting with consumers and other medical professionals. In the 2001 market, practitioners must be able to employ critical reasoning and develop innovative practice models.

Advanced education and training

Continuing education courses and additional training is necessary for practitioners to remain competent within the field; this must be done on a regular basis. Practitioners can utilize AOTA's continuing education courses, online courses, and annual conference and exposition workshops, as well as educational sessions that are offered by leaders in occupational therapy.

In 2000, AOTA's Council on Continued Competence in Occupational Therapy (CCCOT) implemented the Continuing Competence Plan for Professional Development, a comprehensive plan that guides practitioners in developing and maintaining competent skills. The NBCOT, through which practitioners must become certified and eventually recertify, agreed to work in coordination with the AOTA to develop a recertification program that agrees with the principles set forth in the CCCOT's plan.

Future outlook

As health care delivery has changed dramatically with the advent of managed care, the roles of occupational therapists and occupational therapy assistants have expanded, due mostly in the United States to **Medicare** provider payment cutbacks mandated by the Balanced Budget Act (BBA) of 1997. Many jobs were cut in SNFs, leaving occupational therapists out of work. This change forced practitioners to consider other markets that might values their services.

The occupational therapy profession, however, was granted a reprieve when the U.S. Congress made several changes to the Balanced Budget Act. The Balanced Budget Refinement Act of 1999 called for a suspension of a capitation on rehabilitation services. Congress agreed to suspend the capitation because of the controversy surrounding combining occupational therapy, physical therapy, and speech-language pathology.

For occupational therapy to survive, new markets had to emerge. Practitioners proved their worth in less traditional roles and work settings. While therapists still have a place in LTC facilities, they are carving a niche in school systems—the most popular work setting, according to a 2000 survey conducted by AOTA—as well as business-to-business consulting firms that specialize in ergonomics, home modification, and/or assistive devices, wellness education programs, community-based mental health programs, and a variety of specialties in private practice.

It was reported by the U.S. Department of Labor's 2001 *Occupational Outlook Handbook* that the occupational therapy field is expected to grow at a faster rate than any other occupation through 2008. These gains, however, are expected to be made in the years closer to 2008 due to congressional cuts, detailed above.

The increasing demand for occupational therapists is expected, in large part, because of the emerging markets, as well as the increase in those requiring the type of services occupational therapists provide. As baby boomers (those born between 1945 and 1965) age, occupational therapy practitioners will have an even bigger market for home modification, so that the elderly, for example, can remain in their homes longer than normally expected. Advancement in medical technology continues to allow people to live longer, despite serious illness and disability, and occupational therapists can facilitate their independence in daily living and working.

Resources

BOOKS

Punwar, Alice J. and Suzanne M. Peloquin. *Occupational Therapy, Principles and Practice, 3rd ed.* Baltimore: Lippincott Williams & Wilkins, 2000.

PERIODICALS

Bonder, Bette and Charles Christiansen. "Editorial: Coming of Age in Challenging Times." *Occupational Therapy Journal of Research* (Winter 2001): 3-11.

Fidle, Gail S. "Beyond the Therapy Model: Building Our Future." *The American Journal of Occupational Therapy* 54 (January/February 2000): 99-101.

Foto, Mary. "Professional Evolution: Should Health Care Environmental Changes Force OT and PT Practice Into a New Delivery Model?" *OT Week* (9 April 1998): 17–19.

Gourley, Meghan. "Postbaccalaureate Requirement Facilitates Growth." *OT Practice* (17 and 31 July 2000): 9–10.

Gourley, Meghan. "Maintaining Career Competence." *OT Practice* (5 March 2001): 14-16.

Hasselkus, Betty R. "Reaching Consensus." *The American Journal of Occupational Therapy* 54 (March/April 2000): 127–128.

Jacobs, Karen. "Being an Occupation FANATIC." *Administration & Management Special Interest Section Quarterly* 16 (March 2000): 1-4.

Stancliff Walls, Bethany. "What Does Resolution J Mean to the Profession?" *OT Practice* (July/August 1999): 13, 15.

Walker, Kay F. "Adjustments to Managed Health Care: Pushing Against It, Going With It, and Making the Best of It." *The American Journal of Occupational Therapy* 55 (March/April 2001): 17–19.

Wilcock, Anne A. "An Occupational Scientist's Perspective for Future Practice." *OT Week* (28 May 1998): 13-14.

ORGANIZATIONS

The American Occupational Therapy Association, Inc. 4720 Montgomery Lane, Bethesda, MD 20824-1220. (301) 652-2682. <http://www.aota.org>.

The National Board for Certification of Occupational Therapy, Inc. 800 S. Frederick Ave., Ste. 200, Gaithersburg, MD 20877-4150. (301) 990-7979. <http://www.nbcot.org>.

The U.S. Department of Labor, Bureau of Labor Statistics, Division of Information Services. 2 Massachusetts Ave. NE, Room 2860, Washington, DC 20212. (202) 691-5200. <http://www.bls.gov>.

Meghan M. Gourley

Occupational therapy interviews

Definition

The **occupational therapy** interview is the initial fact-finding session between an occupational therapy practitioner and a patient to determine the patient's problem(s) and to discuss possible intervention and treatment.

Purpose

The interview is the first opportunity for the occupational therapy practitioner to get a complete picture of the problems, concerns, and limitations of the patient. All of the information gathered is used toward defining a treatment plan. During the interview, the therapist should learn about how the patient perceives himself or herself in various roles at home, school, work, and during leisure time. The patient also should express goals he or she would like to achieve and what needs should be met.

However, the initial interview should not only be an information-gathering experience for the therapist, but also for the patient. The interviewer should explain his or her role as an occupational therapist and how he or she will facilitate an independent and functional life for the patient. It is the initial interview that helps to set the stage for treatment and becomes the foundation on which the practitioner-patient relationship is based.

Precautions

The therapist should be prepared to gather information about the patient, such as the patient's needs or lifestyles, that the therapist may not agree with. Occupational therapy practitioners need to remain open-minded in any evaluation process and recognize that patients may have differing moral and philosophical views.

KEY TERMS

Assessment—A specific test developed to measure a particular function or role of a patient. In occupational therapy, the words assessment and evaluation are not used interchangeably.

Evaluation—Determination of a person's ability or function using an assessment.

Narrative—A detailed account of an event or experience.

Description

Interviews between the occupational therapy practitioner and patient may begin by the therapist explaining the meaning of the occupational therapy profession and what the therapist hopes to achieve through the rehabilitation process. It is important for the patient to understand what is expected of him or her, and understand that the mission of occupational therapy is to facilitate independence and function within the client's life. The therapist also should cover areas of rehabilitation that pertain directly to the patient's needs, such as physical or mental disability, arthritis, **sexual dysfunction**, or a learning disability.

An effective form of interviewing is the narrative interview where the patient is permitted to speak at length and in depth about his or her life, problems, concerns, or any other topic. This allows the patient to speak freely about whatever topic that troubles or interests him or her most. In any type of interview and throughout the rehabilitation process, the occupational therapy practitioner should employ good listening skills and answer questions with great thought. Therapists should not ignore the use of metaphors during the interviewing process. Studies have shown that it is not uncommon for patients to use symbolic images that represent a feeling in their lives, such as entrapment or fear.

In occupational therapy, several assessments exist in which the patient's occupational performance is measured. They include, but are not limited to, the Canadian Occupational Performance Measure (COPM), the Assessment of Occupational Functioning (AOF), the Occupational Performance History Interview (OPHI), and the Activity Configuration. Each of these assessments yield information on education, work, leisure, activities of daily living, and a patient's satisfaction in his or her performance in daily activities. Several specific areas of the interview should include:

- Education: type of school the patient attended, highest level achieved, grades, social clubs involved in, and career aspirations.
- Work history: past and present jobs, likes and dislikes about job, desirable type of job, preferences of working alone or with others, and plans for future jobs.
- Leisure activities: involvement or interest in sports and hobbies, and whether the patient has a desire to get involved in sports and/or hobbies.
- Culture: what cultural group does the patient identify with, and what customs does the patient engage in, if any.
- Daily schedule: roles and the balance between all roles.

Preparation

In order to sufficiently prepare for the initial interview, the occupational therapy practitioner should plan ahead. The practitioner should arrange for an environment that is conducive to a private interview. Because the therapist's goal is to facilitate openness, the patient should be made to feel comfortable and assured that the information relayed will be kept confidential. The therapist should plan at least several questions in advance that are open-ended and allow for sharing. The practitioner also should plan on taking notes and/or recording the interview. However, they should keep in mind that note-taking and recording can make some clients uncomfortable, so the therapist should explain why it is important to thoroughly document all information shared during the interview so that a comprehensive treatment plan can be formed.

Aftercare

It may be beneficial for the practitioner to seek out the client's family members, friends, or co-workers to gather more information following the initial evaluation with the client.

Results

The occupational therapy practitioner assumes many roles when beginning treatment with a patient: counselor, caregiver, evaluator, researcher, and advocate. The practitioner's comprehensive approach to treatment is imperative to a patient's success.

Health care team roles

A patient seeking occupational therapy services almost always will have contact with other health care professionals who should factor in to the patient's treatment program. Physicians should be kept abreast of ongoing progress. It is always possible that the occupational therapy practitioner will refer a patient for further treatment; for example, mental health counseling that is more specialized. Occupational therapy practitioners must work collaboratively with physical therapists, speech pathologists, and any other health professional the patient has consulted.

Resources

BOOKS

Neistadt, Maureen E., and Elizabeth Blesedell Crepeau. *Willard and Spackman's Occupational Therapy.* Philadelphia: Lippincott-Raven Publishers, 1998.

Reed, Kathlyn L., and Sharon Nelson Sanderson. *Concepts of Occupational Therapy.* Baltimore: Lippincott Williams & Wilkins, 1999.

Williams Pedretti, Lorraine, and Mary Beth Early. *Occupational Therapy, Practice Skills for Physical Dysfunction.* 5th ed. St. Louis: Mosby, 2001.

PERIODICALS

Mallinson, Trudy, Gary Kielhofner, and Cheryl Mattingly. "Metaphor and Meaning in a Clinical Interview." *American Journal of Occupational Therapy* 50 (May 1996): 338–46.

ORGANIZATIONS

The American Occupational Therapy Association. 4720 Montgomery Lane, Bethesda, MD 20824-1220. (301) 652-2682. <http://www.aota.org>.

Meghan M. Gourley

Operating room technology *see* **Surgical technology**

Ophthalmologic ultrasounds

Definition

Ophthalmologic ultrasound is a noninvasive technique that uses high frequency sound to "visualize" structures of the eye. It is the simplest method of imaging the eye in the presence of opacities such as a cataract or vitreous hemorrhaging. Ophthalmologic ultrasound usually employs frequencies of up to 10 million Hertz (10 MHz), but frequencies in the range of 50 to 100 MHz are used in ultrasound biomicroscopy of the eye. Humans cannot hear sounds that emit a frequency of greater than 20,000 Hertz. In order that an ultrasound image can be formed, a transducer or probe transforms electric energy to sound energy, which then penetrates the ocular tissue.

The energy is not absorbed by the tissue as heat, nor is it scattered within the tissue, but is reflected off the tissue, forming the ultrasound image.

Purpose

The purposes of ophthalmologic ultrasound are to study ocular anatomy and to diagnose pathology of the eye. There are many different types of ophthalmologic ultrasound. They include A-scans, B-scans, 3-D scans, duplex ultrasonography, and ultrasound biomicroscopy.

The A-scan ophthalmologic ultrasound is used to measure the axial length of the eye and the thickness of the lens of the eye. The most common use of an A-scan, along with keratometry, which measures the curvature of the anterior surface of the cornea, is to determine the power of the intraocular lens to be implanted following cataract extraction.

A B-scan ophthalmologic ultrasound gives images of the structures throughout the orbit. The B-scan is used by the ophthalmologist in some intraocular surgeries, such as in placement of a radioactive plaque to treat a retinal tumor, and in the extraction of a foreign body that has penetrated the globe. In cryotherapy, the clinical use of low temperatures, ophthalmologic ultrasound imaging helps guide the probe used to treat retinal tears in the presence of vitreous hemorrhaging. It is also used preoperatively in patients with dense **cataracts** to rule out pathology of the posterior pole, and to evaluate resorption of vitreous hemorrhages in diabetic retinopathy. B-scan ultrasonography can locate retinal and choroidal detachments and is used to assess drusen, or **calcium** deposits on the optic nerve and to locate intraocular tumors. The B-scan also can detect changes in structure of the posterior sclera, but because of its limited resolution, anterior scleral pathology is difficult to assess. The new-generation B-scans can assess optic nerve cupping, changes of the optic nerve seen in **glaucoma**.

Color doppler and duplex ophthalmologic ultrasonography are helpful in the assessment of glaucoma, and in diagnosis of ocular tumors and diseases of the anterior segment. Since they evaluate **blood** flow and resistance through the intraocular **blood vessels**, Doppler and duplex ultrasonography can be employed in the diagnosis of a central retinal artery or vein occlusion, and in the diagnosis of temporal arteritis. Temporal arteritis is an inflammation of the temporal artery which can affect **vision**. Restriction of blood flow through other ocular vessels affected in temporal arteritis can also be observed by duplex ultrasonography.

A 3-D ophthalmologic ultrasound gives the eye care practitioner a 3-D image of the eye, facilitating the diag-

KEY TERMS

Adnexa—Structures outside the orbit of the eye that include the lacrymal glands, the lacrymal ducts, the extraocular muscles and the eyelids.

Angle—Part of the eye through which fluid leaves the eye.

Anterior segment—The front part of the eye, that includes the sclera, the cornea, the tear film, the angle of the eye, the iris, and the ciliary body and its processes.

Cataract—Opacification (clouding) of the lens of the eye which occurs as a result of aging, disease, or trauma.

Choroid—Layer of the eye, rich in blood supply, that is found between the retina and the sclera.

Ciliary body processes—Structures of the eye which form the fluid of the anterior chamber and the vitreous.

Cornea—Transparent tissue on the front of the eye that focuses light into the eye through the pupil.

Extraocular muscles—The six muscles which are used to voluntarily move the eye.

Glaucoma—An ocular disease characterized by loss of visual field and damage to the optic nerve. It is often associated with increased intraocular pressure, but not in all cases.

Intraocular—Within the eyeball.

Lens—Intraocular structure in the eye that focuses light onto the retina.

Ophthalmologist—A medical doctor with residency training in medical and surgical management of eye disease.

Optic nerve—Large nerve in the back of the eye through which visual stimuli leave the orbit, to the occipital lobe where vision is processed.

Optometrist—An eye care doctor specifically trained in all aspects of vision and eye care. Optometrists are licensed in all states to diagnose and treat eye disease.

Orbit—The bony cavity of the skull that holds the eyeball.

Posterior pole—The posterior part of the eye that includes the retina and the vitreous.

Radiologist—A physician trained in radiology, the use of radiant energy, to diagnose and treat diseases.

Retina—The inner part of the eye where the photoreceptors are located.

Sclera—Tough white membrane covering the outer part of the eye, not covered by the cornea. It encircles the inside of the eye and is continuous with the optic nerve.

Vitreous—A nonvascular gelatinous material found behind the posterior capsule of the lens.

nosis of a retinal detachment, intraocular tumors, or enlargement of the extraocular muscles. The 3-D ultrasound can be utilized prior to refractive surgery, to assess corneal thickness and irregularities in the corneal surface, and to determine with accuracy the depth of the anterior chamber before implantation of an intraocular lens.

Ultrasound biomicroscopy is employed to assess the normal spatial relationships among anterior segment structures of the eye such as the iris, ciliary processes, and the layers of the cornea. It is also used to assess pathology of the eye and adnexa. Applications of ultrasound biomicroscopy include: calculations of corneal thickness and endothelial cell count, assessment of the cornea after refractive surgery, angle assessment in pupillary block, and elucidation of the causes of glaucoma. Ultrasound biomicroscopy can image the position of implants such as an intraocular lens placed in the eye after cataract surgery, or a filtering bleb, placed intraocu-

larly after glaucoma surgery. It can image tumors of the iris and ciliary body, detect anterior segment abnormalities, and isolate **foreign bodies** that penetrate the globe. With the higher resolution of ultrasound biomicroscopy, scleral pathology, such as scleritis, an inflammation of the sclera, is detectable.

Telesongraphy is a method of using ultrasound to diagnose medical conditions from a remote site. Ophthalmologic ultrasound images can be transmitted via the Internet with this technology.

Description

The images formed by ophthalmologic ultrasound must be resolvable. Resolution is the ability of the eye to distinguish between objects. Resolution can be linear, which determines how far apart two objects are from each other, or contrast, which determines the differences of shades of gray between objects. The higher the frequency employed, the greater the resolution, i.e. smaller objects can be discerned. A frequency of 10 Mhz gives a resolution of 150 micrometers, but resolution as small as 20 micrometers is possible with a 100 Mhz transducer.

An A-scan ophthalmologic ultrasound produces a one dimensional display of intraocular structures. It can employ either applanation or water immersion techniques. The applanation probe, or transducer, touches the cornea of the eye, while the immersion probe is mounted in a water bath surrounding the eye and never compresses the globe. Because the applanation probe applies more pressure to the eye, it can underestimate axial length. Since the probe of the water immersion unit is not in direct contact with the eye, and the sound waves must pass through water before reaching the back of the eye, it is more difficult to judge the layers of the internal eye with this technique, especially when a dense cataract is present.

The B-scan ophthalmologic ultrasound produces a two dimensional real time image. Usually an applanation probe is used, but a water bath technique may give better resolution, important in location of small foreign bodies. In B-scan ultrasound exams the probe is oriented perpendicular to the structure being examined. The images of B-scans are displayed on a video monitor, and can be recorded.

The 3-D ophthalmologic ultrasound produces its image as the probe passes over the eye at numerous angles, and then combines these slices of the eye to produce an image larger than that formed by the B-scan. A 3-D ultrasound can reproduce an image in less than 12 seconds, but it is not a real time image. The anterior segment cannot be imaged well by 3-D ultrasonography.

Doppler ultrasonography assesses blood flow in the eye. Duplex ultrasonography combines the B-scan with the Doppler ultrasonography. The color duplex ultrasound is superimposed with color, allowing the examiner to assess blood flow direction, identify blood vessels, and calculate velocity of blood flow. These techniques, when applied to the eye, assess blood flow through ocular blood vessels.

Ultrasound biomicroscopy uses higher frequencies and thus can image the structures of the eye with greater resolution than a B-scan ultrasound and gives the eye care practitioner a real-time image. Ultrasound biomicroscopy can penetrate the eye only up to 5 mm and thus cannot image the posterior pole. The average length of the eye is 25 mm.

Precautions

Special care is needed when performing an ophthalmologic ultrasound on a ruptured globe.

Preparation

Ophthalmologic ultrasounds are usually performed in the supine position (lying down) and in dim light.

Prior to using the applanation A-scan measurement, an anesthetic drop is instilled in the patient's eye and the patient looks at a target at the end of the probe which gently touches the cornea. An eye cup may keep the eye open or the probe may be held against the eyelid. With the water immersion technique a plastic bag with a hole large enough for the eye and lids to protrude, is placed around the eye.

Prior to a B-scan ultrasonography, an anesthetic is applied to the eye and the patient's eye is held open with an eye cup filled with methyl cellulose. A protective contact lens may be placed on the eye. The patient is given a target on the ceiling on which to fixate, with the eye not being examined. The probe is covered with a coupling gel, and then applied in various directions across the eye, perpendicular to the internal structures of interest. An eye cup, filled with the methyl cellulose, can be held over parts of the ocular adnexa, such as over a closed eye for examination of the lids, when structures external to the globe are examined.

Aftercare

The patient should be instructed not to rub the eyes for 20 to 30 minutes after an ophthalmologic ultrasound and warned that his vision might be slightly compromised for the same time frame.

Complications

There are no known complications from ophthalmologic ultrasound when used for these time periods, and at levels indicated for ultrasound of the orbit and when performed by trained personnel.

Results

The results of ophthalmologic ultrasounds are immediately available to the doctor. Abnormal results indicate an underlying problem and may require further testing and treatment.

Health care team roles

A sonographer, a medical professional trained in sonography, can do an ophthalmologic ultrasound, but in an ophthalmic practice the ultrasound is done by an ophthalmic technician or the doctor. The ultrasound image is always interpreted by a doctor, such as an ophthalmologist, an optometrist, or a radiologist.

Resources

BOOKS

Curry, Reva Arnez and Tempkin, Betty Bates. *Ultrasonography: An Introduction to Normal Structure and Functional Anatomy.* Philadelphia, PA: W.B.Saunders Company, 1995.

Pavlin, Charles J. and Foster, F. Stuart. *Ultrasound Biomicroscopy of the Eye.* Toronto, Canada: Springer-Verlag, 1995.

Williamson, Michael R. *Essentials of Ultrasound* Philadelphia, PA: W.B.Saunders Company, 1996.

PERIODICALS

Bethke, Walter. "An Update on 3-D Ultrasound." *Review of Ophthalmology* (November 2000).

Bohdanecka, Zuzana. "Relationship between Blood Flow Velocities in Retrobulbar Vessels and Laser Doppler Flowmetry at the Optic Disk in Glaucoma Patients." *Ophthalmologica* 213 (1999): 145-149.

Chung, Hak Sung, et. al. "What We Know About Ocular Blood Flow." *Review of Ophthalmology* (April 1999).

Ciou, Hong-Jen, et. al. "Evaluation of Ocular Arterial Changes in Glaucoma with Color Doppler Ultrasonography." *Journal of Ultrasound Medicine* (April 1999): 295-302.

Deramo, V.A, et. al "Ultrasound Biomicroscopy as a Tool for Detecting and Localizing Occult Foreign Bodies After Ocular Trauma." *Ophthalmology* 105 (1999): 2091-2098.

Giovagnorio, Francesco. "Sonography of Lacrimal Glands in Sjorgen Syndrome." *Journal of Ultrasound Medicine* (August 2000): 505-509.

Holladay, Jack T. "Why the A-Scan Is Your Key to Better Cataract Management." *Review of Optometry* (March 1999).

OTHER

Diaz, G. "Telesonography -Telemedicine -Telematics -eHealth." *Telesonography: Ultrasound Remote Diagnosis* 2001. www.drgdiaz.com/telesonography.shtml (July 2, 2001).

Martha S. Reilly, O.D.

Ophthalmoscopic examination *see* **Eye examination**

Opticianry

Definition

Opticianry is the profession where opticians verify and dispense lenses, frames and other optical devices, such as **contact lenses**. In some instances, opticians also grind the lenses for the frames.

Description

Opticians work in tandem with ophthalmologists (M.D.s) and optometrists (O.D.s) to fit eyeglasses and contact lenses. The dispensing opticians use prescriptions determined by eye doctors to assist customers in choosing suitable frames. Part of ensuring a proper fit includes measuring the distance between the centers of the pupils and the distance between the eye surface and the lens.

Opticians help the patient choose frames that are not only fashionable, but will work well with the patient's prescription. For example, some strong prescriptions require thick lenses that cannot fit into a small, wire frame. The optician will recommend thinner, high index lenses if the patient desires smaller frames, or the optician may suggest a larger plastic frame to accommodate the prescription. It is this aspect of the profession that requires the optician to be a skilled technician, a savvy retailer, and a tactful consultant. Patients are also usually asked about their professions or hobbies to see if a special frame or lens is needed. If a patient plays basketball, for example, the optician may recommend polycarbonate lenses in his eyeglasses or protective eyewear.

Once a suitable frame is chosen, opticians create work orders for laboratory technicians who grind and insert lenses into the selected frame. The information includes the prescription, lens material, and lens size. Some opticians, also known as manufacturing opticians or ophthalmic laboratory technicians, produce the lenses. They take the work orders given by the dispensing optician and grind, cut and edge the lenses to the correct prescription, and size for the frame. After the lens is complete, the manufacturing optician inserts it into the correct frame.

The dispensing optician works with the patient to ensure optimal **vision** with the patient's new eyeglasses. The optician may use pliers, files, or screwdrivers to adjust the frame to sit properly on the patient's face. The optician will make sure the lens is sitting in the correct position. If it is not, the patient's vision could be distorted. Before the patient leaves with his new eyeglasses, the optician will direct the patient on proper lens care and cleaning. For example, some anti-reflective coating lenses are to be cleaned only with special cloths and solutions. The patient may return to the optician for eyeglass adjustments as needed.

For customers who prefer contact lenses, opticians measure the size and shape of the eyes, select proper lenses, and give instructions about lens wear and maintenance. Contact lens fitting requires a higher degree of skill, and in some states, opticians are prohibited from this task unless under the immediate supervision of an O.D. or M.D. In many cases, a physician has already recommended the type of contact lens for the patient, and the optician measures the eyes and works with the patient to ensure the proper fit.

Some specialized opticians, called ocularists, help create artificial eyes and shells for patients who may have been injured in accidents or have lost an eye due to disease. Some opticians also specialize in optics, focusing on nonprescription products such as binoculars or microscopes.

Work settings

An optician can work in an ophthalmologist's or optometrist's office, clinic, an optical shop, retail eyeglass chain store, or department store. Other optical shops cater to more elite clientele and are sometimes called "boutiques." These shops feature more expensive, designer frame collections. In these settings opticians are expected to know not only how to correctly fit the lens prescription into the frame, but also be aware of the latest fashion trends.

Because dispensing opticians often work in retail settings, they are required to work weeknights and weekends. Even opticians employed by physicians may have to work evening hours a few nights a week to keep up with patient demand.

Education and training

Some opticians are trained through an apprenticeship under the supervision of a licensed optician, or complete years of on the job training at a clinic or optical shop. In recent years, however, opticians with more formal training are in demand and can command higher salaries.

Community colleges and some universities offer an associate in science degree for opticians. Some technical schools also offer one-year training programs in opticianry. Secondary education opticianry candidates should be proficient in geometry, general sciences, math, and mechanical drawing. The two-year programs include studies in psychology, ophthalmic materials and dispensing, eye anatomy, technical physics, and college level geometry and trigonometry, plus electives.

As of 2001, opticians in 26 states were required to pass the National Opticianry Competency Examination developed by the American Board of Opticianry/National Contact Lens Examiners (ABO/NCLE). Opticians in these states who want to dispense contact lenses must take an additional test, The Contact Lens Registry Examination, before dispensing lenses.

Advanced education and training

Opticians who did not complete a college program may wish to do so, as opticians with more formal education are in higher demand. Certified opticians need to renew their certification every three years. The ABO/NCLE also offers advanced certification that focuses specifically on the advanced level knowledge and skills needed for ophthalmic dispensing: providing spectacle, contact lens, and refraction services.

The ABO also has a master's program which requires candidates to write a technical thesis of at least 2,000 words. Candidates must already have completed the advanced certification program. Once the thesis is completed, it must be reviewed and approved by the masters committee. Upon approval of the thesis by this committee, the title of ABO Master (ABOM) is conferred.

Future outlook

Enrollment in opticianry programs is down as of 2001. There currently is a shortage of dispensing opticians, and that shortage is expected to worsen as the United States' population grows older and has more need of opticianry services. As people age, they need corrective lenses for **presbyopia**, **cataracts**, and other age-related disorders. With these more complicated refractions, opticians with secondary education and a strong knowledge of optics are likely to be in more demand than ever. Also, knowledgeable consumers are more aware of the importance of a good eyeglass and contact lens fit. As this consciousness grows, opticians with more education will be sought out by patients as well as employers.

Current trends also play a part in the demand for opticians. In recent years, eyewear has become more of a fashion statement than ever before. Patients will look to the optician to find the correct frame and lens that will let them see well and look stylish at the same time. Skilled opticians will be able to provide the patient with frames that offer the correct optics for these newer styles.

Opticians who dispense contact lenses will also be in higher demand as the types of lenses available to patients continue to increase. Patients who were once restricted from wearing contact lenses, such as those who need bifocals or have **astigmatism**, now are able to successfully wear contact lenses. These and other innovations will require more experienced contact lens fitters to meet the demands of these patients.

As of 2001, opticians are lobbying in several states to receive permission to increase their scope of practice to include refraction. If they are allowed to do so, the need for new opticians would increase even further. Optical shops would likely grow larger to include tasks that previously only an ophthalmologist or optometrist could perform.

Resources

BOOKS

Belikoff, Kathleen M. *Opportunities in Eye Care Careers.* 2nd ed. Lincolnwood, IL: Contemporary Publishing Company, 1998.

Zinn, Walter J., and Herbert Solomon. *Complete Guide to Eyecare, Eyeglasses & Contact Lenses.* 4th ed. Hollywood, FL: Lifetime Books, 1996.

ORGANIZATIONS

American Board of Opticianry. 6506 Loisdale Rd., Suite 209, Springfield, VA 22150. (703) 719-5800. <http://www.ncleabo.org>.

Commission on Opticianry Accreditation. 7023 Little River Turnpike, Suite 207, Annandale, VA 22003. (703) 941-9110. <http://www.coaccreditation.com>.

National Academy of Opticianry. 8401 Corporate Drive, Suite 605, Landover, MD 20785. (800) 229-4828. <http://www.nao.org/home.htm>.

Opticians Association of America. 7023 Little River Turnpike, Suite 207, Annandale, VA 22003. (703) 916-8856. <http://www.opticians.org>.

OTHER

Gerardi, Steven J. "Is Opticianry Education Important?" *Eyecare Business Online.* <http://www.eyecarebiz.com/archive_results.asp?loc= archive/0300/0300opted.htm>.

Lamperelli, Karlen. "OAA State Leadership Tackles Opticianry Issues." *Vision Monday Online.* <http://www.visionmonday.com>.

"Optician." *Wisconsin Area Health Education Center System Health Care Careers.* <http://www.wihealthcareers.org/disciplines/optician.htm>.

"Opticians, Dispensing." *Bureau of Labor and Statistics, U.S. Department of Labor Occupational Outlook Handbook 2000-01 Edition.* <http://stats.bls.gov/oco/ocos098.htm>.

Mary Bekker

Optometry

Definition

Optometry is the profession of examining the eye for defects, diseases or faults of refraction, and prescribing pharmaceuticals, corrective lenses or exercises to treat these conditions. Doctors of optometry (O.D.s) are trained and licensed to detect and treat ocular symptoms and diseases.

Description

Doctors of optometry are primary health care professionals who examine, diagnose, treat, and manage diseases and disorders of the visual system, the eye, and associated structures, as well as diagnose related systemic conditions. They prescribe glasses, **contact lenses**, low **vision** rehabilitation, vision therapy, and medications, as well as perform certain surgical procedures. O.D.s need eight to 10 years of preparation for their profession—four years to earn the doctor of optometry

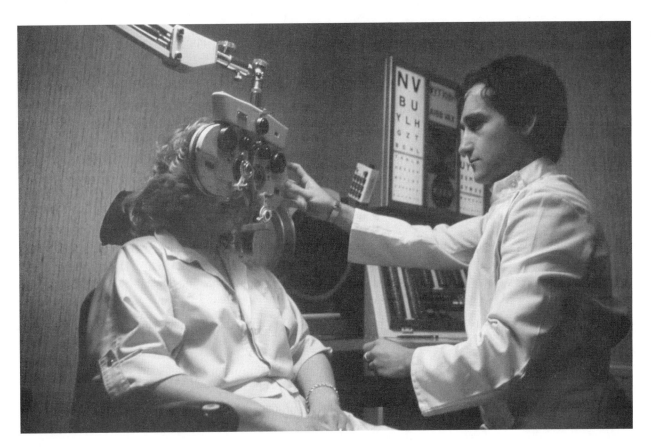

An optometrist uses a refractor to check a patient's eyesight and find the correct prescription. *(Photograph by Andrew McClenaghan. Science Source/Photo Researchers. Reproduced by permission.)*

degree, and one to two years of residency in training. Oklahoma, as of 2001, was the only state where O.D.s were allowed by law to perform laser refractive surgery. Other states also were considering similar measures.

The profession of optometry also routinely includes diagnosing and treating the ocular complications of diseases such as diabetes and **hypertension**; rehabilitating patients with **brain** injury or stroke; providing low vision services for the partially sighted. This includes vision therapy for patients with amblyopia and strabismus (crossed eyes). O.D.s also take an active co-management role with ophthalmologists (M.D.s) in the pre- and post-operative treatment of patients after laser refractive surgery and cataract surgery.

Primary care

All O.D.s treat diseases and dispense corrective lenses for **astigmatism, hyperopia,** and **presbyopia.** They monitor the patient's depth perception and ability to focus and see color. Many optometrists choose primary care or "family practice" because it gives them the biggest diversity of patients.

Some of these primary care O.D.s specialize in contact lens fittings. Recent advances have allowed patients previously restricted from wearing contact lenses to wear a number of types of lenses. Astigmatic and presbyopic patients require more specialized contact lens fitting which these specialists can provide. Sometimes other O.D.s or ophthalmologists will refer their patients to these contact lens specialists. These O.D.s also are more familiar with infections and irritants caused by contact lenses and how best to treat them.

Some O.D.s specialize in certain other areas of optometry, as well as in contact lenses. These specialties include:

Low vision/vision rehabilitation

Some O.D.s focus mainly on low vision services and work in tandem with ophthalmologists, rehabilitation specialists, and government and private agencies. They sometimes work together to determine the best optical devices that improve the quality of life for patients with limited vision. These patients are referred to these optometric specialists usually after a colleague has performed an initial evaluation. The O.D. and members of the spe-

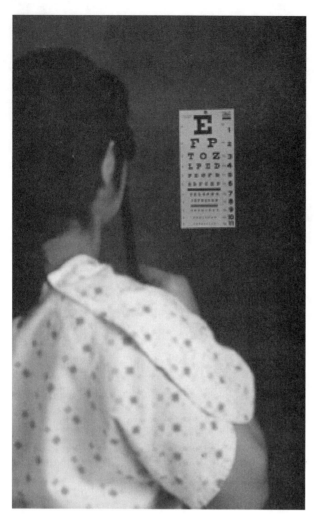

Patient viewing an eye chart. *(Delmar Publishers, Inc. Reproduced by permission.)*

cialized team take the routine exam one step further by utilizing magnifiers, specialized charts, telescopes, colored filters, lenses, prisms, computerized devices, lights, and closed-circuit televisions designed to maximize vision. The low vision specialist is up-to-date on the latest vision aids and treatments so that his patients can lead more productive lives.

Vision therapy (developmental vision)

Vision therapy is a specialty where O.D.s concentrate on how eyesight affects human behavior. Vision therapy specialists work with physicians, psychologists, educators and parents to treat learning disorders, for example, dyslexia, by helping patients with hand-eye and other motor coordination. These specialists also treat patients suffering from amblyopia and strabismus. Some of these patients are adults; many are school-age children.

Pediatric optometry

This is a popular optometric specialty. Common vision problems in children include **myopia**, amblyopia and strabismus. These specialists work with parents and children, and school systems, counseling them on proper treatment as well as **nutrition**.

Geriatric optometry

As patients age, the frequency of ocular disease increases. Specialists can detect and treat **macular degeneration**, **glaucoma** and diabetic eye conditions. They also can detect **cataracts** and co-manage these patients post-operatively with an ophthalmologist.

With the geriatric population expected to increase dramatically due to aging baby boomers, more optometrists will find an expanding need to serve this population, and possibly increase the number of O.D.s who might decide to choose this specialty.

Some O.D.s focus on these patients in an existing practice, while others serve patients in **nursing homes** or clinics with large numbers of elderly patients.

Research and consulting

Some vision companies, especially contact lens manufacturers, seek out optometrists to help them with new product development or to refine existing products. Other optometrists conduct research in a clinical or educational setting.

Work settings

O.D.s may have private, group or partnership practices in hospitals and eye clinics. There are also commissioned posts for optometrists in the military. Government agencies seek advice from O.D.s for health advisory committees, and corporations rely on optometrists for consultation on new products.

Optometrists practice mainly in solo private practices or in a group private practice with other O.D.s. Their offices are located in office buildings, medical parks, storefronts and shopping malls. Some O.D.s opt for working for or franchising chain "superstores" that offer a big selection of frames and quick-turnaround for patients.

With the rise of laser refractive surgery, O.D.s are increasingly becoming a part of ophthalmologists' group practices. In these instances, the O.D. is usually not a co-owner of the practice, but an employee instead. Some refractive laser centers keep O.D.s on staff strictly for co-managing the large volume of refractive surgery patients.

Education and training

O.D.s must complete high school and a bachelor's degree before admission to a four-year optometry school. The pre-optometry student's courses should include physics, organic chemistry, biology or zoology, physiology, statistics, geometry and calculus. These students also need to score in the top percentages of the Optometric Admissions Test before being accepted to an optometry program. Admission to these accredited programs is limited, so it is important for students to maintain a high undergraduate grade point average and achieve a high score on the admissions test to earn a slot at these schools.

The four-year programs focus mainly on clinical and practical teachings. In recent years a few programs have added practice management courses to help optometrists cope with managed care paperwork and increased competition from retail chains. First-year students study **human anatomy** and physiology and the basic principles of optics. Optometric sciences, ocular physiology and pathology, vision anomalies, and instruments of clinical practice are studied in the second year. Third-year students take those same topics to a higher level and begin studying contact lens fitting and general clinical practice. The student's last year of study includes treating patients under the guidance of teaching optometrists, usually at optometry-school run clinics. Student O.D.s during the fourth year prescribe and fit contact lenses, and diagnose and treat visual system conditions.

During the four years, optometry students also are offered a number of electives that include epidemiology, environmental vision, microbiology, and biostatistics.

Optometry schools usually operate clinics where patients need them most—in inner-city neighborhoods, nursing homes or correctional facilities. This enables care for patients in need while offering fourth-year students an opportunity to detect and treat a number of ocular conditions.

After optometry students complete a four year program but before they can begin practice, they must complete a series of written examinations—at least three written and one practical—for a license in order to practice. These licenses are granted by state boards of optometry. Each state has different requirements. While they are similar, graduating optometry students must check with each licensing board for specific requirements.

Advanced education and training

Recent optometry school graduates sometimes complete master's or doctorate degrees in related medical specialties such as physiological optics, visual sciences or **public health**. Some of these doctors enter research or education.

Optometrists who want to specialize in certain areas complete a one-year residency after graduation at educational institutions or hospitals. These internships could include pediatric or geriatric optometry, low-vision rehabilitation or vision therapy.

State boards of optometry require a certain number of continuing education credits for practicing optometrists. This training is completed through specialized courses at meetings, optometry schools, optometric journals and the Internet. Continuing education credits must meet specific requirements of each state. The O.D. must check with the state licensing board for specific details.

Future outlook

More women are becoming optometrists than in years previous. As of 2001, about 25% of practicing optometrists were women. That number should rise since 50% of optometry students as of 2001 are women.

A comprehensive study by the American Optometric Association completed in 1997 predicted that there will be at least 4,000 more optometrists than needed by the year 2015. Several factors could affect that prediction.

- Geriatric population. The increasing number of elderly patients could mean a highly-increased number of office visits for optometrists. These elderly patients need more frequent examinations for myriad eye diseases and conditions.

- Vision plans. Managed care has brought more patients into optometrists' offices in recent years. Before managed care, many patients delayed regular eye exams because of cost. Because comprehensive vision plans routinely pay for regular eye exams, and in some cases contact lenses and eyeglasses, more patients routinely are being seen by O.D.s at a higher rate of frequency.

- Retail chains. More eye care patients are utilizing the convenience of these large "superstores" to fulfill their vision needs. These chains sometimes have several optometrists on staff. The need for "corporate optometrists" is expected to grow in the coming years. These positions do not pay as competitively as private practice; but they also do not incur the large debt that opening or purchasing a practice does.

KEY TERMS

Amblyopia—Decreased visual acuity, usually in one eye, in the absence of any structural abnormality in the eye.

Astigmatism—Asymmetric vision defects due to irregularities in the cornea.

Cataract—A cataract is a cloudiness or opacity in the normally transparent crystalline lens of the eye. This cloudiness can cause a decrease in vision and may lead to eventual blindness.

Glaucoma—Disease of the eye characterized by increased pressure of the fluid inside the eye. Untreated, glaucoma can lead to blindness.

Presbyopia—A condition affecting people over the age of 40 where the system of accommodation that allows focusing of near objects fails to work because of age-related hardening of the lens of the eye.

Refraction—Method of determining the optical status of the eyes. Lenses are placed before the patient's eyes while reading from an eye chart. The result is the eyeglass or contact lens prescription.

Resources

BOOKS

Belikoff, Kathleen, M. *Opportunities in Eye Care Careers,* 2nd ed. Lincolnwood, IL: Contemporary Publishing Company, 1998.

ORGANIZATIONS

American Academy of Optometry 6110 Executive Boulevard, Suite 506 Rockville, MD 20852. (301) 984-1441 Fax (301) 984-4737 aaoptom@aol.com. htttp://www.opt.org.

American Optometric Association. 2420 North Lindbergh Boulevard, St. Louis, MO 63141. (800) 365-2219. <http://www.aoanet.org/>.

Council on Optometric Practitioner Education 4401 East West Highway, Suite 205 Bethesda, MD 20814-4521. (800) 758-COPE (2673) (301) 913-0641 Fax (301) 913-2034. COPE@copeonline.org. <http://www.copeopt.org>.

National Board of Examiners in Optometry. 4340 East West Highway, Suite 1010, Bethesda, MD 20814. (301)652-5192. nbeo@optometry.org. <http://www.optometry.org>.

OTHER

McClure, Lawrence H., Ph.D. "The Evolution of Optometry." *Optometric Management Online.* <http://www. optometric.com/archive_results.asp?loc=article= 70066&sub=1146>.

"Optometry: The Primary Eye Care Profession." *Massachusetts Society of Optometrists Online.* <http://www.massoptom.org/optometry.htm>.

"So You Want to Be an Optometrist." *American Optometric Association Online.*<http://www.aoanet.org/ career-guidance.html>.

Mary Bekker

Optometry assisting

Definition

Optometric assistants aide the optometrist (O.D.) and medical team in a variety of daily duties, including gathering patient history and performing ocular tests.

Description

With the advent of managed care into medicine, O.D.s examine more patients than ever. They are also required to see more patients to keep up with managed care demands and to boost their sagging bottom lines caused by decreased insurance payments. To keep up with the increased office traffic, more O.D.s are turning to their office staff to perform duties only they had handled previously.

An optometric assistant is the first medical staff member the patient meets. Assistants play a critical role in determining the patient's medical problem through recording a detailed patient history and a patient lifestyle questionnaire. During this interview, the assistant will discuss the reason the patient is being examined and any visual difficulties. The assistant makes detailed notes to pass on to the O.D. to help in the diagnosis.

More skilled assistants, called technicians or paraoptometrics, perform testing and other procedures. These include retinal photography, **blood pressure** readings, automated lensometry, automated perimetry, acuities, and corneal topography. High-tech equipment now allows technicians to perform refractions, although these measurements are usually checked by the physician. The technician also may perform pre-testing for **contact lenses**, although with the advances in this technology, many physicians are turning to highly trained contact lens technicians to perform these duties.

Assistants take part in the medical aspects of the practice, but they also handle other duties as well. Assistants perform such tasks as maintaining **medical records**, keeping medical transcriptions, answering telephones, patient recall, and tracking insurance payments. Larger practices may have specific employees for these duties. In smaller practices, assistants are more likely to handle many duties simultaneously.

Work settings

Optometrists either work alone in private practices or in group private practice with other O.D.s. Assistants may be required to handle the responsibilities for more than one physician. O.D. offices are located in office buildings, medical parks, storefronts, and shopping malls. O.D.s who work in chain stores usually do not have assistants, but employees from the parent company. Assistants may also work in hospital settings or clinics.

Optometric assistants may work long hours to meet the needs of patients. Doctors now regularly keep evening and weekend hours. Optometric assistants should also be capable of handling **stress** and many tasks at once. Direct contact with patients, scheduling, and collecting payments require a certain tact.

Education and training

Many assistants receive on-the-job training from other employees or the optometrist. There are certifications available, and a registered optometric assistant is designated by Opt. A., R. The American Optometric Association (AOA) paraoptometric section provides training to optometric assistants. The AOA began certifying paraoptometrics with a new program that instructs assistants on basic optometric terminology, optometric practice operation, anatomy of the eye, and optometric examinations and treatments. Applicants must have a minimum of a high school diploma or equivalent and must be able to verify a minimum of six months employment in the eye care field.

Paraoptometric assistant training certification programs are also available through some universities and community colleges. While these training sessions help develop skills, many optometrists hire assistants with no formal training. More highly trained assistants command higher salaries.

Advanced education and training

Optometric assistants may seek more formal training and become certified ophthalmic medical assistants, technicians or technologists. The Joint Commission on Allied Health Personnel in Ophthalmology (JCAHPO) offers certification that enable assistants to perform everything from clinical optics to assisting an ophthalmologist in the operating room. These positions demand

---

KEY TERMS

Ophthalmology—A medical doctor specializing in diseases of the eye and eye surgery.

Optometry—The profession of examining the eye for defects, diseases, or faults of refraction, and prescribing pharmaceuticals, corrective lenses, or exercises to treat these conditions. Optometrists (O.D.s) are trained and licensed to detect and treat ocular symptoms and diseases.

Polycarbonate—A very strong type of plastic often used in safety glasses, sport glasses, and children's eyeglasses. Polycarbonate lenses have approximately 50 times the impact resistance of glass lenses.

---

much more medical knowledge than optometric assisting. Technicians require a one-year course and technologists must complete a two-year course before being certified.

Future outlook

Optometric assistants will be more in demand as optometrists seek employees that can perform a number of tasks skillfully in their busy offices. This need will become greater as optometrists continue to add patients to their practices because of managed care. They will require more support personnel to perform testing and run their practices efficiently. The number of open positions for optometric assistants is expected to grow at a fast rate in the coming years. Even more importantly, as the population ages the need for qualified eye care professionals will rise to meet their needs.

Resources

BOOKS

Belikoff, Kathleen M. *Opportunities in Eye Care Careers*. 2nd ed. Lincolnwood, IL: Contemporary Publishing Company, 1998.

Zinn, Walter J., and Herbert Solomon. *Complete Guide to Eye Care, Eyeglasses & Contact Lenses*. 4th ed. Hollywood, FL: Lifetime Books, 1996.

ORGANIZATIONS

American Association of Medical Assistants. 20 North Wacker Drive, Suite 1575, Chicago, IL 60606-2903. <http://www.aama.ntl.org>.

American Optometric Association Paraoptometric Section. 243 N. Lindbergh Blvd., St. Louis, MO 63141. (800) 365-2219.

Joint Commission on Allied Health Personnel in
Ophthalmology. 2025 Woodlane Drive, St. Paul, MN
55125-2995. (888) 284-3937. <http://www.jcahpo.org>.

OTHER

"A Rewarding Career." *The Joint Commission on Allied
Health Personnel in Ophthalmology (JCAHPO) Online.*
<http://www.jcahpo.org/Career.pdf>.

"Career Cards: Vision Care: Optometric
Assistants/Technicians." *East Texas AHEC Health Career
Pages.* <http://www.etxahec.org/hcp/20b.htm>.

Kattouf, Richard S., O.D. "Achieving Maximum Efficiency
Without Sacrificing Quality Of Care." *Optometric
Management Online.* <http://www.
optometric.com/archive_results.asp?loc=
articles/03062000121028pm>html

"Medical Assistants." *Bureau of Labor and Statistics, U.S.
Department of Labor Occupational Outlook Handbook
2000-01 Edition.* <http://stats.bls.gov/oco/ocos164.htm>.

"Optometric Technician." *Wisconsin Area Health Education
Center System Health Care Careers.*
<http://www.wihealthcareers.org/disciplines/
optician.htm>.

Mary Bekker

Oral cancer

Definition

Oral **cancer** refers to malignancies in the oral cavity (mouth) and the oropharynx. The oral cavity includes the lips, buccal mucosa (lining of the lips and cheeks), the hard palate, floor of the mouth, teeth, front two-thirds of the tongue, and gingiva (gums). The oropharynx includes the tonsils, soft palate, back third of the tongue, and the back of the throat.

Description

In the United States, oral cancer is diagnosed in approximately 30,000 patients each year and is responsible for about 8,000 deaths. Oral cancer is the sixth most frequently occurring cancer, and the most common sites of oral cavity cancers are the floor of the mouth and the tongue. In the oropharynx the most common sites of cancerous tumors are the tonsils and base of the tongue.

The economic and social impact of this disease is great. Oral cancer may result in serious long-term disabilities such as loss of speech, **hearing**, salivary, and chewing functions, as well as **pain** and disfigurement resulting from head and neck surgery.

Causes and symptoms

Nearly three-quarters of all oral cancers are related to tobacco use—either cigarette, pipe, or cigar smoking, or the use of smokeless tobacco products such as snuff. Tobacco-specific nitrosamines are the carcinogens (cancer-causing substances) implicated in the development of oral cancers. Chronic alcohol consumption is linked to oral cancers, and the use of alcohol and tobacco together poses a greater risk than using either one alone.

Exposure to asbestos or radiation increases the risk of developing oral cancers, and exposure to sunlight is a risk factor for cancer of the lips. A high-fat diet that is also low in fruits, vegetables, and other sources of **vitamins** A and C has been linked to development of oral cancers.

Age, gender, and race affect the risk of developing oral cancers. Oral cancer usually occurs among older adults because they have longer exposure to lifestyle and environmental risk factors. Oral cancer occurs 2.5 times more often in males than females, and blacks are affected more often than whites. The higher rate of oral cancer among black men is attributed to lifestyle, such as nutritional status, tobacco, and alcohol use, rather than genetic differences. Recent research on tobacco and alcohol use, however, has demonstrated comparable rates of oral cancer among blacks and whites.

The signs and symptoms of oral cancer depend upon the site of the tumor. Certain types of lesions in the oral cavity have the potential to become cancerous. Leukoplakias (white lesions) and erythroplakia (red lesions) that do not resolve within two weeks should be evaluated by a healthcare professional. Other possible signs or symptoms include:

- sore throat, hoarseness, or sensation that something is caught in the throat

- lump or thickening in the oral cavity

- difficulty chewing, eating, or swallowing

- difficulty moving the tongue or jaw

- numbness, weakness, or altered sensation in the mouth or tongue

- swelling of the jaw, mouth, or tongue

- changes in hearing, **smell**, or taste

- changes in the fit or feel of dentures or dental appliances

- abnormal odor or discharge from nose, ears, or mouth

- lesions, sores, or thickened patches that do not readily heal or resolve

Diagnosis

An examination to screen for oral cancer may be made by a physician, dentist, or dental hygienist. Though regular self-examination—with attention to inspection for lumps, thickenings, whitish patches, or sores—may detect some oral cancers, it is not a substitute for a thorough professional examination. An oral examination, performed by a physician or dentist using a mirror and lights, identifies abnormalities in the oral cavity. The physician will also palpate the throat, neck, and head for lumps or thickenings. X rays of the mouth, performed by a radiological technologist, may be used to examine suspicious areas.

When an abnormal area is detected in the oral cavity, the definitive diagnostic technique is biopsy—removal of all or part of the suspicious area for examination under the **microscope** by a pathologist. Biopsy is usually performed by an oral surgeon or an ear, nose, and throat specialist, also known as an otolaryngologist. Since squamous cells line the oral cavity, nearly all oral cancers are squamous cell carcinomas.

Staging

Staging refers to the process of determining the extent to which the cancer has metastasized (spread). Since treatment depends upon the stage of the oral cancer, additional diagnostic tests may be performed. These include imaging studies such as **dental x rays** and **CT scans**, and lymph node biopsy. Cancers of the oral cavity are identified as Stages I through IV and recurrent. Stage I cancers are less than three-quarters of an inch (2 centimeters) in size and have not spread to local lymph nodes. Stage II cancers are between three-quarters and one and one-half inches (2-4 centimeters) and have not metastasized to local lymph nodes. Stage III cancers are larger than one and one-half inches (4 centimeters), or are cancers of any size that have spread to a single lymph node on the same side of the neck as the cancer. Stage IV cancers have one or more of the following characteristics:

- spread to surrounding oral cavity tissue
- metastasized to more than one lymph node on the same side of the neck as the cancer
- metastasized to lymph nodes on both sides of the neck
- widespread metastasis throughout the body

Recurrent oral cancers are those that have returned following treatment. Recurrences may present in the oral cavity or elsewhere on the body.

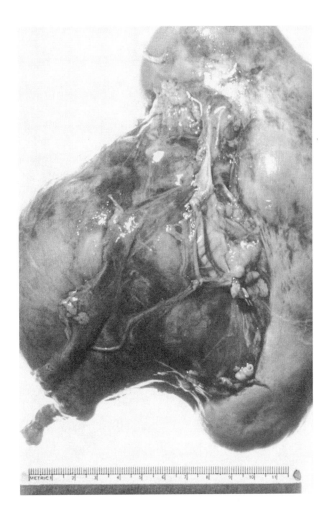

A specimen of a squamous cell carcinoma of the tongue and jaw. *(Custom Medical Stock Photo. Reproduced by permission.)*

Treatment

Treatment depends upon the location and stage of the cancer, as well as the age and overall health of the patient. It generally consists of a combination of surgery to remove as much of the cancer as possible and radiation and/or adjuvant **chemotherapy** (**anticancer drugs**) to kill any remaining cancer cells. Drugs called radiosensitizers are sometimes used to render cancer cells more sensitive to radiation. Most oral cancers are treated with surgery and fractionated (small, measured doses) radiation therapy. Another treatment that is presently being tested is hyperthermia. Since cancer cells are more sensitive to heat than normal cells, hyperthermia treatment involves heating the body in order to kill cancer cells.

Surgical treatment and radiation of the lips and oral cavity may produce disfigurement and difficulty with activities such as eating and talking. Patients recovering from treatment may benefit from rehabilitation with a

KEY TERMS

Adjuvant therapy—Treatment involving radiation, chemotherapy (anticancer drug treatment), or a combination of both.

Biopsy—Surgical removal and microscopic examination of living tissue for diagnostic purposes.

Carcinogen—Any substance or agent capable of causing cancer.

Chemotherapy—Systemic treatment of cancer with synthetic drugs that destroy the tumor either by inhibiting the growth of cancerous cells or by killing them.

Malignant—Cancerous.

Metastasize—The spread of cancer cells from a primary site to distant parts of the body.

Oncologist—A physician who specializes in cancer medicine.

Pathologist—A person who specializes in the diagnosis of disease by studying cells and tissues under a microscope.

Radiation therapy—Treatment using high energy radiation from X-ray machines, cobalt, radium, or other sources.

Stage—A term used to describe the size and extent of spread of cancer.

speech therapist and support from social workers or other mental health professionals.

Prognosis

The prognosis for patients with oral cancer depends, again, upon the location and stage of the cancer, as well as the patient's age, overall health and effectiveness of treatment. Generally, oral cancers detected early, such as Stage I cancers, have the best prognoses. Patients who have had oral cancers are at increased risk for developing another cancer of the mouth, head, or neck; for this reason, all patients require vigilant, regular follow up. Patients who stop smoking or using tobacco products and alcohol also have better outlooks than those who do not.

Health care team roles

Patients with oral cancers may be cared for by oral surgeons, otolarynogologists, oncologists, surgical and oncology nurses, laboratory and radiological technolo-

gists, speech therapists, and mental health professionals. Health educators and behavior modification specialists may be involved in assisting patients with smoking cessation or recovery from alcohol dependency.

Patient education

The objectives of education are to prevent patients from smoking or using tobacco products, and to encourage smokers to quit. Participation in smoking cessation programs should be encouraged, and patients should be informed about the health risks of excessive alcohol consumption. Patient teaching also should describe the role of environmental carcinogens such as asbestos, radiation, and sun exposure in the development of oral cancers.

Prevention

Since tobacco products and alcohol abuse are associated with more than 75% of oral cancers, health education efforts to prevent their use could sharply reduce the incidence of oral cancers. Regular examinations by a dentist or physician are vital for early detection of oral cancers.

Resources

BOOKS

Murphy, Gerald P. et al. *American Cancer Society Textbook of Clinical Oncology.* Second Edition, Atlanta: The American Cancer Society, Inc. 1995, pp. 5, 15, 369-370.

Otto, Shirley E. *Oncology Nursing.* St. Louis: Mosby, 1997, pp. 230-231.

PERIODICALS

Hall, Stephen, et al. "Time to First Relapse as an Outcome and Predictor of Survival in Patients with Squamous Cell Carcinoma of the Head and Neck." *The Laryngoscope* (December 2000): 2041-2046.

Scully, Crispian. and Stephen Porter. "Oral Cancer [Clinical Review: ABC of Oral Health]." *British Medical Journal* (July 8, 2000): 97-100.

Tankere, Frederic, et al. "Prognostic Value of Lymph Node Involvement in Oral Cancers: A Study of 137 Cases." *The Laryngoscope* (December 2000): 2061-2065.

ORGANIZATIONS

American Cancer Society. (800) ACS-2345. <http://www.cancer.org>.

Cancer Care, Inc. (800) 813-HOPE. <http://www.cancercareinc.org>.

Cancer Information Service of the NCI. (800) 4-CANCER. <http://wwwicic.nci.nih.gov>.

Cancer Research Institute. 681 Fifth Avenue, New York, NY 10022. (800) 992-2623.

Centers for Disease Control. <http://www.cdc.gov>.

National Cancer Institute (National Institutes of Health). 9000 Rockville Pike, Bethesda, MD 20892. (800) 422-6237 <http://www.nci.nih.gov>.

National Coalition for Cancer Survivorship. 1010 Wayne Ave., 5th Floor, Silver Spring, MD 20910 (301) 650-8868.

Barbara Wexler

Oral cholecystography *see* **Gallbladder x rays**

Oral contraceptives *see* **Contraception**

Oral debridement *see* **Nonsurgical periodontal therapy**

Oral herpes *see* **Cold sore**

Oral hygiene

Definition

Oral hygiene is the practice of keeping the mouth clean and healthy by brushing, flossing, and using appropriate therapeutic aids to prevent caries (tooth decay) and periodontal disease.

Purpose

The goal of proper oral hygiene is to control plaque, the sticky bacterial film that continually forms on teeth. Plaque adheres to the crevices and fissures of teeth and, when not removed on a regular basis, generates acids that can decay the enamel surface of teeth. Plaque is also a physical and a chemical irritant to the periodontium, the tissues investing and supporting the teeth.

Toothbrushing and flossing remove plaque from teeth, and antiseptic mouthwashes kill some of the **bacteria** in plaque. Fluoride—in toothpaste, drinking water, or dental treatments—also protects teeth by binding with enamel to make it stronger. Despite a patient's best efforts, plaque formation can lead to calculus formation. Calculus, also called tartar, is an adherent, calcified deposit made up of dead bacterial cells from plaque. Calculus does not cause tooth decay, but is a primary cause of periodontal disease. Calculus can only be removed by a dental professional, therefore regular dental visits are essential to good oral hygiene.

Precautions

Brushing should be performed thoroughly and gently with the correct brush, refraining from "scrubbing" at the teeth with too much force. Brushing that is unnecessarily vigorous can cause gum irritation, gum recession, and abrasion of tooth structure. Flossing can also be performed too vigorously. A patient who inserts floss between teeth, then "saws" back and forth with downward force can create fissures in gum tissue that destroy the attachment of gum to tooth.

As deciduous (primary) teeth erupt, caregivers should develop the habit of brushing children's teeth after every meal. Since excess ingested fluoride can cause dental **fluorosis**, a mottled discoloration of tooth enamel, care should be taken that the child does not swallow any toothpaste. A pea-size amount of fluoridated toothpaste is all that is necessary to clean a child's teeth. Fluoride-free toothpaste for children is available.

Patients with full or partial prostheses are not exempt from the need for good oral hygiene. Dentures should be removed daily, cleaned with a brush and rinsed or soaked in a denture cleansing bath. Gum tissue should be brushed and rinsed to remove food particles and bacteria. If possible, dentures should be left out at night to allow the tissues to breathe without pressure from the prosthesis. When not in use, dentures should be covered with water or a denture cleaning solution to prevent drying. Dentures should be adjusted, relined, and replaced when necessary by a dentist.

Fixed prostheses such as bridges and implants require special cleaning tools for proper maintenance and to prevent failure of the prosthesis.

Description

Using a toothbrush

Ideally, patients should brush after every meal and snack with a fluoride toothpaste. Following a set routine ensures that no teeth are missed. A recommended sequence is to start on the upper right outside surfaces, continue to the upper left, switch to the inside left surfaces and return to the inside right. Then brush the occlusal (chewing) surfaces of the back teeth, move to the bottom and repeat the same sequence. The tongue should also be brushed to remove odor-causing bacteria. A thorough tooth brushing should take two to three minutes.

The American Dental Hygienists' Association recommends the following technique:

- Place toothbrush bristles along the gumline at a 45-degree angle. Bristles should contact both the tooth surface and the gum.

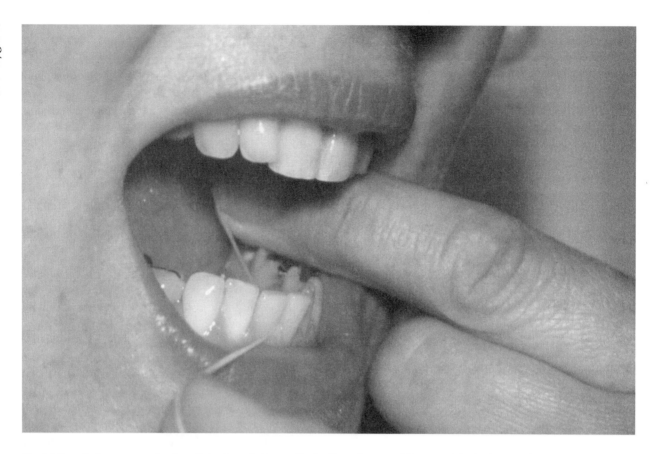

Dental floss helps remove food particles from between the teeth and gums. *(Photograph by Andrew McClenaghan. Science Source/Photo Researchers. Reproduced by permission.)*

- Gently brush the surfaces of two or three teeth using a vibrating, back and forth rolling motion. Lift the brush, move it to the next group of two or three teeth, and repeat.

- Behind anterior teeth, tilt the brush vertically. Make several up and down strokes using the front half of the brush.

- Place the brush against the occlusal (chewing) surface of the teeth and use a gentle back and forth scrubbing motion.

Consumers should look for a toothbrush with soft, nylon, end-rounded bristles in a size and shape that allows them to reach all tooth surfaces easily. Power toothbrushes are available in various styles, and have been proven to be as effective as manual toothbrushes. Research has found no significant differences in plaque reduction between manual and powered tooth brushing.

For those with limited use of their hands, toothbrush handles can be inserted in a small ball, bicycle grip, or sponge hair curler for easier gripping. Children's toothbrushes typically have larger handles, and may be appropriate for adults with less flexibility.

Toothbrushes should be replaced every three to four months, since bristles lose their integrity and don't clean as well after a period of time. In addition, toothbrush bristles and handles collect microbes that can cause colds, the flu, herpes, and periodontal infections. Some brushes have colored bristles that lose their coloration gradually, prompting a patient to replace it when the color is gone.

Using floss

Using dental floss daily to clean between teeth has many benefits. Interproximal (between adjacent teeth) decay is prevented because plaque is removed; interproximal restorations are maintained in healthy condition; and the sulcus surrounding each tooth is kept free from plaque and associated pathogens, ensuring periodontal health. Floss comes in many varieties (waxed, unwaxed, flavored, tape), and may be chosen by personal preference. As with brushing, flossing is easier for a caregiver when he or she is positioned behind the patient.

To begin, one end of an 18-inch piece of floss is wrapped around the middle finger of one hand. Most of the rest of the floss is wrapped around the middle finger of the opposite hand, leaving a one- to two-inch center section that is grasped between the thumb and forefinger of each hand. The floss is eased between two teeth with a gentle back-and-forth motion, then pressed in a c-shape against one tooth, covering as much tooth surface as possible. The floss is worked gently up and down, back and forth, in and out to clean and scrape plaque from the side surface of the tooth, both above and below the gumline. The floss is then lifted over the papilla (raised gum tissue between teeth), and the process is repeated on the opposite tooth. As floss becomes soiled, fresh floss can be released from one hand, and used floss taken up by the other hand.

Using therapeutic aids

Toothpicks, both wooden and plastic, can be used as interdental cleaners. Small interdental brushes are also useful for cleaning wide spaces between teeth and under bridgework. Flossing can be made easier with floss holders. For flossing under fixed bridgework and around implants, floss threaders can be used, or floss with a stiff leader attached to one end.

Complications

Gingivitis is the immediate consequence of poor oral hygiene. An early form of periodontal disease, gingivitis is characterized by inflammation of the gums with painless bleeding during brushing and flossing. This condition is reversible with proper dental care, but if left untreated will progress to **periodontitis**. A professional cleaning by a hygienist or dentist is indicated, followed by home care instruction.

Periodontitis is a disease of the support structures of teeth, the gums, ligaments, and bone. Without support, teeth will loosen and may fall out or have to be extracted. To diagnose periodontitis, a dental professional looks for gums that are red, swollen, bleeding, and shrinking away from the teeth, leaving widening spaces between the teeth and exposed root surfaces vulnerable to decay. Measurements are taken in the sulcus—the space between tooth and gum—to determine the level of attachment of tooth to gum and bone. Studies may be undertaken to measure bacterial load in the sulcus. A general dentist is qualified to treat periodontitis. Some choose to specialize in this area, and are called periodontists. Treatment for periodontitis may include detailed home care instruction, specialized prophylaxis, antibiotic therapy, surgery, or a combination of the above.

Caries, or tooth decay, is a common consequence of poor oral hygiene when acid from bacterial plaque is allowed to form. A dentist will remove the decay, prep the clean cavity, and fill it with an amalgam or resin

---

KEY TERMS

Calculus—An adherent, calcified deposit of bacteria, fungi, desquamated epithelial cells and food debris, formed on the surface of teeth. Also known as tartar.

Caries—Tooth decay.

Fluorosis—Mottled discoloration of tooth enamel, caused by excess systemic intake of fluoride.

Gingivitis—Swollen, bleeding gums, usually not painful.

Periodontitis—A gum disease that destroys the structures supporting the teeth, including gums, ligaments, and bone.

Plaque—A thin, sticky, colorless film of bacteria that forms on teeth.

Sulcus—Pocket space between tooth and gum.

---

restoration. Left untreated, decay can expand, destroying the entire tooth and causing significant **pain**.

Results

With proper home care, oral hygiene may be maintained and oral health problems may be avoided. Older adults no longer assume they will lose all their teeth in their lifetime. Regular oral care preserves appearance, speech, and eating functions, thus prolonging the quality of life. Without proper home care, the patient runs a significant risk of losing teeth prematurely from decay or periodontal disease.

Health care team roles

Dental professionals monitor their patients' oral hygiene practices, making recommendations and providing instruction when necessary. During routine recall visits, a hygienist will typically review home care and make suggestions.

Caregivers such as nurse's aides are critical team members when it comes to oral hygiene. A patient who cannot brush and floss for himself or herself may compromise overall health by exposure to decay or periodontal disease.

Patient education

Patients receive oral hygiene training throughout life, first from parents or caregivers, then from educators, then from dental professionals. A child may be taught to brush by his or her mother, then have that training reinforced by a school health educator. As children begin to visit the dentist regularly, they receive further training at routine visits. Flossing instruction is usually given at the dental office or in school, once permanent teeth have erupted and the child has enough manual dexterity to learn this skill. As the child becomes an adult, the hygienist or dentist can reinforce prior training and make any adjustments necessary.

Training

Health educators and caregivers can receive training from dental professionals to help their students and patients achieve good oral health. In-service programs are available from dental associations and boards, state health boards, and sometimes from local dental offices.

Resources

PERIODICALS

Mantokoudis, D., et al. "Comparison of the Clinical Effects and Gingival Abrasion Aspects of Manual and Electric Toothbrushes." *Journal of Clinical Periodontology* (January 2001): 65-72.

ORGANIZATIONS

American Dental Association. 211 East Chicago Ave., Chicago, IL 60611. (312) 440-2500. <http://www.ada.org>.

American Dental Hygienists' Association. 444 N. Michigan Ave., Suite 3400, Chicago, IL 60611. (800) 243-2342. <http://www.adha.org>.

OTHER

"Gum Disease (Periodontal Disease)." *ADA.org: The Public*. <http://www.ada.org/public/index.asp>.

Healthtouch Online. Medical Strategies Inc. <http://www.healthtouch.com>.

"Oral Health Information." *ADHA Online*. <http://www.adha.org>.

Cathy Hester Seckman, R.D.H.

Oral hygiene aids

Definition

Oral hygiene aids are the tools used in the mouth to remove food residue and plaque, a bacterial film that causes tooth decay (**dental caries**), periodontal disease, and halitosis (bad breath).

Bacterial plaque must be removed daily. The toothbrush and dental floss are the primary oral hygiene aids for this process. The toothbrush is a brush used to clean the teeth by removing plaque from the teeth and stimulating the gums. Dental floss is thin, thread-like material used to clean the areas between teeth and under the gum line. A dental toothpick may be used to clean between teeth.

Also used in conjunction with mouth care are toothpaste and mouthwash. Toothpaste is a preparation used on the toothbrush to clean teeth. Some of the ingredients of toothpaste are as follows:

• polishing agents that aid in cleaning

• fluoride, to prevent dental caries

• antitartar agents, to prevent buildup of calculus

• antiplaque/antigingivitis agents, to control plaque and **gingivitis**

• whiteners, to remove dental stains

• sensitivity agents, to decrease sensitivity to heat, cold, and sweets

Mouthwash is a liquid product that patients gargle or use as a rinse to fight **bacteria**. It is used to control:

• halitosis

• plaque

• gingivitis

• tartar and calculus

Most mouthwashes contain fluoride, which helps to control caries.

Purpose

Oral hygiene aids such as the toothbrush, dental floss, mouthwash, and toothpicks are used in the daily battle against germs that live in the mouth. Plaque is formed when bacteria in the mouth feed on the food residue—particularly sugar residue—and dead epithelial cells (the covering of internal and external body surfaces). Depending on the bacterial pathogen present in the plaque, plaque can cause tooth decay or periodontal disease. When periodontal disease is not treated, it can lead to the loss of teeth when the supporting tissue that keeps teeth in the jaw is destroyed.

Although oral hygiene aids date back thousands of years, many people don't correctly use preventive tools like toothbrushes and interdental aids. In the United States, one-third of people in all age groups have untreated tooth decay, according to *Oral Health 2000*, the United States Surgeon General's report from May 2000. By age 17, 78% of youths have a cavity and 7% have lost at least one tooth, according to the report by Surgeon General David Satcher, M.D.. His report also stated that 48% of adults between the age of 35 and 44 suffer from gingivitis.

Oral hygiene's long history

People have been concerned about oral health for thousands of years. Ancient civilizations used urine as a mouthwash. The earliest record of this usage dates back to China 5,000 years ago when the rinse was used for toothaches and bleeding gums. Although this form of mouth rinse seems disgusting, urine is sterile in a healthy person. Furthermore, historians believe that the urine rinse may have aided in preventing tooth decay.

Ancient civilizations used the toothpick to clean the teeth. The Roman poet, Pliny, wrote in the first century about cleaning the gums with a toothpick made from the bones of puffin fish. Other toothpick materials included gold, ivory, and bronze.

Toothbrushes were in use by the 18th century. While some people cleaned their teeth with small sponges, others used brushes made from the root of a marshmallow. People also brushed their teeth with horsehair bristles.

Contemporary oral hygiene

In modern times, the toothbrush and dental floss are the most important oral cleaning aids. The American Dental Association (ADA) calls brushing and flossing the "dental care twins," the activities crucial to a healthy mouth. The dental toothpick and interdental brush may sometimes be utilized in place of floss, and the household toothpick can be used to remove food from the teeth.

The ADA Seal of Acceptance on products indicates that they were tested for safety and effectiveness.

Contemporary oral hygiene aids are used to remove food residue that can create plaque and cause tooth decay. The residue, especially that from sugar, provide nutrients for germs.

BRUSHING AND INTERDENTAL CLEANING. The toothbrush and dental floss are used to remove plaque. The toothbrush is used to remove plaque from the teeth and stimulates the gums. Dental floss or a dental toothpick is used to remove plaque and food from the areas between teeth. Plaque is a waste product that causes tooth decay. If not removed, it calcifies (hardens) and forms tartar (calculus). This hard, calcified substance must be removed by a dentist or dental hygienist.

MOUTHWASH AND TOOTHPASTE. The ADA recommends that people use mouthwash and toothpaste that contain fluoride, a mineral that helps fight tooth decay. Toothpaste is used on the brush to clean teeth.

Mouthwash is used as a rinse. While a fluoridated toothpaste is essential for daily oral health care, mouthwash can supplement a mouth care regimen and is best recommended on a patient-need basis.

Oral hygiene in the 21st century

In June 2000, the ADA announced that research was under way on new oral hygiene aids, such as chewing gums and mouthwashes that would reverse early tooth decay. In 2000, scientists at the American Dental Association Health Foundation's Paffenbarger Research Center were investigating **calcium** phosphate-based technologies to remineralize hard tooth tissue or possibly slow down caries-producing demineralization. Center director, Frederick Eichmiller, D.D.S., announced in 2000 that other research included the study of toothpaste that strengthened and restored tooth **minerals**.

Description

Within the general categories of toothbrush, interdental aids and mouthwash, the choices can be overwhelming. Because of the vast number of products available, it is important for the dentist and the dental hygienist to advise patients about what type of products to purchase, based on individual needs. Along with that advice, the patient must be reminded to brush and clean interdental areas properly.

Both child and adult patients should use toothpaste and mouthwash containing fluoride, the mineral used to fight tooth decay. Fluoride helps strengthen the tooth's outer surface, and it can stop small areas of decay from spreading.

Proper use of oral hygiene aids will remove plaque, the film of bacteria that forms on teeth. The bacteria creates toxins that irritate the gums and demineralize tooth structure. If left untreated, plaque can initiate damage to the gums and bones supporting the teeth.

Manual toothbrushes

The toothbrush is the oral hygiene aid used to clean teeth. A manual toothbrush is activated by hand and not powered by electricity or batteries. The ADA recommends that people use a toothbrush with soft, rounded filaments (bristles). These brushes are better than those with hard filaments for removing plaque.

A toothbrush with soft bristles is recommended because tooth enamel could be worn away by intense scrubbing. When enamel is worn away, it can promote tooth decay, hypersensitivity, and gum recession. The size of the toothbrush and design of the head are less

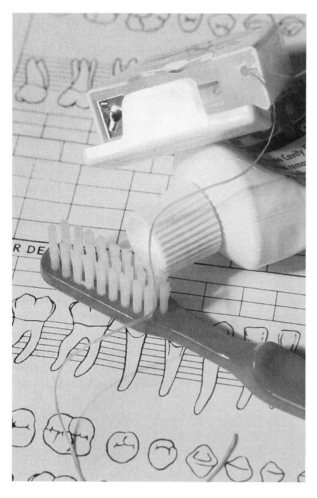

It is important for dentists and dental hygienists to instruct patients in the correct way to brush and floss their teeth. *(P. Stocklein/Custom Medical Stock Photo. Reproduced by permission.)*

important than the patient's commitment to using it properly.

Powered toothbrushes

Powered toothbrushes are operated by batteries or electricity. Powered toothbrushes have heads that move in a counter-rotational, rotary, or up-and-down manner; they work at a speed of 4,200 times per minute. Powered and manual toothbrushes are equally effective in removing plaque if used properly. On the other hand, studies have shown that people with poor oral hygiene or limited dexterity may benefit from using a powered toothbrush. Other studies have shown that some powered brushes are more effective in controlling stain and tartar. For children, this type of brush can be fun to use. For adults, the purchase of a powered-toothbrush could represent a commitment to improving oral hygiene habits.

No matter what type of toothbrush is used, the ADA recommends that patients use a toothpaste containing fluoride.

Toothpaste

Toothpaste is a preparation used to clean the tooth surface and remove plaque. Toothpaste flavor is a matter of consumer preference, and dental professionals advocate any flavor that stimulates people to brush at least twice a day. The ADA and the surgeon general recommend the use of a toothpaste containing fluoride to prevent tooth decay. Other effective ingredients of toothpaste are detergents and abrasives that help to remove plaque when teeth are brushed. Toothpastes that have the ADA Seal of Acceptance have a mild abrasive that is useful for plaque removal.

Tartar-control toothpaste that bear the ADA Seal of Acceptance can reduce tartar formation above the gum line. However, as of spring 2001, these products were not shown to have a "therapeutic effect on periodontal disease."

For people with receding gums and sensitive teeth, the ADA recommends brushing with a toothpaste that includes a desensitizing ingredient. These toothpastes reduce the painful effects of thermal, chemical, and mechanical stimuli on people with dental hypersensitivity.

Dental floss and picks

Dental floss is a thin, thread-like oral hygiene aid used to clean between teeth and under the gum line. Both waxed and unwaxed flosses are effective at fighting plaque. The important criteria when using floss is that it does not shred. Some patients prefer waxed floss, dental tape, or durable diameter floss, believing that they are gentler and easier to manipulate between teeth. For those who find shredding a problem, there are nonshred flosses.

Floss also varies in flavor. Some people find mint-flavored floss refreshing; others say that cinnamon is invigorating. Furthermore, floss widths vary. People with plaque problems may be advised to use the wider "tape" type of dental floss.

Wide spaces between teeth can also be cleaned with dental toothpicks, small pieces of material like soft orangewood, or interdental brushes. In fact, the American Academy of Periodontology recommends the interdental brush when space between the teeth exists.

Mouthwash

A fluoride mouthwash can be used in conjunction with brushing and flossing to help fight tooth decay. A patient may be advised by the dentist to use an antimicrobial mouthwash to control buildup and gingivitis.

Mouthwashes that promise fresher breath provide temporary relief of a condition that may be socially uncomfortable. However, unless these products contain fluoride, these rinses are not effective oral hygiene aids.

Furthermore, the dentist and dental hygienist know that bad breath can be a symptom of gum (periodontal) disease. The odor can be caused by the bacteria created when food particles are not removed from teeth.

Operation

The habit of brushing and flossing is more important than whether a manual or an electric toothbrush, or waxed or unwaxed floss, is used. In addition, many people do not know how to brush or floss correctly, so the dentist and dental hygienist play important roles in preventive patient care. The proper use of oral hygiene aids can be demonstrated and effective products can be recommended by either of these professionals.

Brushing the teeth

Teeth should be brushed at least twice daily, ideally after eating. The dentist and dental hygienist should advise patients to use toothpaste containing fluoride and to spend two minutes brushing their teeth.

BRUSHING THE TEETH MANUALLY. When brushing the teeth, people should use gentle circular motions to massage and scrub the tooth and gums. It is best to have a systematic approach to ensure all teeth are brushed.

The toothbrush is angled 45 degrees so that the bristles touch the teeth and gums. The person moves the brush back and forth with small strokes. Only a few teeth are brushed in this way, and the person brushes several times in one spot until moving on to the next set of teeth. This is done until all teeth are brushed. Then the tongue should be brushed to remove plaque and dead epithelial cells. The next step is to floss the teeth or use the interdental cleaner apropriate for the client.

BRUSHING WITH A POWER TOOTHBRUSH. The power toothbrush, also known as the electric toothbrush, moves the brush with faster strokes than a person can when brushing by hand. However, that speed doesn't contribute to mouth health. The person must brush for two minutes. That is the same amount of time required when brushing manually. However, some power toothbrushes come with two-minute timers, so that people can be aware of how long brushing is needed.

Using oral hygiene aids

Problem	Device/method
Debris removal	Water irrigation Toothbrush
Edentulous (toothless) gingiva under removable denture	Toothbrush (soft nylon) (manual or power assisted)
Exposed furcation maxillary first premolar	Interdental brush and rubber tip
Exposed furcation molars	Floss/yarn in threader Interdental brush and rubber tip
Exposed root surfaces	Fluoride dentifrice Dentifrice containing desensitizing agent
Fixed partial denture	Toothbrush (soft nylon) Floss threader with floss/yarn
Proximal surfaces open contacts	Gauze strip Yarn
Proximal surfaces plaque removal	Floss, or floss with threader Yarn with floss and/or threader Interdental brush or single-tuft brush
Removable denture	Denture brush Clasp brush Chemical cleanser for immersion
Sulcular brushing	Toothbrush with soft end-rounded filaments
Tongue cleaning	Toothbrush (soft nylon)

SOURCE: Alvarez, K.H. *Williams & Wilkins' Dental Hygiene Handbook.* Baltimore: Williams & Wilkins, 1998.

Flossing

Flossing may be done prior to or after brushing. In the dental office, a teeth cleaning appointment may end with the dental hygienist flossing the patient's teeth to remove particles of tartar and abrasive agents that might be left behind by the hygienist. Since flossing is a crucial part of dental health, the hygienist will generally describe this process so that the patient knows how to floss correctly.

DENTAL FLOSS. To clean between teeth with dental floss, the person takes an 18-in (46-cm) length of dental floss and wraps an end around the index or middle finger of each hand. The person inserts the floss in the gap between two teeth and gently moves it back and forth. The floss should rub against the front and back surfaces of each tooth. In addition, the floss up should be worked up and under the gum line to remove food and plaque. When the floss is moved to another area of the tooth, it should be adjusted, so that a clean area of the floss is used. When flossing for the first time, there may be slight gum bleeding. If bleeding persists, the patient should consult a dentist.

TOOTHPICKS. Toothpicks should be regarded as temporary oral hygiene aids. Household toothpicks can be used to remove food from teeth. Dental toothpicks made

KEY TERMS

Calculus—Calcified bacterial plaque.

Caries, dental—The decalcification and destruction of the tooth by microorganisms. Also known as tooth decay.

Cavity—A hole in the tooth.

Fluoride—A mineral that helps fight tooth decay.

Gingivitis—The inflammation of the gingiva (gums).

Periodontitis—The inflammation of the area surrounding the teeth. These areas include the gingiva (gums), the periodontal ligaments that attach teeth to sockets and the alveolar bone, the part of the jaw bone that holds the roots of teeth.

Plaque—A transparent material in the mouth that contains bacteria and causes tooth decay.

Tartar—Plaque that has calcified and hardened on the teeth. Also known as calculus.

of material, such as soft orangewood, can be used to stimulate gums or to reach plaque in the wide spaces between teeth. They can be an effective cleaning device in people with wide spaces between their teeth. However, toothpicks should not be used in place of flossing with dental floss in people with a normal interdental anatomy. Furthermore, patients should be cautioned by dentists and dental hygienists not to chew on toothpicks, as they can damage teeth.

Mouthwash

A fluoride mouthwash used in the morning and evening can help to fight plaque. Patients should be advised to look for products bearing the ADA Seal of Acceptance.

Mouthwash is taken full strength and used as a rinse. The person follows directions on the product. For one ADA-approved rinse, the person measures out 4 tsp (20 ml) of mouthwash and places it in the mouth. The rinse is swirled around for 30 seconds in the mouth and then expelled.

Oral hygiene aids for children

An oral hygiene program should begin when a baby gets his or her first tooth, according to the ADA. At this time, the infant's baby or primary teeth start to surface. Newly erupting teeth can be cared for by the parents,

using an infant toothbrush or a clean washcloth to scrub away any plaque. The ADA recommends that the child's first appointment with the dentist be scheduled by the time the baby is one year old. At this time, the dentist or dental hygienist can provide guidance about proper brushing and flossing.

At age three, most children have 20 primary teeth. By the time children are six years old, their jaws are growing to accommodate permanent or "adult" teeth. Those teeth will grow within the next six years and replace the primary or baby teeth.

TOOTHBRUSHING. For an infant, a parent can use a baby toothbrush or a soft cloth.

Children age six and younger should be supervised brushing their teeth. The parent should place a pea-sized amount of toothpaste on the toothbrush. This small amount helps to minimize the risk of swallowing toothpaste. The parent should still clean the child's mouth once a day to ensure proper cleaning.

When a child is seven and permanent teeth are growing, the ADA advises that children can brush their own teeth. However, an adult should supervise this process. And the dentist or hygienist may recommend that parents set the example by brushing along with the child

FLOSSING. The ADA recommends that children's teeth should be flossed when any two teeth are touching. By age eight, most children are old enough to floss on their own. Children with **orthodontic appliances** may not be able to floss in those areas.

MAKING ORAL HYGIENE EASIER. A disability, an injury, or illness can make it difficult for a person to brush or floss. Patients experiencing difficulty can get recommendations from their dentists or dental hygienists regarding commercial products and self-designed modifications that make the process easier.

When a patient has trouble brushing, the dentist or dental hygienist may advise the patient to purchase a powered toothbrush. If the patient's preference is to brush manually, the ADA recommends self-designed modifications and adaptations; for example, the patient can attach the toothbrush to the hand with an elastic band, using a sponge or rubber ball to widen the handle, and lengthening the handle by attaching a ruler or tongue depressor to it.

If the patient has difficulty flossing due to bridgework, a commercial floss holder or threader can be used to pull floss between teeth. In addition, tiny interdental brushes can be used to clean the area between teeth.

Maintenance

Maintenance is relatively simple for the oral hygiene products used for mouth care.

Toothbrushes

After use, a toothbrush should be allowed to dry in the air. It should not touch other toothbrushes, and people should not share toothbrushes because diseases can be transmitted. For occasional cleaning, the toothbrush can be soaked in a household bleach solution for about 10 minutes and rinsed thoroughly, or can be washed in dishwasher.

The toothbrush should be replaced after three or four months. Since many people do not remember when they bought a toothbrush, they can be told by dentists and dental hygienists to replace the toothbrush when the bristles are worn, bent or at the first sign of wear.

Furthermore, patients should also be advised to dispose of the toothbrush after an illness to prevent the spread of germs. The same procedures should be followed for the brushes used in a powered toothbrush. The brush should replaced after three or four months. Other maintenance will be based on the manufacturer's specifications.

Other hygiene aids

Products such as floss and toothpicks should be disposed of after usage. Toothpaste and mouthwash can be expelled from the mouth after the person rinses or brushes.

Health care team roles

Although oral hygiene aids like the toothbrush, dental floss, mouthwash, and toothpicks are household items, they are not used to fight plaque effectively. As a result, patients may be given instruction about the correct use of these aids by members of the dental team, such as the dentist or dental hygienist. Most dental offices and clinics maintain an inventory of sample products that can be used for demonstration.

A new toothbrush may be used by the dentist to demonstrate effective brushing techniques, such as how to angle the brush. Upon conclusion of the cleaning appointment, the teeth are usually flossed by the dental hygienist to remove particles of tartar and abrasive agents that may be left behind. This process may be described by the hygienist during the flossing.

It is also helpful to give the patient a mirror so that the person can see areas which should be flossed. Another option is to stand in front of the patient and demonstrate the technique for proper flossing or brushing. It is always best to use the patient's own mouth as a model.

The dental professional may then have the patient angle the brush or floss several teeth. The dentist or hygienist then gives the toothbrush or a sample package of floss to the patient. The same process is effective with aids such as floss holders or toothpicks.

Most dental patients rinse their mouths during an appointment. However, the dentist or dental hygienist may need to explain about the types of mouthwash, as well as the amount of time needed for rinsing at home.

Training

Training is required to use oral hygiene aids such as the toothbrush, dental floss, mouthwash, or toothpicks effectively. Since improper use of oral hygiene aid products can lead to tooth decay and gum disease, it is important for the dentist and dental hygienist to provide patients with instructions about the most effective use of these products, their purposes, and techniques for use.

Furthermore, continuing education courses allow dentists, dental hygienists, dental assistants, and others in the dental office to keep informed about advances in dental care, oral hygiene, and new products.

Resources

BOOKS

Alvarez, Kathleen H. *William & Wilkins' Dental Hygiene Handbook*. Philadelphia, PA: Lippincott, Williams & Wilkins, 1998.

Guerini, Vincezo. *A History of Dentistry From the Most Ancient Times Until the End of the Eighteenth Century*. Boston, MA: Longwood Press, 1977.

Leonardi Darby, Michele, ed. *Mosby's Comprehensive Review of Dental Hygiene*. St. Louis, MO: Mosby, Harcourt Health Sciences, 1998.

Nielsen Nathe, Christine. *Contemporary Practice for the Dental Hygienist*. Upper Saddle River, NJ: Prentice Hall, 2000.

Senzon, Sandra. *Hygiene Professional*. Tulsa, OK: PennWell Book, 1999.

Wilkins, Esther M. *Clinical Practice of the Dental Hygienist*. Philadelphia, PA: Lippincott, Williams & Wilkins, 1999.

PERIODICALS

Warren, Paul R.; Smith Ray, Tonya; Cugini, Maryann; Chater, Bernard. "A Practice-Based Study of a Power Toothbrush: Assessment of Effectiveness and Acceptance." *Journal of the American Dental Association* (March 2000), <http://www.ada.org/adapco/prof/pubs/jada/archives/0003/index.html>.

ORGANIZATIONS

American Dental Association. 211 E. Chicago Ave., Chicago, IL 60611. (312) 440-2500. <http://www.ada.org>.

American Dental Hygienists' Association. 444 N. Michigan Ave., Suite 3400, Chicago, IL 60622. (312) 440-8900. <http://www.adha.org>.

Centers for Disease Control and Prevention. National Center for Chronic Disease Prevention and Health Prevention. Division of Oral Health, MS F-10. 4770 Buford Highway, NE. Atlanta, GA 30341. 1-(888)-CDC-2306. <http://www.cdc.gov>.

International Federation of Dental Hygienists. 55 Kemble Road, Forest Hill, London, SE23 2DH, UK. Tel.: +44 208-699-3531. <http://www.ifdh.org>.

National Institute of Dental & Craniofacial Research. National Institutes of Health. Building 45, Room 4AS-18. 45 Center Drive MSC 6400, Bethesda, MD 2089-6400. <http://www.nidr.nih.gov/>.

Liz Swain

Oral hygiene index *see* **Dental indices**

Oral hypoglycemics *see* **Antidiabetic drugs**

Oral medication administration

Definition

Oral medication administration is the process by which drugs are delivered by mouth through the alimentary tract.

Purpose

Drugs are taken by this route because of convenience, absorption of the drug, ease of use, and cost containment. It is, therefore, the most common method used.

Precautions

Other routes are used when a person cannot take anything by mouth, or the drug is poorly absorbed by the gastrointestinal tract. The nurse should check whether the patient has any known **allergies**. It is useful to remember the following checks when administering any medication: the right patient, the right medicine, the right route, the right dose, the right site, and the right time.

Description

Oral drugs are can be prescribed to be taken at different intervals, either before or after food. They can be in either liquid or solid form. Questions about the frequency with which drugs should be taken should be addressed to the primary health care provider.

Preparation

Wash the hands. The patient's order sheet should be checked to ensure that the dose has not already been given. Once that is confirmed, the correct drug and dose should be selected. The appropriate number of pills should be shaken onto the lid of their container and dropped into a small measuring cup to hand to the patient. This should be done immediately prior to giving the drug and not done in advance.

If the medication is liquid, the bottle should be shaken, the cap removed, and the bottle held at eye level with the label turned upwards, to prevent staining. The correct dose should be poured into a measuring cup.

The patient should be informed that his or her doctor has prescribed some medicine for him or her. The nurse should check the drug and dose against the patient's prescription chart again, then confirm the patient's name on his or her wristband. The drug can then be handed to the patient, who should also be offered a drink of water to aid in swallowing pills.

Liquid medicines containing **iron** should be taken through a straw to minimize staining of the teeth.

After ensuring that the drug has been taken, the nurse should record the time and the dose that has been given.

Aftercare

The nurse should monitor the patient's reaction and provide reassurance, if required.

Complications

Possible complications include:

- The drug may interact with other drugs the patient is taking and alter the desired effect.
- The patient may refuse the drug.
- There may be difficulty in swallowing.
- The drug may irritate the gastrointestinal tract.
- The drug may pass quickly through the body, and the benefits of the drug may be lost.

Alimentary—Relating to the system of nutrition.

Alimentary tract—The alimentary tract and the other organs involved in digestion and absorption.

Gastro—Referring to the stomach.

Gastrointestinal tract—The stomach and intestinal tracts involved in digestion and the elimination of waste products.

Intestinal—Referring to the intestine.

Results

Administration of oral medication should result in the patient receiving the proper dose of drug safely, and with no complications. Oral drugs can also interact with other medications that the patient is taking, such as injections. The nurse should check for any adverse reactions if the drug is being administered for the first time.

Health care team roles

The staff should establish whether a patient is taking any drugs prior to being given any additional medication. It is important that a nurse understand the actions, side effects, and incompatibility of drugs, recognize normal doses, and be knowledgeable about any reactions that a patient may experience. The nurse should report any unusual effects to the medical staff and record any side effects or negative reactions to the drug that has been given.

If the medication is to be prescribed regularly for a specific disease, the patient can be directed to a self-help group in which members have the same medical condition. The patient should be helped to feel confident that his or her privacy is ensured.

If the labels on liquid medicine bottles are stained and illegible, the medicine should not be used.

Resources

BOOKS

Denville, N.J. *The Self Help Source Book.* American Self Help Clearinghouse, 1998.

ORGANIZATIONS

American Academy of Nurse Practitioners. AANP, PO Box 12846, Austin, Texas, 78711. (512) 442-4262. admin@aanp.org.

American Nurses Association, 600 Maryland Avenue, SW, Suite 100 West, Washington, DC 20024. (202) 651-7000.

National Association of Clinical Nurse Specialists, 3969 Green Street, Harrisburg, PA, 17110. (717) 234-6799. info@nacns.org.

National League for Nursing, 61 Broadway, 33rd Floor, New York, NY 10006. (212) 363-5555 or (800) 669-1656.

OTHER

"How to Administer Medications." <http://nursing.about.com>.

Margaret A. Stockley, RGN

Orgasmic disorders *see* **Sexual dysfunction**

Orthodontic appliances

Definition

Orthodontic appliances are corrective and supportive braces, designed and prescribed by an orthodontist. The appliances treat malocclusions, including crooked, crowded, and protruding teeth that do not fit properly together.

Purpose

In a controlled manner, dental appliances gently force teeth to move through the supporting bone to a desired position. The purpose of the appliances is to correct tooth crowding, overjet or protruding upper teeth, deep overbite, spacing problems, crossbite and underbite, or lower jaw protrusion.

Precautions

Orthodontists applying orthodontic appliances should make sure that a patient's bones, gums and tooth roots are in a healthy condition. They should also prepare the patient emotionally for the experience of wearing orthodontic appliances. The cooperation of the patient is important in achieving a successful result. Patients with emotional or self-image problems can be difficult to treat.

Description

Orthodontic appliances are custom-made appliances, or braces, which are designed by orthodontists to fix bite problems, or malocclusions. There are two large classifications of these appliances: fixed (cemented and/or bonded to teeth) and removable. Appliances can be active or passive—some actively move the teeth, while others, such as retainers, are designed to keep the teeth where

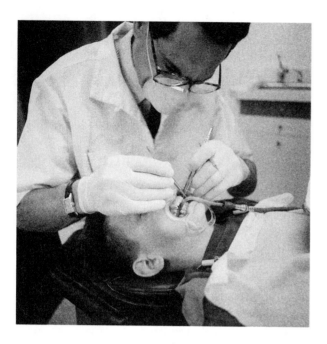

An orthodontist fits a twelve-year-old boy for braces.
(Richard Hutchings Photo. Photo Researchers, Inc. Reproduced by permission.)

they are. Orthodontic appliances, or braces, can be made of metal, ceramic, or plastic. In recent years, there have been advances in the materials used to make braces. The wires used on today's braces are stainless steel, alloys of nickel, titanium, **copper**, and cobalt, and some are heat-activated. They are designed to exert pressure so that results are faster and more comfortable for patients. Clear orthodontic wires are being studied for application in the general population of orthodontic patients. New braces are smaller and more efficient. The wires cause teeth to continue to move during some treatment phases, which can result in a patient having to make fewer appointments for wire adjustments.

Specific examples of orthodontic appliances include headgear, the bionator, Herbst, the Frankel and maxillary expansion appliances. These are orthodontic appliances designed to actively guide the growth and development of the jaw. Headgear or the Herbst appliance can, over the course of treatment, make the lengths of the upper and lower jaw compatible. An upper jaw expansion appliance can significantly widen a narrow upper jaw. One of the newer orthodontic appliances is a plastic aligner, used to move teeth around without requiring brackets. Orthodontists have a wide range of options in selecting an orthodontic appliance for a particular application.

Another advance in the area of orthodontic appliances is that modern braces are less noticeable than those in which a metal band and bracket were placed around each tooth. In many cases, patients have brackets bonded directly to the front teeth, minimizing the "tinsel tooth" appearance. Patients can choose between clear, metal, or colored brackets. Some braces are bonded behind the teeth.

Preparation

Orthodontists have patients undergo diagnostic testing, prior to applying braces, to help plan the best course of treatment. Diagnostic records usually include a medical and dental history, clinical examination, plaster study models of the teeth, photos of the patient's face and teeth, a panoramic or other type of x ray of the teeth, a facial profile x ray, and other x rays. The cephalometric film, or profile x ray, shows the patient's facial form, growth pattern, and front teeth positions. Other x rays, including panoramic x rays, reveal impacted teeth, missing teeth, and shortened or damaged tooth roots.

Aftercare

Patients who have dental appliances have to take special care of their teeth. They must be careful to avoid hard or sticky foods, which can loosen their appliances and therefore diminish the effect. Orthodontic patients must not chew on hard things, such as pencils or nails, because these can damage the appliances. Cleanings must be more thorough than ever. Teeth should be brushed immediately after eating sweet foods. Special floss threaders are available to make flossing easier.

Complications

Successful orthodontic treatment with appliances requires a consistent, cooperative effort by the orthodontist and the patient. A patient's failure to clean his or her teeth, or to wear rubber bands, headgear, or other prescribed appliances, can result in failure of the teeth to move to their desired positions, and can even prolong treatment.

Ankylosis is a condition that in many cases cannot be controlled or detected by the orthodontist. It occurs when the tooth and underlying bone fuse together and become one. Should a patient have this condition, the braces will not be able to move the fused tooth or teeth.

Results

Orthodontic treatment with orthodontic appliances results in improved aesthetics and better function of the teeth and jaws. Left untreated, crooked or crowded teeth can become worse, sometimes requiring costly treatment to address serious problems that can develop over time.

KEY TERMS

Ankylosis—A condition where the tooth fuses to bone.

Bionator—An orthodontic appliance that actively guides the growth and development of the jaw.

Bracket—The braces part that holds the wire.

Crossbite—The condition in which the upper teeth bite inside the lower teeth.

Deep overbite—The condition in which the lower front teeth bite too closely or into the gum tissue behind the upper teeth.

Headgear—An orthodontic appliance, which actively guides the growth and development of the jaw.

Herbst appliance—An orthodontic appliance that actively guides the growth and development of the jaw.

Malocclusion—Misaligned bite.

Maxillary expansion appliances—An orthodontic appliance used to widen a narrow upper jaw.

Overjet—The condition in which the upper front teeth extend beyond normal contact with lower front teeth.

Retainer—A passive orthodontic appliance designed to keep teeth in place.

Orthodontic problems can contribute to conditions that cause tooth decay and gum disease. They also can help to cause abnormal wear of tooth surfaces, inefficient chewing function, excessive stress on gum tissue and supporting bone, as well as jaw misalignment, resulting in headaches and face or neck **pain**.

Health care team roles

The general dentist can identify a **malocclusion** and refer patients to specialists, such as orthodontists. Dental hygienists may help to identify malocclusions during routine **dental hygiene** appointments. Together with dentists, hygienists watch the development of pediatric dental patients. They look at how teeth mesh together, examine the patient's profile, and identify instances of crowding or too much space between teeth. Hygienists in the general or pediatric dental office help patients to maintain healthy teeth and gums while the braces are on, by in-office cleanings and education about proper home-care techniques (brushing, soaking, and removal of

removable appliances) to maintain overall oral health. Dental assistants are ancillary personnel in dentists' or orthodontists' offices who assist in recording data, taking study models, and performing procedures.

Resources

ORGANIZATIONS

Academy of General Dentistry. 211 East Chicago Ave., Chicago, IL 600611. (312) 440-4800. <http://www.agd.org>.

American Association of Orthodontists. 401 N. Lindbergh Blvd. St. Louis, MO 63141-7816. 314-993-1700. <www.aaortho.org>.

American Dental Hygienists' Association. 444 North Michigan Avenue, Suite 3400, Chicago, IL 60611.(312)440-8900. <http://adha.org>.

OTHER

Callahan Barnard, Susan. American Dental Hygienists' Association. Interview with Lisette Hilton, conducted April 16, 2001.

Preis, Frederick (president). American Association of Orthodontists. Interview with Lisette Hilton, conducted April 16, 2001.

Lisette Hilton

Orthopedic tests

Definition

Orthopedic tests are designed to evaluate individuals for musculoskeletal impairment. Orthopedic tests enable the clinician, such as a physician or physical therapist, to identify a specific area of injury and aid in the diagnosis and treatment plan of the injured individual. There is a general plan for physical assessment that includes taking a patient's history; examining how the patient moves and how individual joints move; evaluating sensation and **reflexes**; and, if necessary, administering diagnostic tests to aid in the diagnosis. These are specific orthopedic tests for the upper and lower extremities as well as the spine. The orthopedic tests, or "special tests," help the clinician in the differential diagnosis of the patient.

Purpose

A medical or **health history** taken by the clinician is extremely important in evaluating and diagnosing the patient. A patient's description of the **pain**, weakness, or both will guide the clinician as to what structures to evaluate and which orthopedic tests, if necessary, to complete. After the history has been taken, the clinician may focus on sensory and reflex testing to evaluate the integrity of the nervous system. Depending on where the injury or impairment is on the body, the clinician may opt to evaluate range of motion of the joint(s) of the area of injury or near the injury. For example, if a patient has knee pain, the clinician will more than likely assess how far the patient can bend the knee and straighten the knee. The clinician will compare this movement to the uninvolved side or "good leg." Thus, the clinician has a baseline for the individual and the "good leg" serves as a reference point or goal. It is usually advisable that the "good side" always be evaluated first, so that a true comparison can be made to the affected side. Obviously, if there is bilateral involvement the clinician must use his/her experience with other patients to evaluate and set a plan of care. Also included in an assessment is the evaluation of muscle strength.

Precautions

Most orthopedic tests stress areas to be evaluated in an effort to evaluate pain, joint play, and muscle extensibility. Because of the stress involved during some orthopedic tests, care must be taken to avoid further injury. Before doing any orthopedic tests, an area must be free from fracture or neoplasm (an abnormal growth). Furthermore, any patient with characteristics such as severe spasm, pain with unknown etiology, or pain that awakens the patient at night, should not be evaluated with orthopedic tests until a full medical evaluation can be completed to address these unexplained symptoms.

Description

There are numerous orthopedic tests that help the clinician diagnose impairment. It should be pointed out that these tests alone do not confirm a diagnosis. As stated previously, the medical history and other evaluative tools need to be completed so as to get a total representation of the patient's health and the nature of injury or problem. Furthermore, a positive test does not necessarily indicate a specific problem, and a negative test does not necessarily rule out the problem. Some tests that are frequently used by clinicians to evaluate the spine and extremities will be described below.

Cervical spine

One possible problem associated with the cervical spine could be narrowing of the space occupied by the nerve root. This could be due to many causes, two of which could be injury or **osteoarthritis**. It is possible that as the space occupied by the nerve root closes, there may be impingement on the nerve root. If this occurs there could be pain, changes in sensation, and weakness in the neck, shoulder, and possibly down the arm. Two tests that may help diagnose an individual with this pathology are the distraction and compression tests. The distraction test for the cervical spine is performed by the clinician to assess if there is pressure on the nerve roots. In a positive test, symptoms will decrease or disappear. The compression test is also performed by the clinician to evaluate if there is pressure on the nerve root. If symptoms are provoked down either arm during the test, it would indicate pressure on the nerve root and thus, a positive test.

Shoulder

In the shoulder there are many muscles that act to stabilize and control the humeral head in the glenoid (shoulder socket). Injury can occur to any of these muscles and cause pain in and around the shoulder. The biceps muscle flexes the elbow but has a tendinous attachment that crosses the shoulder. It is commonly involved in overuse injuries. Yergason's test evaluates muscle tendon pathology of the biceps tendon. In this test, a positive result is evidenced by tenderness or pain over the bicipital groove of the shoulder indicating a possible bicipital tendinitis (inflammation of the biceps tendon). Another common test is the Neer impingement test, which evaluates the integrity of the subacromial space (below the highest point of the shoulder blade) as it relates to the supraspinatus muscle (a muscle in the shoulder area). A positive sign is when pain is elicited in the superior shoulder and is usually an indication of some type of injury to the supraspinatus tendon, that is tendinitis. The cause of tendinitis is usually overuse.

Elbow

Tennis elbow test or Cozen's test is used to assess if there is an injury to the lateral epicondyle of the humerus (a bony prominence at the elbow end of the bone). A positive test is indicated by the patient having increased symptoms over the area of the lateral epicondyle. Pain usually indicates involvement of the wrist extensors at their origin. Pain is usually due to inflammation secondary to overuse. Golfer's elbow test or the medial epicondylitis test assesses the integrity of the medial epicondyle and the muscular attachments. A positive sign is pain over the area of the medial epicondyle and is usually indicative of tendinitis of the wrist flexors, also at their origin.

Wrist and hand

A common problem associated with repetitive strain is that of typists who spend hours at a time with the wrist slightly bent in the upward position. Constant stress on the wrist can eventually lead to pain and abnormal sensations, often tingling, of the wrist and hand. The common term is **carpal tunnel syndrome**. Phalen's test is a good test to evaluate the presence of pressure on the median nerve, which is the cause of pain. A positive test occurs when tingling is present in the fingers and is usually indicative of carpal tunnel syndrome. Another common test is the Finkelstein test. It is a test to evaluate the presence of tenosynovitis (inflammation of the tendon sheath) in the thumb. A positive sign is pain across the top and base of the thumb.

Hip

Sometimes individuals who are in sitting positions for extended periods of time, such as being in a wheelchair, may present with tightness of the muscles around the hip. There are three tests that are good tools to evaluate muscle flexibility around the hip. The Thomas test assesses fexibility of the hip flexors. It is a good test to evaluate tightness of the muscles that cross the front of the hip. The Ober test is another common flexibility test to assess the tightness of the tensor fasciae latae (connective tissue that covers the muscle and directs its tightening) and the iliotibial band (connects the pelvis to the leg bone). Ely's test is another test for assessing muscle tightness. It is used for evaluating the tightness of the rectus femoris, which crosses the front of the hip joint.

Knee

The knee is a common area that is frequently involved in pathology. One common problem, especially in the athletic population, is the disruption or tearing of the anterior cruciate ligament (ACL) of the knee. A Lachman test is probably the best orthopedic manual test to evaluate the integrity of the ACL. Other tests that assess the stability of the ligaments and the joint capsule are the Slocum test, lateral pivot shift test, and Hughston's test. The tests mentioned here are termed stress tests, and they assess laxity, or the amount of movement, at the knee joint.

Foot and ankle

The foot and ankle is a complex area that allows for both mobility and stability. There are many flexibility and ligamentous stress tests to evaluate the foot and ankle. Some common tests are the Talar tilt test, Thompson's test, and a test to assess **blood** supply to the lower extremity called Buerger's test.

KEY TERMS

Anatomy—The study of the structural makeup of the human body.

Anterior cruciate ligament—A ligament that attaches the surfaces of the tibia and femur, thus stabilizing the knee joint. This structure prevents anterior translation of the tibia with respect to the femur.

Biomechanics—The study of mechanics pertaining to the human body.

Etiology—The causes of a disease or abnormal condition.

Iliotibial band—A fascial sheath that extends from the upper thigh and traverses down the side of the femur, attaching around the area of the knee joint.

Kinesiology—The study of the principles of biomechanics as it pertains to human movement.

Physiology—The study of the physical and chemical processes as it relates to an organism, i.e. human body.

Rectus femoris—An anterior muscle that, when contracting, can initiate hip flexion, knee extension, or both at the same time.

Spasm—An involuntary and abnormal muscular contraction.

Tensor fasciae latae—A single muscle on the side of the thigh covering the hip joint that, when contracting, aids other muscles in moving the leg away from midline and out to the side.

Preparation

There are many orthopedic tests designed to aid the clinician in better evaluating the patient who has musculoskeletal impairment. Before doing these tests, clinicians must have knowledge of anatomy, biomechanics, kinesiology, and physiology. Furthermore, most of these tests are performed by licensed and experienced clinicians such as physicians, chiropractors, and physical therapists. Before doing these tests, it is important to point out that most of these tests can cause pain and produce symptoms. In fact, some of these tests are termed provocation tests, because they produce or "provoke" onset of symptoms.

Aftercare

Clinicians will focus on specific tests that can best evaluate the joint, limb, or spine. The goal is not to complete as many tests as possible, but to isolate tests that are joint or pathology specific. Clinicians should refrain from over-testing. It is not uncommon that after extensibility tests or stress tests to a joint, the patient may require heat to relax tight tissues or ice to minimize pain and/or inflammation.

Complications

Orthopedic tests are designed to aid the clinician in the determination of a diagnosis. When used sparingly and appropriately, these "special tests" can provide valuable information about the impairment. However, these tests require clinical competencies, and problems can arise when clinicians are not properly trained in certain techniques.

Results

Orthopedic tests will give the clinician some insight into the nature of the patient's complaints, although they may not directly correlate to a specific diagnosis. Imaging studies, such as x rays or an MRI scan, may be done to aid in diagnosis. Once the source of the pain has been determined, a course of treatment will be set. Treatment may include icing and resting the injury and prescribing pain relievers. Surgery is sometimes necessary. **Physical therapy** is often begun as soon as the patient's level of pain permits.

Health care team roles

It is important for the clinician to utilize as many sources as possible when evaluating an individual who presents with musculoskeletal involvement. For example, a physical therapist doing an evaluation needs to take a sound medical history followed by a complete assessment of all systems, i.e. muscular, skeletal, nervous. Furthermore, the physical therapist must be in complete contact with the referring physician and the nursing staff regarding medication, protocols, and diagnostic tests. Other therapies, such as speech, occupational, and respiratory may also be part of the evaluation. If the patient is in a rehabilitation hospital or nursing home, the nursing staff can provide an up-to-date status on the patient. It is quite clear that the evaluation of a patient requires input from the entire healthcare team, including the patient.

Resources

BOOKS

Hertling D., R.M. Kessler. *Management of Common Musculoskeletal Disorders.* Baltimore: Lippincott, Williams & Wilkins, 1996.

Lehmkuhl L.D., L. K. Smith. *Brunnstroms Clinical Kinesiology.* Philadelphia: F.A. Davis Co., 1996.
Magee D. J. *Orthopedic Physical Assessment.* Philadelphia: W.B. Saunders Co., 1997.
Moore K.L., A.F. Dalley. *Clinically Oriented Anatomy.* Baltimore: Lippincott, Williams & Wilkins, 1999.

Mark Damian Rossi, Ph.D., P.T.

Orthopedic x rays *see* **Bone x rays**

Osteoarthritis

Definition

Osteoarthritis (OA) is a progressive disorder of the joints caused by gradual loss of cartilage that may result in the development of bony spurs and cysts at the margins of the joints. The name osteoarthritis comes from three Greek words meaning bone, joint, and inflammation.

Description

OA is one of the most common causes of disability due to limitations of joint movement, particularly in people over the age of 50. It is estimated that 2% of the United States population under the age of 45 also suffers from osteoarthritis; this figure rises to 30% in persons between the ages of 45 and 64, and 63–80% in those over age 70. Approximately 90% of the American population will have some features of OA in their weight-bearing joints by age 40. Men tend to develop OA at earlier ages than women.

OA typically develops gradually, over a period of years. Patients with OA may have joint **pain** on only one side of the body. It primarily affects the knees, hands, hips, feet, and spine.

Causes and symptoms

Osteoarthritis results from deterioration or destruction of the cartilage that normally acts as a protective cushion between bones, particularly in weight-bearing joints such as the knees and hips. As the cartilage is worn away, the bones may form spurs, areas of abnormal hardening, and fluid-filled pockets in the marrow. These are known as subchondral cysts. As the disorder progresses, pain results from deformation of the bones and fluid accumulation in the joints. Pain may be relieved by rest, but worsened by placing weight on, or moving, the joint.

In the early stages of OA, the pain is minor and may take the form of mild stiffness in the morning. In the later stages of OA, inflammation develops; the patient may experience pain even when the joint is not being used; and he or she may suffer permanent loss of the normal range of motion in that joint.

Osteoarthritis typically has been considered by laypeople as an inevitable part of aging caused by simple wear and tear on the joints. This view has been replaced by recent research into cartilage formation and preservation. Osteoarthritis is now considered to be the end result of several different factors that can contribute to cartilage damage, and is classified as either primary or secondary.

Primary osteoarthritis

Primary OA results from abnormal stress on weight-bearing joints, or normal stress affecting weakened joints. Primary OA most frequently affects the finger joints, the hips and knees, the cervical and lumbar spine, and the big toe. Some gene mutations appear to be associated with OA. **Obesity** also increases the pressure on the weight-bearing joints of the body. Finally, as the body ages, there is a reduction in the ability of cartilage to repair itself. In addition to these factors, some researchers have theorized that primary OA may be triggered by enzyme disturbances, bone disease, or **liver** dysfunction.

Secondary osteoarthritis

Secondary OA results from chronic or sudden injury to a joint. It can occur in any joint. Secondary OA is associated with the following factors:

• trauma to the body, including sports injuries

• repetitive stress injuries associated with certain occupations (i.e., the performing arts, construction or assembly line work, computer keyboard operation, etc.)

• repeated episodes of **gout** or septic arthritis

• poor posture or bone alignment caused by developmental abnormalities

• metabolic disorders

Diagnosis

The two most important diagnostic clues in the patient's history are the pattern of joint involvement and the presence or absence of **fever**, rash, or other symptoms outside the joints.

History and physical examination

When taking **vital signs** (i.e., **blood pressure**, weight, temperature), the patient's gait and arm and hand movement should be observed by the nursing staff or physician assistants; if pain is the chief complaint, the affected joint should be examined. After a brief examination, the nurse, nurse practitioner, or physician assistant should ask the length of time the pain has affected the patient and if there have been any limitations in his or her work or home life. The practitioner should record abnormal symptoms on the intake sheet for review by the physician. As part of the **physical examination**, the physician will evaluate swelling, limitations on the range of motion, pain on movement, and crepitus (i.e., cracking or grinding sound heard during joint movement). Osteoarthritis is often similar in presentation to rheumatoid arthritis, but lacks the presence of inflammation (until its very late stages) found in rheumatoid arthritis.

Diagnostic imaging

There is no laboratory test specific to the diagnosis of OA. Laboratory tests are important, however, in ruling out other diseases that may be responsible for the symptoms the patient is presenting. Treatment is usually based on the results of diagnostic imaging, which is conducted by a radiologic technician or radiologist. The features of the disease are a loss of joint space, the presence of subchondral cysts, and evidence of new bone formation (i.e., bone spurs). The patient's symptoms, however, do not always correlate with x-ray findings. **Magnetic resonance imaging** (MRI) and computed tomography (CT), or computed axial tomography (CAT) scans can be used to more precisely determine the location and extent of cartilage damage.

Prognosis

Osteoarthritis is a progressive disorder without a permanent cure. In some patients, the rate of progression can be slowed by weight loss, appropriate **exercise**, surgical treatment, and the use of alternative therapies.

Health care team roles

Early detection and diagnosis are key factors that affect the outcome of the progression of OA. Patients may present with vague symptoms of joint pain and stiffness, which should be noted when taking the patient history. The patient should be asked when these symptoms began. Co-morbid conditions such as **heart** disease, **hypertension**, or other disease should be considered. After ongoing observation and consultation with the patient, a more complete diagnosis can be made.

As with other painful conditions, understanding of the patient's lifestyle changes and physical condition is of the highest priority. **Patient education** and follow-up

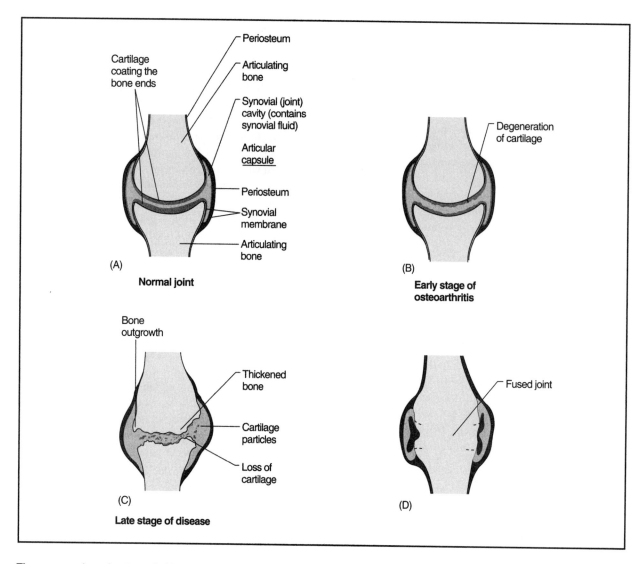

Periosteum

Cartilage
coating the
bone ends

Articulating
bone

Synovial (joint)
cavity (contains
synovial fluid)

Articular
capsule

Periosteum

Synovial
membrane

Articulating
bone

(A)
Normal joint

Degeneration
of cartilage

(B)
**Early stage of
osteoarthritis**

Bone
outgrowth

Thickened
bone

Cartilage
particles

Loss of
cartilage

(C)
Late stage of disease

Fused joint

(D)

The progression of osteoarthritis. *(Illustration by Hans & Cassidy.)*

support can assist with the mental health treatment, if necessary. Health care staff should counsel the patient on the basic facts of OA, make themselves available for follow-up phone consultation, and track the patient's visits to other health care providers. If the patient seems especially distressed about the condition, staff may recommend to the physician that the patient seek mental health support.

Should a rheumatologist or other subspecialist be consulted by the patient, members of the health care team should coordinate and monitor the treatment prescribed outside of the team's environment.

Patient contact has been shown to be a valuable aspect of the management of OA. Optimal follow-up consists of staff members (i.e., nurses, nurse practitioners, physicians assistants) making phone calls to patients and recording changes in symptoms, compliance with treatment regimen,

and any decline of condition. Nursing parameters can include pain control, assessment of medication efficacy, exercise, diet, means of joint protection, and awareness of psychosocial factors of depression/anxiety.

Knowledge of over-the-counter medications for OA can assist the patient in avoiding **drug interactions** or undue financial burden. Patients with limited range of motion may require special accommodations in waiting and treatment rooms; they may need an entrance to the building or a bathroom that is specially made to accommodate the handicapped, or a modified examination table.

Treatment

Treatment of patients with OA is tailored to the needs of each individual. Patient's symptoms vary widely due to the location of the joints involved, the rate of progression, the severity of symptoms, the degree of disability, and individual response to specific forms of treatment. Most treatment programs include several forms of therapy and include the participation of the entire health care team.

Patient education and psychotherapy

Patient education is an important part of OA treatment because of the highly individual nature of the disorder and its potential impact on the patient's life. Patients who are depressed because of changes in employment or recreation usually benefit from participation in self-help groups, or counseling. The patient's family or friends should be involved in discussions of coping, household reorganization, and other aspects of the patient's disease and treatment regimen.

Medications

Patients with mild OA may be treated only with pain relievers such as acetaminophen (i.e., Tylenol). Most patients with OA, however, are given **nonsteroidal anti-inflammatory drugs** (NSAIDs). These include compounds such as ibuprofen (e.g., Motrin, Advil), ketoprofen (e.g., Orudis), and naproxen (e.g. Naprosyn). NSAIDs have the advantage of relieving slight inflammation as well as pain. Patients taking NSAIDS, however, may experience side effects, including **stomach** ulcers, sensitivity to sun exposure, kidney disturbances, and nervousness/anxiety or depression. Topical capsaicin cream (e.g., AthriCare) may provide relief when applied to affected areas.

Some OA patients are treated with **corticosteroids**, which are injected directly into the joints to reduce inflammation. As of 2001, studies were being conducted regarding the use of hyaluronic acid, which is more commonly injected into the knee. Because the joint naturally contains some hyaluronic acid (for joint lubrication), the addition of extra hyaluronic acid can protect the joint, in some cases, for six months to one year.

Physical therapy

Patients with OA are encouraged to exercise as a way of keeping joint cartilage lubricated and mobile. Consultation with a physical therapist is highly recommended, as it can ensure patient compliance and safety while exercising. Low-impact exercises to increase balance, flexibility, and range of motion are also recommended. These exercises may include walking, swimming or other water activities, **yoga**, and other stretching exercises, or isometric exercises (i.e., a program of exercises in which a muscle group is tensed against another muscle group or an immovable object so that the muscles may contract without shortening).

Physical therapy may also include massage, the application of moist hot packs, or soaks in a hot tub. Prescriptions may be written for protective devices. Instructions for their use would be given to patients by physical therapy staff.

Surgery

Surgical treatment of OA may include the replacement of a damaged joint with an artificial part or appliance, surgical fusion of spinal bones, scraping or removal of damaged bone from the joint, or the removal of a piece of bone in order to realign the bone.

Protective measures

Support staff will be required to educate the patient on the correct use of any protective measure, the length of time it will be needed, and counsel on the correct way to bend, lift or move the affected joint. The consequences of not using protective measures should be outlined (i.e., exacerbation of symptoms, additional muscle strain, undue pain from noncompliance). Depending on the location of the affected joint, patients with OA may be advised to use neck braces or collars, crutches, canes, hip braces, knee supports, bed boards, or elevating chairs and toilet seats. Patients would also be advised to avoid unnecessary bending, stair climbing, or lifting of heavy objects.

Potential treatments

Several methods of treatment for OA are being investigated. They include:

- Disease-modifying drugs. These compounds may be useful in assisting the body to form new cartilage or improve its repair of existing cartilage.

- Hyaluronic acid. This treatment is well supported in theory.

- Electromagnetic therapy. This treatment is viewed with skepticism by mainstream medicine.

- Gene therapy. This is a promising area of treatment, although it may not be available for several years.

Alternative treatment

DIET. Food intolerance can be a contributing factor to OA, although this is more significant in rheumatoid arthritis. Dietary suggestions that may be helpful for people with OA include emphasizing high-fiber, complex-carbohydrate foods, while minimizing **fats**.

NUTRITIONAL SUPPLEMENTS In recent years, a combination of glucosamine and chondroitin sulfate has been studied as a dietary supplement to help the body maintain and repair cartilage. These substances are nontoxic and do not require prescriptions, but studies continue to be conducted to evaluate their effectiveness. Other supplements that may be helpful in the treatment of OA include the antioxidant **vitamins** A, C, and E, and **minerals** selenium and **zinc**.

Resources

BOOKS

Hellman, David B. "Arthritis & Musculoskeletal Disorders." In *Current Medical Diagnosis and Treatment,* edited by Lawrence M. Tierney, Jr., et al. Stanford, CT: Appleton & Lange, 1998.

Neustadt, David H. "Osteoarthritis." In *Merck Manual of Diagnosis and Theory,* edited by Robert E. Rakel. Philadelphia: W. B. Saunders Company, 1998.

PERIODICALS

Gelber A.C., et al. "Joint injury in young adults and risk for subsequent knee and hip osteoarthritis." *Annals of Internal Medicine* 133 (2000): 321-328.

Manek, N.J., and N. Lane. "Osteoarthritis." *Current Concepts in Diagnosis and Management* 61 (2000): 1796-1804.

OTHER

National Library of Medicine. *Medline Plus Health Information.* <http://www.nih.gov/medlineplus/druginfo/antiinflammatorydrugsnonsteroi202743.html>. (May 8, 2001).

Michele R. Webb

Osteogenic sarcoma *see* **Sarcomas**

Osteoporosis

Definition

The word osteoporosis literally means "porous bones." It occurs when bones lose an excessive amount of their protein and mineral content, particularly **calcium**. Over time, bone mass, and therefore bone strength, is decreased. As a result, bones become fragile and break easily. Even a sneeze or a sudden movement may be enough to break a bone in someone with severe osteoporosis.

Description

Osteoporosis is a serious **public health** problem. Some 28 million people in the United States are affected by this potentially debilitating disease, which is responsible for 1.5 million **fractures** (broken bones) annually. These fractures, which are often the first sign of the disease, can affect any bone, but the most common locations are the hip, spine, and wrist. Breaks in the hip and spine are of special concern because they almost always require hospitalization and major surgery, and may lead to other serious consequences, including permanent disability and even death.

To understand osteoporosis, it is helpful to understand the basics of bone formation. Bone is living tissue that is constantly being renewed in a two-stage process (resorption and formation) that occurs throughout life. In the resorption stage, old bone is broken down and removed by cells called osteoclasts. In the formation stage, cells called osteoblasts build new bone to replace the old. During childhood and early adulthood, more bone is produced than removed, reaching its maximum mass and strength by the mid-30s. After that, bone is lost at a faster pace than it is formed, so the amount of bone in the skeleton begins to slowly decline. Most cases of osteoporosis occur as an acceleration of this normal aging process—a form referred to as primary osteoporosis. The condition can also be caused by other disease processes or prolonged use of certain medications that result in bone loss—a form called secondary osteoporosis.

Osteoporosis occurs most often in older people and in women after **menopause**. It affects nearly half of all men and women over the age of 75. Women, however, are five times more likely than men to develop the disease. They have smaller, thinner bones than men to begin with, and they lose bone mass more rapidly after menopause (usually around age 50), when they stop producing a bone-protecting hormone called estrogen. In the five to seven years following menopause, women can lose about 20% of their bone mass. By age 65 or 70, though, men and women lose bone mass at the same rate. As an increasing number of men reach an older age, they are becoming more aware that osteoporosis is an important health issue for them as well.

Causes and symptoms

A number of factors increase the risk of developing osteoporosis. They include:

- Age. Osteoporosis is more likely as people grow older and their bones lose tissue.

- Gender. Women are more likely to have osteoporosis because they are smaller and so start out with less bone. They also lose bone tissue more rapidly as they age. While women commonly lose 30–50% of their bone mass over their lifetimes, men lose only 20–33% of theirs.

- Race. Caucasian and Asian women are at higher risk for the disease than women of African or Hispanic ethnicities.

- Figure type. Women with small bones and those who are thin are more liable to have osteoporosis.

- Early menopause. Women who stop menstruating early because of heredity, surgery or a lot of physical **exercise** may lose large amounts of bone tissue early in life. Conditions such as anorexia and bulimia may also lead to early menopause and osteoporosis.

- Lifestyle. People who smoke or drink too much, or do not get enough exercise have an increased chance of getting osteoporosis.

- Diet. Those who do not get enough calcium or protein may be more likely to have osteoporosis. People who constantly diet are more prone to the disease. It has been shown that adolescent girls (but not boys) have insufficient calcium intake levels in the diet. This calcium deficiency occurs during a period of rapid bone growth, stunting the peak bone mass ultimately achieved; thus, these individuals are at greater risk of developing osteoporosis.

- Genetics. People with a family history of osteoporosis are more likely to contract the disease.

- Chronic use of medication. Certain types of medication, such as steroids, interfere with the body's ability to absorb calcium or accelerate calcium depletion, damaging bone density.

Osteoporosis is often called the "silent" disease, because bone loss occurs without symptoms. People often do not know they have the disease until a bone breaks, frequently in a minor fall that would not normally cause a fracture. A common occurrence is compression fractures of the spine. These can happen even after a seemingly normal activity, such as bending or twisting to pick up a light object. The fractures can cause severe back **pain**, but sometimes they go unnoticed—either way, the vertebrae collapse down on themselves, and the person actually loses height. The hunchback appearance of many elderly women, sometimes called "dowager's hump" or "widow's hump," is due to this effect of osteoporosis on the vertebrae.

Diagnosis

Certain types of doctors may have more training and experience than others in diagnosing and treating people with osteoporosis. These include geriatricians, who specialize in treating the aged; endocrinologists, who specialize in treating diseases of the body's **endocrine system** (glands and hormones); and orthopedic surgeons, who treat fractures, such as those caused by osteoporosis.

Before making a diagnosis of osteoporosis, the doctor usually takes a complete medical history, conducts a physical exam, and orders x-rays, as well as **blood** and urine tests, to rule out other diseases that cause loss of bone mass. The doctor may also recommend a bone density test. This is the only way to determine if osteoporosis is present. It can also show how far the disease has progressed.

Several diagnostic tools are available to measure the density of a bone. The most accurate and advanced of the densitometers uses a technique called DEXA (dual energy x-ray absorptiometry). With the DEXA scan, a double x-ray beam takes pictures of the spine, hip, or entire body. It takes about 20 minutes to do, is painless, and exposes the patient to only a small amount of radiation—about one-fiftieth that of a **chest x ray**. The ordinary x ray is one, though it is the least accurate for early detection of osteoporosis, because it does not reveal bone loss until the disease is advanced and most of the damage has already been done. Other tools that are more likely to catch osteoporosis at an early stage are computed tomography scans (**CT scans**) and machines called densitometers, which are designed specifically to measure bone density. The CT scan, which takes a large number of x rays of the same spot from different angles, is an accurate test, but uses higher levels of radiation than other methods.

People should talk to their doctors about their risk factors for osteoporosis and if, and when, they should get the test. A woman should have bone density measured at menopause, and periodically afterward, depending on the condition of their bones. Men should be tested around age 65. Men and women with additional risk factors, such as those who take certain medications, may need to be tested earlier.

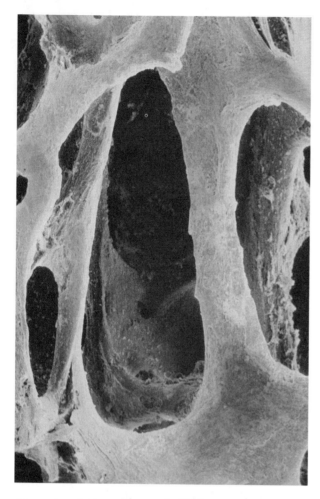

A scanning electron micrograph (SEM) of cancellous (spongy) bone from an osteoporosis patient. Osteoporosis is characterized by increased brittleness of the bones and a greater risk of fractures. This is reflected here in the thin appearance of the bony network of the cancellous bone that forms the core of the body's long bones *(Photograph by Professor P. Motta, Photo Researchers, Inc. Reproduced by permission.)*

Treatment

There are a number of good treatments for primary osteoporosis, most of them medications. In addition, calcium (0.5 to 2 g/day) and **vitamin D** (400 to 800 IU/day) supplementation can reduce the rate of bone loss in women who are more than five years postmenopausal. Fracture reduction efficacy of calcium and vitamin D supplementation, administered independently, has been demonstrated in women older than 75 years of age.

For people with secondary osteoporosis, treatment may focus on curing the underlying disease.

Drugs

For most women who have gone through menopause, the best treatment for osteoporosis is hor-

mone replacement therapy (HRT). Many women participate in HRT when they undergo menopause, to alleviate symptoms such as hot flashes, but hormones have other important roles as well. They protect women against **heart** disease, the number one killer of women in the United States, and they help to relieve and prevent osteoporosis. HRT increases a woman's supply of estrogen, which helps build new bone, while preventing further bone loss.

Some women, however, do not want to take or are not candidates for hormones, because some studies show they are linked to an increased risk of **breast cancer** or uterine **cancer**. Other studies reveal that risk is due to increasing age. (Breast cancer tends to occur more often as women age.) Whether or not a woman takes hormones is a decision she should make carefully with her doctor. Women should talk to their doctors about personal risks for osteoporosis, as well as their risks for heart disease and breast cancer.

Novel delivery systems of HRT have been developed. For example, Vivelle is a estradiol transdermal system that is used for prevention of osteoporosis. It uses a "patch" to continously deliver the hormone estradiol through the skin.

Studies have shown women who started taking HRT within five years of menopause show significantly reduced rates of hip fractures than women who began HRT more than five years postmenopausal. However, even while taking HRT, 10 to 20% of women continue to lose bone density and therefore may require additional intervention.

For people who cannot or will not take estrogen, other agents can be good choices. These include:

- bisphosphonates
- calcitonin
- selective estrogen receptor modulators
- sodium fluoride
- androgens

Although there are a number of bisphosphonates used for the treatment of various forms of osteoporosis and resorptive bone diseases, alendronate (sold under the brand name Fosamax), etidronate (sold under the brand name Didronel), and risedronate (sold under the brand name Actonel) are some of the agents most commonly used for therapeutic treatment of postmenopausal osteoporosis. Biphosphonates act by decreasing bone resorption or breakdown. For example, alendronate attaches itself to bone that has been targeted by bone-eating osteoclasts. It protects the bone from these cells. Osteoclasts help the body break down old bone tissue.

Alendronate has shown to be an effective agent in preventing bone loss and building bone in recently post-menopausal women and is especially useful in women who have contraindications for HRT. It has been licensed for the treatment and prevention of vertebral and nonvertebral postmenopausal osteoporosis. Alendronate has proven safe in very large, multi-year studies, but not much is known about the effects of its long-term use. Side effects are generally minimal with abdominal pain, nausea, dyspepsia, constipation and **diarrhea** occurring in 3% to 7% of patients treated with alendronate. It can be taken daily, and now a new formulation has been developed that can be taken weekly.

Etidronate has been shown to reduce the rate of new vertebral and nonvertebral fractures. It appears to be well tolerated in clinical studies.

Calcitonin is a hormone that has been used as an injection for many years. It is also marketed as a nasal spray. It also slows down bone-eating osteoclasts. Side effects are minimal, but calcitonin builds bone by only 1.5% a year, which may not be enough for some women to recover the bone they lose.

Selective estrogen receptor modulators (SERMs) such as raloxifene, droloxifene, idoxifene, and tamoxifen are used as alternatives to hormone replacement therapy (HRT) which commonly use estrogen. SERMs have been shown to protect against postmenopausal bone loss without the estrogenic side effects. Raloxifene was the first SERM to be approved in the osteoporosis market for prevention and treatment of osteoporosis. Raloxifene binds to estrogen receptors and mimics estrogen's action on bone by preventing bone loss, and improving cholesterol **metabolism**, therefore acting as an agonist. It also acts as an estrogen antagonist in the uterus and the breasts, by not imitating the action of estrogen. These drugs may thus improve blood lipid profiles and protect against breast cancer. There is an enhanced risk of venous thromboembolic events during raloxifene therapy, especially during the first four months of therapy. It also has a propensity to induce hot flashes, and leg pain.

Sodium fluoride has been used as an anabolic agent to stimulate bone formation. However, a high incidence of side effects, mainly gastrointestinal symptoms and lower extremity pain syndrome have occurred in clinical trials.

Androgens have been used for reducing bone loss. Androgens are classified as anabolic steroids, which include nandrolone, stanozolol and testosterone, are used as antiresorptive agents. Androgens are important for postmenopausal women as they serve as a substrate for the peripheral production of estrogens.

The treatments currently available are antiresorptive, which limits the ability to increase bone mass. Other bone-building agents are under investigation including parathyroid hormone which has been clinically evaluated but is still awaiting FDA approval as of March 2001. The biphosphonates have demonstrated the most dramatic reduction in fracture rates and may be the best choice for women with severe osteoporosis. Estrogen's effect may be similar, but has not been established in large randomized trials. Raloxifene may be particularly useful in women who wish to benefit from a breast cancer risk reduction. Calcitonin may be the least potent but may be useful in women who cannot tolerate other therapies.

Surgery

Unfortunately, treatment for osteoporosis is usually tied to fractures that result from advanced stages of the disease. For complicated fractures, such as broken hips, hospitalization and a surgical procedure are required. In hip replacement surgery, the broken hip is removed and replaced with a new hip made of plastic, or metal and plastic. Though the surgery itself is usually successful, complications of the hip fracture can be serious. Those individuals have a 5%–20% greater risk of dying within the first year following that injury than do others in their age group. A large percentage of those who survive are unable to return to their previous level of activity, and many end up moving from self-care to a supervised living situation or nursing home. Getting early treatment and taking steps to reduce bone loss are vital.

Alternative treatment

Alternative treatments for osteoporosis focus on maintaining or building strong bones. A healthy diet low in **fats** and animal products and containing whole grains, fresh fruits and vegetables, and calcium-rich foods (such as dairy products, dark-green leafy vegetables, sardines, salmon, and almonds), along with nutritional supplements (such as calcium, magnesium, and vitamin D), and weight-bearing exercises are important components of both conventional prevention and treatment strategies and alternative approaches to the disease. In addition, alternative practitioners recommend a variety of botanical medicines or herbal supplements. Herbal supplements designed to help slow bone loss emphasize the use of calcium-containing plants, such as horsetail (*Equisetum arvense*), oat straw (*Avena sativa*), alfalfa (*Medicago sativa*), licorice (*Glycyrrhiza galbra*), marshmallow (*Althaea officinalis*), and yellow dock (*Rumex crispus*). Homeopathic remedies focus on treatments believed to help the body absorb calcium. These remedies are likely to include such substances as *Calcarea carbonica* (calcium carbonate) or silica. In traditional Chinese medicine,

KEY TERMS

Alendronate—A nonhormonal drug used to treat osteoporosis in postmenopausal women.

Anticonvulsants—Drugs used to control seizures, such as in epilepsy.

Biphosphonates—Compounds (like alendronate) that slow bone loss and increase bone density.

Calcitonin—A hormonal drug used to treat post-menopausal osteoporosis.

Estrogen—A female hormone that also keeps bones strong. After menopause, a woman may take hormonal drugs with estrogen to prevent bone loss.

Glucocorticoids—Any of a group of hormones (like cortisone) that influence many body functions and are widely used in medicine, such as for treatment of rheumatoid arthritis inflammation.

Hormone replacement therapy (HRT)—Also called estrogen replacement therapy, this controversial treatment is used to relieve the discomforts of menopause. Estrogen and another female hormone, progesterone, are usually taken together to replace the estrogen no longer made by the body. It has the added effect of stopping bone loss that occurs at menopause.

Menopause—The ending of a woman's menstrual cycle, when production of bone-protecting estrogen decreases.

Osteoblasts—Cells in the body that build new bone tissue.

Osteoclasts—Cells that break down and remove old bone tissue.

Selective estrogen receptor modulator—A hormonal preparation that offers the beneficial effects of hormone replacement therapy without the increased risk of breast and uterine cancer associated with HRT.

practitioners recommend herbs thought to slow or prevent bone loss, including dong quai (*Angelica sinensis*) and Asian ginseng (*Panax ginseng*). Natural hormone therapy, using plant estrogens (from soybeans) or progesterone (from wild yams), may be recommended for women who cannot or choose not to take synthetic hormones.

It should be noted, however, that very few clinical trials are conducted on alternate therapies and therefore efficacy cannot be established.

Prognosis

There is no cure for osteoporosis, but it can be controlled. Most people who have osteoporosis fare well once they get treatment. The medicines available now build bone, protect against bone loss, and halt the progress of this disease.

Health care team roles

Doctors, nurses, physical therapists, radiation technologists, and dietitians all play roles in the process of controlling osteoporosis. Because osteoporosis is treatable but not curable, the main responsibility for controlling the progress of the disease rests with the patient. All of these team members play an important role in identifying risk of osteoporosis before it strikes and in convincing the patient to take appropriate steps (including lifestyle modification) to minimize the dangers of fracturing major bones.

Prevention

Building strong bones, especially before the age of 35, and maintaining a healthy lifestyle are the best ways of preventing osteoporosis. To build as much bone mass as early as possible in life, and to help slow the rate of bone loss later in life:

Get calcium in foods

Experts recommend 1,500 milligrams (mg) of calcium per day for adolescents, pregnant or breast-feeding women, older adults (over 65), and postmenopausal women not using hormone replacement therapy. All others should get 1,000 mg per day. Foods are the best source for this important mineral. Milk, cheese, and yogurt have the highest amounts. Other foods that are high in calcium are green leafy vegetables, tofu, shellfish, Brazil nuts, sardines, and almonds.

Take calcium supplements

Many people, especially those who do not like or cannot eat dairy foods, do not get enough calcium in their diets and may need to take a calcium supplement. Supplements vary in the amount of calcium they contain. Those with calcium carbonate have the most amount of useful calcium. Supplements should be taken with meals and accompanied by six to eight glasses of water a day. Calcium supplements and **antacids** interfere with absorption of alendronate and should be taken at least one half hour later.

Get vitamin D

Vitamin D helps the body absorb calcium. People can get vitamin D from sunshine with a quick (15–20 minutes) walk each day or from foods such as **liver**, fish oil, and vitamin-D fortified milk. During the winter months it may be necessary to take supplements (400–800 IU/day).

Avoid smoking and alcohol

Smoking reduces bone mass, as does heavy drinking. To reduce risk, do not smoke and limit alcoholic drinks to no more than two per day. An alcoholic drink is 1.5 oz (44 mL) of hard liquor, 12 oz (355 mL) of beer, or 5 oz (148 mL) of wine.

Exercise

Exercising regularly builds and strengthens bones. Weight-bearing exercises—where bones and muscles work against gravity—are best. These include aerobics, dancing, jogging, stair climbing, tennis, walking, and lifting weights. People who have osteoporosis may want to attempt gentle exercise, such as walking, rather than jogging or fast-paced aerobics, which increase the chance of falling. Try to exercise three to four times per week for 20–30 minutes each time. As physical activity improves muscle strength and coordination it may also aid in reducing the risk of fall-related fractures.

Those at risk should avoid medications known to compromise bone density, such as glucocorticoids, thyroid hormones and chronic heparin therapy.

Resources

BOOKS

Adams, John S. and Barbara P. Lukertet. *Osteoporosis: Genetics, Prevention and Treatment.* Boston: Kluwer Academic, 1999.

Kessler, George J., et al. *The Bone Density Diet: 6 Weeks to a Strong Body and Mind.* New York: Ballantine Books, 2000.

Krane, Stephen M., and Michael F. Holick. "Metabolic Bone Disease: Osteoporosis." In *Harrison's Principles of Internal Medicine.* 14th ed. Ed. by Anthony S. Fauci, et al. New York: McGraw-Hill, 1998.

Lane, Nancy E., ed. *The Osteoporosis Book.* New York: Oxford University Press, 1998.

McIlwain, Harris, et al. *Osteoporosis Cure: Reverse the Crippling Effects With New Treatment.* New York: Avon Books, 1998.

Notelovits, Morris, et al. *Stand Tall! Every Woman's Guide to Preventing and Treating Osteoporosis.* 2nd ed. Gainesville, FL: Triad Publishing Co., 1998.

PERIODICALS

Feder, G., et al. "Guidelines for the Prevention of Falls in People over 65." *British Medical Journal* 321 (2000): 1007-1011.

McClung, Michael R., et al. "Effect of Risedronate on the Risk of Hip Fracture in Elderly Women." *The New England Journal of Medicine* 344, no. 5 (2001): 333-40.

ORGANIZATIONS

Arthritis Foundation, 1330 W. Peachtree St., PO Box 7669, Atlanta, GA 30357-0669. (800) 283-7800. <http://www.arthritis.org>.

National Center for Complementary and Alternative Medicine (NCCAM), 31 Center Dr., Room #5B-58, Bethesda, MD 20892-2182. (800) NIH-NCAM. Fax: (301) 495-4957. <http://nccam.nih.gov>.

National Osteoporosis Foundation, 1150 17th Street, Suite 500 NW, Washington, DC 20036-4603. (800) 223-9994. <http://www.nof.org>.

Osteoporosis and Related Bone Diseases-National Resource Center. 1150 17th St., NW, Ste. 500, Washington, DC 20036-4603. (800) 624-BONE. <http://www.osteo.org>.

Crystal Kaczkowski, MSc

Otoscope

Definition

An otoscope is a hand-held device for visual examination of the auditory canal, inner ear, and tympanic membrane.

Purpose

An otoscope is designed to enable the health care professional to view the auditory canal, inner ear, and tympanic membrane as part of a normal **physical examination**. It is also used if **infection** of the auditory canal is suspected, if there is a blockage due to the presence of a foreign object or build up of wax, and to inspect the tympanic membrane for signs of rupture, puncture, or **hearing loss**.

Description

An otoscope consists of a handle with power source, an optical head with fiberoptic strands, a lens, specula, a small light bulb, a polished reflector, and may have pneumoscopy bellows as an option. The unit is designed to be operated by one hand, enabling the other hand to manipulate the patient's ear.

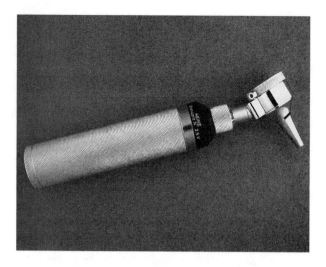

An otoscope shines light into the ear and allows a health care practitioner to view the inside of the ear through an opening in the otoscope. *(Photograph by Wolfgang Weinhäupl. Science Source/Photo Researchers. Reproduced by permission.)*

Batteries, either disposable or rechargeable, can power the unit and are often stored in the handle of the otoscope. Alternatively, the unit can be recharged using a transformer to enable it to be used from a 110V power supply mounted on a wall. Some units have other options available for the power source, including a clip-on battery unit with a two-pronged cord that can be attached to a pocket or table, and a cord with batteries that is attached to the otoscope and hangs around the health care professional's neck.

An optical head is attached to the handle and contains fiberoptic strands, a bulb, a swivel-headed magnifying lens, and the reflector, allowing the health care professional to view the patient's auditory canal via an attached speculum. The lens is constructed of scratch-resistant optical glass. Specula may be disposable or autoclavable and can range in size from 2.5–8mm. This enables the appropriate-sized speculum to be selected for the patient's ear offering comfort for the patient during the otoscopy procedure, while providing a positive ear seal for pneumoscopy. An otoscope bulb provides light that shines through the tip of the speculum while a reflector increases the amount of forward light given off by the device. The bulb is usually halogen to give off a clear light that will not affect the color of the ear canal, potentially altering the diagnosis. The illuminated canal is viewed through the magnifying lens.

Pneumoscopy bellows are made of plastic or rubber and are attached to the otoscope via a thin plastic tube. When the bellows are squeezed, a small puff of air is forced through the tubing, striking the tympanic membrane. The action of the air striking the membrane is viewed through the otoscope. Signs of oscillation are normal.

Each otoscope has different features depending on the manufacturer and the cost of each unit.

Operation

The patient will be asked to sit with the head tipped slightly toward the shoulder so that the ear to be examined is pointing up. After selecting the appropriate sized speculum for the patient's ear, the speculum is attached to the optical head of the otoscope and gently inserted into the patient's ear. The doctor or nurse may hold the ear lobe as the speculum of the otoscope is inserted into the ear. Both ears are usually examined, even if there seems to be a problem with just one ear, and the procedure takes no more than a few minutes to perform.

Maintenance

The otoscope should be maintained by ensuring the bulb light is bright and extends from the tip of the speculum to the eardrum. Bulbs should be replaced every six months, and rechargeable batteries changed every two years. The fiberoptic strands in the optical head may crack over prolonged use, and if the light remains dim, the unit should be repaired. The device should be checked for air leaks that prevent an adequate seal to be formed around the ear or permit air to escape from around the lens or where attachments fit the unit. A poor seal will also allow moisture to enter behind the lens and fogging will occur.

Health care team roles

The otoscope enables the professional to detect signs of infection, obstruction, and injury in the ear canal and eardrum. It is most often used by physicians and **advanced practice nurses**.

Training

The person using the scope should know how to recognize signs of inflammation and disease, including pressure behind the eardrum and be thoroughly familiar with the normal appearance and anatomy of the ear. Training hospitals may offer otoscopy programs.

Resources

OTHER

"Hotchkiss Otoscope." <http://www.preferredproduct.com>.

Schwartz, Richard H. "The Maintenance of the Office Otoscope." *Slack Incorporated Newspaper.* Apr. 2001. <http://www.slackinc.com>.

KEY TERMS

Auditory canal—The ear canal.

Ear speculum—A cone or funnel-shaped attachment for an otoscope that is inserted into the ear canal to examine the eardrum.

Otoscope—A hand-held instrument with a tiny light and a funnel-shaped attachment called an ear speculum, which is used to examine the ear canal and eardrum.

Pneumoscopy—An examination using air.

Tympanic membrane—The ear drum.

"Welch Allyn 3.5v Diagnostic with Convertible Handle."
    <http://www.nurses.com>.

Margaret A Stockley, RGN

Otoscopic examination

Definition

An otoscopic examination is the visual examination of the auditory canal and tympanic membrane using an **otoscope**.

Purpose

An otoscopic examination is a procedure that examines the auditory canal and tympanic membrane for **infection** or blockage due to the presence of a foreign object or build up of wax, the tympanic membrane for signs of rupture, puncture, or **hearing loss**, and the canal for any variations from normal. Some otoscopes can deliver a small puff of air to the eardrum to determine if the eardrum will vibrate (which is normal). An otoscopic examinations is also part of a normal **physical examination**.

Precautions

No special precautions are required. However, if an ear infection is present, an ear examination may cause some discomfort or **pain**.

Description

An otoscopy is an ear examination with an otoscope, a handheld instrument with a tiny light and a cone-shaped attachment called an ear speculum. A physician or nurse usually performs an otoscopic examination as part of a complete physical examination. The ears may also be examined if an ear infection is suspected, or if the patient has a **fever**, ear pain, or **hearing** loss. The patient will be asked to sit with the head tipped slightly toward the shoulder so the ear to be examined is pointing up. The doctor or nurse may hold the ear lobe as the speculum of the otoscope is inserted into the ear. Both ears are usually examined, even if the problem seems to affect just one ear, and the procedure takes no more than a few minutes to perform.

Preparation

No special preparation is required prior to an ear examination with an otoscope. The ear speculum, which is inserted into the ear, is cleaned and sanitized before it is used. Specula come in various sizes, and the doctor or nurse will select the size that will be most comfortable for the patient's ear.

Aftercare

If an ear infection is diagnosed, the patient may require treatment with **antibiotics**. If there is a buildup of wax in the ear canal, it might be rinsed or scraped out.

Complications

This type of ear examination is simple and generally harmless. Caution should always be used any time an object is inserted into the ear. This process could irritate an infected external ear canal and could rupture an eardrum if performed improperly or if the patient moves.

Results

The ear canal is typically skin-colored and covered with tiny hairs. It is normal for the ear canal to have some yellowish-brown earwax. The eardrum is typically thin, shiny, and pearly-white to light gray in color. The tiny bones in the middle ear can be seen pushing on the eardrum membrane like tent poles. The light from the otoscope will reflect off of the surface of the eardrum. Abnormal results such as a red or swollen ear canal may indicate an ear infection is present. In cases where the eardrum has ruptured, there may be fluid draining from the middle ear. A doctor may also see scarring, retraction of the eardrum, or bulging of the eardrum.

Health care team roles

The health care team should be aware of the physiology of the auditory canal to detect any deviations

KEY TERMS

Auditory canal—Ear canal.

Ear speculum—A cone- or funnel-shaped attachment for an otoscope that is inserted into the ear canal to examine the canal and the eardrum.

Otoscope—A handheld instrument with a tiny light and a funnel-shaped attachment called an ear speculum.

Tympanic membrane—Ear drum.

from normal. A knowledge of the function and care of the otoscope is important to ensure the light is bright, there are no loose parts, and if disposable speculums are not used, the speculums are sterilized between patients. Hospitals may offer training programs in the use of otoscopes and their detection of abnormalities of the auditory canal.

Resources

ORGANIZATIONS

American Academy of Otolaryngology—Head and Neck Surgery. One Prince Street, Alexandria, VA 22314. (703) 836-4444.

Ear Foundation. 2000 Church Street, Box 111, Nashville, TN 37236. (615) 329-7807. (800) 545-HEAR.

National Institute on Deafness and Other Communication Disorders. 1 Communication Avenue, Bethesda, MD 20892-3456. Voice: (301) 496-7243. TTY: (301) 402-0252.

OTHER

"Ear Test." <http://www.healthanswers.com>.

Hearing Health Information. <http://www.hei.org>.

Schwartz, Richard H. "The Maintenance of the Office Otoscope." *Slack Incorporated Newspaper* April 2001. <http://www.slackinc.com>.

Margaret A. Stockley

Outlays *see* **Dental crowns, inlays, and bridges**

Ova & parasites collection *see* **Stool O & P test**

Overdose

Definition

An overdose is the accidental or intentional use of a drug or medicine in an amount that is higher than normally used or prescribed.

Description

All drugs have the potential to be misused, whether legally prescribed by a doctor, purchased over the counter at the local drug store, or bought illegally on the street. Taken in combination with other drugs or with alcohol, even drugs normally considered safe do cause death or serious long-term consequences. Children are particularly at risk for accidental overdose, accounting for more than one million poisonings each year from drugs, alcohol, and other chemicals and toxic substances. People who suffer from depression and who have suicidal thoughts are also at high risk for drug overdose.

Causes and symptoms

Accidental drug overdose may be the result of the misuse of prescription medicines or commonly used medications such as **pain** relievers and cold remedies. Symptoms differ depending on the drug taken. Some of the drugs commonly involved in overdoses are listed below along with symptoms and outcomes.

Acetaminophen is the generic name for the commonly used pain reliever Tylenol. An overdose of this drug can cause **liver** damage with symptoms that include loss of appetite, tiredness, nausea and vomiting, paleness, and sweating. The next stage of symptoms indicates liver failure and includes abdominal pain and tenderness, swelling of the liver, and abnormal **blood** tests for liver enzymes. In the last stage of this **poisoning**, liver failure advances and patients become jaundiced, with yellowing of the skin and whites of the eyes. They may also experience kidney failure, **bleeding disorders**, and encephalopathy (swelling of the **brain**).

Salicylates are found in aspirin and some creams or ointments used for muscle and joint pain such as Ben-Gay and for psoriasis, a skin condition. Initial symptoms are gastrointestinal irritation, **fever**, and vomiting, possibly with blood in the vomit. An overdose of salicylates will cause metabolic acidosis and respiratory alkalosis, conditions in which the body's pH (acid/base balance) malfunctions. Symptoms include rapid **heart** beat and fast breathing. Nervous system symptoms include confusion, hallucinations, tiredness, and ringing in the ears. An increased tendency to bleed is also common. Serious complications include acute renal failure, **coma**, and **heart failure**. Acute salicylate poisoning can lead to death.

Anticholinergic drugs that block the action of acetylcholine, a neurotransmitter include atropine, scopolamine, belladonna, **antihistamines**, and antipsychotic agents. They cause the skin and moist tissues such as in the mouth and nose to become dry and flushed. Dilated pupils, an inability to urinate, and mental disturbances are also symptoms. Severe toxicity can lead to seizures, abnormal heart rhythms, extremely high **blood pressure**, and coma.

Cholinergic drugs that stimulate the parasympathetic nervous system, such as carbamate and pilocarpine, cause nausea, **diarrhea**, increased secretion of body fluids such as sweat, tears, saliva, and urine, fatigue, and muscle weakness. Convulsions are possible. Death can occur due to **respiratory failure** and heart failure.

Antidepressant drugs such as amitriptyline, desipramine, and nortriptyline can cause irregular heart rate, vomiting, low blood pressure (hypotension), confusion, and seizures. An overdose of antidepressants also causes symptoms similar to those seen with anticholinergic drug overdoses.

Depressant drugs such as tranquilizers, **antianxiety drugs**, and sleeping pills cause sleepiness, slowed or slurred speech, difficulty walking or standing, blurred **vision**, impaired ability to think, disorientation, and mood changes. Overdose symptoms can include slowed breathing, very low blood pressure, stupor, coma, **shock**, and death.

Cocaine and crack cocaine overdoses cause seizures, high blood pressure, increased heart rate, paranoia, and other changes in behavior. Heart attack or stroke are serious risks within three days after cocaine overdose.

Heroin, morphine, and codeine are narcotic or opiate drugs. Clonidine and diphenoxylate (Lomotil) are also in this category. Overdose with opiate drugs causes sedation (sleepiness), low blood pressure, slowed heart rate, and slowed breathing. Pinpoint pupils, where the black centers of the eyes become smaller than normal, are common in opiate overdose. However, if other drugs are taken at the same time as the opiates, they may counteract this effect on the pupils. A serious risk is that the patient will stop breathing (respiratory arrest).

Digoxin, a drug used to regulate the heart, can cause irregular heartbeats, nausea, confusion, loss of appetite, and blurred vision.

Diagnosis

Diagnosis of a drug overdose may be based on the symptoms that develop; however, the drug may do extensive damage to the body before significant symptoms develop. If the patient is conscious, the physician may be able to find out what drugs were taken and in what amounts. The patient's recent medical and social history may also help in a diagnosis. Information such as a list of medications that the patient takes, whether or not alcohol was consumed recently, or whether the patient had eaten in the last few hours can be valuable in determining how fast the overdosed drug will be absorbed into the system.

Different drugs have varying effects on the body's pH and on certain elements in the blood such as potassium and **calcium**. Blood tests can be used to detect changes in body chemistry that may give as clues to what drugs were taken. Blood can also be screened for various drugs in the system. Once the overdose drug is identified, blood tests can be used to monitor how fast the drug is being cleared out of the body. Urine tests are another way to screen for some drugs and to detect changes in the body's chemistry. Blood and urine tests may show if there is damage to the liver or **kidneys** as a result of the overdose.

Treatment

Immediate care

If a drug overdose is discovered or suspected, and the person is unconscious, having convulsions, or not breathing, emergency help must be called immediately. If the person who took the drug is not having symptoms, it is recommended not to wait to see if symptoms develop, but to call a poison control center immediately. Providing as much information as possible to the poison control center can help determine what the next course of action should be.

The poison control center, paramedics, and emergency room staff will want to know the following:

- what drug(s) were taken
- how much of the drug was taken
- when was the drug taken
- if the drug was taken with alcohol or any other drugs or chemicals
- what the age of the patient is
- what symptoms the patient is experiencing
- if the patient is conscious
- if the patient is breathing

KEY TERMS

Gastric lavage—The inside of the stomach is rinsed with a saline (salt water) solution or regular tap water; also called a stomach pump.

Hypotension—Having a low blood pressure: less than 90/60 mmHg.

Intubation—A procedure in which a tube is inserted through the mouth or nose and into the trachea to keep the airway open and to help the patient breathe.

The poison control center may recommend a liquid called **ipecac** syrup, which is used to induce vomiting. Ipecac syrup is an over-the-counter medication available from pharmacies, and no prescription is required. Pediatricians may advise families to keep ipecac syrup on hand in households with children. This medication should be used only on the advice of a medical professional. An important caveat is that vomiting should not be induced if the patient is unconscious as there is serious risk of choking.

Emergency care

Emergency medical treatment may include:

- Assessment of the patient's airway and breathing to make sure that the trachea, the passage to the **lungs**, is not blocked. If needed, a tube may be inserted through the mouth or nose and into the trachea to help the patient breathe. This procedure is called endotracheal (in the trachea) intubation.

- Assessment of the patient's **vital signs**, including heart rate, blood pressure, body temperature, respiratory rate, and other physical signs that might indicate the effects of the drug.

- Blood and urine samples may be collected to test for the presence of the suspected overdose drug, and other drugs or alcohol that might be present.

- Attempt to eliminate the whatever of the drug that has not yet been absorbed. Vomiting may be induced using ipecac syrup or other drugs that cause vomiting. Ipecac syrup should not be given to patients who overdosed with tricyclic antidepressants, theophylline, or any drug that causes a significant change in mental status.

- Gastric lavage, also known as pumping the **stomach**, may be attempted. For this procedure, a large flexible tube is inserted through the nose or mouth, down the throat, and into the stomach. The contents of the stomach are then suctioned out through the tube. A solution of saline (salt water) or regular tap water is pushed down into the tube to rinse out the stomach. The saline solution or water is then suctioned out. This process is repeated several times until the suctioned fluid is clear.

- Activated charcoal to absorb the drug is sometimes given through a stomach tube or by having the patient swallow it.

- Medication to stimulate urination or defecation may be given to try to flush the excess drug out of the body faster.

- Intravenous (IV) fluids may be given. An intravenous line, a needle inserted into a vein, may be put into the arm or back of the hand. Fluids, either sterile saline (salt water solution) or dextrose (sugar water solution), can be administered through this line. Increasing fluids can help to flush the drug out of the system and to reestablish balance of fluids and **minerals** in the body. The pH of the body may need to be corrected by administering electrolytes such as sodium, potassium, and bicarbonate through the IV line. If drugs need to be administered quickly, they can also be injected directly into the IV line.

- Hemodialysis is a procedure in which blood is circulated out of the body, pumped through a dialysis machine, then reintroduced back into the body. This process can be used to filter some drugs out of the blood and can clean the blood. It may also be used temporarily or long term if the kidneys are damaged due to the overdose.

- Antidotes that are available for some drug overdoses may be administered. An antidote is another drug that counteracts or blocks the overdose drug.

- Psychiatric evaluation is performed if the drug overdose was taken deliberately. If the overdose is determined to be a deliberate act, further psychiatric care is provided while the patient is hospitalized.

Prognosis

While many victims of drug overdose recover without long-term effects, there can be serious consequences. Some drug overdoses cause the failure of major organs like the kidneys or liver, or failure of whole systems like the respiratory or circulatory systems. Patients who survive drug overdose may need **kidney dialysis**, kidney or liver transplant, or ongoing care as a result of heart failure, stroke, or coma. Death can occur in almost any drug overdose situation, especially if treatment is not started immediately.

Health care team roles

Nurses play a vital role in helping victims of drug overdoses. The emergency room nurses perform the gastric lavage procedure on the patient who has overdosed, as well as administrating antidotes or other medications ordered by the doctor. Nurses are responsible for monitoring the patient and recording important assessment findings. Nurses should be cognizant of the importance of careful monitoring of drug levels.

Another important assessment done by the nurse, either in the emergency room or on the psychiatric unit, is the evaluation of patient support systems. A deliberate overdose can be a devastating event for the entire family, and the nurse can help foster communication between the patient and family members. When a family tries to minimize the intentional overdose, the nurse must strongly emphasize that any suicidal threat or act ought to be regarded as critical.

Prevention

To protect children from accidental drug overdose, all medications should be stored in containers with child-resistant caps. All drugs should be out of sight and out of reach of children, preferably in a locked cabinet. The person to whom medication is prescribed should take it according to the directions. Threats of suicide need to be taken seriously, and appropriate help sought for people with depression or other mental illness that may lead to suicide.

Resources

BOOKS

Haddad, Lester M. *Clinical Management of Poisoning and Drug Overdose, 3rd ed.* Philadelphia: W. B. Saunders, 1998.

PERIODICALS

Borowsky, I. W. "Adolescent Suicide Attempts: Risks and Protectors." *Pediatrics* 107 (2001): 485-93.

OTHER

Anker, Anthony. *Drug Overdose from AAEM Emergency Medical and Family Health Guide/Poisioning.* <http://www.emedicine.com/aaem/topic169.htm>.

Graber, Mark A. "Emergency Medicine: Overdose and Toxindromes." *University of Iowa Family Practice Handbook, 3rd ed.* <http://www.vh.org/Providers/ClinRef/FPHandbook/Chapter01/20-1.htm>.

"Poisoning." *The Merck Manual of Diagnosis and Therapy, 17th ed.* <http://www.merck.com/pubs/mmanual/section23/chapter307/307a.htm>.

"Poisoning." *The Merck Manual Home Edition.* <http://www.merck.com/pubs/mmanual_home/sec24/286.htm>.

"Suicidal Behavior." *The Merck Manual Home Edition.* <http://www.merck.com/pubs/mmanual_home/sec7/85.htm>.

Lori Beck

Oxygen chamber therapy *see* **Ventilation assistance**

Oxygen mask application *see* **Nasal cannula/face mask application**

Oxygen therapy

Definition

Oxygen may be classified as an element, a gas, and a drug. Oxygen therapy is the administration of oxygen at concentrations greater than that in room air to treat or prevent hypoxia. Oxygen delivery systems are classified as stationary, portable, or ambulatory, and oxygen can be administered by mask, nasal cannula, and tent. Hyperbaric oxygen therapy involves placing the patient in an airtight chamber with oxygen under pressure.

Purpose

The body is constantly taking in oxygen and releasing carbon dioxide. If this process is inadequate, oxygen levels in the **blood** decrease, and the patient may need supplemental oxygen. Oxygen therapy is a key treatment in respiratory care. The purpose is to increase oxygen saturation in tissues where the saturation levels are too low due to illness or injury. Oxygen therapy is frequently ordered in the **home care** setting, as well as in acute care.

Some of the conditions that oxygen therapy is used for include:

• documented hypoxemia

• severe respiratory distress (e.g., acute **asthma** or **pneumonia**)

• severe trauma

• acute **myocardial infarction**

• short-term therapy, such as post-anesthesia recovery

Hyperbaric oxygen therapy is used in the following conditions:

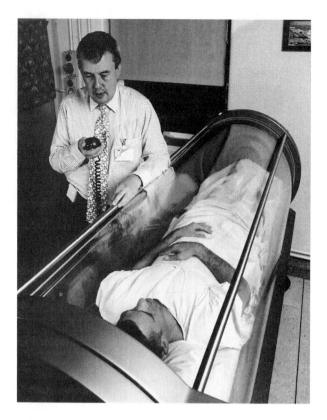

A doctor communicates with a patient lying in a pressure chamber and undergoing hyperbaric oxygen therapy.
(James King-Holmes/Science Photo Library. Photo Researchers, Inc.)

- gas gangrene
- decompression sickness
- air embolism
- smoke inhalation
- carbon monoxide poisoning
- cerebral hypoxic event

Precautions

Oxygen supports combustion, therefore no open flame or products that are combustible should be permitted when oxygen is in use. These include petroleum jelly, oils, and aerosol sprays. A spark from a cigarette, electric razor, or other electrical device could easily ignite oxygen-saturated hair or bedclothes around the patient. Explosion-proof plugs should be used for vaporizers and humidifier attachments.

Care must be taken with oxygen equipment used in the home or hospital. Cylinders should be kept in carts, or have collars for safe storage. If not stored in a cart, smaller canisters may be lain on the floor. Knocking cylinders together can cause sparks, so bumping them

should be avoided. In the home, the oxygen source must be placed at least 6 ft (1.8 m) away from flames or other sources of ignition, such as a lit cigarette. Oxygen tanks should be kept in a well-ventilated area. Oxygen tanks should not be kept in the trunk of a car. Use "No Smoking—Oxygen in Use" signs to warn visitors not to smoke near the patient.

Special care must be given when administering oxygen to **premature infants**, because of the danger of high oxygen levels causing retinopathy of prematurity or contributing to the construction of ductus arteriosis. PaO_2 (partial pressure of oxygen) levels greater than 80 mm Hg should be avoided.

Patients who are undergoing a laser **bronchoscopy** should have concurrent administration of supplemental oxygen to avoid **burns** to the trachea.

Description

The procedure discussed is the administration of oxygen therapy other than with mechanical **ventilators** and hyperbaric chambers.

In the hospital, oxygen is supplied to each patient room and is available via an outlet in the wall. Oxygen is delivered from a central source through a pipeline in the facility. A flow meter attaches to the wall outlet to access the oxygen. A valve regulates the oxygen flow and attachments may be connected to moisturize the oxygen flow. In the home, the oxygen source is usually an oxygen canister or an air compressor. Whether in home or hospital, plastic tubing connects the oxygen source to the patient. Oxygen is most commonly delivered to the patient via a nasal cannula or mask attached to the tubing. Another delivery option is transtracheal oxygen therapy, which involves a small flexible catheter inserted in the trachea or windpipe through a tracheostomy tube. In this method, the oxygen bypasses the mouth, nose, and throat, and a humidifier is required at flow rates of 2.1 pt (1 l) per minute and above. Other oxygen delivery methods include tents and specialized infant oxygen delivery systems.

Preparation

A physician's order is required for oxygen therapy except in emergency use. The need for supplemental oxygen is determined by inadequate oxygen saturation, as determined by blood gas measurements, pulse oximetry, or clinical indications. No special preparation of the patient is required to administer oxygen therapy.

Aftercare

Once oxygen therapy is initiated, periodic assessment and documentation of oxygen saturation levels is required. If the patient is using a mask or a cannula, gauze can be tucked under the tubing to prevent irritation of the cheeks or the skin behind the ears. Water-based lubricants can be used to relieve dryness of the lips and nostrils.

Complications

Complications from oxygen therapy used in appropriate situations are infrequent. Respiratory depression, oxygen toxicity, and absorption atelectasis are the most serious complications with overuse of oxygen.

Delivery equipment may present other problems. Perforation of the nasal septum as a result of using a nasal cannula and non–humidified oxygen has been reported. In addition, bacterial contamination of nebulizer and humidification systems can occur, potentially leading to the spread of pneumonia. High-flow systems that employ heated humidifiers and aerosol generators, especially when used by patients with artificial airways, also pose a risk of **infection**.

Results

The patient demonstrates adequate oxygenation through pulse oximetry, **blood gases**, and clinical observation. Signs and symptoms of inadequate oxygenation include **cyanosis**, drowsiness, confusion, restlessness, **anxiety**, or slow, shallow, difficult, or irregular breathing. Patients with obstructive airway disease may exhibit "aerophagia" or "air hunger," as they work to pull air into the **lungs**. In cases of carbon monoxide inhalation, the oxygen saturation can be falsely elevated.

Health care team roles

Team members include the physician, nurse, and respiratory therapist. **Respiratory therapy** technicians and nursing assistants who are adequately trained may check and document that oxygen therapy is being used appropriately and the oxygen flow is as ordered.

- Physicians are responsible for ordering oxygen therapy. The prescription must include the flow rate and when the patient will need to use the oxygen.

- Nurses are responsible for assessing patients, ensuring that oxygen therapy is initiated as prescribed, monitoring oxygen delivery systems, and recommending changes in therapy.

KEY TERMS

Combustion—Burning or fire. Objects that are combustible ignite easily.

Cyanosis—Blue, gray, or dark purple discoloration of the skin caused by a deficiency of oxygen.

Flow meter—Device for measuring the rate of a gas, especially oxygen, or liquid.

Hypoxic—Oxygen deficient.

Oxygen—A non-metallic element occurring free in the atmosphere as a colorless, odorless, tasteless gas.

Oxygenation—Saturation with oxygen.

- Respiratory therapists may assess patients, initiate and monitor oxygen delivery systems, and recommend changes in therapy.

Patient education

Patient education involves instructing patients regarding the safe use of oxygen. Patients must be advised not to change the flow rate of oxygen unless directed to do so by the physician. Patients in the home setting are directed to notify the suppliers when replacement oxygen supplies are needed.

A physician should be notified and emergency services may be required if the following develop:

- frequent headaches
- anxiety
- cyanotic (blue) lips or fingernails
- drowsiness
- confusion
- restlessness
- slow, shallow, difficult, or irregular breathing

Resources

BOOKS

Branson, Richard, et al. *Respiratory Care Equipment.* 2nd ed. Philadelphia: Lippincott, 1999.

Burton, George G., et al. *Respiratory Care: A Guide to Clinical Practice.* 4th ed. Philadelphia: Lippincott, 1997.

Dunne, Patrick J., and Susan L.McInturff. *Respiratory Home Care: The Esentials.* Philadelphia: F. A. Davis Company, 1998.

Pagana, Kathleen D., and Timothy J. Pagana. *Diagnostic Testing and Nursing Implications.* 5th ed. St. Louis: Mosby, 1999.

Wilkins, Robert, et al. *Clinical Assessment in Respiratory Care.* 4th ed. St. Louis: Mosby, 2000.

PERIODICALS

Crockett, A. J., and J. M. Cranston et al. "A review of long-term oxygen therapy for chronic obstructive pulmonary disease." *Respiratory Medicine* 95 (June 2001): 437-443.

Eaton, T. E., et al. "An evaluation of short-term oxygen therapy: the prescription of oxygen to patients with chronic lung disease hypoxic at discharge." *Respiratory Medicine* 95 (July 2001): 582-587

Kelly, Martin G., et al. "Nasal septal perforation and oxygen cannulae." *Hospital Medicine* 62, no. 4 (April 2001): 248.

Ruiz-Bailen M, M. C. Serrano-Corcoles and J. A. Ramos-Cuadra. "Tracheal injury caused by ingested paraquat." *Chest* 119, no. 6 (June 2001): 1956-7

ORGANIZATIONS

American Association for Respiratory Care 11030 Ables Lane, Dallas, Texas 75229. <http://www.aarc.org>.

American Lung Association 1740 Broadway, New York, NY 10019-4374. (800) LUNG-USA. <http://www.lungusa.org>.

Maggie Boleyn, RN, BSN

Oxytocin *see* **Uterine stimulants**